Nursing Now!

Nursing Now!

Today's Issues, Tomorrow's Trends

fourth edition

Joseph T. Catalano, PhD, RN
Department Chair
Professor of Nursing
East Central University
Ada, Oklahoma

F. A. DAVIS COMPANY • Philadelphia

F. A. Davis Company
1915 Arch Street
Philadelphia, PA 19103
www.fadavis.com

Printed in the United States of America

Last digit indicates print number: 10 9 8 7 6 5 4 3 2 1

Acquisitions Editor: Lisa B. Deitch
Developmental Editor: Anne-Adele Wight
Project Editor: Ilysa H. Richman
Art Manager: Carolyn O'Brien

As new scientific information becomes available through basic and clinical research, recommended treatments and drug therapies undergo changes. The author(s) and publisher have done everything possible to make this book accurate, up to date, and in accord with accepted standards at the time of publication. The author(s), editors, and publisher are not responsible for errors or omissions or for consequences from application of the book, and make no warranty, expressed or implied, in regard to the contents of the book. Any practice described in this book should be applied by the reader in accordance with professional standards of care used in regard to the unique circumstances that may apply in each situation. The reader is advised always to check product information (package inserts) for changes and new information regarding dose and contraindications before administering any drug. Caution is especially urged when using new or infrequently ordered drugs.

Library of Congress Cataloging-in-Publication Data

Catalano, Joseph T.
    Nursing now: today's issues, tomorrow's trends / Joseph T. Catalano—4th ed.
      p. ; cm.
    Includes bibliographical references and index.
    ISBN-13: 978-0-8036-1447-5
    ISBN-10: 0-8036-1447-0
    1. Nursing—Vocational guidance—United States.   2. Nursing—Social
aspects—United States.   3. Nursing—Philosophy.   I. Title.
    [DNLM: 1. Nursing—trends.   WY 16 C357n 2006]
  RT82.C33 2006
  610.7306′9—dc22

                                    2005026211

To all those hard-working students with high stress levels who are the future leaders of the nursing profession.

The events of the past few years have permanently altered some aspects of the social fabric of the world, but other elements have remained discouragingly constant. The health-care industry is reflective of this dichotomy. Although new technological advances have pushed health care forward at a fevered pace, the number of our citizens who do not have health insurance has increased to an all-time high. Newly developed medications and therapies hold out hope of cure for many deadly diseases, but medical errors continue to take a distressingly high toll of life. Schools of nursing are turning out record numbers of graduates, but the projections for future nursing shortages remain high.

You might be asking yourself about now, "Do I really want to get into this profession?" The answer is resounding "YES!" There could not be a better time to be a professional nurse. Society, as well as the medical community, is finally recognizing the vital role nurses play in the health-care system. Graduates from today's nursing programs have opportunities for professional practice and advancement that could only be dreamed about a few years ago. Yes, the demands are many, but the rewards are great. Today's nursing students must learn more, do more, and be more. Students entering nursing schools today come from diverse cultural, personal, and educational backgrounds, yet they must master a tremendous amount of information and learn a wide variety of skills so that they can successfully pass the licensure exam and become highly skilled registered nurses.

The fourth edition of *Nursing Now! Today's Issues, Tomorrow's Trends* is a first step in meeting the challenges of the future health care system. It incorporates many of the suggestions that our faithful readers have made over the past three years since the last edition was published. We are very excited about the revised text and believe its quality and content meet the high standards demanded by our readers.

Two new chapters have been added based on our readers' suggestions. Chapter 22, "Develop-ments in Current Nursing Practice," discusses some of the new and emerging roles in which nurses can practice, and Chapter 23, "Nursing Research and Evidence-Based Practice," discusses some of the key issues in nursing research. The chapter on the NCLEX exam was completely revised to reflect the recent changes by the NCSBN, and the test-taking skills section was revised and expanded into its own chapter (Chapter 10). This was done in response to our readers who feel that test-taking skills are important not only for the NCLEX, but throughout their nursing programs. All other chapters were revised with the addition of current content and resources.

We worked hard to retain and enhance the interactive format of the text. In addition to the journal layout, current issues boxes, and integrated questions throughout, we have added pictures and cartoons to increase the visual appeal of the book. We have increased the overall size of the book and increased the amount of "white-space" throughout to break up the long text sections. There is also a newly expanded interactive Web site available for students with a number of interactive learning activities.

The book's primary purpose remains the same as past editions. It presents an overview and synthesis of the important issues and trends that are basic to the development of professional nursing and affect nursing both today and into the future. Our readers tell us that the book can be used both at the beginning of the student's educational process as an "Introduction to Nursing" course and toward the end of the process as an "Issues and Trends" course. Some instructors even use it throughout their programs, incorporating chapters as the content is reflected in their course presentations. Nursing students remain the primary intended audience for *Nursing Now!* However, practicing nurses have reported that there is a sufficiently wide range of current issues and topics covered in enough depth to be useful for their practice.

Another dichotomy that nurses face on a daily basis is the ability to hold onto unchanging principles while working in a constantly changing environment. Simply stated, a nurse's ability to adapt to changes in the health-care system while remaining focused on providing high-quality care is the basis for successful professional practice. The only way nurses will be able to effectively practice their profession in a demanding health-care system is to remain firmly rooted in those values and beliefs that have always served as their source of strength. Even more than in the past, nurses need to look to each other for the inspiration and the strength that allows them to succeed. Professional organizations still serve as the most powerful force for nurses, and membership in professional organizations is becoming increasingly important.

It is our belief that this book will help future nurses become familiar with the important issues and trends that affect the profession and health care. The nursing profession needs highly skilled nurses who can teach, do research, solve complicated client problems, provide highly skilled care, and obtain advanced degrees. The leaders of the profession will come from those students who have a clear understanding of what it means to be a professional nurse and are willing to invest the effort in attaining their goals.

Joseph T. Catalano, PhD, RN

Acknowledgments

I would like to express my thanks to all of my students and colleagues who have over the years shaped my thoughts and ideas about the nursing profession. I also thank all the nurses who have contributed chapters to this book on such short notice. Your willingness to write well and write quickly is reflected in the quality of the chapters you produced.

Tonia Aiken, RN, BSN, JD
President and CEO
Aiken Development Group
New Orleans, Louisiana

Kristy Baker, MS, RN
Instructor, School of Nursing
Southwestern Oklahoma State University
Weatherford, Oklahoma

Barbara Bellfield, MS, RNP-C, RN
Family Nurse Practitioner
Ventura County Public Health
Loma Vista Road
Ventura, California

Lydia DeSantis, RN, PhD, FAAN
University of Miami
School of Nursing
Miami, Florida

Mary Evans, JD, RN
316 N. Tejon
Colorado Springs, Colorado

Donna Gentile O'Donnell, RN, MSN
Deputy Health Commissioner (Retired)
Philadelphia, Pennsylvania

Nicole Harder, RN, BN, MPA
Coordinator, Learning Laboratories
Helen Glass Centre for Nursing
Faculty of Nursing
University of Manitoba
Winnipeg, Manitoba
Canada

Roberta Mowdy, MS, RN
Instructor
Department of Nursing
East Central University
Ada, Oklahoma

Mary Ann Remshardt, EdD, RN
Assistant Professor
Department of Nursing
East Central University
Ada, Oklahoma

Kathleen Mary Young, RN, C, MA
Instructor
Western Michigan University
Kalamazoo, Michigan

Contents

Unit 1   The Growth of Nursing   1

    1 The Development of a Profession   3
    2 Historical Perspectives   23
    3 The Evolution of Licensure, Certification, and Nursing Organizations   37
    4 Theories and Models of Nursing   54
    5 The Process of Educating Nurses   77
    6 Critical Thinking   99

Unit 2   Making the Transition to Professional   113

    7 Ethics in Nursing   115
    8 Bioethical Issues   135
    9 Nursing Law and Liability   161
    10 Taking and Passing Tests   186
    11 NCLEX: What You Need to Know   202
    12 Reality Shock in the Workplace   222

Unit 3   Leading and Managing   245

    13 Principles of Leadership and Management   247
    14 Communicating Successfully   266
    15 Delegation and Supervision in Nursing   290
    16 Collective Bargaining and Governance   303
    17 Health Care Delivery Systems   323
    18 Nursing Informatics   343

Unit 4   Issues in Delivering Care   365

    19 The Politically Active Nurse   367
    20 Spirituality and Health Care   393
    21 Cultural Diversity   413
    22 Developments in Current Nursing Practice   431
    23 Nursing Research and Evidence-Based Practice   447
    24 Alternative and Complementary Healing Practices   465

Glossary   497
Appendix Specialty Nursing Organizations   511
Index   515

Nursing is an art.

Florence Nightingale (1820–1910)
British nurse, educator

Every one of us needs to show how much we care for each other and, in the process, care for ourselves.

Diana, Princess of Wales
(1961–1997)

1

The Growth of Nursing

1

The Development of a Profession

Joseph T. Catalano

Learning Objectives

After completing this chapter, the reader will be able to:

- Define the terms *position, job, occupation,* and *profession.*
- Compare the three approaches to defining a profession.
- Analyze those traits defining a profession that nursing has attained.
- Evaluate why nursing has failed to attain some of the traits that define a profession.
- Correlate the concept of power with its important characteristics.

WHAT IS A PROFESSION?

Since the time of Florence Nightingale, each generation of nurses, in their own way, has fostered the movement to professionalize the image of nurses and nursing. The struggle to change the status of nurses from that of female domestic servants to one of high-level health-care providers who base their protocols on scientific principles has been a primary goal of nursing's leaders for many years. Yet some people, both inside and outside of the profession of nursing, question whether the search for and attainment of professional status is worth the effort and price that must ultimately be paid.

At some levels in nursing, the question of **professionalism** takes on immense significance. However, to the busy **staff nurse**—who is trying to allocate client assignments for a shift; distribute the medications at 9 A.M. to 24 clients; and supervise two aides, a licensed practical nurse (LPN) or licensed vocational nurse (LVN), and a nursing student—the issue may not seem very significant at all.

Indeed, when nurses were first developing their identity separately from that of physicians, there was no thought about their being part of a **profession.** Over the years, as the scope of practice has expanded and the responsibilities have increased, nurses have increasingly begun to consider what they do as professional activities.

This chapter presents some of the current thought concerning professions and where nursing stands in relationship to these viewpoints.

> *Over the years, as the scope of practice has expanded and the responsibilities have increased, nurses have increasingly begun to consider what they do to be professional activities.*

What Do You Think?

Do you really care if nursing is a profession? How will it affect the way you practice nursing?

APPROACHES TO DEFINING A PROFESSION

In common usage, terms such as *position, job, occupation, profession, professional,* and *professionalism* are often used interchangeably and incorrectly. The following definitions will clarify what is meant by these terms within this text.

Position: A group of tasks assigned to one individual.
Job: A group of positions that are similar in nature and level of skill that can be carried out by one or more individuals.
Occupation: A group of jobs that are similar in type of work and that are usually found throughout an industry or work environment.
Profession: A type of occupation that meets certain criteria (discussed later in this chapter) that raise it to a level above that of an occupation.
Professional: A person who belongs to and practices a profession. (The term *professional* is probably the most misused of all these terms when describing people who are clearly involved in jobs or occupations, such as a "professional truck driver," "professional football player," or even a "professional thief.")
Professionalism: The demonstration of high-level personal, ethical, and skill characteristics of a member of a profession.[1]

Experts in social science have been attempting to develop a "foolproof" approach to determine what constitutes a profession for almost 100 years, but with only minimal success. Three common models are the process approach, the power approach, and, most widely accepted, the trait approach.

Process Approach
The process approach views all occupations as points of development into a profession along a continuum ranging from position to profession.

Continuum of Professional Development:
Position ⟷ Profession

Using this approach, the question becomes not whether nursing and truck driving are professions, but where they are located along the continuum. Occupations such as medicine, law, and the ministry are widely accepted by the public as being closest to the professional end of the continuum.[2] Other occupations may be less clearly defined.

The major difficulty with this approach is that it lacks criteria on which to base judgments. Final determination of the status of an occupation or profession depends almost completely on public perception of the activities of that occupation. Nursing has always had a rather poor public image when it comes to being viewed as a profession.

Power Approach
The power approach uses two criteria to define a profession:

1. How much independence of practice does this occupation have?
2. How much power does this occupation control?

The concept of power is discussed later in this chapter, but in this context it refers to political power and the amount of money that the person in that occupation earns.[3]

Using this determinant, occupations such as medicine, law, and **politics** would clearly be considered professions. The members of these occupations earn high incomes, practice their skills with a great deal of independence, and exercise significant power over individuals, the public, and the political community, both individually and in organized groups. The ministry is generally perceived as having power and influence. However, most persons in this group, except for a few individuals such as television evangelists, have relatively low income levels. Nursing, of course, with its relatively poor salaries, low membership in organizations, and perceived lack of political power, would clearly not meet the power criteria for a profession.

The question that comes to mind is whether power, independence of practice, and high incomes are the only elements that determine professional status. Although those three factors confer status in our culture, other elements can be considered significant in how a profession is viewed. For example, for many, members of the clergy have a great deal of power when they act as counselors, speakers of the truth, and community leaders.

Trait Approach

Of the many researchers and theorists who have attempted to identify the traits that define a profession, Flexner,[4] Bixler,[5] and Pavalko[6] are most widely accepted as the leaders in the field. These three social scientists have determined that the following common characteristics are important:

- High intellectual level
- High level of individual responsibility and **accountability**
- Specialized body of knowledge
- Knowledge that can be learned in institutions of higher education
- Public service and altruistic activities
- Public service valued over financial gain
- Relatively high degree of **autonomy** and independence of practice
- Need for a well-organized and strong organization representing the members of the profession and controlling the quality of practice
- A **code of ethics** that guides the members of the profession in their practice
- Strong professional identity and commitment to the development of the profession

- Demonstration of professional competency and possession of a legally recognized license

NURSING AS A PROFESSION

How does nursing compare with other professions when measured against these widely accepted professional traits? The profession of nursing meets most of the criteria but falls short in a few areas.

High Intellectual Level of Functioning

In the very early stages of the development of the practice of nursing, this criterion did not apply. Florence Nightingale raised the bar for education, and graduates of her school were considered to be highly educated compared with other women of that time. However, most of the tasks performed by these early nurses are generally considered by today's standards to be menial and routine.

On the other hand, as health care has advanced and made great strides in technology, pharmacology, and all branches of the physical sciences, a high level of intellectual functioning is required for even relatively simple nursing tasks, such as taking a client's temperature or blood pressure using automated equipment. Nurses use **assessment** skills and knowledge, have the ability to reason, and make routine judgments based on clients' conditions daily. Without a doubt, professional nurses must and do function at a high intellectual level.

High Level of Individual Responsibility and Accountability

Not too long ago, a nurse was rarely, if ever, named as a **defendant** in a malpractice suit. The public, in general, did not view nurses as having enough knowledge to be held accountable for errors that were made in client care. This is not the case in the health-care system today. Nurses are often the primary, and frequently the only, defendants named when errors are made that result in injury to the client. Nurses must be accountable and demonstrate a high level of individual responsibility for the care and services they provide.

The concept of accountability has legal, ethical, and professional implications that include accepting responsibility for actions taken to provide **client** care as well as accepting responsibility for the consequences of actions that are not performed. Nurses can no longer state that "the physician told me to do it" as a method of avoiding responsibility for their actions.

Specialized Body of Knowledge

Most early nursing skills were based either on traditional ways of doing things or on the intuitive knowledge of the individual nurse. As nursing developed into an identifiable, separate discipline, a specialized body of knowledge called "nursing science" was compiled through the research efforts of nurses with advanced educational degrees. Although this body of specialized nursing knowledge is relatively small, it forms a theoretical basis for the practice of nursing today. As more nurses obtain advanced degrees, conduct research, and develop philosophies and theories about nursing, this body of knowledge will increase in scope.

Evidence-Based Practice

In professional nursing today, there is an increasing emphasis on evidence-based practice. Almost all the currently used nursing theories address this issue in some way. Simply stated, evidence-based practice is the practice of nursing in which interventions are based on data from research that demonstrates that they are appropriate and successful. It involves a systematic process of uncovering, evaluating, and using information from research as the basis for making decisions about and providing client care. Many nursing practices and interventions of the past were performed merely because that was the way it was always done (accustomed practice) or because of deductions from physiological or pathophysiological information. Clients are now more sophisticated and knowledgeable about health-care issues and demand a higher level of knowledge and skill from their health-care providers.

The development of information technology has made evidence-based practice in nursing a reality. In the past, nurses relied primarily on units within their own facilities for information about the success of treatments, decisions about health care, and outcomes for clients. Nursing education now requires nursing students to perform Web-based research for papers and projects, so that by the time of graduation, they feel comfortable accessing a wide range of the most current and highest quality of information through electronic sources. Of course, one of the key limiting factors of evidence-based practice is the quality of the information on which the practice is based. Evaluating the quality of information on the Web can be difficult at times.

The first step in developing an evidence-based practice is to identify exactly what the intervention is supposed to accomplish. Once the goal or client outcome is identified, the nurse needs to evaluate current practices to determine whether or not they are achieving the desired client outcomes. If they are unsuccessful, or if the nurse feels they can be more efficient with fewer complications, then research sources need to be collected. These can be from published journal articles (either electronic or hard copy) and from presentations at research or practice conferences, which often present the most current information. Then a plan should be developed to implement the new findings. This process can be applied to changing policy and procedures or developing training programs for facility staff. Research data should always be used when initiating new practices or modifying old ones (see Chapter 23).

> " *Evidence-based practice is the practice of nursing in which interventions are based on data from research that demonstrates that they are appropriate and successful.* "

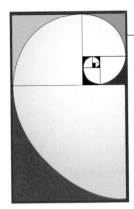

Issues Now

Web Sites: Friend or Foe?

Have a paper or report to do for class? Need information on pheochromocytoma, posttraumatic stress disorder, Kawasaki's disease? No problem, look it up on the Web, right? Well, yes and no. Without any question, there is a tremendous amount of information about almost any subject available just a few mouse clicks away. But the bigger question is: how good is that information? The truth of the matter is that anyone can post almost anything on-line these days, and there are no organizations or agencies that oversee or review the information for quality, accuracy, or objectivity. So how are you supposed to know what is good and what is not? Although there is no foolproof method for determining the quality of any given Web site, there are some telltale markers that can point you in the right direction when you are rating the quality of the information you are seeking.

Marker 1: Peer Review

All major professional journals have a peer review process that requires any manuscripts submitted to be reviewed by two or three professionals who are considered experts or at least knowledgeable in the subject matter. Peer review is one of the key elements in ensuring the accuracy of the information in the manuscript. When considering a Web source, look for a clear statement of the source of the information and how that information is reviewed. If the information is from an established source, such as a recognized professional journal, then it has been peer-reviewed and has a higher degree of accuracy. Examine the format and writing style of the document. If it seems to be very choppy, or the style, tone, or person the article is written in changes throughout the article, it is an indication that it was not well edited and probably not peer-reviewed. Use the information with caution.

Marker 2: Author Credentials

The name of the author and his or her titles and credentials should be listed. Be cautious if no author or publisher is listed. Of course, anyone can use another person's name as the author, but it is relatively easy to cross-check authors' names through other databases, such as those found in libraries. Before accepting the information as gospel, it is probably worth looking up the author and seeing what other articles or books he or she has written. Another key to establishing author credentials is to establish to whom the Web site belongs. In general, personal Web pages are less likely to contain authoritative information. You can also look at the last three letters in the Web site address. The ones that end in ".gov," ".org," or ".edu" will tend to have higher-quality information. Also, see whether the information has a copyright. If the information is copyrighted, then the person felt strongly enough about what he or she was posting to go to the effort to make sure no one else can use it as their original information.

Marker 3: Prejudice and Bias

Although there is almost always a small degree of prejudice and bias in all written material, most legitimate authors will strive to be as objective as possible. Many times if you read a document with a critical eye, you can discern obvious prejudicial

(continued)

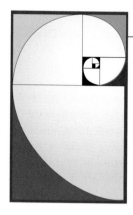

Issues Now continued

viewpoints. See if the author has a vested interest in the content of the document. You can be pretty sure that an article about the effects of tobacco use on the respiratory system written by a scientist who was hired by the R. J. Reynolds Company would have a decidedly different viewpoint than an article written by a scientist who was employed by the National Health Information Center. See if contact information is provided by the author and who the sponsor or publisher of the document is. If these are not provided, be suspicious about the information.

Marker 4: Timeliness

Of course all of us want the most recent information we can find and sometimes mistakenly make the assumption that because it is on the Web, it is new. In reality, professional journals that post their partial-text or full-text articles on their Web sites usually take anywhere from 6 to 9 months to do so. If you want the absolutely most current information, the hard-copy journal texts found in the library still are your best bet. Some forms of the Web have been around for as many as 10 years now, so some of the material can be very outdated. See if you can determine when the site was last updated and how extensively the information was revised. It is also a good practice to look to other sources (Web, journals, books, etc.) to compare the material for currency. Many Web sites have links where you can access other related information. If those links have messages such as "Page discontinued" or "Link no longer available" be extremely cautious with the information. Good links should connect you to other reliable sites.

Marker 5: Presentation

Although the old saying is that "you can't tell a book by its cover," experienced Web-surfers can often tell a lot about a Web site by its presentation. Some look well developed and professional, and others look very amateurish. There is no guarantee that the slick-looking Web sites are better, but it is one factor to consider in the overall evaluation of the information you are seeking. Take a look at the graphics. They should be balanced with the text and help explain or demonstrate information in the text. If the graphics seem to be just decorative, it should raise a red flag about the content of the site. Some sites use a compressed format that requires special programs such as Adobe Acrobat to view them. If you do not have access to these programs, then the information in the site is unusable. Move on to the next site.

In summary, the Internet can be a very valuable source of information about a wide variety of subjects. However, each source of information needs to be evaluated carefully. Following the five markers discussed here will place you on the path to deciding the quality of the information presented in any Web site.

Sources: Thurmond, VA: Considering theory in assessing quality of Web-based courses. Nurse Educator 27(1):20–24, 2002.
DeBourgh, GA: Using Web technology in a clinical nursing course. Nurse Educator 26(5):227–233, 2001.
Timmons, S: Use of the Internet by patients: Not a threat to nursing, but an opportunity? Nurse Education Today 21(2):104–109, 2001.
Take a byte: Evaluating Web sites. American Nursing Student 5(1):1, 2001.
www.mlanet.org/resources/medspeak/topten.html

Public Service and Altruistic Activities

Almost all major nursing theorists, when defining nursing, include a statement that refers to a goal of helping clients adapt to illness and achieve their highest level of functioning. The public (variously referred to as consumers, patients, clients, individuals, or humans) is the focal point of all nursing models and nursing practice. The public service function of nursing has always been recognized and acknowledged by society's willingness to continue to educate nurses in public, tax-supported institutions as well as in private schools. In addition, nursing has been viewed universally as being an altruistic profession composed of selfless individuals who place the lives and well-being of their clients above their personal safety. In the earliest days, dedicated nurses provided care for victims of deadly plagues with little regard for their own welfare. Today, nurses are found in remote and often hostile areas, providing care for the sick and dying, working 12-hour shifts, being "on call," and working rotating shifts.

Few individuals enter nursing in order to become rich and famous. It is likely that those who do so for these reasons quickly become disappointed. Although the pay scale has increased tremendously since the 1990s, nursing is, at best, a middle-income occupation. Surveys among students entering nursing programs continue to indicate that the primary reason for wishing to become a nurse is to "help others" or "make a difference" in someone's life and to have "job security." Rarely do these beginning students include "to make a lot of money" as their motivation.[7]

Well-Organized and Strong Representation

Professional organizations represent the members of the profession and control the quality of professional practice. The National League for Nursing (NLN) and the American Nurses Association (ANA) are the two major national organizations that represent nursing in today's health-care system. The NLN is primarily responsible for regulating the quality of the educational programs that prepare nurses for the practice of nursing, whereas the ANA is more concerned with the quality of nursing practice in the daily health-care setting. These and other organizations are discussed in more detail in Chapter 3.

Both these groups are well organized, but neither can be considered powerful when compared with other professional organizations, such as the American Medical Association (AMA) or the American Bar Association (ABA). One reason for their lack of strength is that fewer than 15 percent of all nurses in the United States are members of any professional organization at the national level.[3] Many nurses do belong to specialty organizations that represent a specific area of practice, but these lack sufficient political power to produce changes in health-care laws and policies at the national level.

Nurses' Code of Ethics

Nursing has several codes of ethics that are used to guide nursing practice. The ANA Code of Ethics for Nurses, the most widely used in the United States, was first published in 1971, updated in 1985, and last updated in 2001. The current ANA Code of Ethics, while maintaining the integrity found in earlier versions, is now more relevant to current health-care and nursing practices. This code of ethics is recognized by other professions as a standard with which others are compared. The nurses' code of ethics and its implications are discussed in greater detail in Chapter 7.

Competency and Professional License

Nurses must pass a national licensure examination to demonstrate that they are qualified to practice nursing. Only after passing this examination are nurses allowed to practice. The granting of a nursing **license** is a legal activity conducted by the individual state under the **regulations** contained in that state's nurse practice act.

WHEN NURSING FALLS SHORT OF THE CRITERIA

Before Florence Nightingale practiced nursing, people considered it to be unnecessary, if not outright dangerous, to educate nurses through independent nursing programs in publicly supported educational institutions. As nursing has developed, particularly in the United States, the recognition of the intellectual nature of the practice, as well as the vast amount of knowledge required for the job, has led to a belief by some nursing leaders that college education for nurses is now a necessity.

Nursing is the only major discipline that does not require its members to hold at least a baccalaureate degree in order to obtain licensure. Although the number of diploma programs in nursing has decreased tremendously since 1990, associate degree programs continue to maintain high enrollment and graduate large numbers of individuals. Whether a baccalaureate degree nursing program should be the minimum requirement for entry-level nurses remains a hotly debated issue.[1,6,7,10]

Autonomy and Independence of Practice

Historically, the handmaiden or servant relationship of the nurse to the physician was widely accepted. It was based on several factors, including social norms. For example, women became nurses, whereas men became physicians; women were subservient to men, the nature of the work being such that nurses cleaned and physicians cured. In terms of the relative levels of education of the two groups, the average nursing program lasted for 1 year, whereas physician education lasted for 6 to 8 years.

Unfortunately, despite efforts to expand nursing practice into more independent areas through updated nurse practice legislation, nursing retains much of its subservient image. In reality, nursing is both an independent and interdependent discipline. Nurses in all health-care settings must work closely with physicians, hospital administrators, pharmacists, and other groups in the provision of care. In some cases, nurses in **advanced practice** roles, such as **nurse practitioners,** can and do establish their own independent practices. Most state **nurse practice acts** allow nurses more independence in their practice than they realize. To be considered a true profession, nursing will need to be recognized by other disciplines as having practitioners who practice nursing independently.

Professional Identity and Development

The issue of job versus career is in question here. A job is a group of positions that are similar in nature and level of skill that can be carried out by one or more individuals. There is relatively little commitment to a job, and many individuals move from one job to another with little regard to the long-term outcomes. A career, in contrast, is usually viewed as a person's major lifework, which progresses and develops as the person grows older. Careers and professions have many of the same characteristics, including a formal education, full-time employment, requirement for lifelong learning, and a dedication to what is being achieved. Although an increasing number of nurses view nursing as their life's work, many still treat nursing more as a job.

The problem becomes circular. The reason nurses lack a strong professional identity and do not consider nursing a lifelong career is because nursing does not have full status as a profession. Until nurses are fully committed to the profession of nursing, identify with it as a profession, and are dedicated to its future development, nursing will probably not achieve professional status.

MEMBERS OF THE HEALTH-CARE TEAM

The health-care delivery system employs large numbers of diagnosticians, technicians, direct care providers, administrators, and support staff (Table 1.1). It is estimated that there are more than 300 job titles used to describe health-care workers. Among these are nurses, physicians, physician assistants, social workers, physical therapists, occupational therapists, respiratory therapists, clinical psychologists, and pharmacists. All these individuals provide services that are essential to daily operation of the health-care delivery system in this country.

Of particular importance among this array of health-care workers are various types of nurses: registered nurses, licensed practical (vocational) nurses, nurse practitioners, case managers, and clinical nurse specialists. Each of these requires a different type of educational background, clinical expertise, and, sometimes, professional credentialing. In general, all nurses make valuable contributions within the health-care delivery system. There has been an increased demand for nurses who are

Table 1.1 Other Key Health-Care Team Members

Title	Credential	Practice
Physician (MD)	License–Medical	Medical—limited only by specialization Some serve as primary care providers
Physician (DO)	License–Osteopath	Medical, with focus on body movement and holistic health—similar to MD Can serve as primary care providers
Physician (DC)	License–Chiropractor	Limited—focus on spinal column and nervous system Unable to prescribe medications
Physician (DPM)	License–Podiatry	Limited—foot problems Can prescribe medications, perform foot surgery
Physician Assistant	Certification–no individual license	Practice on physician's license Practice limited by medical practice act and wishes of supervising physician
Social Workers	License	Increasingly important as health care becomes more complex Resolve financial, housing, psychosocial, and employment problems; do discharge planning and assist clients in transfer between facilities. May serve in case management roles to coordinate services.
Physical Therapists	License	Focus on helping clients maintain or regain the highest level of function possible after strokes, spinal cord injury, arthritis, or residual effects of traumatic accidents. Help prevent physical decline and regain the ability to groom, eat, and walk through individualized range of motion and exercise programs. Therapy occurs in hospitals, clinics, or in the community
Respiratory Therapists	License	Strive to restore normal or as near normal pulmonary functioning as possible by conducting diagnostic tests and administering treatments that have been prescribed by a physician
Clinical Psychologists	License	Assist clients to manage mental health problems Private practice, clinics
Pharmacists	License	Distribute prescribed and over-the-counter medications, educate clients, monitor appropriate medication selections, detect interactions and untoward responses in community pharmacies and institutional settings Valuable resource for nurses

educated to deliver care in the community setting and in long-term health-care settings rather than in the hospital. There has also been a need for nurse case managers who are prepared to coordinate care for vulnerable populations requiring costly services over extended periods. Nursing education programs are attempting to meet these needs by preparing individuals who can practice independently and autonomously, network, collaborate, and coordinate services. These programs also offer more clinical experiences in rehabilitation, nursing home, and community settings.

Registered Nurses, Licensed Practical Nurses, and Unlicensed Assistive Personnel

Registered nurses (RNs) who have been educated at the associate, diploma, or baccalaureate level have traditionally been considered the cornerstone of the current health-care delivery system. In the past, most RNs worked within hospital settings and provided direct client care and nursing administration functions within these facilities. Owing to past trends in health-care funding, there were fewer hospital admissions, which temporarily decreased the demand for RNs in acute care facilities and increased the need for well-prepared nurses who could function autonomously within the community. However, current trends in population and health care have demonstrated a need for RNs in both acute care and community settings. The need still remains within institutional settings for licensed practical nurses (LPNs) and unlicensed assistive personnel (UAP) who work under the supervision of an RN. This pattern of care is particularly evident in nursing homes and other long-term care facilities.[2]

Advanced Practice Nurses

For individuals who are unfamiliar with the health-care delivery system, it is sometimes difficult to understand the similarities and differences between nursing titles and roles. This confusion is particularly evident in the case of clinical nurse specialists (CNSs) and nurse practitioners (NPs), who are sometimes collectively referred to as advanced practice nurses (APNs).

The nurse practitioner. In general, NPs are prepared to provide direct client care in primary care settings, focusing on health promotion, illness prevention, early diagnosis, and treatment of common health problems. Their educational preparation varies, but in most cases individuals successfully complete a graduate nurse practitioner program and are certified by the American Nurses Credentialing Center (ANCC) or an appropriate professional nursing organization. Depending on the individual state practice act, NPs have a range of responsibility for diagnosing diseases and prescribing both treatments and medications. A growing number of states now grant NPs direct third-party reimbursement for their services without a physician.

The clinical nurse specialist. Clinical nurse specialists usually practice in secondary or tertiary care settings and focus on care of individuals who are experiencing an acute illness or an exacerbation of a chronic condition. In general, they are prepared at the graduate level and are ANCC certified. CNSs are highly skilled practitioners who are comfortable working in high-tech environments with seriously ill individuals and their families. Because of the nature of their work, they are excellent health-care educators and physician collaborators.

Attempts have been made to combine the roles of the CNS and NP so that the best qualities of both roles are preserved. The goal of this combination is to provide high-quality care to individuals in a wide array of health-care settings who have a wide range of health problems. Advocates of this movement include the NLN, the American Association of Colleges of Nursing (AACN), and the ANA. Titling for this new blended role is unconfirmed, and state legislatures may make the final decisions through their licensing laws. As such, titling, educational preparation, and practice privileges will probably vary from one state to another.

Case Managers

One argument for the blended NP–CNS role is the need for case managers who possess the expertise of both levels of preparation. Case managers coordinate services for clients with high-risk or long-term health problems who have access to the full continuum of health-care services. Case managers provide services in various settings, such as acute care facilities, rehabilitation centers, and community agencies. They also work for managed-care companies, insurance companies, and private case management agencies. Their roles vary depending on the circumstances of their employment; however, their overall goal is to coordinate the use of health-care services in the most efficient and cost-effective manner possible.

Case management is the glue that holds health-care services together across practitioners, agencies, funding sources, locations, and time. Titling, educational preparation, and certification of nurse case managers are now available. The ANCC has developed certification eligibility criteria for nurse case managers, and an examination is available. At this time, case managers can be physicians, social workers, registered nurses, and even well-intentioned laypersons with little health-care education.

EMPOWERMENT IN NURSING

One of the concerns that has plagued nurses and nursing almost from its development as a separate health-care specialty is the relatively large amount of personal responsibility shouldered by nurses combined with a relatively small amount of control over their practice. Even in the more enlightened atmosphere of today's society, with its concerns about equal opportunity, equal pay, and collegial relationships, many nurses still seem uncomfortable with the concepts of power and control in their practice. Their discomfort may arise from the belief that nursing is a helping and caring profession whose goals are separate from issues of power.

Historically, nurses have never had much power, and previous attempts at gaining power and control over their practice have been met with much resistance from groups who benefit from keeping nurses powerless. Nevertheless, all nurses use power in their daily practice, even if they do not realize it. Until nurses understand the sources of their power, how to increase it, and how to use it in providing client care, they will be relegated to a subservient position in the health-care system.

The Nature of Power

The term *power* has many meanings. From the standpoint of nursing, power is probably best defined as the ability or capacity to exert influence over another person or group of persons. In other words, power is the ability to get other people to do things even when they do not want to do them. Although power in itself is neither good nor bad, it can be used to produce either good or bad results.

Power is always a two-way street. By its very definition, when power is exerted by one person, another person is affected; that is, the use of power by one person requires that another person give up some of his or her power. Individuals are always in a state of change, either increasing their power or losing some; the balance of power rarely remains static. **Empowerment** refers to the increased amount of power that an individual or group is either given or gains.

Origins of Power

If power is such an important part of nursing and the practice of nurses, where does it come from? Although there are many sources, some of them would be inappropriate or unacceptable for those in a helping and caring profession. The following list includes some of the more accessible and acceptable sources of power that nurses should consider using in their practice.[3,8,9] These sources are:

- Referent
- Expert
- Reward
- Coercive
- Legitimate
- Collective

Referent Power

The referent source of power depends on establishing and maintaining a close personal relationship with someone. In any close personal relationship, one individual often will do something he or she would really rather not do because of the relationship. This ability to change the actions of another is an exercise of power.

Nurses often obtain power from this source when they establish and maintain good therapeutic relationships with their clients. Clients take medications, tolerate uncomfortable treatments, and participate in demanding activities that they would clearly prefer to avoid because the nurse has good relationships with them. Likewise, nurses who have good collegial relationships with other nurses, departments,

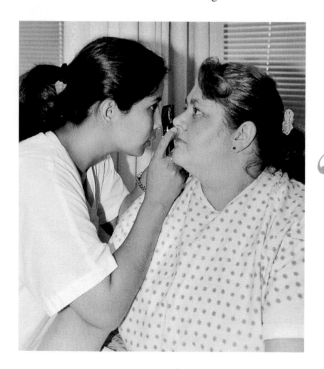

edge may increase the amount of respect they are given by physicians. Nurses access this expert source of power when they use their knowledge to teach, counsel, or motivate clients to follow a plan of care. Nurses can also use expert power when dealing with physicians.

> *By demonstrating their knowledge of the client's condition, recent laboratory tests, and other elements that are vital in the client's recovery, nurses demonstrate their expert power. This knowledge may increase the amount of respect that they are given by physicians.*

and physicians are often able to obtain what they want from these individuals or groups in providing care to clients.

Expert Power

The expert source of power derives from the amount of knowledge, skill, or expertise that an individual or group has. This power source is exercised by the individual or group when knowledge, skills, or expertise is either used or withheld in order to influence the behavior of others. Nurses should have at least a minimal amount of this type of power because of their education and experience. It follows logically that increasing the level of nurses' education will, or should, increase this expert power. As nurses attain and remain in positions of power longer, the increased experience will also aid the use of expert power. Nurses in advanced practice roles are good examples of those who have expert power. Their additional education and experience provide these nurses with the ability to practice skills at a higher level compared with nurses prepared at the basic education level.

By demonstrating their knowledge of the client's condition, recent laboratory tests, and other elements that are vital in the client's recovery, nurses demonstrate their expert power. This knowl-

Power of Rewards

The reward source of power depends on the ability of one person to grant another some type of reward for specific behaviors or changes in behavior. The rewards can take on many different forms, including personal favors, promotions, money, expanded privileges, and eradication of punishments. Nurses, in their daily provision of care, can use this source of power to influence client behavior. For example, a nurse can give a client extra praise for completing the prescribed range-of-motion exercises. There are many aspects of the daily care of clients over which nurses have a substantial amount of reward power. This reward source of power is also the underlying principle in the process of behavior modification.

Coercive Power

The coercive source of power is the flip side of the reward source. The ability to punish, withhold rewards, and threaten punishment is the key element underlying the coercive source of power. Although nurses do have access to this source of power, it is probably one that they use minimally, if at all. Not only does the use of the coercive source of power destroy therapeutic and personal relationships, but it can also be considered unethical and even illegal in certain situations. Threatening clients with an injection if they do not take their oral medications may

Issues in Practice

Kasey is an RN who has worked on the busy surgical unit of a large city hospital for the past 6 years. As one of three RNs on the unit's day shift, she often serves as the charge nurse when the assigned charge nurse has a day off. She is hard working, caring, and well organized and provides high-quality care for the often very unstable postoperative clients they receive on a daily basis.

Approximately 2 weeks ago, Kasey's mother was admitted for a high-risk surgical removal of a brain tumor that was not responding to chemotherapy or radiation therapy. The surgery did not go well, and Kasey's mother was admitted to the surgical unit after the procedure. During the past 2 weeks, she has shown a gradual but steady decline in condition and is no longer able to recognize her family, speak, or do any self-care. It is believed she will probably not live more than a week longer.

Per hospital policy, Kasey is not assigned to care for her mother; however, during her shifts, Kasey is spending more and more time with her mother, sometimes to the detriment of her assigned clients. She is also beginning to make more demands on the unit nursing staff, often overseeing their care and requesting that only certain nurses care for her mother. One of the other nurses on the unit suggested that Kasey's mother be moved to a less specialized unit. When Kasey heard about the suggestion, she became livid and loudly scolded the nurse for her insensitivity in the middle of the nurses station.

QUESTIONS FOR THOUGHT

1. Is the practice of not allowing nurses to provide care for their relatives evidence-based or accustomed practice?

2. Identify the steps in making this policy evidence based.

3. Do you think nurses should be allowed to care for relatives? Why? Why not?

motivate them to take those medications, but it is generally not considered to be a good example of a therapeutic communication technique.

Legitimate Power

The legitimate source of power depends on a legislative or legal act that gives the individual or organization a right to make decisions that they might not otherwise have the authority to make. Most obviously, political figures and **legislators** have this source of power. This power can also be disseminated and delegated to others through legislative acts. In nursing, the state board of nursing has access to the legitimate source of power because of its establishment under the nurse practice act of that state. Similarly, nurses have access to the legitimate source of power when they are licensed by the state under the provisions in the nurse practice act or when they are appointed to positions within a health-care agency. Nursing decisions made about client care can come only from individuals who have a legitimate source of power to make those decisions—that is, licensed nurses.

Collective Power

The collective source of power is often used in a broader context than individual client care and is the underlying source for many other sources of power. When a large group of individuals who have similar beliefs, desires, or needs become organized, a collective source of power exists. For

individuals who belong to professions, the professional organization is the focal point for this source of power. The main goal of any organization is to influence policies that affect the members of the organization. This influence is usually in the form of political activities carried out by politicians and **lobbyists.**

Professional organizations that can deliver large numbers of votes have a powerful means of influencing politicians. The use of the collective source of power contains elements of reward, coercive, expert, and even referent sources. Each source may come into play at one time or another.

How to Increase Power in Nursing

Despite some feelings of powerlessness, nurses really do have access to some important, and rather substantial, sources of power. What can nurses, either as individuals or as a group, do to increase their power?

Professional Unity

Probably the first, and certainly the most important, way in which nurses can gain power in all areas is through professional unity. The most powerful groups are those that are best organized and most united. The power that a professional organization has is directly related to the size of its membership. According to the ANA, there are approximately 2.7 million nurses in the United States. It is not difficult to imagine the power that the ANA could have to influence legislators and legislation if all of those nurses were members of the organization rather than the 250,000 who actually do belong. This point—that nurses need to belong to their national nursing organization—cannot be emphasized too much.

Political Activities

A second way in which nurses can gain power is by becoming involved in **political action.** Although this produces discomfort in many, nurses must realize that they are affected by politics and political decisions in every phase of their daily nursing activities.

The simple truth is that if nurses do not become involved in politics and participate in important legislation that influences their practice, someone other than nurses will be making those decisions for them. Nurses need to become involved in political activities from local to national levels. The average legislator knows little about issues such as clients' rights, national health insurance, quality of nursing care, third-party reimbursement for nurses, and expanded practice roles for nurses, yet they make decisions about these issues almost daily. It would seem logical that more informed and better decisions could be made if nurses took an active part in the legislative process.

> *Probably the first, and certainly the most important, way in which nurses can gain power in all areas is through professional unity. The most powerful groups are those that are best organized and most united.*

Accountability and Professionalism

A third method of increasing power is by demonstrating the characteristics of accountability and professionalism. Nursing has made great strides in these two areas in recent years. Nurses, through professional organizations, have been working hard to establish standards for high-quality client care. More important, nurses are now concerned with demonstrating competence and delivering high-quality client care through processes such as peer review and evaluation. By accepting responsibility for the care that they provide and by setting the standards to guide that care, nurses are taking the power to govern nursing away from non-nursing groups.

Networking

Finally, nurses can gain power through establishing a nurse support network. It is common knowledge that the "old boy" system remains alive and well in many segments of our seemingly enlightened twenty-first century society. The old boy system, which is found in most large organizations ranging from universities to businesses and governmental agencies, provides individuals, usually men, with the encouragement, support, and nurturing that allow them to move up quickly through the ranks in the organization to achieve high administrative positions. Nursing and nursing organizations have never had this type of system for the advancement of nurses. An important element in making this system work involves never criticizing another "old boy" in public, even though

there may be major differences of opinion in private. Presentation of a united front is extremely important in maintaining power within this system.

Part of the difficulty in establishing a nurse support network arises from the fact that nurses have not been in high-level positions for very long. The framework for a support system for nurses is now in place; with some commitment to the concept and some activity, it can grow into a well-developed network to allow the brightest, best, and most ambitious people in the profession to achieve high-level positions.

Future Trends in the Nursing Profession

Clearly, it would be difficult to make an airtight case for nursing as a profession, yet nursing does meet many of the criteria proposed for a profession. Although it would probably be most accurate to call nursing a developing or aspiring profession, for the purposes of this book, nursing will be referred to as a profession. Only when nurses begin to think of nursing as a profession, work toward raising the educational standards for entry level, and begin practicing independently as professionals, will the status of profession become a reality for nursing. The movement of any discipline from the status of occupation to one of profession is a dynamic and ongoing process with many considerations.

All the experts now predict a severe shortage of professional nurses, ranging from between 200,000 to 800,000, by the year 2020. In the past, the way that nursing shortages were handled was to use a quick-fix method of producing more nurses in a shorter period of time by reducing the educational requirements. The current nursing education system is producing approximately 40,000 graduates from diploma and associate degree programs every year.[10] Although this number may help alleviate the nursing shortage, the more critical question to ask is whether this level of education is going to prepare nurses to meet the challenges of a rapidly changing and demanding health-care system into the twenty-first century.

As the national employment picture continues to evolve for registered nurses from bedside caregivers to coordinators of care, and financial resources become stressed, perhaps more nurses will begin to look on what they do as a lifelong commitment. Professional commitment is a complicated issue, but little doubt exists that nurses will not have increased independence of practice until they begin to demonstrate that they are professionals committed to the field of nursing.

Conclusion

Ongoing changes in the health-care system will have a major impact on how, where, and even who practices nursing. Unless nurses become involved in decisions about the direction in which health care is going, band together as a profession, and exert some of the tremendous potential power that they have, politicians, physicians, hospital administrators, and insurance companies will ultimately be shaping their future. The move toward mandated staffing ratios is one way that nurses are demonstrating their power to achieve a goal when they band together and exert power as a group.

Nursing has taken great strides forward in achieving professional status in the health-care system.

Currently, many nurses accept the premise that nursing is a profession and therefore are not very concerned about furthering the process. Even as nursing has matured and evolved into a field of study with an identifiable body of knowledge, the questions and problems that have plagued this profession persist. In addition, advances in technology, management, and society have raised new questions about the nature and role of nursing in the health-care system. Only by understanding and exploring the issues of professionalism will nurses be prepared to practice effectively in the present and meet the complex challenges of the future.

Issues in Practice

Mandatory Staffing Ratios: The California Experience

California was the first state that approved laws that mandate nurse-to-client staffing ratios (Table 1.2). Guidelines were developed in January 2002 and went into effect in January 2004.

Initial studies of the effects of the mandatory staffing ratios in California have disproved the California Hospital Association's claim that they would be too costly and cause the closing of hospital units if not entire institutions. The estimated cost to meet the mandated ratios was between 1 and 1.7 percent, or approximatley $217,000 per hospital. Although the cost estimates seem to be fairly accurate, the overall effect was only marginal for hospitals' bottom lines. It did not improve the profit margin but it did not significantly decrease it either.

It has been more difficult to come up with explanations of why this has occurred. Nursing groups claim that the better staffing ratios produce better client care, which in turn results in reduced costs for insurance and settlements from malpractice law suits. Others believe that hospitals, in meeting the mandatory staffing

Table 1.2 California Proposed Nurse-to-Client Ratios (April 2002)

Hospital Unit	Ratio
ICU	1:2*
Operating room	1:1*
Neonatal ICU	1:2*
Intermediate care nursery	1:4*
Well-baby nursery	1:8*
Postpartum (multiple births never to exceed 8 per nurse)	1:8 (1:4 couplets; 1:6 mothers only)
Labor and delivery	1:2
Postanesthesia care unit (recovery room)	1:2
Emergency departments	1:4 (1:2 critical; 1:1 trauma)
Burn unit	1:2
Pediatrics	1:4
Step-down/telemetry	1:4
Specialty care (oncology)	1:5
Telemetry unit	1:5
General medical/surgical	1:6 initially 1:5 phased in
Behavioral health psychiatric units	1:6
Mixed units	1:6 initially 1:5 phased in

(continued)

Issues in Practice continued

levels, are using fewer of the very expensive agency nurses. All groups seem to agree that increased staffing levels increase nurses' moral and as a result, there is a reduction in turnover rates. Replacing RNs who quit because of poor staffing is very expensive. An average estimated cost to recruit and train a medical surgical nurse is approximately $46,000.00 and for a specialty nurse, such as ICU or ER, it may run as high as $64,000.00.

A slowly growing body of research demonstrates the connection between staffing levels and positive or negative health-care outcomes for hospitalized clients. Nursing associations and consumer groups feel that the quality of care is increased along with client safety with higher levels of RNs in the health-care setting. Although in the short run, mandatory staffing levels may seem to increase the nursing shortage, the long-term view is that it will help reduce the nursing shortage by addressing one of the leading causes of attrition among nurses—burnout from poor working conditions. If the health-care industry can keep more nurses in health care rather than having them leave for less stressful work settings, a major contribution will have been made to address the nursing shortage.

QUESTIONS FOR THOUGHT

1. Do you think the proposed staffing ratios are a good thing? Why or why not? How would they affect health care in your town?

2. Does your state have any proposed legislation regarding mandatory staffing ratios? If so, obtain copies of the bills, read them, and discuss them with your class.

3. Do you know who your legislator is? Have you contacted him or her about how you feel about mandatory staffing ratios? If not, call him or her today!

Sources: Garretson, S: Nurse to patient ratios in American health care. Nursing Standard 19(14):33–37, 2004; Spetz, J: California's minimum nurse-to-patient rations: The first few months. Journal of Nursing Administration 34(12):571–578, 2004; Bochum, K: Ratio rationale: RNs exxplain why rations matter. California Nurse 100(10):9–11, 2004.

Critical Thinking Exercises

- Distinguish between an occupation and a profession.
- Is nursing a profession? Defend your position.
- Discuss four ways in which nursing can improve its professional status.
- Name the three sources of power to which nurses have the most access. Discuss how nurses can best use these sources of power to improve nursing, nursing care, and the health-care system.

References

1. Karp, M, Jacobs, J, Hughes, Katherine: Credentials, curriculum and access. Institute on Education and the Economy 5, 2000.
2. Kennedy, M: APNs: Improved outcomes at lower costs. Am J Nurs 104:9, 19, 2004.
3. Smith, GR: Power and health care reform. J Nurs Educ 33:194–197, 1994.
4. Bellack, JP, and O'Neil, EH: Recreating nursing practice for a new century. Nursing and Health Care Perspectives 21(1):14–24, 2000.
5. Lindeman, CA: The future of nursing education. J Nurs Educ 39(1):5–12, 2000.
6. Lusk, M, and Decker, I: Moving towards a model of nursing education and practice. Nursing and Health Care Perspectives 22(2):81–84, 2001.
7. Gatxke, H, and Ransom, JE: New skills for a new age: Preparing nurses for the 21st century. Nursing Forum 36(3):18–28, 2001.
8. Fitzpatrick, ML: Prologue to Professionalism. Robert J. Brady, Bowie, MD, 1983.
9. O'Grady, ET: Health policy and politics. Nursing Economics 18(2):88–90, 2001.
10. American Nurses Association: Nursing Social Policy Statement. ANA, Washington, DC, 1999.

Bibliography

Burke, RJ: The ripple effect: Staffing post restructuring. Nursing Management 33(2):41–43, 2002.

Callister, J, et al.: Inquiry in baccalaureate nursing education: Fostering evidence-based practice. Nursing Education 44(2):59–65, 2005.

Carter, M: The ABCs of staffing decisions. Nursing Management 35(6):16, 2004.

Ferguson, L, Day R: Evidence-based nursing education: Myth or reality. Nursing Education 44(3):107–116, 2005.

Freeman, LH, et al.: New curriculum for a new century. Nursing Education 41(1):38–40, 2002.

Irving, JA, and Sniper, J: Preserving professional values. J Prof Nurs 18(1):5, 2002.

Kinsman, L, and James, EL: Evidence based practice needs evidence based implementation. Lippincott's Case Management 6(5):208–219, 2001.

Kovner, C, Harrington, C, CMS Study: Correlation between staffing and quality. AJN 102(9):65–66, 2002.

Manojlovich, M: Predictors of professional practice behaviors in hosptial settings. Nurs Res 54(1):41–47, 2005.

Manthey, M: Continuing the case for the baccalaureate. J Prof Nurs 18(1):7, 2002.

Narayan, MC, et al.: Searching for nursing's future. Nursing Management 33(1):26–30, 2002.

O'Bryan, L, et al.: Rework the workload. Nursing Management 33(3):38–40, 2002.

Thompson, D, and Burns, H: Work environment for nurses and the impact on protecting patients from health care errors. J Prof Nurs 20(3):145–147, 2004.

2

Historical Perspectives

Joseph T. Catalano

Learning Objectives

After completing this chapter, the reader will be able to:

- Explain why studying the history of health care and nursing is important to the profession of nursing.
- Name three "historical threads" found in the study of nursing history and discuss why they are important.
- Discuss Christian influences on health care and nursing.
- Discuss the influences of the Renaissance and Reformation on health care and nursing.
- Describe the major changes in health care and nursing that occurred during and immediately after World War II.

UNDERSTANDING OUR HISTORY

Knowledge about the profession's past can help us understand how nursing developed and even suggest solutions to problems that face the profession today. Several threads run throughout the history of nursing, including society's beliefs about the causes of illness, the value placed on individual life, and the role of women in society. The wars of modern history have also had a significant impact on nursing, particularly in influencing the development of technology and guiding the direction of health care. This chapter is not a treatise on the history of health care and nursing, but presents some key historic milestones that helped to form the foundations of health and nursing care.

ORIGINS OF NURSING

Before Nursing

Current nursing practice is a relatively recent development. The major concern of most early civilizations was the survival of the group, and because illness and injury threatened this survival, many primitive health-care practices grew from processes of trial and error. In prehistoric times, women tended to care for the ill and injured. Evil spirits were thought to be the cause of illness, and the medicine men and women who practiced witchcraft were considered religious figures.

Driving Out Demons

In ancient eastern civilizations, starting from about 3500 B.C., health care was intertwined with religion. Taoism emphasized balance and

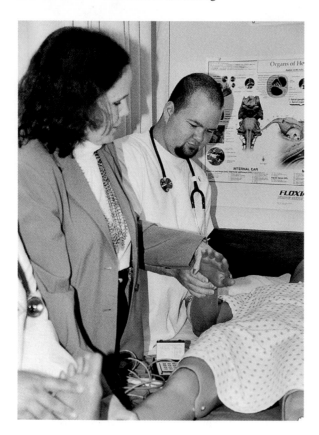

group, and because illness and injury threatened this survival, many primitive health-care practices grew from processes of trial and error.

Ancient Sciences

During the same period, the ancient Egyptians' belief that all disease was caused by evil spirits and punishing gods was changing. Health-care providers from that time showed a well-developed understanding of the basis of disease. Writings from 1500 B.C. refer to surgical procedures, the role of the midwife, bandaging, preventive care, and even birth control. Women enjoyed a higher status in Egyptian society and even worked in hospitals.[1] Physicians, however, were still men, who served in multiple roles as surgeons, priests, architects, and politicians.

The Babylonian Empire, united in 2100 B.C., was a civilization that focused on astrology. Its health-care practices included special diets, massage therapy, and rest to drive evil spirits from a body. People would go to the marketplace to seek advice on how to treat their ailments. During the height of the empire, strict guidelines governed doctors' fees and responsibilities in medical practice. There is also

the driving of demons out of the ailing body. Acupuncture developed over the next several thousands of years, and medicinal herbs were used in preventive health care.

In Southeast Asia, Hinduism emphasized the need for good hygiene, and written records would soon chronicle a number of surgical procedures. This was also the first culture to document medical treatment outside the home, although women were prohibited from working. The rise of Buddhism around 530 B.C. caused a surge in health care, with public hospitals and high standards for doctors and other hospital workers and an emphasis on hygiene and prevention of disease. The development of medical knowledge was hindered to a degree by the refusal of the physicians to come in contact with blood and infectious body secretions and the prohibition against dissection of the human body.

The major concern of most early civilizations was the survival of the

What Do You Think?

Is the study of history really necessary for nursing students? Why or why not?

_____

_____

_____

_____

_____

_____

_____

_____

_____

_____

_____

_____

_____

evidence from this period of child care and treatment for some diseases, but most care still took place in the home.

By 1900 B.C., the Hebrews had formed a nation along the Mediterranean and adopted many of the health practices of their neighbors. They integrated elements of the Egyptian sanitary laws to form the Mosaic Code that, as in many other cultures, mixed religion and medicine. Caring for widows, orphans, and other strangers in need was part of daily life. Hebrews had good knowledge of anatomy and physiology, especially the circulatory system. Physician-priests routinely performed operations such as cesarean sections (named later by the Romans), amputation, and circumcisions. They also enforced rules of purification, performed sacrifices, and conducted rituals related to food preparation.

The Father of Medicine

Ancient Greece was a culture that focused on appeasing the gods, and its medical practice was no exception. The god Apollo was devoted to medicine and good health. The Greeks performed sacrifices to appease the gods and practiced abortion and infanticide in an attempt to control the population. People took hot baths at spas to improve health, but the sick and injured were cared for at clinics. Although women were held in high esteem, they were not permitted to provide any health care outside the home. Around 400 B.C., the writings of Hippocrates began to change medical practice in Greece. One of a roving group of physician-priests, Hippocrates was called "the father of medicine." His beliefs focused on harmony with the natural law instead of on appeasing the gods. He emphasized treating the whole client—mind, body, spirit, and environment— and making diagnoses on the basis of symptoms rather than on an isolated idea of a disease. He was also concerned with ethical standards for physicians, expressed in the now-famous Hippocratic oath.

Health Care in the Roman Empire

Ancient Romans clung to superstitions and polytheism as the foundations for medical as well as religious practices. This dominant empire ruled from around 290 B.C. and absorbed useful elements of whatever culture they conquered—including the Greeks and Hebrews—into their own. They developed a quite advanced system of medicine and a pharmacology that included more than 600 medications derived from herbs and plants. Roman physicians were eventually able to distinguish between various conditions and performed many surgeries. They also did physical therapy for athletes; diagnosed symptoms of infections; identified job-related dangers of lead, mercury, and asbestos; and published medical textbooks.

The Romans' advances in creating an unlimited supply of clean water via aqueducts were critical in maintaining the good health of its citizens, as were central heating, spas and baths, and more advanced systems for sewage disposal.

Because the great Roman armies were so crucial to the empire, they developed early hospitals to care for sick and injured soldiers. These were mobile and were staffed by female as well as male attendants, who performed duties that would today be thought of as nursing care: cleaning and bandaging wounds, feeding and cleaning clients, and providing comfort to the wounded and dying. In many ways, women enjoyed an equal place in society, and they provided home health care as well as midwifery.

> " *The term* nurse *is thought to have originated in this period, from the Latin word* nutrire, *meaning to nourish, nurture, or suckle a child.* "

Early Efforts at Nursing

The Sanctity of Life

The rise of Christianity, starting from 30 A.D., brought with it a strong belief in the sanctity of all human life. Christians considered practices such as human sacrifice, infanticide, and abortion—which had been common in Roman society—to be murder. Following the teachings of Jesus meant that caring for the sick, poor, and disadvantaged was of primary importance, and groups of believers soon organized to offer care for those in need.

Early writings of the Christian period record women's important role in ministering to the sick and providing food and care for the poor and homeless. Wealthy Roman women who had converted to Christianity established hospital-like institutions and residences for these caregivers in their homes. The term *nurse* is thought to have originated in this period, from the Latin word *nutrire,* meaning to nourish, nurture, or suckle a child. The majority of care was still provided by a family member in the home. Most early Christian hospitals were roadside houses for the sick, poor, or destitute, who were cared for by male and female attendants alike. The attendants learned from a process of trial and error and by observing others.

A Time of Disease

The Dark Ages, from roughly 500 to 1000 A.D., were marked by widespread poverty, illness, and death. Plagues and other diseases such as smallpox, leprosy, and diphtheria ravaged the known world and killed large segments of populations. Health care at this time was almost nonexistent.

However, the strong beliefs of the Catholic Church, which was based in Rome, produced monasteries and convents that became centers for the care of the poor and the sick. By 500 A.D., there were several religious nursing orders in what is today England, France, and Italy. Men and women worked there and also traveled to rural areas where they were needed, combining religious rituals with home remedies as well as treatments such as bandaging, cautery, bloodletting, enemas, and leeching.

The biggest contribution to health care in this period may have been the insistence on cleanliness and hygiene, which lessened the spread of infections. Medieval nurses did not have any formal schooling but learned through apprenticeships with older monks or nuns. Eventually hospitals came to be built outside of monastery grounds. Secular orders were also established, which could provide a wider range of services to the sick because they were not limited by religious restrictions and obligations.

> *Medieval nurses did not have any formal schooling but learned through apprenticeships with older monks or nuns.*

Early Military Hospitals

At the end of the Dark Ages, there were a series of holy wars and invasions, including the Crusades, which produced many sick and injured who were far from home. Military nursing orders developed to care for the soldiers, but these were made up exclusively of men who wore suits of armor to protect themselves and their hospitals against attacks. These orders, with the emblem of the red cross, were extremely well organized and dedicated, and they existed well into the Renaissance.

Development of the Modern Nurse

Health Care in the Renaissance

In the intellectual reawakening of the Renaissance in Europe, starting in about 1350, nursing emerged in a recognizable form, although it did not grow steadily as a profession during this period. Inventions from this time include the microscope and thermometer, but the use of more modern diagnoses and treatment was viewed with skepticism. Monastic hospitals still regarded the restoration of health as secondary to the salvation of the soul.

Major political changes initiated by the Protestant Reformation in 1517 had the greatest effect on the health care of the period. In Catholic nation-states, including Italy, France, and Spain, health care remained generally unchanged from that of the Middle Ages, although the number of male nursing orders gradually decreased. By 1500, the majority of health care was provided by female religious orders.

What Do You Think?

Imagine yourself living in one of the historical periods discussed in this chapter. Given your or your family's health-care problems, how would your lives be different?

_____

_____

_____

_____

_____

_____

_____

_____

_____

_____

_____

_____

A Nursing Hierarchy

In the nation-states that broke away from the Catholic Church, such as England, Germany, and the Netherlands, health care soon degenerated to a point that was even worse than that of the Middle Ages. The role of women was reduced under Protestant leadership, and the male nurse all but disappeared. Secular nursing orders gradually took over the duties of the many substandard hospitals that had been established in metropolitan areas. The most famous of these was the Sisters of Charity, established in 1600.

These orders were the first to establish a nursing hierarchy. Primary nurses were called sisters and those assisting them were called helpers and watchers. It is at this time that people began to recognize the benefit of skilled nursing care. The first nursing textbooks appeared, and the use of midwives became widespread. Although hospitals were gaining importance, most clients still received health care at home.

The Industrial Revolution (1850–1950) caused a flood of people from rural areas throughout Europe into cities, and cramped living situations caused very bad health conditions and the spread of disease and plagues. Factory owners supported some forms of health care to keep their workers on the job, and this led to an early form of community health nursing. The Sisters of Charity expanded their care to include home care. Only a few male nursing orders survived the Protestant Reformation and Industrial Revolution, and several non-Catholic nursing orders were founded, including the famous Quaker Society of Protestant Sisters of Charity, which provided care primarily for prisoners and children.

NURSING IN THE UNITED STATES

Five hospitals existed in America before the Revolutionary War, housing the homeless and the poor and including rudimentary infirmaries. However, there were no identifiable groups of nurses for these infirmaries.[2] Health care in America at this time reflected that of the European countries the settlers had come from. Infant mortality rates were very high, ranging between 50 and 75 percent. One of the first schools of nursing was established in 1640 by the Sisters of St. Ursula in Quebec, and Spanish and French religious orders would establish hospital-based training schools in the New World over the next 100 years.

In Colonial Times

During the Revolutionary War, there was no organized medical or nursing corps, but small groups of untrained volunteers cared for the wounded and sick in their homes or in churches or barns. Benjamin Franklin founded Pennsylvania Hospital, the first U.S. hospital dedicated to treating the sick, in 1751.

Between the Revolutionary and the Civil Wars, health care in the United States increased markedly with the influx of religious nursing orders from Europe. More early schools of nursing developed at this time. Despite the rapid increase in the number of hospitals, most nursing care was still given at home by family members. Hospitals were considered a last resort and still had very high mortality rates.

When the States Went to War

The Civil War caused more death and injury than any war in the history of the United States, and the demand for nurses increased dramatically. Women volunteers (as many as 6000 for the North and 1000 for the South) began to follow the armies to the battlefields to provide basic nursing care, although many of them were untrained. Navy Nurses, the American Red Cross, and the Army Nurse Corps all date from this period. Large numbers of women came out of their homes to work in the hospitals, and a number of African-American volunteers in the North paved the way for others to enter the health-care field in the future.

> *Large numbers of women came out of their homes to work in the hospitals, and a number of African-American volunteers in the North paved the way for others to enter the health-care field in the future.*

Technological developments in the nineteenth century included medications such as morphine and codeine for pain and quinine to treat malaria. The arrival of 30 million immigrants in this century meant that the need for health care increased accordingly. Hospitals sprang up, and many instituted their own schools of nursing. Still, home care was the preferred type of nursing.

After 1914

Untrained Nurses

At the beginning of World War I, there were only about 400 nurses in the Army Nurse Corps, but by 1917 that number swelled to 21,000. Because many hospitals were recruiting untrained women to provide basic care, a committee on nursing was formed to establish standards, and eventually the Red Cross began a training program for nurse's aides. This was supported by physicians but opposed by many nursing leaders, who were concerned that it relegated nursing to "women's work," which would be seen as something anyone could do with minimal training. Because nurse's aides were a cheap source of labor, they began to replace more trained nurses in hospitals. Unfortunately this also resulted in a lower quality of care.

Between Wars

After the war, a segment of the nursing profession began to focus intensely on improving the educational standards of nursing care. At this time, 90 percent of nursing care was still given at home, but nurses began to practice in industry and in branches of government outside of the military. The standards of nursing care were low, and external quality controls were nonexistent.

The Great Depression took its toll on health care and nursing, as jobs became scarce and many nursing schools closed. At this time, the federal government became one of the largest employers of nurses. The newly organized Joint Committee on Nursing recommended that jobs should go to more qualified nurses and that the work day be reduced from 12 to 8 hours, although these measures were not widely implemented. During this period, hospitals became the primary source of health care, supported by hospital insurance programs. As the size of hospitals increased, more nursing jobs became available.

Establishing Standards

World War II produced another nursing shortage, and in response, Congress passed the Bolton Nurse Training Act, which shortened hospital-based training programs from 36 to 30 months. The new Cadet Nurse Corps established minimum educational standards for nursing programs and forbade discrimination on the basis of race, creed, or sex.[2] Many schools revised and improved their curriculums to meet these new standards.

To encourage more nurses to enter the military, the U.S. government granted women full commissioned status and gave them the same pay as men with the same rank. By the end of the war, African-American and male nurses were also admitted to the armed services.

> " *The Civil War caused more death and injury than any war in the history of the United States, and the demand for nurses increased dramatically.* "

Modern Times: Emerging Specialties

A Team of Nurses

The advancements in health care made during World War II required that nurses receive more highly specialized education to meet clients' unique needs. After the war, many nurses left the profession to raise families, and the spaces were filled by graduates of new programs that trained licensed practical nurses (LPNs) and licensed vocational nurses (LVNs) in just 1 year. At this time, the concept of team nursing came to be widely accepted, although it removed the registered nurses (RNs) from direct client care, requiring them to serve as team leaders.

A Growing Need

Technical nursing programs, which granted associate degrees (associate degree nurse [ADN]) at 2-year community colleges, were developed to help with the nursing shortage. With the baby boom, the need for nurses continued to grow, and what had been a quick-fix solution began to take a stronger hold. By the mid-1960s, ADNs outnumbered the nurses with baccalaureate degrees (BSN) and the technical LPNs. ADNs also won the right to take the same licensing examinations as RN graduates from diploma and BSN programs.

Still, as the health-care system became increasingly complicated, some nursing leaders questioned whether 1- or 2-year LPN and ADN programs were adequate to meet the needs of the profession. Slowly the number of BSN programs and graduate-level programs began to increase.

Vietnam: Traveling Hospitals

The mobile army surgical hospital (MASH) units that had been developed during the Korean War were replaced during the Vietnam War with medical unit, self-contained transportable (MUST) hospitals, which were staffed by nurses as well as physicians. Some 5000 nurses served in this war, and for the first time, graduates of 2-year ADN programs were commissioned into the armed services. Several Navy nurses were injured in the line of duty, and one Army nurse was killed. Only recently have the efforts of these and other women who served been recognized at the Vietnam Women's War Memorial in Washington, dedicated in 1993.

NURSING LEADERS

The nursing profession as it is practiced today owes a great deal to a number of outstanding nurses who had a vision for the future. The few discussed here are representative of the great drive and dedication of the many individuals who created change and influenced the development of the nursing profession, even to this day.

Florence Nightingale (1820–1910)

Universally regarded as the founder of modern nursing, Florence Nightingale dedicated her long life to improv-

ing health care and nursing standards. Raised in England, Nightingale was considered highly educated for her time. Through travels with her family, she became aware of the substandard health care in many countries in Europe. In 1851, she attended a 3-month nurses training program at the church-run hospital in Kaiserwerth, Germany. She was impressed with the program but came to believe that this brief training was insufficient. She later ran a private nursing home and realized that the only way to improve health care was to educate women to be reliable, high-quality nurses.

Volunteering Under Fire

Plans to develop a school of nursing in England were interrupted in 1854 by a cholera epidemic. Nightingale volunteered her services and learned a great deal about how to prevent the spread of disease. When the Crimean War broke out that same year, she obtained permission to take a group of 37 volunteer nurses into the battlefield area. British medical officers initially refused their assistance, but as conditions worsened they were admitted to the hospital.

After just 6 months of the nurses' cleaning and bandaging wounds, cooking, and cleaning the wards, the mortality rate dropped from 42 to 2 percent.[3] Nightingale expanded her reform to include supplies, a military post office, convalescent camps for long-term recovery, and residences for soldiers'

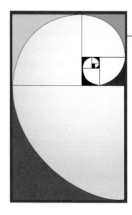

Issues Now

Nurses on the Front Line in Disaster Response

The profession of nursing has a long history of going where health care is needed, whether it is around the corner or half way around the world. Nurses have provided much-needed health care in natural disasters, such as the Southeast Asian tsunami in 2004, and in man-made disasters, such as the strife produced by revolutionary war in Africa or the September 11 terrorist attacks in New York City.

How the Team Works

Although there are several disaster response teams located throughout the United States, the International Medical Surgical Response Team (IMSRT) working out of Massachusetts General Hospital in Boston was the first one organized and remains one of the best known. The IMSRT operates under the Department of Homeland Security of the U.S. State Department and Emergency Management Agency.

The initial charter of the IMSRT called for a team of highly qualified nurses and physicians available to respond rapidly to disasters anywhere in the world. Their goal was to be able to reach a disaster site within 2 or 3 days maximum, provide basic life-saving care, and then evacuate the critically ill to health care facilities where more advanced care could be provided. Because of the success of the team's initial efforts, IMSRT has become a 24-7 on-call organization that will respond quickly to disasters anywhere in the world. They are flown to these locations on military cargo planes.

The nurses working with the IMSRT are experts at multitasking and must be willing to do whatever is necessary to accomplish the task. These tasks include setting up tents, moving supplies and equipment, picking up trash, and a variety of health-related tasks that generally are not considered nursing functions. The team carries a mobile tent hospital that includes a holding area, an ICU, a surgical suite, and an ER-type resuscitation area.

Special Functions

In addition to what would be considered "normal" nursing functions, the highly trained nurses of the IMSRT are often called upon to serve as pharmacists, OR, OB, and ER nurses—often all at the same time. They must also be able to deal with the tremendous psychological needs of large groups of people who have been through a major trauma. After the team finishes its work, they often donate their mobile hospital and medical supplies to the country of need, providing an often much-needed, if only temporary, acute care facility.

The team may range between 25 and 60 health-care providers depending on the size of the disaster and the needs of the population to be served. Usually about half of the team is composed of nurses, many of whom have critical care or emergency room experience. The type of care given by these nurses is a reflection of what is best in nursing—providing care to people because they need it and because nurses want to help.

Sources: D'Antonio, P: Moments when time stood still: Nursing in disaster. AJN 104(11):66–72. Nurses Have Key Role in International Response Team, AACN News. 21(3):1, 12.

families. She also began to help with the care given at the front lines. At the height of her work in the war, she supervised 125 nurses in several large hospitals, and her accomplishments were recognized by the Queen of England with an Order of Merit, the highest award given to English civilians.

What Do You Think?

What would current nursing practice and nursing education be like without the influences of Florence Nightingale?

_____

_____

_____

_____

_____

_____

_____

_____

_____

_____

_____

_____

A Health-Care Reformer

The war experience strengthened Nightingale's convictions that nursing education required major reform. Believing that nursing schools should be run by nurses and be independent of hospitals and physicians, she advocated a program of at least 1 year that included basic biological science, techniques to improve nursing care, and supervised practice. She regarded nursing as a lifelong endeavor and felt that nurses should be in direct contact with clients rather than doing menial jobs such as cooking and cleaning. She worked tirelessly for the reform of health care and nursing and was appointed to many related committees and commissions. A prolific writer, she wrote extensively about improving hospital conditions, sanitation, nursing education, and health care in general.

Her famous Nightingale Training School for Nurses opened in 1860 and began to train nurses who were in great demand throughout Europe and the United States. At this school, she advocated health maintenance and the concept that nursing was both an art and a science. She taught that each person should be treated as an individual and that nurses should meet the needs of clients, not the demands of physicians.

The school flourished, although it faced strong opposition from physicians who felt that nurses were already overtrained. Many early graduates went on to become important nursing leaders. Nightingale's ideas were somewhat diluted during the first half of the twentieth century, but they have since resurfaced and are now evaluated in the light of a rapidly changing health-care system.

> " *The war experience strengthened Nightingale's convictions that nursing education required major reform. Believing that nursing schools should be run by nurses and be independent of hospitals and physicians, she advocated a program of at least 1 year that included basic biological science, techniques to improve nursing care, and supervised practice.* "

Isabel Adams Hampton Robb (1860–1910)

Isabel Adams Hampton Robb started out as a teacher in her home province of Ontario, Canada, but in 1881 she went to New York City to train to be a nurse. After graduation, she moved to Rome and became a superintendent of a hospital there. She had always focused on the academic rather than the clinical side of nursing, but in Italy her conviction grew that nurses needed a solid theoretical education—a belief that was not well accepted by the medical community of the time. From that point on, she dedicated her life to raising the standards of nursing education in the United States, first as director of the Illinois Training School for Nurses, a school that was unique for its time in that it was university-based and emphasized academic learning. She later headed the new Johns Hopkins Training School for Nurses and would implement her ideas there as well.

Hampton Robb brought together leaders from key nursing schools to form the American Society of Superintendents of Training Schools for Nurses, and she served as its chairman. The group was the precursor to the National League for Nursing, which was dedicated to improving the standards for nursing education.

In 1896, Hampton Robb became the first president of a group for staff nurses in active practice, called the Nurses Associated Alumnae of the United States and Canada, which would later become the American Nurses Association (ANA), dedicated to the improvement of clinical practice. She later helped develop the *American Journal of Nursing,* the first professional journal dedicated to the improvement of nursing, which is still the official journal of the ANA.

Lillian Wald (1867–1940)

Lillian Wald was raised in Ohio and graduated from the New York Hospital School of Nursing in 1901. After working as a hospital nurse, she entered medical school, but encounters with New York's poor and sick caused her to change direction. She instead opened the Henry Street Settlement, a storefront health clinic in one of the poorest sections of the city, which organized nurses to make home visits, focusing on sanitary conditions and children's health. Wald became a dedicated social reformer, an efficient fundraiser, and an eloquent speaker. Although women still did not have the right to vote, her political influence was felt worldwide.

Under Wald's auspices, Columbia University developed courses to prepare nurses for careers in public health. Wald also advocated wellness education, which the medical community did not value at the time. The Metropolitan Life Insurance Company saw the value in her beliefs, however, and asked her to organize its nursing branch. She is also credited with founding the American Red Cross's Town and Country Nursing Service and with initiating the concept of school nursing. In 1912, she founded and became the first president of the National Organization of Public Health Nursing. Many child health and wellness programs in use today are based on her efforts. Current proposals for health-care reform often include her ideas about public health nursing, independent clinics, and health maintenance.

What Do You Think?

Who is your favorite historical nursing leader? What are some of that person's characteristics that attracted you? Are there any current nurses or nurse educators who provide you with a role model? What are some of that person's characteristics that attract you?

Lavinia Lloyd Dock (1858–1956)

Lavinia Lloyd Dock left her home in Pennsylvania to attend New York's Bellevue Training School for Nurses in 1885. She noticed that many of her fellow students struggled to learn about all the medications that were becoming available, and she would later write the first medication textbook for nurses. She worked alongside Lillian Wald at the Henry Street Settlement and Isabel Hampton Robb at Johns Hopkins Hospital.

Like Wald, Dock believed that poverty and squalor contributed to poor health, and she dedicated herself to social reform to address these problems. However, she soon learned that she was limited in her influence because she was a woman, and she spent most of her career dedicated to the pursuit of equal rights. For 20 years she lobbied legislators at all levels about women's right to vote, believing that this was the only way to influence social reform and health care. An excellent example of the diverse ways that nurses can help achieve higher-quality health care, she is considered one of the most influential leaders in the early twentieth century.

Annie W. Goodrich (1866–1954)

Annie Goodrich provided nursing care at Lillian Wald's Henry Street Settlement in New York after receiving her nursing degree. She was known as an outstanding nursing educator and ran a number of nursing schools in New York. In 1910, she was appointed a state inspector of nursing schools, a position that up to that time had been held only by physicians. After the U.S. Army asked her to survey its hospital nursing departments, Goodrich proposed that it organize its own nursing school. The school opened later that year, with her as its dean, and this school would serve as the model for others established at Army hospitals during World War I.

To respond to the need for nurses in the war, Goodrich also established a nursing training program at Vassar College, and after the war other colleges and universities slowly began to develop their own nursing programs. She had demonstrated that learning theoretical information in a classroom was just as important in training highly skilled nurses as clinical practice. When the war was over, Goodrich returned to the Henry Street Settlement and then became a nursing educator, eventually serving as dean at the Yale University School of Nursing. Her many writings about nursing education and her experiences with military nursing have been a great contribution to the nursing profession.[4]

Conclusion

Many of the problems and difficulties with today's health-care system, and those of nursing in particular, are based in the historical development of the profession. Knowledge of these historic roots can help us understand why the profession of nursing is the way it is and even suggest solutions to problems that may seem unsolvable. For example, nursing today appears to be a profession with a high level of responsibility but a low level of power.

How did this situation develop? What can be done about it? A great deal of confusion exists about the education of nurses, unlike the situation in other health-care professions. Why does nursing have this problem, and how can this confusion be addressed? Those who belong to the nursing profession have a responsibility not only to learn about how these and other conditions developed, but also to relate that knowledge to nursing's possibility for growth in the future.

Issues in Practice

Case Study

Clara, who is 108 years old, is admitted through the hospital emergency room (ER) for nonspecific complaints of chest pain and dizziness. This is the third time that she has come to the hospital with this complaint in the past month. Although previous examinations and tests have shown no acute disease process, the ER physician thought that because of her age and long history of coronary artery disease, Clara should be monitored and evaluated more closely. Clara has no private insurance, but she is covered under Medicare, Parts A and B, with supplemental coverage from a small insurance company in her state.

Despite her age, Clara is mentally alert and competent. She lives by herself in a small apartment and manages basic daily care, including shopping and cleaning, with only minimal assistance from friends. She has no living family members, except for a few aging cousins in a distant state. She takes several medications at home: diltiazem (Cardizem) for her heart problems, ranitidine (Zantac) for a hiatal hernia, and papaverine (Pavabid) to increase her general circulation.

After a complete physical examination, including several laboratory tests and an electrocardiogram (ECG), she is scheduled for a cardiac catheterization. A significant block is seen in one of the major coronary arteries, and the physicians decide to perform an angioplasty on the artery. She is admitted to the intensive care unit (ICU) after the procedure, where she also receives two units of blood because she is anemic. She recovers without incident and is discharged 5 days after her admission. The total cost for her hospitalization, including tests and angioplasty, is more than $15,000.

Clara is not a typical client for her age group. Many medical experts would categorize the treatment given her as overtreatment because of the current emphasis on quality of life, death with dignity, and the futility of treating the hopelessly ill. Yet, as people in the United States continue to age, it is more likely that Clara will become the norm rather than the exception. Many issues—ethical, financial, and others—surround this case.

Critical Thinking Questions

1. As a general rule, should a complicated and expensive procedure, such as an angioplasty, always be approved for a 108-year-old client? If not, what should be the exceptions?
2. From a historical perspective, how would a client with Clara's health-care problems be treated in the Roman Empire? The Middle Ages? The United States in the 1800s? The United States in the 1950s?
3. The state where Clara lives has a severe budget shortfall, and substantial cuts in Medicaid benefits have taken place. The entire budget for immunizations of the state's children is only $10,000. What would you do as administrator of the state's Medicaid program if faced with the option of immunizing the children or paying for Clara's angioplasty?
4. The elderly, through various entitlement programs, consume a large proportion of the national budget. This cost is borne mainly by young and middle-aged workers through their taxes. Is it fair that the young be required to carry the burden for the care of the old?
5. Is the government ever justified in rationing health care and/or limiting access to health care?

References

1. Jenson, DM: History and Trends in Professional Nursing. CV Mosby, St. Louis, 1959.
2. Kalisch, PA, and Kalisch, BJ: The Advance of American Nursing. JB Lippincott, Philadelphia, 1995.
3. Woodham-Smith, C: Florence Nightingale. McGraw-Hill, New York, 1957.
4. Mason, DJ: Policy and Politics for Nurses. WB Saunders, Philadelphia, 1993.

Bibliography

Cristy, T: The first fifty years. Am J Nurs 9(9):1778–1784, 1971.
Cristy, T: Portrait of a leader: Lavinia Lloyd Dock. Nurs Outlook 17(6):72–75, 1969.
Cristy, T: Portrait of a leader: M. Adelaide Nutting. Nurs Outlook 17(1):20–24, 1969.
Cristy, T: Portrait of a leader: Isabel Hampton Robb. Nurs Outlook 17(3):26–29, 1969.
Cristy, T: Portrait of a leader: Isabel Maitland Stewart. Nurs Outlook 17(10):44–48, 1969.
D'Antonio, P. Women, nursing and baccalaureate education in 20th century America. Journal of Nursing Scholarship. 36(4): 379–384, 2004.
Grypma, S, Critical issues in the use of biographic methods in nursing history. Nurs Hist Rev 13:171-187, 2005.
Jamieson, EM, et al.: Trends in Nursing History. WB Saunders, Philadelphia, 1968.
Holder, V: From handmaiden to right hand: World War I and advancements in medicine. AORN J 80(5):911–923, 2004.
Lewenson, S: Integrating nursing history into the curriculum. J Professional Nursing 20(6):374–381.
Murphy-Ende, K: Advanced practice nursing: Reflections on the past, issues for the future. Oncol Nurs Forum 29(1):26–33, 2002.
Newlson, S: The rhetoric of rupture: Nursing as a practice with a history? Nurs Outlook 52(5):255–261, 2004.
Selanders, LC: Florence Nightingale: Perseverance, power, possibilities. Maryland Nurse 4(3):1–2, 2001.
Smoyak, SA: Florence Nightingale, insane nurse. J Psychosoc Nurs Ment Health Serv 39(10):6–8, 2001.

3

The Evolution of Licensure, Certification, and Nursing Organizations

Joseph T. Catalano

Learning Objectives

After completing this chapter, the reader will be able to:

- Identify the purposes and needs for nurse licensure.
- Distinguish between permissive and mandatory licensure.
- Explain why institutional licensure is unacceptable in today's health-care system.
- Evaluate the importance of nurse practice acts.
- Analyze the significance of professional certification.

MEETING EXPECTATIONS

Almost from the inception of nursing, societal needs and expectations have been the driving forces behind the establishment of the standards that guide the profession. In the early days of nursing, when health care was relatively primitive and society's expectations of nurses were low, there was little demand for regulations or controls over and within the profession. However, as technology and health care have advanced and become more complex, there has been a corresponding increase in societal expectations for nurses. All nurses now accept **licensure** and **certification** examinations as a given in today's health-care system. Where did these examinations come from, and what do they mean to the profession? This chapter explores the answers to these questions.

Rather than looking on the advent of sophisticated telecommunications, growing information technologies, redesigned health-care organizations, and increasing **health-care consumer** demands with fear and trepidation, nurses should consider this an exciting time of growth and opportunity. In today's health-care system, nurses have an almost unlimited number of ways to provide new and creative nursing care for clients in all settings. As society's needs and expectations change, so will the regulations and standards that help define nursing practice. Through their professional nursing organizations, nurses can help shape health-care regulations that establish the most freedom to provide effective care while maintaining the goal of protection of the public. It is likely that in the future state boards of nursing will look much different, just as the profession of nursing will differ from that of its past.

THE DEVELOPMENT OF NURSE PRACTICE ACTS

A nurse practice act is state legislation regulating the practice of nurses that protects the public, defines the scope of practice, and makes nurses accountable for their actions. Nurse practice acts establish state boards of nursing (SBN) and define specific SBN powers regarding the practice of nursing within the state. Rules and regulations written by the SBNs become **statutory laws** under the powers delegated by the state **legislature.**

> *Rather than looking on the advent of sophisticated telecommunications, growing information technologies, redesigned health-care organizations, and increasing health-care consumer demands with fear and trepidation, nurses should consider this an exciting time of growth and opportunity.*

Regulatory Powers

Although nurse practice acts differ from one state to another, the SBNs have many powers in common. All SBNs have the power to grant licenses, to approve nursing programs, to establish standards for nursing schools, and to write specific regulations for nurses and nursing practice in general in that state.

Of particular importance is the SBNs power to deny or revoke nurse licenses[1] (Box 3.1). Other functions of nurse practice acts include defining nursing and the scope of practice, ruling on who can use the titles registered nurse (RN) and licensed practical nurse/licensed vocational nurse (LPN/LVN), setting up an application procedure for licensure in the state, determining fees for licensure, establishing requirements for renewal of licensure, and determining responsibility for any regulations governing expanded practice for nurses in that particular state.

The Need for Licensure

Imagine what the quality of health care would be if anyone could walk into a hospital, claim to know

Box 3.1

Reasons the State Boards of Nursing May Revoke a Nursing License

- Conviction for a serious crime
- Demonstration of gross negligence or unethical conduct in the practice of nursing
- Failure to renew a nursing license while still continuing to practice nursing
- Use of illegal drugs or alcohol during the provision of care for clients or use that carries over and affects clients' care
- Willful violation of the state's nurse practice act

how to care for clients, and be given a job as a nurse. This situation might sound impossible in today's health-care system, but not too long ago it was the norm rather than the exception.

Throughout the last half of the nineteenth century and the first half of the twentieth century, rapid growth in health-care technology led to the increasing use of hospitals as the primary source of

OOPS!

health care. Individuals who were qualified to provide this care, however, were in short supply. There were wide variations both in the abilities of those who claimed to be nurses and in the quality of the care they provided. Paradoxically, nursing leaders who had always advocated some type of **credentialing** for nurses to ensure competency found that their attempts to initiate registration or licensure met with strong opposition from physician groups, hospital administrators, and practicing nurses themselves.

Early Attempts at Licensure

Although the idea of registering nurses had been in existence for some time, Florence Nightingale was the first to establish a formal register for graduates of her nursing school. In the United States and Canada, there was widespread recognition of the need for some type of credentialing of nurses as far back as the mid-1800s. The first organized attempt to establish a credentialing system was initiated in 1896 by the Nurses Associated Alumnae of the United States and Canada (later to become the American Nurses Association). As with other early attempts at licensure, it was met with resistance and eventually failed.[2]

Several early American nursing leaders, including Lillian Wald and Annie Goodrich, recognized the inconsistent quality of nursing care and the need for licensure to protect the public. In 1901, after an extensive and lengthy campaign to educate the public, physicians, hospital administrators, and nurses themselves about the need for licensure, the International Council of Nurses passed a resolution that required each state to establish a licensure and examination procedure for nurses. It took 3 years before the state of New York, through the New York Nurses Association, developed a licensure bill that passed the legislature (Box 3.2).

Other states that followed New York's lead were North Carolina, New Jersey, and Virginia. Although these states had bills that were weaker than New York's nurse practice act, passage of such legislation was considered a major accomplishment for several reasons. Women did not even have the right to vote in general elections at the time these bills were passed. In addition, few requirements and regulations for licensure existed during this period in the history of the United States, even for the medical profession.

Box 3.2

Key Points in the New York State Licensure Bill (1904)

- Established minimum educational standards
- Established the minimum length of basic nursing programs at 2 years
- Required all nursing schools to be registered with the state board of regents (who oversee all higher education)
- Established a state board of nursing (SBN) with five nurses as members
- Formulated rules for the examination of nurses
- Formulated regulations for nurses that, if violated, could lead to the revocation of licensure

Sources: Hirsh, IL: Statement on nursing's scope describes how two levels of nurses practice. American Nurse 20:13, 1988.

The Importance of Licensure Examinations

The thought of having to take an examination that can determine whether or not one can practice nursing can make even the best student anxious. Adding to the tension is the fact that the examination is given outside of the academic setting, by computer, and is created by individuals other than the students' teachers. (See Chapters 10 and 11 for a detailed discussion of NCLEX-RN, CAT.)

A Measure of Competency

Some type of objective method, however, is necessary to prove that the individual is qualified to practice nursing safety; otherwise the public is not protected from unqualified practitioners. Early attempts at creating licensure examinations for nurses were met with resistance. Although all states had some form of licensure examination by 1923, the format and length of the examinations varied widely. Some states required both written and practical examinations to demonstrate safety of practice; others added an oral examination.

Although licensure was and is a state-controlled activity, the major nursing organizations in the United States eventually realized that to have some consistency of quality across the country, a single examination that all nurses needed to pass should be devised. The American Nurses Association (ANA) Council of State Boards of Nursing was organized in 1945 to oversee development of a uniform examination for nurses that could be used by all state boards of nursing.

The NCLEX-RN, CAT

The National League for Nursing Testing Division developed a test that was implemented in 1950. Originally the test was simply called the State Board Examination, but it was renamed the National Council Licensure Examination (NCLEX) in 1987. In 1994, the computerized version of the examination was implemented—the National Council Licensure Examination Computerized Adaptive Testing, for Registered Nurses (NCLEX-RN, CAT).

Licensure for nurses has undergone a major change. States are currently in the process of implementing the Mutual Recognition Model for Nursing Licensure, which will allow nurses licensed in one state to practice nursing in other states that belong to their regional agreement. The eventual goal is to have a "universal" nursing license that will allow nurses to practice in all states without having to become relicensed each time they cross a state border.

REGISTRATION VERSUS LICENSURE

The terms *registration* and *licensure* are often used interchangeably, although they are not synonymous. They serve a similar purpose, but some technical differences exist.

Registration

Registration is the listing, or registering, of names on an official roster after certain pre-established criteria have been met. Before mandatory licensure by the states was accepted, any health-care institution could call an applicant's school to find out whether the applicant had met the standards for a position by graduating from a school of nursing or by passing an examination. The school would tell the institution whether the applicant's name appeared on the official roster or register, hence the origin of the term *registered nurse*. With the advent of state board examinations, an institution merely has to call the SBN to find out whether the individual is registered or licensed.

Licensure

Licensure is an activity conducted by the state through the enforcement powers of its regulatory boards to protect the public's health, safety, and welfare by establishing professional standards. Licensure for nurses, as for other professionals who deal with the public, is necessary to ensure that everyone who claims to be a nurse can function at a minimal level of competency and safety. There are several different types of licensure.

Permissive Licensure

Permissive licensure allows individuals to practice nursing as long as they do not use the letters "RN" after their names. Basically, permissive licensure only protects the "registered nurse" title but not the practice of nursing itself. Under a permissive licensure law, anyone could carry out the functions of an RN, regardless of their level of education, without having to pass an examination indicating competency.

Health-care administrators seem to support the concept of permissive licensure because it allows them to employ less-educated and lower-paid employees rather than the more highly educated and paid RNs. However, they also recognize that the quality of care decreases when the education level of health-care providers is lower. Although most early licensure laws were permissive, all states now have mandatory licensure.

Mandatory Licensure

Mandatory licensure requires anyone who wishes to practice nursing to pass a licensure examination and become registered by the SBN. Because different levels of nursing practice exist, different levels of licensure are necessary. At the technical level, the individual must take and pass the LPN/LVN examination; at the professional level, the individual must take and pass the RN examination.

Mandatory licensure forced SBNs to distinguish between the activities that nurses at different levels could legally perform. The scope of practice defines the boundaries for each of the levels: advanced practice nurse (APN), RN, and LPN/LVN. As more levels of nursing education (e.g., the associate degree in nursing [ADN]) have been added, however, lines dividing the different scopes of practice have become blurred. In the current health-care system, it is not unusual to find LPNs/LVNs performing activities that are generally considered professional.

A particularly confusing element in today's health-care system is the use of unlicensed individuals to provide health care. The advent of certified nursing assistants (CNA) and unlicensed assistive personnel (UAP) has led to widespread use of such individuals in all health-care settings. Although they must be supervised by an RN or LPN/LVN, these individuals are sometimes illegally assigned nursing tasks much more advanced than their levels of training. (See Chapter 14 for a more detailed discussion of delegation.) Even though permissive licensure is no longer legal, CNAs and UAP appear to fall under an unofficial type of permissive licensure.

Institutional Licensure

Cut Corners, Cut Costs

Although universally rejected by every major nursing organization, **institutional licensure** has become a reality for many other types of health-care workers, such as respiratory therapists and physical therapists. In some state legislatures, bills have been introduced to allow **foreign graduate nurses** and nurses who are licensed in foreign countries to work in specific institutions without taking the U.S. licensure examination. Up to this point, these bills have been stopped by the state nursing organizations before they could become law. Institutional licensure has been proposed periodically over the years as an alternative to governmental licensure.

Institutional licensure allows individual health-care institutions to determine which individuals are qualified to practice nursing within general guidelines established by an outside board. Although this type of licensure appeals to hospitals and nursing homes because it would allow them to hire individuals with less education at a reduced cost, some serious difficulties are associated with it.

A Lack of External Control

Probably the most critical problem is the lack of any external control to determine a minimal level of competency. The designations of RN and LPN/LVN would be virtually meaningless under institutional licensure. These nurses would not be under the control of a state licensing board and thus would not be held to the same standards of practice as nurses who were licensed by the states.

A second problem is that nurses who wished to move to a new place of employment would have to undergo whatever licensure procedure the new institution had established before being allowed to work there. Currently, nurses who move from one state to another can obtain licensure by endorsement by having the state recognize their nursing license from the original state of licensure. This process is generally referred to as reciprocity.

CERTIFICATION

At first glance, it may appear that there is not much difference between certification and licensure. Strictly defined, licensure can be considered a type of legal certification. In the more widely accepted use of the term, however, certification is a granting of credentials to indicate that an individual has achieved a level of ability higher than the minimal level of competency indicated by licensure.[3] As technology increases and the health-care environment becomes more complex and demanding, nurses are finding a need to increase their knowledge and skill levels beyond the essentials taught in their basic nursing courses.

Certification acknowledges the attainment of increased knowledge and skills and provides nurses with a means to validate their own self-worth and competence. Some certification also carries with it a legal status, similar to licensure; but in many cases, certification merely indicates a specific professional status. The public, employers, and even nurses themselves have difficulty understanding what certification means.

Another element that adds confusion to the understanding of the process of certification is that a large number of groups can offer certification. These are usually professional specialty groups like the National Association of Pediatric Nurse Associates and Practitioners (NAPNAP) and the American Association of Critical-Care Nurses (AACN), but they can also be national organizations like the National League for Nursing (NLN) or the ANA.

Individual Certification

The most common type of certification is called individual certification. When a nurse has demonstrated that he or she has attained a certain level of ability above and beyond the basic level required for licensure in a defined area of practice, that nurse can become certified. Usually some type of written and practical examination is required to demonstrate this advanced level of skill.

The ANA has its own certifying organization, the American Nurses Credentialing Center (ANCC) that offers widely recognized certifications in more than 40 areas. Almost all nurses with individual certification are required to maintain their skills and competencies through continuing education and a specified number of continuing education units (CEU). Recertification may be achieved through CEUs or retaking of the certification examination.

Organizational Certification

Organizational certification is the certification of a group or health-care institution by some external agency. It is usually referred to as accreditation and indicates that the institution has met standards established by either the government or by a nongovernmental agency. Often the ability of the institution to collect money from insurance companies or the federal government depends on whether or not the institution is certified by a recognized agency. Most hospitals are accredited by the Joint Commission on Accreditation of Healthcare Organizations (JCAHO) as a minimum level of accreditation.

Advanced Practice

Some state governments may either award or recognize certification granted to nurses in areas of advanced practice. In these cases, the certification becomes a legal requirement for practice at the APN level. Depending on the individual state's nurse practice act, nurses thus certified fall under regulations in the state's practice act that control the type of activities nurses may legally carry out when they perform advanced roles.

For example, many states recognize the position of **nurse midwife** as an advanced practice role for nurses. In these states, a nurse midwife is allowed to practice those skills allowed under the nurse practice act of that state after obtaining certification. Generally nurse midwives are allowed to conduct prenatal examinations, do prenatal teaching, and deliver babies vaginally in uncomplicated pregnancies. They are not usually allowed to perform cesarean sections.

Varying Standards

An independent certification center was proposed in 1978 to establish uniform criteria and standards and to oversee all certification activities. Although it would eliminate much of the current confusion about certification and would help with the legal recognition of APNs, this proposal has not yet been acted upon because of opposition from physician and health-care administration groups.

Unfortunately, there is no uniformity among states in the recognition of certification of APNs. Some states recognize almost all certifications and have provisions in their nurse practice acts to help guide these practices. Other states have very little legal recognition of certification levels and thus few guidelines for

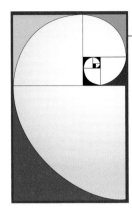

Issues Now

Study Shows Nurse Practitioners Lower Health-Care Costs and Improve the Quality of Care at the Same Time

A number of studies have been conducted over the past few years on how Advanced Practice Nurses (APNs) fit into the health-care system and their overall effect on the quality of care. Initially, many physicians were opposed to APNs because they felt their level of training was inadequate to provide high-quality care and because they would be "cutting into" their practice and source of income.

These concerns have proven to be unwarrented. APNs tend to serve segments of the population that physicians generally do not treat, and the quality of care has been consistently judged to be at least at the level of physician care if not higher.

The University of Pennsylvania Study

The University of Pennsylvania conducted a study of hospitalized older adults suffering from congestive heart failure (CHF). Nationwide, CHF is a leading cause of morbidity and mortality among the elderly population. It is estimated that treatment of this disorder costs the health-care industry some $24 billion per year. It is logical to conclude if this group of elderly could avoid exacerbations of CHF requiring hospitalization, the costs for their care should decrease.

A group of master-degree prepared APNs received 2 months' additional training centered on care of the elderly population with cardiac-related problems. The elderly subjects were divided into two groups: a control group that received the usual hospital-based care and the test group that received care by the specially trained APNs. The study was conducted over a 1-year period. At the end of the year, the test group cared for by APNs had a 13.7% lower rate of death or hospitalization and an average reduction of cost of care of $4,845.00 per client. Also, the test group went an average of 110 days longer without major complications associated with CHF than the control group.

Although there has not been any hard analysis of why these results occurred, there seems to be several underlying factors. First, as nurses, APNs have a basic orientation toward holistic and preventative care, rather than the narrow sick care model taught in most medical schools. By approching clients' health care needs from a broad focus that includes such elements as lifestyle, diet, and envirionment, the APNs' care not only treats the clients' present problems but also affects those things that contribute to it.

Second, many clients, particularly the elderly, will delay medical help in a hospital setting, particularly if they have to go through the emergency room, until they are severely ill. APN care is easier to access, and treating symptoms before they become acute is more cost effective and better for the client.

Third, APNs do not charge as much per visit as physicians do. They are inherently more cost-effective for primary health care.

In the end, the same old problem still plagues nursing, even at the advanced practice level: lack of respect from the medical community. Studies

(continued)

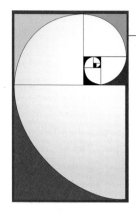

Issues Now continued

such as the University of Pennsylvania study will help erase the underlying predjudices and increase the level of respect for nurses throughout the medical community.

Sources: Levine, S, and Marek, A: Nurses step to the front. U.S. News and World Report 138(4):67–71, 2004.
Gearon, C: Medicine's turf wars: Specialists without M.D.'s are pushing for more medical power. U.S. News and World Report 138(4):57–62.
Sole, M: How do you define the clinical nurse specialist? AACN News 21(1):5, 2004.
Kennedy, M: APNs: Improved outcomes at lower costs. AJN 104(9):19, 2004.

practice. This confusion may result from so many organizations offering certification in different areas. In some advanced practice specialties, such as nurse practitioner, two or more organizations may offer certification for the same title. The certification standards vary from organization to organization, and the method of determining certification may also be different.

A More Significant Role

It is expected that advanced practice nurses will play a larger role in the rapidly evolving health-care system of the future. What that role will be depends on how well governmental organizations and the public understand the contributions practitioners can make as **primary care providers.** Without a uniform definition of this specialty, such nurses will not be utilized to their full potential.

Licensure and certification are both methods of granting credentials to demonstrate that an individual is qualified to provide safe care to the public. Without proof of competency, the profession of nursing would become chaotic, disorganized, and even dangerous. It is important for nurses to keep a watchful eye on pending legislation and practices that health-care institutions are initiating. Many of these proposals and practices are covert ways of reintroducing permissive and institutional licensure.

NURSING ORGANIZATIONS AND THEIR IMPORTANCE

Strength in Numbers

The establishment of a professional organization is one of the most important defining characteristics of

a profession. Many professions have a single major professional organization to which most of its members belong and several specialized suborganizations that members may also join. Professions with just one major organization generally have a great deal of political power.

Nurses need and use power in every aspect of their professional lives, ranging from supervising nonlicensed personnel to negotiating with the administration for increased independence of practice. Clearly, an individual nurse probably does not have much power; but for nurses as a group, the potential is increased exponentially by the organization. The dedication to high-quality nursing standards and improved methods of practice by the major nursing organizations has led to improved care and increased benefits to the public as a whole.[4]

> *Clearly, an individual nurse probably does not have much power; but for nurses as a group, the potential is increased exponentially by the organization.*

Speaking With One Voice

National nursing organizations need the participation and membership of all nurses in order to claim that they are truly representative of the profession. A large membership allows the organization to speak with one voice when making its values about health-care issues known to politicians, physicians' groups, and the public in general.

The National League for Nursing

Purposes

The primary purpose of the National League for Nursing (NLN) is to maintain and improve the standards of nursing education. The NLN is also a strong force in community health nursing, occupational health nursing, and nursing service activities. Its bylaws state that its purpose is to foster the development and improvement of hospital, industrial, public health, and other organized nursing services and of nursing education through the coordinated action of nurses, allied professional groups, citizens, agencies, and schools so that the nursing needs of the people will be met.

Membership

Although membership is open to individual nurses, the primary membership of the NLN comes in the form of agency membership, usually through schools of nursing. One of the major functions of this organization, through the National League for Nursing Accrediting Commission (NLNAC), is to accredit schools of nursing through a self-study process. The schools are given a set of criteria, or **essentials for accreditation,** and are then required to evaluate their programs against these criteria. After the evaluation report is written and sent to the NLNAC, site representatives visit the school to verify the information in the report and see whether the school has met the criteria. If the school meets the evaluation criteria, it is accredited for up to 8 years.

Accreditation of a school of nursing by the NLNAC indicates that the school meets national standards. In some work settings, it is a requirement that a nurse be a graduate of an NLNAC-accredited school of nursing before the nurse can be hired or accepted into many master's level nursing programs.

Other services and activities that the NLN carries out include testing, evaluating new graduate nurses, supplying career information and continuing education workshops and conferences for all levels of nursing, publishing a wide range of literature and videotapes covering current issues in health care, and compiling statistics about nursing, nurses, and nursing education.

The American Association of Colleges of Nursing

Purposes

The American Association of Colleges of Nursing (AACN) was established to help colleges with schools of nursing work together to improve the standards for higher education for professional nursing. The AACN, through the Commission on Collegiate Nursing Education (CCNE), has developed standards for the accreditation of baccalaureate schools of nursing and is poised to become a major accreditation agency, competing with the NLNAC. The AACN has developed and published a set of guidelines for the education of professional nursing students that is widely used as the theoretical basis for baccalaureate curricula.

Membership

Only deans and directors of programs that offer baccalaureate or higher degrees in nursing with an upper-division nursing major are permitted membership in the AACN.

The American Nurses Association

Purposes

The American Nurses Association (ANA) grew out of a concern for the quality of nursing practice and the care that nurses were providing. The major purposes for the existence of the ANA, as stated in its bylaws, include improvement of the standards of health and access to health-care services for everyone, improvement and maintenance of high standards for nursing practice, and promotion of the professional growth and development of all nurses, including economic issues, working conditions, and independence of practice.[5]

The American Association of Colleges of Nursing (AACN) was established to help colleges with schools of nursing work together to improve the standards for higher education for professional nursing.

Membership

Membership in the ANA is limited to 52 constituents: 50 state organizations, Washington, DC, and Puerto Rico. An individual joins a state organization and through the state organization indirectly is a member of the ANA. Certain discounts in membership are offered for new members and new graduate nurses. Various levels of membership are available for nurses who work part-time or those who are retired. The ANA makes every effort to encourage individual nurses to join the organization. Unfortunately, most nurses do not belong to this potentially powerful, politically active, and very influential organization.

Each state has the opportunity to determine what is needed from each member to run the state association; the amount of the dues that is sent to ANA is predetermined. Although dues are not inexpensive (they change a little from year to year, but are about $200 per year), the ANA offers various plans for payment, such as three equal payments over the course of a year or monthly payroll deductions. Because of the efforts of the ANA, nurses' salaries have risen to a point where this sum is affordable.

Other Services

When nurses pursue advanced education and levels of practice, as many are doing today, the ANA ANCC is essential for testing and certification of many of these practice levels. Although other organizations offer advanced practice certification, without the ANCC, there would be even less standardization for and less recognition of these practitioners by the public, physicians, or lawmakers.

Entry into practice. Another important issue that the ANA has been involved in is the entry-level education requirement for professional nurses. The ANA has supported the baccalaureate degree as the minimum educational requirement for nurses for the last 25 years. The ANA is in the forefront of the debate over **entry into practice,** which has continued into the twenty-first century.

Standards of practice. Additional functions carried out by the ANA include the establishment and continual updating of standards of nursing practice. These standards are the yardstick against which nurses are measured and held accountable by **courts of law.** The ANA also established the official code of ethics that guides professional practice.

Legislation and Economics

Many of the political and economic activities of the ANA are carried out in the halls of legislatures and offices of legislators. The ANA Political Action Committee (ANA-PAC) is one of the most powerful in Washington, DC. (See Chapter 19 for a more detailed discussion.) Such activities have a profound effect on the role that nurses play and will continue to play in health care well into the twenty-first century.

Successful PAC activities require money and the power of a large, unified membership. The ANA-PAC seeks to influence legislation about nurses, nursing, and health care in general. It has been and will be a strong voice in the formulation of current national health-care reform.

Another important function of the ANA is economic. In many states, the ANA is the official **bargaining agent** for nurses in the negotiation of **contracts** with hospitals, nursing homes, and other health-care agencies that employ nurses. However, **collective bargaining** is done on a state-to-state basis—some states are **collective bargaining units** and others are not. (See Chapter 16 for a more detailed discussion.) Professional organizations represent professional groups better than a labor union that has little knowledge of professional activities or needs.

The National Student Nurses' Association

Purposes

The National Student Nurses' Association (NSNA) is an independent legal corporation established in 1953 to represent the needs of nursing students. Working closely with the ANA, which offers services, an official publication, and close communication, the NSNA consists of state chapters that represent student nurses in those particular states.

The main purpose of the NSNA is to help maintain high standards of education in schools of nursing, with the ultimate goal of educating high-quality nurses who will provide excellent health care. Students' ideas, concerns, and needs are extremely important to nursing educators. Most nursing programs have committees in which students are asked to participate, including curriculum development and evaluation techniques. It is important that students belong to these committees and actively participate in the committees' activities.

Membership

Membership consists of all nursing students in registered nurse programs. Students can join at the local, state, or national level or at all levels if desired. Dues are low, with a discount for the first year's membership.

Other Services

Additionally, the NSNA is concerned with developing and providing workshops, seminars, and conferences that deal with current issues in nursing and health care, with a wide range of subjects, from ethical and legal concerns to recent developments in pharmacology, test-taking skills, and professional growth. Student nurses who belong to the NSNA and who take an active part in its functions are much more likely to join the ANA after they graduate. Professional identity and professional behavior are learned. By beginning the process during the formal school years, student nurses develop professional attitudes and behaviors that they will maintain for the rest of their lives.

Benefits for Students

Many benefits exist for student nurses who belong to the NSNA. A number of scholarships are available through this organization to members of the NSNA. Members receive the official publication of the organization, *Imprint,* and the *NSNA News,* which keep the student nurse current on recent developments in health care and nursing.

The student member also has political representation on issues that may affect the student now or in the future. Some of these issues include educational standards for practice, standards of professional practice, and health insurance. The NSNA is also concerned with the difficulty that many nursing students from minority groups experience in the educational process. The Breakthrough Project is an attempt by the NSNA to help such students enter the profession of nursing.

Practicing Professionalism

Student nurses who join the NSNA experience firsthand the operation, activities, and benefits of a professional organization. In schools with active memberships, the NSNA can be a very exciting and useful organization for students.

Many NSNA chapters are involved in community activities that provide services at a local level and allow the student to practice "real" nursing. These services include providing community health screening programs for hypertension, lead poisoning, vision, hearing, and birth defects; setting up information and education programs; giving immunizations; and working with groups concerned with drug abuse, child abuse, drunken driving, and teen pregnancy. All nursing students should be encouraged to belong to this organization.

The International Council of Nurses

Membership in the International Council of Nurses (ICN) consists of national nursing organizations, and it serves as the international organization for professional nursing. The ANA is one member among 104 nursing associations around the world. Each member nation sends delegates and participates in the international convention held every 4 years. The quadrennial conventions, or congresses, are open to all nurses and delegates from all nations.

The goal of the ICN is to improve health and nursing care throughout the world. The ICN coordinates its efforts with the United Nations and other international organizations when appropriate in the pursuit of its goals.

Some issues that have been the focus of concern of the ICN are social and economic welfare of nurses, the changing role of nurses in the present health-care environment, the challenges being faced by the various national nursing organizations, and how government and politics affect the nursing profession and health care. Overseeing the ICN is the Council of National Representatives. This body meets every 2 years and serves as the governing organization. ICN headquarters is located in Geneva, Switzerland.

Sigma Theta Tau

Sigma Theta Tau is an honorary organization that was established in colleges and universities to recognize individuals who have demonstrated leadership or made important contributions to professional nursing. It is international, and candidates are selected from among senior nursing students or graduate or practicing nurses.

The organization has its headquarters in Indianapolis, where it has a large library open to members to use for scholarly activities and research. It also boasts the first on-line nursing journal, which can be accessed by any nurse with a computer anywhere in the world. Local chapters of Sigma Theta Tau collect and distribute funds to nurses who are conducting nursing research. The organization also holds educational conferences and recognizes those who have made contributions to nursing.

Grassroots Organizations

A growing trend in contemporary nursing has been the formation of grassroots nursing organizations. In reality, all nursing organizations start as the grassroots efforts of local nursing groups that are trying to solve a particular problem. Over time, these small grassroots organizations become more structured, larger, and eventually become national or international when they spread to other areas across the country or around the world. Unfortunately, the large organizations tend to lose sight of the fundamental issues they were originally formed to solve, or they are unable to deal effectively with local problems.

Working to Bring About Change

Grassroots organizations usually have relatively small memberships; are localized to a town, city, or sometimes a state; and attempt to solve a problem or deal with an issue that the members feel is not being adequately handled by a large national organization. They may be created as a completely new and separate organization, or they may break away from a larger, established group. Because all the members of grassroots organizations are passionately concerned about only one or two issues at a time that affect them directly, they tend to work hard to effect change and can bring a great deal of concentrated power to bear upon people, such as legislators, who make the decisions about the issues.

Grassroots groups use a number of techniques that are often frowned upon by the more established organizations to attain their goals. In addition to the traditional techniques of writing letters, sending e-mail, and calling legislators, members of grassroots groups actively seek media attention, march on capitol buildings and state houses, introduce resolutions, and testify before committee hearings. Their success varies from issue to issue and location to location.

Successful Grassroots Efforts

Two examples of successful grassroots efforts are found in California and Pennsylvania. The California Nurses Association decided to break away from the ANA because it was not addressing some key state issues such as length of hospital stays, reduction in professional nursing staffs, and **managed care's** preoccupation with profit. The grassroots group in Pennsylvania formed a completely new organization, the Nurses of Pennsylvania (NPA), and focused their energies on the trend to replace licensed registered nurses with unlicensed technicians, sometimes called "downskilling."

Special-Interest Organizations

Why Do They Exist?

The historical origins of special-interest organizations in nursing are even older than those of the main national organizations. For example, the Red Cross, established in 1864, is one of the oldest special-interest organizations that nurses have been involved with. Like the Red Cross, most specialty organizations in nursing were founded when a group of nurses with similar concerns sought professional and individual support. These organizations usually start out small and informal, then increase in size, structure, and membership over a number of years. There were relatively few of these organizations until 1965, when an explosion in specialty organizations in nursing took place. During the next 20 years, almost 100 new organizations were formed, with the associated effect of diminishing membership levels in the ANA.

Clinical practice. Specialty organizations are usually organized according to clinical practice area. Organizations exist for almost every clinical specialty and subspecialty known in nursing, such as obstetrics/gynecology, critical care, operating room, emergency department, and occupational health, as well as less known areas such as flight nursing, urology, and cosmetic surgery.

Education and culture. Another focal area for these organizations is education and ethics. Organizations such as the American Association of Colleges of Nursing and the Western Interstate Commission for Higher Education fall into this category. Often organizations focus on the common **ethnic group,** cultural, or religious backgrounds of nurses. The National Association of Hispanic Nurses and the National Black Nurses Association represent this type of specialty organization.

Education and standards. Although many of these organizations promote the personal and professional growth of their membership, they also carry out many other activities. Particularly important among these activities is establishing the standards of practice for the particular specialty area. Much as the ANA establishes overall standards of practice for nursing in general, the specialty organizations establish standards for their particular clinical areas. Providing educational services for their members is another important activity of specialty organizations. Conferences, workshops, and seminars in the clinical area represented are important venues for nurses to keep current on new developments and to maintain high standards of practice.

Should They Matter to You?

How many of these specialty nursing organizations are there? No one really knows. Many such organizations are informal and run by volunteers. Organizations are continually being formed, and others are being disbanded.

Should nurses belong to these organizations? The answer is yes, but only after they belong to the ANA. Many of the larger specialty organizations have recognized this fact and have established close ties with the ANA. The ANA, in its turn, is well aware of the membership bleed-off from the specialty organizations and has initiated efforts to become more involved in the specialty nursing areas.

Before nurses join a specialty organization, they should determine whether its purposes are at odds with those of the ANA. Many of the large specialty organizations have their own lobbyists in both state and national legislatures. Because the legislators really do not know the differences between the various nursing organizations, they can easily become confused over health-care issues if they are receiving pressure from two nursing groups representing opposing sides of the same issue. At this point, legislators may simply surmise that nurses really do not know what they want and vote on an important issue without regard to nurses and nursing.

Conclusion

Nursing, in its journey toward professionalism, has been propelled and shaped by its nursing organizations, which were the main vehicles for the development of educational and practice standards, initiation of licensure, promotion of advanced practice, and general improvement in the level of care nurses provided.

From their beginnings, nursing organizations have served as channels of communication between nurses, consumers of health care, and other health-care professionals. In many cases, the nursing organizations have served as a focus of power for the profession to influence those important health policies

Issues in Practice

Juanita R, an RN at a large, inner-city hospital, has been working on her off-hours as a volunteer in a storefront clinic to treat the indigent and underserved population of that part of the city. The clinic clientele is primarily Mexican-American, as are the majority of the 20 nurses working at the clinic. Because all the nurses, including a family nurse practitioner, volunteer their time and receive no pay, the small private grant that Juanita had managed to secure was adequate to cover the cost for rental of the building, basic supplies for the clinic, and a few medications. However, the grant is about to run out and is nonrenewable.

Juanita first tried to obtain money from the hospital to keep the clinic going, but she was told that the hospital was having its own financial problems because of managed care demands and could not spare any money. At a staff meeting of the nurses from the clinic, the nurses decided to band together and form a grassroots organization called the Store-Front Clinic Nurses to focus their efforts on obtaining funds to keep the clinic open. They printed and passed out flyers, called local and city politicians, encouraged the patrons of the clinic to talk to people they knew, and even called the local television station for an interview about their plight.

Although most of the nurses' effort went unrewarded, a large pharmaceutical company became aware of their plight and wanted to provide a sizable financial stipend to the clinic, in addition to supplying free medications, for a period of at least 5 years. In addition to their philanthropic interests, the pharmaceutical company also wanted to gather long-term data about a newly developed antihypertensive medication. The company would provide the medication free to the clients at the clinic, the majority of whom had some degree of hypertension, and all the nurses would have to do is take and record the clients' blood pressure readings and complete "reported side effects" forms on each client. Client identifier codes, rather than names, would be used to maintain confidentiality. Juanita, as the group's coordinator, would be responsible for coordinating and preserving the data.

Although Juanita saw it as an answer to her prayers, she was concerned about the medication project. The pharmaceutical company said that no research consent forms were needed because the medication had already been through clinical trials and had received approval by the Food and Drug Administration. Juanita called another meeting of her nurses to discuss the issue. Without the grant, the clinic would close, but if they accepted the grant, they would have to participate in a medication research project that made Juanita feel uncomfortable.

1. What are the main issues in this case study?
2. What ethical principles are being violated? What is the ethical dilemma that Juanita is facing?
3. Are there any other solutions to this problem?

that affect the whole nation. That continued unity is essential for the survival of nursing.

The tendency toward specialization has led to an ever-increasing number of nursing organizations, however, each focusing on a particular practice field within the profession. This trend has diluted the unity and ultimately lessened the power that nursing as a profession can exert in health-care issues. Although it is important to recognize the complexity of today's health-care system and the pluralism inherent in nursing, unity of opinion on major issues is essential if nursing is to have any influence on the future of the profession.

The challenge for nurses in the future is to use the diversity in the profession as a positive force and to unite as a group on important issues. Awareness of earlier development of nursing organizations provides a perspective for the current situation and can act as a framework for planning the future.

What Do You Think?

What type of power does the individual nurse have? Cite examples of individual nurses who have used their power to effect changes in health care and nursing.

Critical Thinking Exercises

- Develop a strategy for increasing the membership of the ANA.
- A labor union is attempting to organize the nurses at your hospital. Is it better for the professional nursing organization to represent the nurses? Why?
- A new graduate nurse is working in the intensive care unit (ICU) of a large hospital. She wants to join a nursing organization but only has a limited amount of money to spend. Her coworkers in the ICU want her to join the AACN, but she would also like to join the ANA. Basing her decision on economic and professional issues, which organization should she join?
- Compare and contrast certification and licensure. Should certification be legally recognized? Justify your answer.

References

1. Mikos C: Legal checkpoints: Beware the consequences of license relinquishment. Nurse Manager 35(10):16, 18, 2004.
2. Simpson R: Small bytes for busy people. Multistate licensure: Regulating cross-country care. Journal of Clinical System Management 6(8/9):14, 2004.
3. Mills, AC, and McSweeny, M: Nurse practitioners and physician assistants revisited. J Prof Nurs 18(1):36–46, 2002.
4. Manton, A, and Chamberlain, B: The importance of joining professional nursing organiazations. Imprint 51:5, 38–40, 2004.
5. American Nurses Association: Nursing's Social Policy Statement. ANA, Washington, DC, 1995.

Bibliography

Adams, D, and Miller, BK: Professionalism in nursing behaviors of nurse practitioners. J Prof Nurs 17(4):203–210, 2001.
Barkley, TW, et al.: Practice issues: Credentialing, perscriptive authority, and liability. Nurse Practitioner Forum 2001 12(2):106–114, 2001.
Clowney J: Moving ahead: Learning from experience. Renewing your vigour. NURS TIMES 101(2):75, 2005.
Garnero, T: On solving the nursing shortage. Nurse Week (Special Edition) Feb 4, 2002, p 11.
Gingerich B: Accreditation actions. Certification and licensure: CAM services providers. Home Health Care Management Practice, 16(6):531–533, 2004.
Martin B: Are you ready for certification, the mark of excellence? AACN NEWS, 21(11):10, 2004.
Martin, SA: Network to promote advanced practice mentoring relationships. AACN News 19(3):5, 2002.
Mikos C: Legal checkpoints: Inside the Nurse Practice Act. Nurse Manager 35(9):20, 22, 91, 2004.
Results of a multistate licensure survey. AJN-2005 Career Guide: 40, 2005.
Poe L: Eleven answers about the Nurse Licensure Interstate Compact. Utah Nurse 13(3):18, 2004.
Salladay S: Ethical problems. Nursing credentials: What's in a name (badge)? Nursing 34(8):11, 2004.
Sofer D: Mandatory BSNs? New New York nurses could be required to eventually obtain baccalaureates. AJN 104(10):22, 2004.
Tahan H: Guest column. Certification helps CMs meet today's challenges: Skills, knowledge, competency enhanced. Hospital Case Management 13(2):22, 31–32, 2005.
Whelan, J: "A necessity in the nursing world." The Chicago Nurses Professional Registry 1913–1950. Nurs Hist Rev 13:49–75, 2005.
Your guide to certification: Here's what you need to know to pursue recognition of your expertise. AJN 2005 Career Guide: 56–69, 2005.

4

Theories and Models of Nursing

Joseph T. Catalano

Learning Objectives

After completing this chapter, the reader will be able to:

- Explain why theories and models are important to the profession of nursing.

- Analyze the four key concepts found in nursing theories and models.

- Interrelate systems theory as an important element in understanding nursing theories and models.

- Evaluate how the four parts of all systems interact.

- Synthesize three nursing theories, identifying how the different nursing theorists define the key concepts in their theories.

CARING FOR REAL PEOPLE

For many nurses, and for most nursing students, the terms *theory* and *model* evoke images of textbooks filled with abstract, obscure words, and convoluted sentences. The visceral response is often "Why is this important? I want to take care of real people!" The simple answer is that understanding and using nursing theories or models will help you be a better nurse and provide better care to real people.

DIFFERENCES BETWEEN THEORIES AND MODELS

What is a Theory?

Although the terms *theory* and *model* are not synonymous, in nursing practice they are often used interchangeably. Strictly speaking, a theory refers to a speculative statement involving some element of reality that has not been proved. For example, the theory of relativity has never been proved, although the results have often been observed.

The nursing profession tends to use the term *theory* when attempting to explain apparent relationships between observed behaviors and their effects on a client's health. In this nursing context, the goal of a theory is to describe and explain a particular nursing action to make a **hypothesis** or predict its effect on a client's outcome, such as improved health or recovery from illness. For example, the action of turning an unresponsive client from side to side every 2 hours should help prevent skin breakdown and improve respiratory function.

In recent years, nursing has been moving toward using research findings to guide nursing practice. This approach, called evidence-based practice, is an important element in improving nursing care and proving many of the long-standing theories that the nursing profession has developed over the years.[1]

> *In recent years, nursing has been moving toward using research findings to guide nursing practice. This approach, called evidence-based practice, is an important element in improving nursing care and proving many of the long-standing theories that the nursing profession has developed over the years.*

What Is a Model?

A model is a hypothetical representation of something that exists in reality. The purpose of a model is to attempt to explain a complex reality in a systematic and organized manner. For example, a hospital organizational chart is a model that attempts to demonstrate the interrelationships of the various levels of the hospital's administration.[2]

What Do You Think?

Do you consider yourself to be healthy? What factors make you healthy? What factors are indicators of illness?

_____

_____

_____

_____

_____

_____

_____

_____

_____

_____

_____

_____

_____

What Do Nurses Do?

Although a model tends to be more concrete than a theory, they both help explain and direct nursing actions. This ability, using a systematic and structured approach, is one of the key elements that raises nursing from a task-oriented job to the level of a real profession. With the use of a **conceptual model,** nurses can provide intelligent and thoughtful answers to the question "What do nurses do?" Consider this scenario:

> Mr. X had surgery for intestinal cancer 4 days ago. He has a colostomy and needs to learn how to take care of it at home because he is going to be discharged from the hospital in 2 days. When the nurses attempt to teach him colostomy care, he looks away, makes sarcastic personal comments about the nurses, and generally displays a belligerent and hostile attitude.

Without an understanding of the underlying dynamics involved, the nurses' reactions to this client's behavior might be to become sarcastic and scold the client about his behavior or simply to minimize the amount of contact with him.[2] This type of response will not improve Mr. X's health status. If the nurses knew about, however, and understood the dynamics of the grief theory, they would realize that Mr. X was probably in the anger stage of the grief process. This understanding would direct the nurse to allow, or even to encourage, Mr. X to express his anger and **aggressiveness** without condemnation and to help him deal with his feelings in a constructive manner. Once Mr. X gets past the anger stage, he can move on to taking a more active part in his care and thus improve his health status. The **client goals** would then be achieved.

If a researcher were to stop 10 people at random on the street and ask the question, "What do nurses do?" he or she would likely get 10 different answers, but the confusion about nurses' activities extends far beyond the public at large. What if the researcher asked 10 hospital administrators, 10 physicians, or even 10 nurses the same question? It could be anticipated that the answers would vary almost as much as the answers from laypeople.

The Iowa Project

In an attempt to identify what exactly it is that nurses do, J.C. McCloskey and G.M. Bulechek, two nurse researchers at the University of Iowa, have been conducting a research project since 1990 to develop a **taxonomy** of the **interventions** that nurses use in their practice (Box 4.1). This research has been called Nursing Interventions Classification (NIC), the Iowa Interventions Project, or simply the Iowa Project.[3–5]

The first results, published in 1994, categorized and ranked 336 interventions that nurses use when they provide care to clients. A follow-up study was conducted about 2 years after the original and published in 1996. This study categorized and ranked 433 interventions used by nurses. McCloskey and Bulechek[6] also investigated what nursing interventions were commonly used by nurses in specialty settings. Forty specialty areas responded, and the researchers were able to develop a table that lists what core skills are used by each organization.

This type of research helps identify the important contributions made by nursing to the health and well-being of clients. It also demonstrates the complex and demanding nature of the nursing profession. Although additional research has been conducted into this topic, the findings of McCloskey and Bulechek[4–6] continue to be considered the standard for all subsequent studies.

KEY CONCEPTS COMMON TO NURSING MODELS

Although nursing models vary in terminology and approach to health care, four concepts are common to almost all of them: client or patient (individual or collective), health, environment, and nursing. Each nursing model has its own specific definition of these terms, but the underlying definitions of the concepts are similar.

> *Although nursing models vary in terminology and approach to health care, there are four concepts that are common to almost all of them: client or patient (individual or collective), health, environment, and nursing.*

Client

The concept of client (or patient) is central to all nursing models, because it is the client who is the primary recipient of nursing care. Although the term *client* is usually used to refer to a single individual, it can also refer to small groups or to a large collective of individuals (for community health nurses, the community is the client).

A complex relationship. The concept of client has changed over the years as the knowledge and understanding of human nature has developed and increased. A client constitutes more than a person who simply needs **restorative care** and comes to a health-care facility with a **disease** to be cured. Clients are now seen as complex entities affected by various interrelating factors, such as the mind and body, the individual and the **environment,** and the person and the person's family. When nurses talk about clients, the term *biopsychosocial* is often used to express the complex relationship between the body, mind, and environment.

> *Nursing models tend to be holistic; they are concerned with curing disease and restoring a client's health, but they also focus on prevention of disease and maintenance of health. A healthy person is just as important to many nursing models as the person with a disease.*

Modeling a healthy client. A client, in many of the nursing models, does not have to have an illness to be the central element of the model (this explains the current preference of using the term *client* over the term *patient*). This is also one of the clearest distinctions between medical models and nursing models. Medical models tend to be restrictive and are almost exclusively devoted to curing diseases and to restoring health. Nursing models tend to be **holistic;** they are concerned with curing disease and restoring a client's health, but they also focus on prevention of disease and maintenance of health. A healthy person is just as important to many nursing models as the person with a disease.

Health

Like the concept of client, the concept of health has undergone much development and change over the years as knowledge has increased. Originally

Box 4.1
What Constitutes Care?

At first glance, it would seem that everybody knows that nurses take care of clients. But what constitutes care? A study conducted by the faculty of the University of Iowa, called the Nursing Interventions Classification (NIC) or simply the Iowa Project, has identified 336 tasks or interventions that nurses are responsible for in their care of patients. Not all nurses carry out all 336 of these tasks all the time, but during an average career, a nurse would likely be involved in the majority of these tasks. Although this project was undertaken in the mid-1990s, it remains the benchmark study. Since the original study, several additional studies have been conducted that reaffirm the findings of the Iowa Project, and several researchers have undertaken projects to use the data generated by the Iowa Project in actual client care situations.

This project is an excellent example of how a nursing theory led to a research project that developed information that can be used by nurses in their daily practice. Based on the belief that nursing interventions are specific actions that a nurse can perform to bring about the resolution of a potential or actual health-care problem, the NIC attempted to identify and classify nursing interventions. It also attempted to rank those interventions according to the number of times a nurse was likely to perform one during a working day. The goal of the project was to develop a nursing information system that could be incorporated into the current information systems of all clinical facilities. By using the NIC system, hospital administrators, physicians, nurses, and even the public should be better able to recognize and evaluate the multiple interventions that nurses are responsible for in their daily work.

It is a generally acknowledged fact that nurses, as the largest single group of health-care providers, are essential to the welfare and care of most clients. Yet, in an age of health-care reform, nurses are finding it increasingly difficult to delineate the specific contributions they make to health care. If nurses are unable to define the care they provide, how are the reformers, politicians, and the public going to be able to identify the unique contribution made by nursing?

Unfortunately, many of the contributions that nurses make to health care are currently invisible because there is no method of classification for them in the computerized database systems now in use. Commonly used nursing interventions such as active listening, emotional support, touch, skin surveillance, and even family support cannot be measured and quantified by most current information systems.

The large number of interventions used daily by nurses demonstrates the complex and demanding nature of the profession. The breadth and depth of knowledge and skills demanded of nurses on a daily basis is much greater than is found in many other health-care professions. One study found that nurses working in general medical/surgical units during a 6-month period were likely to care for 500 clients with more than 600 individual diagnoses (many clients have multiple diagnoses). These researchers also found that the physical demands of the work were actually less difficult and tiring than dealing with the emotional and technical demands of handling the huge amounts of information generated by the care given.

Sources: Moorhead S. Nursing outcomes classification (NOC): Iowa outcomes project. Mosby, Inc., 2004, ed. 3.
Haugsdal C: Using the Nursing Interventions Classification to describe the work of the nurse practitioner. Journal of American Academy of Nurse Practitioners 15(2):87–94, 2003.
Hansen M: Iowa Patient Safety Project update. Iowa Nurse Reporter. 15(2):17, 2002.
Bulechek, GM, et al: Nursing interventions used in nursing practice. Am J Nurs 94(10):59–61, 1994.

thought of as an absence of disease, a more current realistic view is that of health as a continuum, ranging from a completely healthy state where there is no disease to a completely unhealthy state, which results in death. At any given time in their lives, everyone is located somewhere along the health continuum and may move closer to one side or the other depending on circumstances and health status.[7]

Health is difficult to define because it varies so much from one individual to another. For example, a 22-year-old bodybuilder who has no chronic diseases perceives health differently than an 85-year-old who has diabetes, congestive heart failure, and vision problems. The perception of health also varies from one culture to another and at different historical periods within the same culture. In some past cultures, a sign of health was pure white skin, whereas in the modern American culture, a dark bronze suntan has been more desirable as a sign of health—although there is an increasing recognition of the harmful effects of ultraviolet light on the skin.

Environment

The concept of environment is another element in most current nursing models. Nursing models often broaden the concept of environment from the simple physical environment to include elements such as living conditions, public sanitation, and air and water quality. Factors such as interpersonal relationships and social interactions are also included.

Some internal environmental factors that affect health include personal psychological processes, religious beliefs, sexual orientation, personality, and emotional responses. It has long been known that individuals who are highly self-motivated and internally goal directed (i.e., type A personality) tend to develop ulcers and have myocardial infarctions at a higher rate than the general population. Medical models, which are primarily illness oriented, although acknowledging this factor, may not consider it to be treatable. Nursing models that consider personality as one of the environmental factors that affect health are more likely to attempt to modify the individual's behavior (internal environment) to decrease the risk of disease.

Like the other key concepts found in nursing models, the concept of environment is used so that it is consistent within a particular model's overall context. Nursing models try to show how various

aspects of environment interrelate and how they affect the client's health status. In addition, nursing models treat environment as an active element in the overall health-care system and assert that positive alterations in the environment will improve the client's health status.

Nursing

The Concept of Nursing

The culminating concept in all the various nursing models is nursing itself. After consideration of what it means to be a client, what it means to be healthy, and how the environment influences the client's health status either positively or negatively, the concept of nursing delineates the function and role nurses have in their relationships with clients.

Historically, the profession of nursing has been interested in providing basic physical care (i.e., hygiene, activity, nourishment), psychological support, and relief of discomfort for clients. Modern nursing, although still including these basic elements of client care, has expanded into areas of health care that were only imagined a generation ago.

> *The culminating concept in all the various nursing models is nursing itself. After consideration of what it means to be a client, what it means to be healthy, and how the environment influences the client's health status either positively or negatively, the concept of nursing delineates the function and role nurses have in their relationships with clients.*

Client as Partner

In the modern nurse–client relationship, the client is no longer the passive recipient of nursing care. The relationship has been expanded to include clients as key partners in curing and in the health maintenance process. In conjunction with the nurse, clients set goals for care and recovery, take an active part in achieving those goals, and help in evaluating whether or not those actions have achieved the goals.[8]

What Do You Think?

How do you define nursing? What activities are important for the nurse to carry out?

Because of the broadened understanding of environment, several nursing models include manipulation of environmental elements that affect health as an important part of the nurse's role. The environment may be directly altered by the nurse with little or no input from the client, or the client may be taught by the nurse to alter the environment in ways that will contribute to curing disease, increasing comfort, or improving the client's health status.[9]

Four key concepts. To analyze and understand any nursing model, it is important to look for these four key concepts: client, health, environment, and nursing. These concepts should be clearly defined, closely interrelated, and mutually supportive. Depending on the particular nursing model, one element may be emphasized more than another. The resultant role and function of the nurse depend on which element is given greater emphasis.

GENERAL SYSTEMS THEORY

A widely accepted method for conceptualizing and understanding the world and what is in it is derived from a systems viewpoint. Generally understood as an organized unit with a set of components that interact and affect each other, a system acts as a whole because of the interdependence of its parts.[10]

As a result, when part of the system malfunctions or fails, it interrupts the function of the whole system rather than affecting merely one part. Humans, plants, cars, governments, the health-care system, the profession of nursing, and almost anything that exists can be viewed as a system. The terminology and principles of systems theory pervade U.S. society.

A Basis in Thought

Manageable Fragments

Although general systems theory in its pure form is rarely, if ever, used as a nursing model, its process and much of its terminology underlie many nursing models. Elements of general systems theory in one form or another have found their way into many textbooks and much of the professional literature. General systems theory often acts as the unacknowledged **conceptual framework** for many educational programs. An understanding of the mechanisms and terminology of general systems theory is helpful in providing an orientation to understanding nursing models.

General systems theory, sometimes referred to simply as **systems theory,** is an outgrowth of an innate intellectual process. The human mind has difficulty comprehending large, complex entities as a single unit. As a result, the mind automatically divides that entity into smaller, more manageable fragments and then examines each fragment separately. This is similar to the process of deductive reasoning, in which a single complex thought or theory is broken down into smaller, interrelated pieces. All scientific disciplines, from physics to biology and the social sciences (e.g., sociology and psychology), use this method of analysis.

Reassembling the Fragments

Systems theory takes the process a step further. After analyzing or breaking down the entity, systems theory attempts to put it back together by showing how the parts work individually and together within the system. This interrelationship of the parts makes the system function as a unit. Often, particularly when the system involves biological or sociological entities, the system that results is greater than the sum of its parts.

For example, a human can be considered to be a complex, biosocial system. Humans are made up of a large number of smaller systems such as the endocrine system, neurological system, gastrointestinal system, urinary system, and so forth. Although each of these systems is important, in and of themselves they do not make a human. Many animals have the same systems, yet the human is more than the animal and more than the sum of the systems.

A Set of Interacting Parts

Although the early roots of general systems theory can be traced as far back as the 1930s, von Bertalanffy is usually credited with the formal development and publication of general systems theory around 1950.[11] His major achievement was to standardize the definitions of the terms used in systems theory and make the concept useful to a wide range of disciplines. Systems theory is so widely applicable because it reflects the reality that underlies basic human thought processes.

Very simply, a system is defined as a set of interacting parts. The parts that comprise a system may be similar or they may vary a great deal from each other, but they all have the common function of making the system work well to achieve its overall purpose.

A school is a good example of how the dynamics and interrelatedness of a system work. A school as a system consists of a large number of units including buildings, administrators, teachers, students, and various other individuals (e.g., counselors, financial aid personnel, bookkeepers, and maintenance persons). Each of these individuals has a unique job but also contributes to the overall goal of the school, which is to provide an education for the students and to further the development of knowledge through research.

All systems consist of four key parts: the system itself (i.e., whether it is an open system or a closed system), input and output, throughput, and a feedback loop.

Open and Closed Systems

A system is categorized as being either open or closed. Very few systems are completely open or completely closed. Rather, they are usually a combination of both open and closed systems.

Open Systems

Open systems are those in which relatively free movement of information, matter, and **energy** into and out of the system exists. In a completely open system, there would be no restrictions on what moves in and out of the system, thus making its boundaries difficult to identify. Most systems have some control over the movement of information, energy, and matter around them. This control is maintained through the semipermeable nature of their boundaries, which allows some things in and keeps some things out, as well as allowing some out while keeping others in. This control of input and output leads to the dynamic equilibrium found in most well-functioning systems.

Closed Systems

Theoretically, a **closed system** prevents any movement into and out of the system. In this case, the system would be totally static and unchanging. Probably no absolutely closed systems exist in the real world, although there are systems that may tend to be closed to outside elements. A stone, for example, considered as a system, seems to be very nearly a perfectly closed system. It does not take anything in or put anything out. It does not change very much over long periods. In reality, though, it is affected by a number of elements in nature. It absorbs moisture when it is damp, freezes when cold, and becomes hot in the summer. Over long periods, these factors may cause the stone to crack, break down, and eventually become topsoil.

Systems that nurses deal with frequently are relatively open. Primarily, the client can be categorized as a highly open system that requires certain input elements and has output elements also. Other systems that nurses commonly work with (e.g., hospital administrators and physicians) are generally considered to be open systems, although their degree of openness may vary widely.

Input and Output

The processes by which a system interacts with elements in its environment are called *input* and *output*. Input is defined as any type of information, energy, or material that enters the system from the environment through its boundaries. Conversely, output is defined as any information, energy, or material that leaves the system and enters the environment through the system's boundaries. The end product of a system is a type of output that is not reusable as input. Open systems require relatively large amounts of input and output.

Throughput

A third term sometimes used in relationship to the system's dynamic exchange with the environment is *throughput*. Throughput is a process that allows the input to be changed so that it is useful to the system.

For example, most automobiles operate on some form of liquid fossil fuel (input) such as gasoline or diesel fuel. However, going to the gas station and pouring liquid fuel on the roof of the car will not produce the desired effects. If the fuel is put into the gas tank, it can be transformed by the carburetor or fuel injection system into a fine mist, which when mixed with air and ignited by a spark plug burns rapidly to produce the force necessary to propel the car. Without this internal process (throughput), liquid fuel is not a useful form of energy.

Feedback Loop

The fourth key element of a system is the *feedback loop*. The feedback loop allows the system to monitor its internal functioning so that it can either restrict or increase its input and its output and maintain the highest level of functioning.

Positive feedback. Two basic types of feedback exist. Positive feedback leads to change within the system, with the goal of improving the system. Students in the classroom, for example, receive feedback from the teacher in several ways; it may be in the form of direct verbal statements such as "good work on this assignment" or feedback by examination and homework grades. Feedback is considered positive if it produces a change in a student's behavior, such as motivating him or her to study more, spend more time on assignments, or prepare more thoroughly for class.

Negative feedback. Negative feedback maintains stability; that is, it does not produce change. Negative feedback is not necessarily bad for a system. Rather, when a system has reached its peak level of functioning, negative feedback helps it maintain that level. For example, an athlete who has reached his or her peak level of performance through long hours of practice knows what type of practice is required to stay at that level of ability. Negative feedback—in the form of optimal times in the case of runners or number of pounds lifted in the case of weightlifters—indicates that no changes in practice patterns are required.

The feedback loop is an important element in systems theory. It makes the process circular and links the various elements of the system together. Without a feedback loop, it is virtually impossible for the system to have any meaningful control over its input and output.

> " *The feedback loop is an important element in systems theory. It makes the process circular and links the various elements of the system together.* "

Feedback loops are used at all levels in a hospital. Nurses get feedback about the care they provide both from clients and from their supervisors. The hospital administration gets feedback from clients and accrediting agencies. Physicians get feedback from clients, nurses, and the hospital administration. Systems theory is present, if sometimes unseen, in almost all health-care settings. Professional nurses need to be able to understand and identify the components of systems theory when they are encountered to improve their nursing practice and quality of care.

MAJOR NURSING THEORIES AND MODELS

At least 15 published nursing models (or theories) have been used to direct nursing education and nursing care.[12] The six nursing models discussed here (Table 4.1) have been selected because they are the most widely accepted and are good examples of how the concepts of client, health, environment, and nursing are used to explain and guide nursing actions.

Discussion of these theories is not intended to be exhaustive, but rather to provide an overview of the main concepts of the nurse theorist. It is important to understand the terms used in the theories as defined by their authors and to see the interrelationship between the elements in each theory as well as the similarities and differences among the various different models.

The Roy Adaptation Model

As developed by Sister Callista Roy, the Roy Adaptation Model of nursing is very closely related to systems theory.[13] The main goal of this model is to allow the client to reach his or her highest level of functioning through adaptation.

Client

The central element in the Roy Adaptation Model is man (a generic term referring to humans in general, or the client in particular, collectively or individually). Man is viewed as a dynamic entity with both input and output. As derived from the context of the four modes in the Roy Adaptation Model, the client is defined as a biopsychosocial being who is affected by various stimuli and displays behaviors to help adapt to the stimuli. Because the client is constantly being affected by stimuli, adaptation is a continual process.[13]

Inputs are called stimuli and include internal stimuli that arise from within the client's environment as well as stimuli coming from external environmental factors such as physical surroundings, family, and society. The output in the Roy Adaptation Model is the behavior that the client demonstrates as a result of stimuli that are affecting him or her.

Output, or behavior, is a very important element in the Roy Adaptation Model, because it provides the **baseline data** about the client that the nurse obtains through assessment techniques. In this model, the output (behavior) is always modified by the client's internal attempts to adapt to the input, or stimuli. Roy has identified four internal adaptational activities that clients use and has called them the four adaptation modes:

1. The physiological mode (using internal physiological process)
2. The self-concept mode (developed throughout life by experience)
3. The role function mode (dependent on the client's relative place in society)
4. The interdependence mode (indicating how the client relates to others)

Table 4.1 Comparison of Selected Nursing Models

Nursing Theory	Client	Health	Environment	Nursing
Roy Adaption Model	Human being—a dynamic system with input and output	A continuum with the ability to adapt successfully to illness	Both internal and external stimuli that affect behaviors	Multistep process that helps the client adapt and reach the highest level of functioning
Orem Self-Care Model	Human being—biological, psychological, social being with the ability for self-care	Able to live life to the fullest through self-care	The medium through which the client moves	Assistance in self-care activities to help the client achieve health
King Model of Goal Attainment	Person—exchanges energy and information with the environment to meet needs	Dynamic process to achieve the highest level of functioning	Personal, interpersonal, and social systems and the external physical world	Dynamic process that identifies and meets the client's health-care needs
Watson Model of Human Caring	Individual—has needs, grows, and develops to reach a state of inner harmony	Dynamic state of growth and development leading to full potential as a human being	The client must overcome certain factors to achieve health	Science of caring that helps clients reach their greatest potential
Johnson Behavioral System Model	Person—a behavioral system; an organized, integrated whole composed of seven subsystems	A behavioral system able to achieve a balanced, steady state	All the internal and external elements that affect client behavior	Activities that manipulate the environment and help clients achieve the balanced state of health
Neuman Health-Care Systems Model	An open system that constantly interacts with internal and external environment	An individual with relatively stable internal functioning of a high state of wellness (stability)	Internal and external stressors that produce change in the client	Identifies boundary disruption and helps clients in activities to restore stability

Health

In the Roy Adaptation Model, the concept of health is defined as the location of the client along a continuum between perfect health and complete illness. Health, in this model, is rarely an absolute. Rather, "a person's ability to adapt to stimuli, such as injury, disease, or even psychological stress, determines the level of that person's health status."[13] For example, a client who was in an automobile accident, had a broken neck, and was paralyzed but who eventually went back to college, obtained a law degree, and became a practicing lawyer would, in the Roy Adaptation

Model, be considered to have a high degree of health because of the ability to adapt to the stimuli imposed.

Environment

The Roy Adaptation Model's definition of environment is synonymous with the concept of stimuli. The environment consists of all those factors that influence the client's behavior, either internally or externally. This model categorizes these environmental elements, or stimuli, into three groups: (1) focal, (2) contextual, and (3) residual.

Focal stimuli are environmental factors that most directly affect the client's behavior and require most of his or her attention. **Contextual stimuli** form the general physical, social, and psychological environment from which the client emerges. **Residual stimuli** are factors in the client's past, such as personality characteristics, past experiences, religious beliefs, and social norms that have an indirect effect on the client's health status. Residual stimuli are often very difficult to identify because they may remain hidden in the person's past memory or may be an integral part of the client's personality.

Nursing

Assessment

In the Roy Adaptation Model, nursing becomes a multistep process, similar to the nursing process, to aid and support the client in the attempt to adapt to stimuli in one or more of the four adaptive modes. To determine what type of help is required to promote adaptation, the nurse must first assess the client.

The primary nursing assessments are of the client's behavior (output). Basically, the nurse should try to determine whether the client's behavior is adaptive or maladaptive in each of the four adaptational modes previously defined. Some first-level assessments of the pneumonia client might include a temperature of 104°F, a cough productive of thick green sputum, chest pain on inspiration, and signs of weakness or physical debility, such as the inability to bring in wood for the fireplace or to visit friends.

A second-level assessment should also be made to determine what type of stimuli (input) are affecting the client's health-care status. In the case of the client with pneumonia, this might include a culture and sensitivity of the sputum to identify the invasive bacteria, assessment of the client's clothes

to determine whether they were adequate for the weather outside, and an investigation to find out whether any neighbors could help the client when he or she is discharged from the hospital.

Analysis

After performing the assessment, the nurse analyzes the data and arranges them in such a way as to be able to make a statement about the client's adaptive or maladaptive behaviors; that is, the nurse identifies the problem. In current terminology, this identification of the problem is called a **nursing diagnosis.** The problem statement is the first part of the three-part PES (problem–etiology–signs and symptoms) formulation that completes the nursing diagnosis (Fig. 4.1).

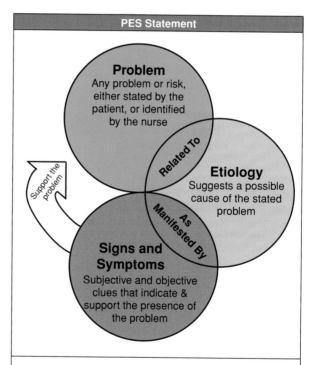

Together, these components make up the **PES** (**P**roblem, **E**tiology, **S**igns/symptoms) statement, which is demonstrated below

Pain, acute, may be related to *surgical wound,* as manifested by *facial grimacing, increased heart rate* and *verbal complaints* of pain at the incision site

Figure 4.1 Together, these components make up the PES (problem–etiology–signs and symptoms) statement: *Pain,* acute, may be related to *surgical wound,* as manifested by *facial grimacing, increased heart rate,* and *verbal complaints* of pain at the incision site.

Setting Goals

After the problem has been identified, goals for optimal adaptation are established. Ideally, these goals should be a collaborative effort between the nurse and the client. A determination of the actions that need to be taken to achieve the goals is the next step in the process. The focus should be on manipulation of the stimuli to promote optimal adaptation. Finally, an evaluation is made of the whole process to evaluate whether the goals have been met. If the goals have not been met, the nurse must determine why, not how, the activities should be modified to achieve the goals.[11]

The Orem Self-Care Model

Dorothea E. Orem's model of nursing is based on the belief that health care is each individual's own responsibility. The model is aimed at helping clients direct and carry out activities that either help maintain or improve their health.[14]

Client

As with most other nursing models, the central element of the Orem model is the client, who is a biological, psychological, and social being with the capacity for self-care. Self-care is defined as the practice of activities that individuals initiate and perform on their own behalf to maintain life, health, and well-being. Self-care is a requirement both for maintenance of life and for optimal functioning.

Health

In the Orem Self-Care Model, health is defined as the person's ability to live fully within a particular physical, biological, and social environment, achieving a higher level of functioning that distinguishes the person from lower life forms.

Quality of life is an extremely important element in this model of nursing. A person who is healthy is living life to the fullest and has the capacity to maintain that life through self-care. An unhealthy person is an individual who has a self-care deficit. This group of unhealthy individuals also includes adults with diseases and injuries, young and dependent children, the elderly, and the disabled. This deficit is indicated by the inability to carry out one or more of the key health-care activities. These activities have been categorized into six groups:

> *The primary goal of nursing in the Orem model is to help the client conduct self-care activities in such a way as to reach the highest level of human functioning.*

- Air, water, and food
- Excretion of waste
- Activity and rest
- Solitude and social interactions
- Avoiding hazards to life and well-being
- Being normal mentally under universal self-care

Universal Self-Care

In the Orem model, self-care is a two-part concept. The first type of self-care is called universal self-care and includes those elements commonly found in everyday life that support and encourage normal human growth, development, and functioning. Persons who are healthy, according to the Orem model, carry out the activities listed in order to maintain a state of health. To some degree, all these elements are necessary activities in maintaining health through self-care.[15]

The second type of self-care comes into play when the individual is unable to conduct one or more of the six self-care activities. This second type of self-care is called health deviation self-care. Health deviation self-care includes those activities carried out by individuals who have diseases, injuries, physiological or psychological stress, or other health-care concerns. Activities such as seeking health care at an emergency room or clinic, entering a drug **rehabilitation** unit, joining a health club or weight control program, or going to a physician's office fall into this category.

Environment

Environment, in the self-care model, is the medium through which clients move as they conduct their daily activities. Although less emphasized in this model, the environment is generally viewed as a negative factor in a person's health status because many environmental factors detract from the ability to provide self-care. Environment includes social interactions with others, situations that must be resolved, and physical elements that affect health.

Nursing

The primary goal of nursing in the Orem model is to help the client conduct self-care activities in such a way as to reach the highest level of human functioning. Because there is a range of levels of self-care ability, three distinct levels, or systems, of nursing care are delineated, based on the individual's ability to undertake self-care activities. As clients become less able to care for themselves, their nursing care needs increase.

Wholly Compensated Care

A person who is able to carry out few or no self-care activities falls into the wholly compensated nursing care category in which the nurse must provide for most or all of the client's self-care needs. Examples of clients who require this level of care include comatose and ventilator-dependent clients in an intensive care unit, clients in surgery and the immediate recovery period, women in the labor and delivery phases of childbirth, and clients with emotional and psychological problems so severe as to render them unable to conduct normal activities of daily living.

Partially Compensated Care

Clients in the partially compensated category of nursing care can meet some to most of their self-care needs but still have certain self-care deficits that require nursing intervention. The nurse's role becomes one of identifying these needs and carrying out activities to meet them until the client reaches a state of health and is able to meet the needs personally. Examples of this level of nursing care include postoperative clients who can feed themselves and do basic activities of daily living (ADL) but are unable to care for a catheter and dressing and clients with newly diagnosed diabetes who have not yet learned the technique of self-administered insulin injections.

Supportive Developmental Care

Clients who are able to meet all of their basic self-care needs require very little or no nursing interventions. These clients fall in the supportive developmental category of nursing care, in which the nurse's main functions are to teach the client how to maintain or improve health and to offer guidance in self-care activities and provide emotional support and encouragement.

What Do You Think?

Based on your experiences with the health-care system, write your own definition of client (patient). What factors led you to this definition?

_____

_____

_____

_____

_____

_____

_____

_____

_____

_____

_____

Also, the nurse may adjust the environment to support the client's growth and development toward self-care or may identify community resources to help in the self-care process.[15] Conducting prenatal classes, arranging for discharge planning, providing child screening programs through a community health agency, and organizing aerobic exercise classes for postcoronary clients all are nursing actions that belong in the supportive developmental category of care.

A Three-Step Process

Nursing care is carried out through a three-step process in the Orem model. Step 1 determines whether nursing care is needed. This step includes a basic assessment of the client and identification of self-care problems and needs. Step 2 determines the appropriate nursing care system category and plans nursing care according to that category. Step 3 provides the indicated nursing care or actions to meet the client's self-care needs.

Five Methods

In the Orem model, step 3—the provision of nursing care (implementation phase)—is carried out by helping the client through one or a combination of five nursing methods:[12]

- Acting for or doing for another person
- Guiding another person
- Supporting another person (physically or psychologically)
- Providing an environment that promotes personal

[...text obscured by lottery ticket images...]

...stablishing
...g client care
...King Model
...e M. King.
...del.[16]
...nursing
...ound in the
...social. The
...onal sys-
...l is the main
...rovide care
...h they deal
...activities
...notion
...at the social
...programs in
...f nursing at
...l to include
...e an effect

...int of care in
...The client is
...es energy and
...rsonal sys-
...ectual needs
...of life.
...pletely by
...re developed
...ling on the
...cations with
...and tension
in the environment.

Environment

Environment is an important concept in the King model and encompasses a number of interrelated elements. The personal and interpersonal systems or groups are central to King's conception of environment. They are formed at various levels according to internal goals established by the client.

Personal systems. At the most basic level are the personal systems, where an interchange takes place between two individuals who share similar goals. An example of such a personal system is a client–nurse relationship.

Interpersonal systems. At the intermediate level are the interpersonal systems that involve relatively small groups of individuals who share like goals, for example, a formal weight-loss program in which the members have the common goal of losing weight. Human interactions, communications, role delineation, and stress reduction are essential factors at this level.

Social systems. At the highest level are social systems, which include the large, relatively homogeneous elements of society. The health-care system, government, and society in general are some important social systems. These social systems have as their common goals organization, authority, power, status, and decision. Although the client may not be in direct interaction with the social systems, these systems are important because the personal and interpersonal systems necessarily function within larger social systems.

Evoking the principle of nonsummativity,* whenever one part of an open system is changed, all the other parts of the system feel the effect. For example, a decision made at the governmental level to reduce Medicare or Medicaid payments may affect when and how often a client can use health-care services such as doctor's office visits, group therapy, or emergency room care.

The King model also includes the external physical environment that affects a person's health and well-being. As the person moves through the world, the physical setting interacts with the personal system to either improve or degrade the client's health-care status.

Health

Viewed as a dynamic process that involves a range of human life experiences, health exists in people

*Nonsummativity is the degree of interrelatedness among the systems parts. The higher the degree of nonsummativity, the greater the interdependence of parts.

when they can achieve their highest level of functioning. Health is the primary goal of the client in the King model. It is achieved by continually adjusting to environmental stressors, maximizing the use of available resources, and setting and achieving goals for one's role in life. Anything that disrupts or interferes with people's ability to function normally in their chosen roles is considered to be a state of illness.

Nursing

The King model considers nursing to be a dynamic process and a type of personal system based on interactions between the nurse and the client. During these interactions, the nurse and the client jointly evaluate and identify the health-care needs, set goals for fulfillment of the needs, and consider actions to take in achieving those goals. Nursing is a multifaceted process that includes a range of activities such as the promotion and maintenance of health through education, the restoration of health through care of the sick and injured, and preparation for death through care of the dying.[11]

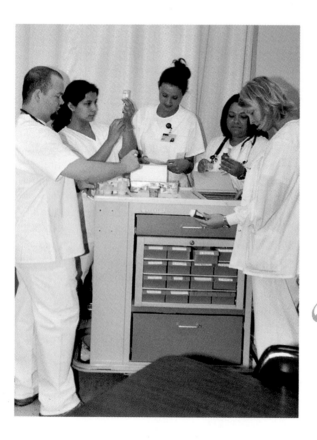

The process of nursing in the King model includes five key elements considered central to all human interactions:

- Action
- Reaction
- Interaction
- Transaction
- Feedback

The Watson Model of Human Caring

Although the concept of caring has always been an important, if somewhat obscure, element in the practice of nursing, the Watson Model of Human Caring defines caring in a detailed and systematic manner. In the development of her model, Jean Watson used a philosophical approach rather than the systems theory approach seen in many other nursing models. Her main concern in the development of this model was to balance the impersonal aspects of nursing care that are found in the technological and scientific aspects of practice with the personal and interpersonal elements of care that grow from a humanistic belief in life. Watson is also one of the very few theorists who openly recognize the client's and family's spirituality and spiritual beliefs as an essential element of health.[17]

Client

The concept of client or person in the Watson model is not well developed as separate from the concept of nursing. The individuality of the client is a key concern. The Watson model views the client as someone who has needs, who grows and develops throughout life, and who eventually reaches a state of internal harmony.

The client is also seen as a gestalt, or whole, who has value because of inherent goodness and capacity to develop. This gestalt, or holistic, view of the human being is a recurring theme in the Watson model; it emphasizes that the total person is more important to nursing care than the individual injury or disease process that produced the need for care.

> *The Watson model views the client as someone who has needs, who grows and develops throughout life, and who eventually reaches a state of internal harmony.*

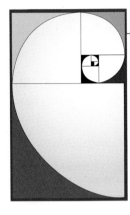

Issues Now

Looking to the Future: The Pew Commission Final Report

Projected estimates of the nursing shortage based on data collected by the U.S. Bureau of the Census Current Population Survey, Division of Nursing, the Pew Commission, and the Buerhaus and Staiger data collection agency in 1998 are now considered woefully inadequate. Current projections of the nursing shortage range from 400,000 to as many as 1,000,000 by the year 2010. The Pew Commission's final report addressed the competencies that nurses in the future will need:

Twenty-One Competencies for the Twenty-First Century

1. Embrace a personal ethic of social responsibility and service.
2. Exhibit ethical behavior in all professional activities.
3. Provide evidence-based, clinically competent care.
4. Incorporate the multiple determinants of health in clinical care.
5. Apply knowledge of the new sciences.
6. Demonstrate critical thinking, reflection, and problem-solving skills.
7. Understand the role of primary care.
8. Rigorously practice preventive health care.
9. Integrate population-based care and services into practice.
10. Improve access to health care for those with unmet health needs.
11. Practice relationship-centered care with individuals and families.
12. Provide culturally sensitive care to a diverse society.
13. Partner with communities in health-care decisions.
14. Use communication and information technology effectively and appropriately.
15. Work in interdisciplinary teams.
16. Ensure care that balances individual, professional, system, and social needs.
17. Practice leadership.
18. Take responsibility for quality of care and health outcomes at all levels.
19. Contribute to continuous improvement of the health-care system.
20. Advocate for public policy that promotes and protects the health of the public.
21. Continue to learn and help others to learn.

The Pew Commission also went on to identify five key areas for professional education:

1. Change professional training to meet the demands of the new health-care system.
2. Ensure that the health professions workforce reflects the diversity of the nation's population.
3. Require interdisciplinary competence in all health professionals.
4. Continue to move education into ambulatory practice.
5. Encourage public service of all health professional students and graduates.

The changes that will occur over the next decade may threaten some health-care professionals, but they will also open up a vista of opportunities for those willing to look creatively into the future. Nursing has to recognize that it will grow only to the extent that it is able to contribute to the needs of an evolving health-care system.

(continued)

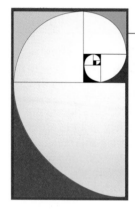

ISSUES NOW continued

These needs will change with time. The Pew Report, although broad in scope, provides the nursing profession with a blueprint for dealing with these changes as they occur. It is a call to action that nurses and the nursing profession need to hear.

Sources: Critical Challenges: Revitalizing the Health Professions for the 21st Century. Pew Health Professions Commission, San Francisco, 1995.
Bellack, JP, and O'Neil, EH: Recreating nursing practice for a new century: Recommendations of the Pew Health Professions Commission's Final Report. Nursing and Health Care Perspectives 21(1):14–21, 2000.
Brady, M, et al: A proposed framework for differentiating the 21 Pew Competencies by level of nursing education. Nursing and Health Care Perspectives 22(1):30–36, 2001.
Pontious, M: Where have all the nurses gone? The Oklahoma Nurse 47(1):1, 18, 2002.
More than one million new nurses needed by 2010. The American Nurse 34(1):5, 2002.

Environment

Environment in the Watson model is a concept that is also closely intertwined with the concept of nursing. Viewed primarily as a negative element in the health-care process, the environment consists of those factors that the client must overcome to achieve a state of health. The environment can be both external physical and social elements and internal psychological reactions that affect health.

Health

To be healthy according to the Watson model, the individual must be in a dynamic state of growth and development that leads to reaching full potential as a human. As with other nursing models, health is viewed as a continuum along which a person at any point may tend more toward health or more toward illness.

Illness, in the Watson model, is the client's inability to integrate life experiences and the failure to achieve full potential or inner harmony. In this model, the state of illness is not necessarily synonymous with the disease process. If the person reacts to the disease process in such a way as to find meaning, then that response is considered to be healthy. A failure to find meaning in the disease experience leads to a state of illness.

Nursing

Watson makes a clear distinction between the science of nursing and the practice of curing (medicine).[12] She defined nursing as the science of caring in which the primary goal is to assist the client to reach the greatest level of personal potential. The practice of curing involves the conduct of activities that have the goal of treatment and elimination of disease.

The process of nursing in the Watson model is based on the systematic use of the scientific problem-solving method for decision making. To best understand nursing as a science of caring, the nurse should hold certain beliefs and be able to initiate certain caring activities.

Values. Basic to the beliefs necessary for the successful practice of nursing in the Watson model is the formation of a humanistic altruistic system of values based on the tenet that all people are inherently valuable because they are human. In addition, the nurse should have a strong sense of faith and hope in people and their condition because of the human potential for development.

Caring. A number of activities are important when practicing nursing according to Watson's caring way. These activities include establishing a relationship of help and trust between the nurse and the client; encouraging the client to express both positive and negative feelings with acceptance; manipulating the environment to make it more supportive, protective, or corrective for the client with any type of disease process; and assisting in whatever way is deemed appropriate to meet the basic human needs of the client.

The Johnson Behavioral System Model

By integrating systems theory with behavioral theory, Dorothy E. Johnson has developed a model of nursing that considers client behavior to be the key to preventing illness and to restoring health when illness occurs. Johnson holds that human behavior is really a type of system in itself that is influenced by input factors from the environment and has output that in its turn affects the environment.[12]

Client

Drawing directly on the terminology of systems theory, the Johnson model describes the person, or client, as a behavioral system that is an organized and integrated whole. The whole is greater than the sum of its parts because of the integration and functioning of its subsystems. In the Johnson model, the client as a behavioral system is composed of seven distinct behavioral subsystems. In turn, each of these seven behavioral subsystems contains four structural elements that guide and shape the subsystem.

Security. The first behavioral subsystem is the attachment, or affiliate, subsystem, which has security as its driving force. The type of activity that this subsystem undertakes is, for the most part, inclusion in social functions, and the behavior that is observed from this subsystem is social interaction.

Dependency. The second behavioral subsystem is the dependency subsystem, which has as its initiating force the goal of helping others. The primary type of activity involved is nurturing and promoting self-image. The observable behaviors that are a result of this activity include approval, attention, and physical assistance of the person.

Taking In. The third behavioral subsystem is called the ingestive subsystem, which has as its driving force the meeting of the body's basic physiological needs of food and nutrient intake. Correspondingly, its primary activity is seeking and eating food.

Eliminative Behavior. The fourth behavioral subsystem is the eliminative; its goal is removal of waste products from the system. Its primary activity is means of elimination, which is observed as the behavior of expelling waste products.

Sexual Behavior. The fifth behavioral subsystem is sexual behavior, which is found in the Johnson model's description of the person. The sexual subsystem has gratification and procreation of the species as its goals. It involves the complex activities of identifying gender roles, sexual development, and

actual biological sexual activity. It manifests itself in courting and mating behaviors.

Self-Protection. The sixth behavioral subsystem is called the aggressive subsystem, and its driving force is the goal of self-preservation. All the actions that individuals undertake to protect themselves from harm, either internal or external, derive from this subsystem and are shown in actions toward others and the environment in general.

Achievement. The seventh, and final, behavioral subsystem is identified as achievement. Achievement has as its driving force the broad goal of exploration and manipulation of the environment. Gaining mastery and control over the environment is the primary activity of this subsystem; it can be demonstrated externally when the individual shows that learning has occurred and higher-level accomplishments are being produced.[18]

As with all open systems, the behavioral system that makes up the person seeks to maintain a dynamic balance by regulating input and output. This regulation process takes the form of adapting to the environment and responding to others. However, the Johnson model sees human behavior as being goal directed, which leads the person to constant growth and development beyond the maintenance of a mere steady state.

Health

A state of health exists, according to the Johnson model, when balance and steady state exist within the behavioral systems of the client. Under normal circumstances, the human system has enough inherent flexibility to maintain this balance without external intervention. At times, however, the system's balance may be disturbed to such a degree by physical disease, injury, or emotional crisis as to require external assistance. This out-of-balance state is the state of illness.

Environment

In the Johnson model, the environment is defined as all those internal and external elements that have an effect on the behavioral system. These environmental elements include obvious external factors, such as air temperature and relative humidity; sociological factors, such as family, neighborhood, and society in general; and the internal environment, such as bodily processes, psychological states, religious beliefs, and political orientation.

All seven behavioral subsystems of the client are involved with his or her relationship to the environment through the regulation of input and output. The client is continually interacting with the environment in the attempt to remain healthy by maintaining an internal dynamic balance.

Nursing

In the Johnson model, nursing is an activity that helps the individual achieve and maintain an optimal level of behavior (state of health) through the manipulation and regulation of the environment.[11] Nursing has functions in both health and illness. Nursing interventions to either maintain or regain health involve four activities in the regulation of the environment:

- Restricting harmful environmental factors
- Defending the client from negative environmental influences
- Inhibiting adverse elements from occurring
- Facilitating positive internal environmental factors in the recovery process

As a professional, the nurse in the Johnson model provides direct services to the client. By interacting with, and sometimes intervening in, the multiple subsystems that are found in the client's environment, the nurse acts as an external regulatory force. The goal of nursing is to promote the highest level of functioning and development in the client at all times.

Nursing actions include helping the client act in a socially acceptable manner, monitoring and aiding with biological processes necessary for maintenance of a dynamic balance, demonstrating support for medical care and treatment during illness, and taking actions to prevent illness from recurring. In this model, nursing makes its own unique contribution to the health and well-being of individuals and provides a service that is complementary to that provided by other health-care professionals.

> *In the Johnson model, nursing is an activity that helps the individual achieve and maintain an optimal level of behavior (state of health) through the manipulation and regulation of the environment.*

The Neuman Health-Care Systems Model

As envisioned by Betty Neuman, the Health-Care Systems Model focuses on the individual and his or her environment and is applicable to a variety of health-care disciplines apart from nursing. Drawing from systems theory, the Neuman model also includes elements from stress theory with an overall holistic view of humanity and health care.[19]

Client

In this model, the client is viewed as an open system that interacts constantly with internal and external environments through the system's boundaries. The client-system's boundaries are called lines of defense and resistance in the Neuman model and may be represented graphically as a series of concentric circles that surround the basic core of the individual. The goal of these boundaries is to keep the basic core system stable by controlling system input and output.

Neuman classifies these defensive boundaries according to their various functions. The internal lines of resistance are the boundaries that are closest to the basic core and thus protect the basic internal structure of the system. The normal lines of defense are outside the internal lines of resistance; they protect the system from common, everyday environmental stressors. The flexible line of defense surrounds the normal line of defense and protects it from extreme environmental stressors. The general goal of all these protective boundaries is to maintain the internal stability of the client.

Health

Health, then, in the Neuman model is defined as the relatively stable internal functioning of the client. Optimal health exists when the client is maintained in a high state of wellness or stability.

As in other nursing models, health is not considered an absolute state, but rather a continuum that reflects the client's internal stability while moving from wellness to illness and back. It takes a considerable amount of physical and psychological energy to maintain the stability of the person who is in good health.

The opposite of a healthy state, illness exists when the client's core structure becomes unstable through the effects of environmental factors that overwhelm and defeat the lines of defense and resistance. These environmental factors, whether internal or external, are called stressors in this model.

Environment

The environment is composed of internal and external forces, or stressors, that produce change or response in the client. Stressors may be helpful or harmful, strong or weak.

Stressors are also classified according to their relationship to the basic core of the client-system. Stressors that are completely outside the basic core are termed extrapersonal stressors and are either physical, such as atmospheric temperature, or sociological, such as living in either a rural or an urban setting. Interpersonal stressors arise from interactions with other human beings. Marital relationships, career expectations, and friendships are included in this group of interpersonal stressors. Those stressors that occur within the client are called intrapersonal and include involuntary physiological responses, psychological reactions, and internal thought processes.

Nursing

Identifying Stressors

The nurse's role in the Neuman model is to identify at what level or in which boundary a disruption in the client's internal stability has taken place and then to aid the client in activities that strengthen or restore the integrity of that particular boundary. The Neuman model expands the concept of client from the individual to include families, small groups, the community, or even society in general.

Nursing's main concern in this model is either to identify stressors that will disrupt a defensive boundary in the future (prevention) or to identify a stressor that has already disrupted a defensive boundary, thereby producing instability (illness).[19] The Neuman model is based on the nursing process and identifies three levels of intervention: primary, secondary, and tertiary.

Types of Intervention

A **primary intervention** has as its main goal the prevention of possible symptoms that could be caused by environmental stressors. Teaching clients about stress management, giving immunizations, or encouraging aerobic exercise to prevent heart disease are examples of primary interventions.

A **secondary intervention** is aimed at treating symptoms that have already been produced by stressors. Many of the actions that nurses perform in the hospital or clinic (e.g., giving pain medications or teaching a client with cardiac disease about the benefits of a low-sodium diet) fall into this secondary intervention category.

Tertiary care actions seek to restore the client's system to an optimal state of balance by adapting to negative environmental stressors. Teaching a client how to care for a colostomy at home after discharge from the hospital is an example of nursing activities at the tertiary level.

TRENDS FOR THE FUTURE IN NURSING THEORY

Although the search for the perfect nursing model continues, the emphasis in recent years has shifted from developing new theories to applying existing theories to nursing practice. Also, the new theorists seem to be more interested in expanding existing nursing theories by including such concepts as cultural diversity, spirituality, family, and social change rather than starting all over again from the beginning. A good example of this trend is the cultural meaning–centered theory that was published by Mendyka and Bloom.[20] This theory expands the King model by adding a cultural perspective.

> *Although the search for the perfect nursing model continues, the emphasis in recent years has shifted from developing new theories to applying existing theories to nursing practice.*

A More Recent Theory

One of the more recent of the established nursing theories is the Man-Living-Health Model proposed by Rosemary Rizzo Parse. Although her original work started in 1981, a more developed form of her theory was published in 1987.[21-23] Parse's theory stresses the elements of experience, personal **values,** and lifestyle choices in the maintenance of health.

A Matter of Choice

In this theory, the client can be any person or family who is concerned with the quality of their life situation.

The client is viewed as an open, whole being who is influenced by past and present life experiences. The ability to make free choices is essential in this theory. The client, through choices he or she makes, interacts with the environment to influence health either positively or negatively.

Health, for Parse, is an ongoing process. By making free choices, the client's health status is continually unfolding. In addition, health is determined by lived experiences, synthesis of values, and the way the client lives.[24]

Finding Meaning

The main role of nursing in the Parse model is to guide clients in finding and understanding the meaning of their lives. Once the client chooses a healthy life situation, the nurse can further increase the quality of the client's life and improve his or her health status. The ability to change the client's health-related values is an important skill for nurses to master in this model.

Parse never really defines the concept of environment in relationship to her theory. Specifically, it seems to be any health-related setting, but it can also be expanded to include past and present experiences.

New Challenges to Nursing Theory

As with any developing science, nursing will continue to change and respond to the dynamic trends of society. Older nursing models will either be replaced by new ones or modified to include developing concepts. Indeed, one of the hallmarks of a sound nursing theory or model is its flexibility and ability to adapt to new discoveries.

The increasing number of **independent nurse practitioners** and other advanced practice nurses are testing nursing theories as they have never been tested before. The theories that are flexible, realistic, and usable in practice will survive and remain as the pillars of professional nursing.[24] Those that are too theoretical or rigid will fall by the wayside and become mere footnotes in nursing texts.

One of the hallmarks of a sound nursing theory or model is its flexibility and ability to adapt to new discoveries.

Conclusion

As nursing takes its rightful place among the other helping professions, nursing theory will take on additional importance. Nursing theory and models are the systematic conceptualizations of nursing practice and how it fits into the health-care system. Nursing theories help describe, explain, predict, and control nursing activities to achieve the goals of client care. By understanding and using nursing theory, nurses will be better able to incorporate theoretical information into their practice to provide new ways of approaching nursing care and improving nursing practice.

The development of nursing theory and models indicates a maturing of the profession. As the knowledge associated with the profession increases and becomes unique, more complex, and better organized, the general body of nursing science knowledge also increases. Only when nursing has a well-developed body of specialized knowledge will it be fully recognized as a separate scientific discipline and a true profession.

Critical Thinking Exercises

rs. M, an 88-year-old woman, has been a resident of St. Martin's Village, a lifetime care community, since her husband died 8 years ago. Her health status is fair. She has adult-onset diabetes controlled by oral medication and a scar from a tumor behind her left ear that was removed surgically. The wound from this tumor removal has never healed completely, and it has continuously oozed a serous fluid requiring a dressing.

At St. Martin's Village, Mrs. M has her own apartment, which she maintains with minimal assistance, receives one hot meal each day in a common dining room, and has access to a full range of services such as a beauty shop, recreational facilities, and a chapel. She is generally happy in this setting. She has no immediate family nearby, and the cost of the facility was covered by a large, one-time gift from her now deceased husband. Recently, she has become much weaker and has had difficulty walking, attending activities including meals, and changing the dressing on her ear. The nurse at St. Martin's Village is sent to evaluate this client.

• Select two nursing models and apply their principles to this case study. Make sure you include the concepts of client, health, environment, and nursing.

References

1. Ferguson, L, Day, R: Evidence-based nursing education: Myth or reality. Nursing Education. 44(3): 107–116, 2005.
2. Algase, DL, et al.: Nursing theory across curricula. J Prof Nurs 17(5):248–255, 2002.
3. Rice, B: CIC work in year 2: Data gathering, analysis, and work force modeling. Colleagues in Caring Newsletter, October 1997, pp. 3–4.
4. Titler, MG, et al: Use of the nursing interventions classification by critical care nurses. Critical Care Nurse 16(4):38–54, 1996.
5. Felton, G, et al: How does the NLNAC support the Pew Health Commission competencies? Nursing and Health Care Perspectives 21(1):53, 2000.
6. McCloskey, JC, et al.: Nursing interventions core to specialty practice. Nurs Outlook 46(3):67–76, 1998.
7. Mitchell, PR, and Grippando, GM: Nursing Perspectives and Issues. Delmar, Albany, NY, 1993.
8. McCann-Flynn, JB, and Heffron, PB: Nursing: From Concept to Practice. Robert J. Brady, Bowie, MD, 1984.
9. Riehl-Sisca, JP: Conceptual Models for Nursing Practice. Appleton & Lange, E. Norwalk, CT, 1989.
10. Putt, A: General Systems Theory Applied to Nursing. Little, Brown, Boston, 1978.
11. Stevens, BJ: Nursing Theory: Analysis, Application, Evaluation. Little, Brown, Boston, 1984.
12. Fawcett, J: Analysis and Evaluation of Conceptual Models of Nursing. FA Davis, Philadelphia, 1989.
13. Roy, C, and Andrews, HA: The Roy Adaptation Model: The Definitive Statement. Appleton & Lange, E. Norwalk, CT, 1991.
14. Orem, DE: Nursing: Concepts of Practice. Mosby–Year Book, St. Louis, 1991.
15. Leininger, MM (ed): Cultural Care Diversity and Universality: A Theory of Nursing. National League for Nursing, New York, 1992.
16. King, IM: King's theory of goal attainment. Nursing Science Quarterly 5:19–25, 1992.
17. Watson, J: Nursing: Human Science and Human Care: A Theory of Nursing. Appleton-Century-Crofts, E. Norwalk, CT, 1985.
18. Schaefer, KM, and Pond, JB: Levine's Conservation Model: A Framework for Nursing Practice. FA Davis, Philadelphia, 1991.
19. Neuman, B: The Neuman Systems Model. Appleton & Lange, E. Norwalk, CT, 1989.
20. Davidson, AW: Research issues. Person-environment mutual process: Studying and facilitating healthy environments from a nursing science perspective. Nursing Science Quarterly 14(2):101–108, 2001.
21. Parse, RR: Man-Living-Health: Theory of Nursing. Wiley, Philadelphia, 1987.
22. Parse, RR: The lived experience of contentment: A study of the Parse Research Method. Nursing Science Quarterly 14(4):330–338, 2001.
23. Fawcett, J: Scholarly dialogue. The nurse theorists: 21st-century update: Rosemarie Rizzo Parse. Nursing Science Quarterly 14(2):126–131, 2001.
24. Gaudine, AP: Demonstrating theory in practice: Examples of the McGill Model of Nursing. Journal of Continuing Education in Nursing 32(2):77–85, 2001.

Bibliography

Algase, DL, et al.: Nursing theory across curricula. J Prof Nurs 17(5):248–255, 2002.
Baldwin A: Wagging the dog: An analysis of year 2000 workforce and education outcomes from recommendations of the 1995 Pew Commission report. J Allied Health 30(3):160–167, 2001.
Determining cost of nursing interventions: Iowa Intervention Project. Nursing Economics 19(4):146–160, 2001.
More than one million new nurses needed by 2010. The American Nurse 34(1):5, 2002.
Narayan, MC, et al.: Searching for nursing's future? Nursing Management 33(1):26–30, 2002.
Nightingale, F: Notes on Nursing: What It Is and What It Is Not. Harrison, London, 1859 (Reprinted by JB Lippincott, Philadelphia, 1966).
Nursing shortage puts patients at risk and creates liability problems. Health Care Risk Management 23(6):61–65, 2002.
O'Connor, NA, et al.: Documenting patterns of nursing interventions using cluster analysis. J Nurs Meas 9(1):73–90, 2001.
Pontious, JM: Where have all the nurses gone? The Oklahoma Nurse 47(1):1, 18, 2002.
SREB Study Indicates Serious Shortage of Nursing Faculty. Council On Collegiate Education for Nurses, 2002.
Stafford, J. Nursing students turned away: Faculty shortage limits enrollment nationwide. The Oklahoman. August 25, 2005, 2B

5

The Process of Educating Nurses

Joseph T. Catalano

Learning Objectives

After completing this chapter, the reader will be able to:

- Compare the major differences between the diploma, associate degree nursing, and bachelor of science in nursing educational programs.

- Discuss at least three types of advanced nursing degrees.

- Distinguish between the different types of doctoral degrees available to nurses.

- Explain the concept of advanced practice for nurses.

EDUCATIONAL PATHWAYS

Unlike many other professions, nursing has several related, but unique, educational pathways that lead to licensure and professional status. Indeed, the current system of nursing education creates a great deal of confusion about nursing, not only among the public, but among nurses themselves. Perhaps the belief that "a nurse is a nurse is a nurse" developed because even though registered nurses may be prepared in educational programs that vary in length, orientation, and content, the graduates all take the same licensing examination, and, superficially, all seem to be able to provide the same level of care. The licensure examination measures knowledge at the minimal level of safe practice. The workplace has not provided pay differences to distinguish levels of education despite studies showing performance differences.

PARADIGM SHIFTING

As we progress into the twenty-first century, nursing faces many difficult challenges and extraordinary opportunities. Current and future trends in health care are being driven by a number of powerful societal forces that are producing an inevitable reshaping of health-care delivery. Traditionally somewhat insulated from the forces of change, nursing educators have been forced to recognize that graduates need to be prepared with knowledge and skills that are in tune with a rapidly evolving health-care system. The most powerful of these forces of change are:

- The movement toward a market-driven health-care economy
- The wider use of capitated managed care for financing coverage
- The increasing age and diversity of the U.S. population
- A shortage of registered nurses
- A shortage of qualified nursing faculty
- The rapid leaps forward in health-care and information technology

According to the Department of Health and Human Services, Division of Nursing, in a report on the basis of a survey conducted in 2001, slightly less than 60 percent of registered nurses remained employed in hospitals, about the same as in 1998, and down from 66 percent in 1992.[1] The remainder were employed in a wide variety of settings, including private practice, public health agencies, home health care, primary nursing school–operated nursing centers, **ambulatory care centers,** insurance and managed care companies, education, and health-care research. There is also an ever-growing group of **emerging health occupations** that have not yet been officially recognized by professional organizations.

What Do You Think?

Does an individual prepared in a technical course of study have enough knowledge to be a provider of professional nursing care in today's more complex health-care system? Do you think that the American Nurses Association (ANA) position statement on nursing education advocates a valid position? If yes, what can be done to bring nursing education into line with it?

_____

_____

_____

_____

_____

_____

_____

_____

_____

_____

_____

B o x   5 . 1

Johnson & Johnson Promotes Nursing

The "Discover Nursing" ad campaign was initiated by the Johnson & Johnson Company in response to the nursing shortage in 1999 and is still a very active campaign. The goal is to bring more people into nursing. Working with nursing leaders and other concerned health-care organizations, the ad campaign is running a series of high-quality and catchy television commercials that feature nurses, both women and men, speaking about their work, its effect on society, and the rewards of a career in nursing.

A second element of the campaign is an associated Web site (www.discovernursing.com). The site has several sections that include answers to the question of "Why Nursing?"; details about the nursing market, benefits, and salaries; and nursing specialties. Under the "How?" section of the site, there is information concerning nursing basics, a nursing program search with links to nursing programs across the country, a scholarship search program, and information about additional funds for nursing education.

The site also has profiles of nurses who share their stories of why they became nurses and elements of their careers that they find most rewarding.

Johnson & Johnson initially committed $25 million to this campaign for the television ads, maintenance of the Web site, and scholarship money for nursing students. Additional money has been added since that time. The campaign is an excellent example of how private industry, with the encouragement of the nursing profession, can work with nurses to benefit the health-care system.

The Pew Report

The Pew Health Professions Commission Report, sometimes referred to as the Pew Report, was a major study of health care and nursing education that also reinforces the belief that there is a need for reform in nursing education.[2,3] Its 21 recommendations for all schools preparing health-care professionals are comprehensive and include:

- Expanding the scientific basis of the programs
- Promoting interdisciplinary education
- Developing cultural sensitivity
- Establishing new alliances with managed care companies and government
- Increasing the use of computer technology and interactive software

The Pew Report also recommended a differentiated practice structure to simplify and consolidate the titles that are used for the different practitioner levels so that there is just one title for each level.

As more and more health care shifts to ambulatory and community-based settings, nursing educators need to re-evaluate whether the graduates of their programs are adequately prepared to meet the demands of these areas of care and whether their own educational and skill preparation is sufficient.

> *Perhaps the belief that "a nurse is a nurse is a nurse is a nurse" developed because even though registered nurses may be prepared in educational programs that vary in length, orientation, and content, the graduates all take the same licensing examination, and, superficially, all seem to be able to provide the same level of care.*

NURSES OF THE FUTURE

Nurses of the future will need to practice with self-reliance, independence, and flexibility. They will be required to have well-developed decision-making skills on the basis of critical thinking ability, a working knowledge of community resources, and computer and technical competencies. Just as important,

they will need to deliver high-quality client education and care while working within the constraints of a managed care system with tight cost control measures.

Will nursing education ever be able to prepare a graduate who fulfills all the qualities required of nurses of the future? Nursing education responds with a "yes," but only with curricular changes that provide graduates with the tools to continue to learn as they advance in their careers.

Hospital Skills and More

Hospital-based acute care nursing practice will always have an important place in any health-care system. Highly skilled acute care nurses will always find a place to practice. It is generally accepted that the older population requires more health care of all types—acute, chronic, and community based. Although the current system experienced a decrease in the use of acute care beds, a gradual reverse in this trend is beginning as the "baby boomers" become the senior citizens who require more care for acute problems.

Paradigm shifting in nursing education does not need to be an either/or proposition. It is sometimes felt that nursing education is either acute care focused or it is community focused. Nursing education needs to combine the two so that the graduate can practice with competence in either or both settings. The skills are similar, but the emphasis may be different. Although some hospital skills are being done by non-nurses at a cheaper cost, nursing education must still teach such important skills as critical thinking, therapeutic relationship, **primary care** and **case management,** as well as how to be comfortable with a consumer-driven health-care system.

Critical Thinking

Critical thinking has been an important element in nursing practice for many years. It is generally recognized as the ability to use basic core knowledge and decision-making skills in deciding and resolving situations with a relatively small amount of data and a high degree of risk and ambiguity. Although it has not always been called critical thinking, nursing has long been concerned with the ability to make good judgments and decisions about client care. (See Chapter 6 for a fuller discussion of critical thinking.)

Issues Now

Ten Health-Care Trends to Watch

Nursing students and nurse educators need to remain in tune with the unprecedented transformations that are and will be taking place in health-care delivery and professional nursing. These trends have a number of driving forces, including technological advancements, financial restructuring, shifts in social structure, and consumer demands.

Ten Trends That Will Affect Health Care

1. Changing demographics and increasing cultural diversity. Increasing numbers of minority groups as well as an aging population are trends that will have a major effect on health care for many years to come. It is projected that by the year 2020, more than 20 percent of the population will be 65 and older, with those older than 85 constituting the most rapidly increasing segment of the population. Other projections indicate that by the year 2050, the white population of the United States will no longer be the majority.

2. Explosion of technology. Telehealth, telemedicine, nanotechnology, electronic medical records, and health-oriented Internet databases all are a common part of today's health-care system that were unheard of even a few years ago. Nurses of the twenty-first century will not only need the basic computer skills that many children currently master by the time they reach high school, but will also need to have a high degree of technological sophistication.

3. Economic and social globalization. Although globalization may seem to many nurses to be an abstract concept concerning events that happen "out there," events such as those of 9/11 have a way of bringing the reality home in a very dramatic way. Information technology and communications, international travel and commerce, multinational corporations, and political changes everywhere all contribute to the trend to globalization.

4. Better-educated consumers, the Genome Project, alternative health-care practices, and palliative care. Clients in today's health-care system are consumers who want to actively participate planning the care they are to receive. Through the Internet, clients now have access to information that was formerly available only to health-care practitioners. A better-educated consumer is more likely to be interested in health promotion and maintenance, resulting in a greater interest in alternative health-care practices.

Only recently have new settings for and types of care—such as hospice, pain management, support groups, bereavement counseling, and spiritual practices—been advocated as valid parts of total client care. Nurses need to not only understand and feel comfortable when providing care to clients who use these settings, but be prepared for an active role in the provision of care.

5. Increasingly complex health care and shift to population-based care. Although more and more health care is being provided outside the traditional hospital setting, clients who are admitted to hospitals are much more seriously ill than in the

(continued)

Issues Now continued

past. Currently, there is a ratio of one critical care or specialty unit care bed to each general care bed in hospitals across the country. This means that fully half of the clients admitted to the hospital are in need of high-level, complex health care such as is provided in critical care units.

6. Managed health care and out-of-control health-care costs. Over the past decade, managed care has become a reality of life. Despite the promise of flexible financing, prevention of illness, and promotion of health when it first started, managed care still remains an illness-based, fee-for-service system with all the problems associated with that process.

Health-care costs now approach 15 percent of the gross national product (GNP). More than 40 million Americans have no health insurance. Cost concerns will continue to influence almost every aspect of nursing practice, from staffing, work assignments, and use of unlicensed personnel to increased out-of-pocket cost of health-care services and medications not covered by insurance.

7. Governmental health-care regulations and policies. Complex and sometimes contradictory health-care regulations from both the federal and state levels add to the confusion found in nursing practice. It is imperative that nurses belong to their professional nursing organizations and participate actively in political activities to move the health-care system in a direction that is more nurse and client friendly.

8. Collaborative practice. Health care has been a team effort for many years. As the health-care system becomes more complex in the future, and clients have increasingly more complex health-care problems, the need for collaborative practice will only increase.

9. Nursing shortage. Over the years, there have been cycles of nursing shortages coupled with nursing surpluses; however, current projections are for a very severe nursing shortage that will peak somewhere around 2020. Despite the problems produced by the shortage, there are opportunities too. There has already been an upward trend in salaries, and many facilities are offering more flexibility in working hours. Nurses are also finding new opportunities for advancement, interesting work settings, increased demand for advanced practice nurses (APNs), and careers in case management.

10. Advances in nursing research. One of the key characteristics of a profession is the development of a unique body of knowledge through research. The growing body of research provides a scientific basis for client care practices. As nursing research advances in the future, client outcomes will improve, the health of communities will be promoted, and the most vulnerable of the population will be protected.

Sources: Lindeman, CA: The future of nursing. Nursing Education 39(1):5–12, 2000.
Heller, BR, et al: 10 Trends to watch. Nursing and Health Care Perspectives 21(1):9–14, 2001.

At a fundamental level, the nursing process is a type of critical thinking. Unfortunately, in the health-care system of the future, a nurse's critical thinking skills will have to go far beyond those of the basic nursing process. Nursing education will need to prepare students for more advanced critical thinking by exposing them to real-life situations that require the use of creativity, intuition, analysis, and deductive and inductive reasoning. These situations are introduced in the classroom as case studies and are reinforced in the clinical setting through guided experiences and mentoring.

> *Nursing education will need to prepare students for more advanced critical thinking by exposing them to real-life situations that require the use of creativity, intuition, analysis, and deductive and inductive reasoning.*

The Therapeutic Relationship

Trust Is Essential

Therapeutic relationship skills have been long stressed by mental health nursing faculty as a key element in the treatment of psychiatric problems. In reality, therapeutic relationship skills are essential for all nurses to fulfill their roles as health-care providers and healers. Although these skills are currently being taught in a limited and focused way in most schools of nursing, they need to be expanded to involve directed services and relationship-centered nursing care.

Relationship-centered nursing care is client focused and revolves around the client's trust in, value of, and understanding of the nurse's skills and role in the healing process. The client must be able to feel comfortable with the nurse and share his or her understanding of both illness and health.

Follow-up Care

Currently, in many licensed practical nurse/licensed vocational nurse (LPN/LVN) programs and schools offering the associate degree in nursing,

clinical experiences consist of one-time, 8-hour provision of care for an acute or chronically ill client. Little time is spent in follow-up care. However, many bachelor of nursing science (BSN) programs and some associate degree nursing (ADN) programs have expanded clinical experiences to include **discharge planning** and follow-up home health care experiences.

To meet the demands of the future health-care system, all nursing education programs must be able to develop learning experiences for students that involve care for selected individuals or families over extended periods of time, perhaps ranging from several weeks to several semesters.

Case Management

A New Entity

Care management is a general term that refers to a method of coordinating care either with an individual client or on a system-wide basis. **Case management,** a new entity in a health-care system driven by the demand for cost-effective care, usually is associated with coordinating care for an individual client as he or she moves from one level to another through the health-care system. Case management is now a certified specialty. Almost all the proposals for revisions in the health-care system include the **case manager** as an important element in the overall management of care.

Currently, case managers do not have to be registered nurses. Many individuals with degrees in social work and human resources as well as registered nurses are serving in the capacity of case managers. Perhaps the ideal situation would be to function as a **health-care team,** with both a registered nurse and a social worker coordinating all aspects of the client's care.

A Wide Range of Skills

As case managers, nurses are responsible for developing **clinical pathways** and for directing and guiding the overall health care of a specific group of clients. Case management includes not only overseeing the clients' care while they are in the hospital but also following clients through their rehabilitation at home, long-term follow-up, health-care practices, and developmental stages.

The knowledge and thinking required by an effective case manager go far beyond what is currently required of new graduates. Nurses must be able to understand not only the immediate disease process but also the long-term outcomes and factors that influence the disease. Case managers must also practice health-focused nursing and primary levels of intervention. Decisions will need to be made about care from a broad **database** as well as an understanding of the client's abilities, knowledge level, and even financial status.

Nursing education will be severely challenged to provide experiences to prepare students for this role. Students must be allowed to experience the authority, accountability, and responsibility of guiding a client's health care over an extended period. It might be beneficial to combine the learning experiences mentioned earlier in establishing the therapeutic relationship with the managed care experience.

The Consumer in Authority

A consumer-driven health-care system is at one and the same time the nurse's dream and nightmare. Many widely used nursing models or theories claim to be client centered, which translates into being consumer driven. Yet, when these models are put into practice, the care given is more provider driven than anything else.

Care as Requested

A client/consumer-driven health-care system means that the care given is defined by the consumer and the outcomes are also determined by the consumer. The nurse must be able to accept the authority of the group or community as a determinant of health care. The nurse's role becomes one of a partner in guiding, implementing, and overseeing ways to deliver requested health care for a given community.

> *A consumer-driven health-care system is at one and the same time the nurse's dream and nightmare.*

Many nursing programs, particularly baccalaureate programs, include a course in community health and home-health-care nursing. A requirement of these courses is often to have the students per-

form a community survey in which they determine the needs of the community as they perceive them. Many of these courses have been modified so that the students learn from the community members what they perceive to be their own needs.

Paradigm shifting is never easy. Major paradigm shifts in thinking and acting are even more difficult. Nursing education is currently dealing with a huge paradigm shift. How educators are meeting these challenges will, to a large extent, shape the future of professional nursing.

ANA POSITION PAPER ON EDUCATION FOR NURSES

A Historical Perspective

After evaluating the changes that occurred in the health-care system during the 1950s and studying the projected educational needs for nurses, the American Nurses Association (ANA) published a paper in 1965 that took a stand on an issue that was, and still is, highly controversial. Although written almost 40 years ago, this document is still relevant to many of the issues in nursing education today.

For full appreciation of the significance of this paper, it must be examined from a historical perspective. The overall purpose of the ANA has always been to ensure high-quality nursing care to the public by fostering high standards of nursing practice. In addition, the ANA was concerned with furthering the professional and educational advancement of nurses as well as protecting the occupational welfare of nurses. To achieve these goals, the ANA took responsibility for establishing the scope of practice for nurses and for guaranteeing the competence of those who claim the title of nurse.

After World War II, there was an explosion of scientific and technological knowledge that was used in health care. The educational level of the population was also increasing, resulting in greater public demand for higher-quality health care. In re-evaluating the nature and scope of nursing practice, and the type and level of quality of education needed to meet these new demands, the ANA reached the conclusions that are presented in its position paper.

Support for the Bachelor's Degree

Since 1965, the ANA has upheld the belief that baccalaureate education should be the basic level of preparation for professional nurses. Specifically, the ANA concluded that:

> The education for all those who are licensed to practice nursing should take place in institutions of higher education; minimum preparation for beginning professional nursing practice at the present time should be the baccalaureate degree education in nursing; minimum preparation for beginning technical nursing practice at the present time should be associate degree education; education for assistants in the health care service occupations should be short, intensive pre-service programs in vocational education institutions rather than on the job training.[4]

There were several assumptions on which the ANA based this position paper:

- Nursing is a helping profession and, as such, provides services that contribute to people's health and well-being.
- Nursing is of vital significance to the individual receiving services; it meets needs that cannot be met by the client, the family, or other persons in the community.
- The demand for the services of nurses will continue to increase.
- The professional practitioner is responsible for the nature and quality of all nursing care that clients receive.
- The services of professional practitioners of nursing will continue to be supplemented and complemented by the services of nurse practitioners who will be licensed.
- Education for those in the health-care professions must increase in depth and breadth as scientific knowledge expands.
- The health care of the public, in the amount and to the extent needed and demanded, requires the services of large numbers of health occupation workers, in addition to those licensed as nurses, to function as assistants to nurses. These workers are presently designated nurses' aides, orderlies, assistants, and attendants.
- The professional association must concern itself with the nature of nursing practice, the methods for improving nursing practice, and standards for membership in the professional association.[4]

Specialization and Interdependence

The rationale for taking such a strong stand on the future of nursing education derived from recognition by the profession of its heritage, its immediate problems, emerging social issues and trends, the nature of nursing practice, and the extent to which nurses could realistically enact changes for continued professional progress. The ANA drew on Florence Nightingale's vision of nursing and nursing education, which emphasized the value of education for the development of the profession. It was important to Nightingale that schools of nursing be independent of hospitals and have a strong theoretical component on which to base clinical practice.

By recognizing the increasing complexity of society, the ANA realized that nursing was not only becoming more specialized but was also moving toward greater interdependence with other groups in society. One of these key groups was the U.S. federal government. As the government began increasing aid for nursing education, educational facilities expanded, providing greater opportunities for professional advancement. Larger numbers of students with more varied backgrounds were recruited into the profession, requiring greater flexibility in nursing education programs to accommodate their needs.

Schools of nursing were, at the same time, also hard pressed to meet the attendant demands of science and technology that were changing the traditional role of nurses. In addition to expanding roles for nurses, greater consumer awareness and expectations were placing new demands on nurses' abilities.

Even in 1965, the ANA recognized that nurses were required to master a very large and extremely complex body of knowledge. In addition, nurses were being increasingly called upon to make critical and independent decisions about client care.

Effects of the ANA Paper

The implications of this paper were far-reaching and highly controversial. The ANA paper affected many different elements of society and the health-care industry.

A changing role for hospitals. Hospitals recognized that they would no longer retain their traditional role of preparing nurses for practice. Even though pressure to move nursing education from hospital-based diploma schools to institutions of higher education had been building for some time, in the mid-1960s,

75 percent of the graduating nurses were from hospital-based diploma programs.[5]

Colleges under pressure. Colleges and universities were hard pressed to quickly develop undergraduate and graduate curricula for increasing numbers of nursing majors. The relatively few baccalaureate programs in existence at the time were generally small and found it difficult to expand rapidly. It also became evident that a clear distinction between technical and professional programs needed to be made.

The Debate Continues

To this day, the ANA remains firmly committed to its stand that all nursing education should be housed in institutions of higher learning. Over 40 years have elapsed since this statement was made, and the profession of nursing is still trying to reach a consensus on the issue of basic educational preparation for entry into practice.

An examination of the current entry into practice debate from an educational perspective reveals a number of similarities in the social and political pressures felt by nursing in 1965. Not only do these same challenges exist in today's health-care system, but many new challenges have developed because of fast-paced technology developments and social changes.

Defining a Profession

A similar resolution defining entry into practice was proposed by the ANA in 1985, but it also met strong opposition and was never enacted. In 1996, the American Association of Colleges of Nursing (AACN) presented its own position paper emphasizing the belief that the baccalaureate degree should be the minimal requirement for entry into the nursing profession. The discussion remains ongoing with seemingly little hope for resolution. The most influential reasons these proposals have not been adopted are economic, not conceptual. Although some experts believe it is time to leave the old debate behind and work toward developing a better-educated profession in general, many others see the issue as important to the definition of nursing as a profession.

Continuing discussion and efforts to bring about collaborative agreement on nursing education is a goal that the profession must work toward. Only after the issue of basic entry-level education for professional nursing is resolved, and when nurses, like all other professionals, obtain their knowledge from recognized schools of higher education, will nursing as a profession be able to resolve its other important problems. Advancement of clinical practice, preparation for advanced practice roles, and an increased body of nursing knowledge all depend on baccalaureate entry-level education for professional nurses.

> *Continuing discussion and efforts to bring about collaborative agreement on nursing education is a goal that the profession must work toward.*

DIPLOMA SCHOOLS

No Academic Degree

The Nightingale School of Nursing was a diploma school in the strict use of the term. When nurses graduated from this school they were given a certificate or diploma noting their graduation, but no academic degree. The first graduates from the Nightingale School soon began to establish their own schools of nursing based on the Nightingale model and adhered to her philosophy of nursing education. These were also diploma schools.

An Improvement in Care

After an initial period of uncertainty and trepidation, both physicians and hospital administrators began to recognize that when the education of nurses improved, so too did the overall quality of the care provided by their hospitals. They also understood that these types of schools that were closely associated with hospitals could provide a source of free, or inexpensive, labor in the form of nursing students.

Diploma schools sprang up throughout Europe so that, in time, each hospital had its own school of nursing. Many of Nightingale's principles and concerns about nursing education were abandoned during this period of growth.

Catching up to Europe

In the United States, developments in nursing education, as with health care in general, lagged behind those in Europe. It was not until the mid-1870s that the first school of nursing was established in the United States. This was a diploma school attached to the New England Hospital for Women.[6]

As in Europe, the idea of diploma schools quickly caught on, and within 10 years almost every large hospital in the United States had its own diploma school of nursing. These schools had very little in common with the Nightingale School of Nursing. There was no uniformity in curriculum, length of program, or requirements. To guarantee adequate enrollment, candidates were again being recruited from the lowest levels of society.

Learning on The Job

A Source of Cheap Labor

In early hospital-based diploma schools of nursing, hospitals used the student nurses as a major source of free labor for their facilities. There was little or no classroom or theoretical study. The students learned exclusively by hands-on experience during their 12- to 14-hour, 7-days-a-week work shifts.

Most of the students were young, single women recruited just after they graduated from high school. They were confined to dormitories on the hospital property. The dormitories were monitored closely by a housemother who enforced the rigorous rules of behavior covering all aspects of the students' lives and dismissed students for even minor infractions of the rules. The early diploma schools of nursing were organized and administered on a model that was similar to the strictest of the religious orders.

> *In early hospital-based diploma schools of nursing, hospitals used the student nurses as a major source of free labor for their facilities. There was little or no classroom or theoretical study.*

Submission to Authority

The nurses who graduated from these schools were proficient in basic nursing skills and could assume positions in the hospital where they were trained or in home nursing, where they worked on a case-by-case basis without any additional orientation or education. Because of the 24-hour-a-day, 7-day-a-week socialization process administered by these schools, diploma graduate nurses tended to be very submissive to authority and willing to carry out any duty to please the physician, administrator, or head nurse. Before the advent of licensure examinations and standardization of practice, nurses from diploma schools were often limited to employment in their own training institutions or in home-health-care settings.

A Move Toward Accreditation

Diploma schools of nursing remained relatively unchanged in the United States until 1949, when the National Nursing Accrediting Service, working under the guidance of the National League for Nursing Education, became the licensing body for all schools of nursing that voluntarily sought accreditation. The first formal accreditation of nursing schools occurred in the early 1950s. In 1952, the National League for Nursing (NLN) assumed accrediting responsibilities for all schools of nursing.[7] Accreditation by the National League for Nursing Accrediting Commission (NLNAC) has always been and remains a voluntary undertaking.

Outcome Criteria

To be accredited by the NLN, schools of nursing had to meet specific outcome criteria and teach specific content in their curricula. Many of the diploma schools of nursing could not or would not comply with these criteria and eventually closed. Some of the requirements for the schools that did choose to comply with the NLN included:

- Implementing a 3-year course of study meeting the criteria established by the state board of nursing using only faculty with baccalaureate or higher degrees in nursing
- Developing a unique philosophy and demonstrating how that philosophy was implemented through learning objectives, course objectives, and outcome criteria
- Showing an adequate pass rate on the State Board or National Council Licensure Examination (NCLEX)

A Jump in Expense

One of the key factors that all state boards of nursing were concerned about was that the school be able to demonstrate that the students were not being used as unpaid hospital personnel while they were in their education and training programs. When students could no longer be used as free labor, diploma nursing schools went from being virtually free to the hospital to being very expensive.

Not only did the hospitals still have to pay for the room and board of the students, but they also now had to hire and pay additional staff because the students could no longer be included in the overall staff numbers. Even more diploma schools closed because of the financial burdens to the hospitals. The

schools that stayed open began increasing their tuition rates to the point that they were as expensive as programs granting academic degrees.

CONVERTING THE CURRICULUM

During the 1960s and 1970s, many diploma schools became associated with universities and converted their curricula into degree-granting programs. According to the 2001–2002 statistics published by the NLN, there are only 115 accredited diploma programs still functioning. They are of universally high quality and meet all the standards necessary for NLN accreditation. The main emphasis remains preparing nurses who are highly competent in technical nursing skills through extensive hands-on practice in the clinical setting, but elements of leadership, humanities, and general sciences are also included in the classroom setting.[8]

ASSOCIATE DEGREE NURSING

The **associate degree nursing (ADN) program** was developed by Mildred Montague as a short-term solution to the nursing shortage experienced after World War II.[9] Originally designed to prepare students for technical nursing practice, the 2-year ADN programs were offered through community colleges with an emphasis on developing the skills necessary to provide high-quality bedside care in less time than BSN programs.

Technical Orientation

A successful pilot program for ADNs was conducted by Montague at Teachers' College in Columbia University in New York City in 1952 to prepare technical nurses who could assist professional nurses. It demonstrated that community college–based programs could attract large numbers of students, prove cost effective, and produce skillful technical nurses in half the time required for BSN programs.[10]

Which exam to take? Early on, there was some heated debate concerning licensure and titling for this group of nurses. The technical orientation of the curriculum was, and is, very similar to that found in programs that prepare LPNs, but the location of the programs in the community college setting and the increased theoretical orientation seemed to elevate these programs to a higher educational plane. It was finally decided that the ADN graduates should take the registered nurse (RN) licensure examination rather than the LPN/LVN examination.

A Proven Track Record

The emphasis on technical skills of the ADN programs met a need in the health-care system of the 1960s and 1970s. By the early 1980s, there were more than 800 ADN programs across the United States; as of 2002, the number was close to 900, with more than 63,000 students attending.[11] Graduates from these programs soon exceeded the number of graduates from all the BSN and LPN/LVN programs combined.

Although it is possible to complete the requirements for an ADN in 2 academic years, most programs take at least 3 years to complete for a new student who has no prior college credit.[11] ADN graduates have a proven track record for providing safe bedside care for clients from the first day they are hired. They function well as team members and, after a period of orientation, can assume responsibility for the care of clients who are more acutely ill.

BACCALAUREATE EDUCATION

A Slow Increase

The development of schools of nursing in the university and college setting was a gradual process that extended over several decades. Only a few collegiate nursing programs were established during the years when the diploma programs were expanding. Some of these early collegiate programs were a hybrid mixture of college-level classes and diploma school clinical experiences that still granted only a diploma rather than an academic degree.

Early attempts at college-level nursing programs sometimes took the form of "pre-nursing" courses over a 1- or 2-year period that prepared students to enter upper division schools of nursing. Generally acclaimed as the first university program to be completely conducted in the higher education setting, the University of Minnesota School of Nursing was opened in 1909. In 1923, the Yale School of Nursing began accepting students; it is considered the first autonomous college of nursing in the United States.

The number of university-based nursing programs gradually increased over the years, and by the beginning of World War II there were 76 programs granting baccalaureate degrees in nursing.

These programs tended to specialize in preparing nurses for public health nursing, teaching, administration, and supervisory positions in hospitals. Although all these programs included a clinical component, the emphasis was more on theoretical knowledge, development of decision-making skills, and leadership.

Universities in general enjoyed rapid growth immediately after World War II, and higher-education nursing programs expanded along with the universities. Many military nurses, prepared by the Cadet Nurse Corps during World War II, went back to school under the G. I. Bill to complete their baccalaureate degrees.

Training for a Profession

During this rapid growth period, these **baccalaureate degree nursing programs** were plagued with problems similar to those found in the diploma programs during their own rapid expansion period. Primarily, the lack of uniformity in content, curriculum, and even length of programs was problematic. It was difficult to find qualified faculty because most of the nurses up to this time had received their education in diploma programs. No doctorate degrees existed in nursing, few nurses had master's degrees, and only a smattering of nurses had baccalaureate degrees.

During the late 1940s and early 1950s, awareness began to develop that there was a need to stratify nursing education programs into technical levels and professional levels. It became apparent that all health-care professionals should have, at minimum, a baccalaureate degree.[12]

> *During the late 1940s and early 1950s, awareness began to develop that there was a need to stratify nursing education programs into technical levels and professional levels. It became apparent that all health-care professionals should have, at minimum, a baccalaureate degree.*

The NLN began to develop strict criteria for the accreditation of baccalaureate nursing programs. These criteria included courses in general education, general sciences, humanities, and language as well as specific nursing courses. They required a certain number of hours to be spent in the clinical setting practicing nursing skills, a faculty prepared at the master's degree level, and the availability of laboratory and library facilities for the students. Faculty-to-student ratios were limited, particularly in the clinical setting, and outcome criteria were required for the students.[13]

Different Approaches
Although all university-level baccalaureate degrees in nursing have the same number of required credit hours and educational requirements for baccalaureate degrees, there are three avenues for attaining this degree.

The professional degree. The BSN degree fulfills the criteria of a professional degree. It meets the overall requirements for a college baccalaureate degree (124 credit hours, 65 hours of nursing major, and most of the general education requirements), but does not meet all the general education requirements for an academic bachelor of science (BS) degree. Although this degree is usually obtained in a traditional college setting, it can also be obtained through an **external degree** program where the student has to meet the criteria for the BSN.

The full academic degree. The second approach is found in programs that offer a bachelor of science degree with a major in nursing (BS Nursing). This degree is the full academic college degree and guarantees that the person holding it has met all of the general education, science, and major subject requirements. According to statistics published by the NLN for academic year 2001–2002, there were more than 530 accredited programs offering baccalaureate degrees in nursing.

A third avenue that may be pursued is sometimes called the career ladder program (see section on ladder programs in this chapter).

PRACTICAL/VOCATIONAL NURSING

The practical/vocational nurse, in one form or another, has been a part of the health-care system in the United States for more than 100 years. Although the earliest formal schools of practical/vocational nursing were started around 1890, informal training programs for this level of nursing probably existed well before that time—for example, in the Young Women's Christian Association (YWCA), particularly in New York City.

A Useful Trade
These programs took uneducated girls who had migrated from rural areas and farms to the cities in search of employment and taught them a useful trade with which they could support themselves. With no regulation or accreditation for the early practical/vocational nurse programs, there were wide variations in the quality, length, and focus of what was being taught. Generally, the students were taught to provide home care, similar to that given by private duty nurses, for clients ranging from newborns to the elderly and invalids.

The number of **practical/vocational nursing programs** gradually increased over the next 50 years. Graduates of these 3-month programs were beginning to find employment in hospitals and nursing homes as well as in areas of private duty. During the nurse shortage after World War I, many hospitals found that these relatively undereducated nurses, after receiving on-the-job training in the hospital, could function at a fairly high level of skill, and at a much reduced cost. The word got around, and soon the number of these unlicensed nurses grew.

Compulsory Licensure

By the late 1930s, the ANA saw the need to regulate the quality of the practical/vocational nursing programs to protect public safety. It was not until 1938 that the state of New York took seriously the ANA's recommendation for compulsory licensure for practical/vocational nurses and enacted the first law requiring such licensure.

In 1960, all practical/vocational nurses were required to pass a licensure examination before they could practice. These nurses are now referred to as licensed practical nurses (LPNs). In Texas and California, these nurses are called licensed vocational nurses (LVNs).

The Importance of Technique

Although education for LPNs and LVNs varies slightly from one state to another, there are some common characteristics. Most of the programs are from 9 to 12 months and are measured in clock hours rather than academic hours. They are often offered in hospitals, high schools, vocational schools, or trade schools, although some programs are conducted in community colleges or even in universities.

Orientation of the curricula in these programs is highly technical and emphasizes the learning of skills in the setting of a hospital or nursing home with less emphasis on theoretical knowledge. Because they are **technicians,** it is much more important for practical/vocational nurses to learn how to do something than why it is being done.

> *The practical/vocational nurse, in one form or another, has been a part of the health-care system in the United States for more than 100 years.*

Filling a Shortage

The stated scope of practice for the practical/vocational nurse involves providing care for clients in hospitals,

nursing homes, or the home setting for those who have stable conditions. LPNs/LVNs are to be under the supervision of an RN or a licensed physician.

However, in the real world, LPNs/LVNs are often required to provide care well outside of their scope of practice, often functioning in leadership roles or providing care in acute settings with highly unstable clients. LPNs/LVNs are often hired when there are shortages of RNs to fill the gaps in client care.

Many associate degree RN programs have developed a ladder curriculum whereby an LPN/LVN can go back to school for a shorter period, often receiving credit for years of experience, complete the program in 1 year, and then take the RN licensure examination.

LADDER PROGRAMS

Upward Mobility

Career ladder, educational ladder, **articulation,** or educational mobility programs have become increasingly popular as a result of an interest in **upward mobility,** educational articulation, and **career mobility.** A ladder program allows nurses to upgrade their education and move from one educational level to another with relative ease by granting credit for previous course work and experience and without loss of credits from previous education.

Each ladder program is developed according to the philosophy of the particular nursing school, may use any one of a number of curricular patterns, uses one of several means of **advanced placement** or credit granted for previous education, and must meet NLNAC accreditation standards.

Ladder programs take several different forms. Some ladder programs provide a **competency-based education** that allows the students to proceed at their own pace as long as they fulfill required educational outcomes. Ladder programs have become increasingly popular as colleges move toward Web-based courses and programs.

The Associate Ladder

The LPN/LVN-to-ADN ladder allows individuals who have been licensed as LPNs/LVNs to take a minimal number of courses in an associate degree program to obtain their ADN and then take the NCLEX-RN, CAT to become licensed as registered nurses. Programs vary widely as to how many credits they will accept from the LPN/LVN programs and how many courses the students take to complete the degree. Some of the requirements for number of hours are out of the control of the nursing programs, because they have been established as general education requirements of the college or are state regents requirements. These programs are highly compatible because of the similarity of curricula and the technical orientation of both types of programs.

The Baccalaureate Ladder

There are also LPN/LVN-to-BSN ladder programs that either allow licensed LPNs/ LVNs to challenge a number of courses or grant them credit for nursing courses based on previous experience and demonstrated competency. Students who enter these types of ladder programs usually spend more time in school than those in the LPN/LVN-to-ADN programs. In addition to meeting the requirements of the BSN, they also have to meet the general education requirements for a baccalaureate degree and complete 124 hours of college-level courses. One problem in developing these types of ladder programs is that many states' boards of regents do not recognize courses taken at the vocational-technical level as higher education courses and therefore will not transfer them into the college setting.

Two Plus Two

Nursing education has seen a marked increase in the number of ADN-to-BSN and diploma-to-BSN ladder programs sometimes called **two plus two (2 + 2) programs.** These programs admit individuals who are already licensed as registered nurses but who have either a diploma or associate degree.

These programs may take several different forms. Upper division baccalaureate programs work exclusively with ADN-RNs, have no generic students, and are designed exclusively to meet the educational needs of students who are already RNs.

Other programs accept ADN or diploma graduates as students, in addition to generic students. These schools often have separate programs for ADNs or diploma RNs that allow them to take examinations to prove educational knowledge and nursing proficiency **(challenge examinations)** in specific classes, thus granting credit for their nursing experience. The RNs then take advanced-level nursing

courses such as Community Health/Home Health Care, Leadership, and Critical Care, which are not commonly found in diploma or ADN programs.

In either case, on completion of the degree requirements, these nurses are granted a baccalaureate degree. Some of these programs have an **open curriculum** that allows students to enter and leave the program freely. There are 418 such programs accredited by the NLNAC.[11]

The Master's Ladder

For the ADN

A growing trend in educational ladder programs is the ADN-to-MSN programs. Schools that offer this type of ladder must have an MSN program in place. The ADN students who enter these programs are given credit for prior classes and work experience and take both undergraduate and graduate level courses, receiving a BSN along the way to obtaining the MSN.

These programs vary a great deal from school to school and may require from three to five semesters of classes. Often they are offered on a part-time basis, with many evening and weekend classes or Web-based classes to meet the needs of working students.

For the Nurse Practitioner

Another type of educational ladder program that is less common is the nurse practitioner (NP)-to-MSN program. These programs admit nurse practitioners who graduated from programs that allowed the student to become certified but did not include enough credit hours for a master's degree. Again, the students are granted credit for past classes and work experience and often are allowed to challenge a certain number of core courses. Then they take the remaining required courses and are granted an MSN at graduation.

MASTER'S- AND DOCTORAL-LEVEL EDUCATION

The baccalaureate degree is considered a generalist degree that exposes a student to a wide range of subjects during the 4 years spent in college. The master's degree, on the other hand, is a specialist's degree.[14] Students who pursue a master's degree concentrate their study in one particular subject area and become expert in that given area.

Master's Degree Programs

Master's degree nursing programs have been in existence almost from the time baccalaureate-level nursing programs were started. These early master's degree in nursing programs were designed for students who had baccalaureate degrees in other majors, such as biology, and wanted to become nurses. After completion of an additional 36 to 42 credit hours in nursing courses only, these students were awarded the MSN, and could then take the licensure examination for registered nurses.

Experience Required

Today, most master's degrees in nursing programs are restricted to registered nurses who have the baccalaureate degree. Many of these programs require at least 1 year of clinical practice after the BSN and require an additional 36 to 46 college credit hours. Most students who enter master's degree programs attend classes on a part-time basis while they are working and may take up to 5 years to complete the requirements. Many universities have recognized this trend and have tailored their programs to meet the needs of these part-time students; universities now offer courses over the Internet, by distance education in the evening, on weekends, or 1-day-a-week programs. There are 296 accredited master's degree programs in the United States.[11]

There are a number of available areas of study for those pursuing master's degrees in nursing. Some of the more popular areas include nursing administration, community health, psychiatric mental health, adult health, maternal–child health, gerontology, rehabilitation care, nursing education, and some more advanced areas of practice, such as anesthesiology, pediatric nurse practitioner (PNP), family nurse practitioner, geriatric nurse practitioner (GNP), and obstetrical–gynecological nurse practitioner.[15] Most of these programs require the student to pass a comprehensive written or oral examination, and some courses require the student to write an extensive research thesis before graduation.

Professional and Academic Degrees

There are two basic types of master's degrees in nursing. The master's of science in nursing (MSN) is the professional degree, and the master's of science with a major in nursing degree (MS Nursing) is the formal academic degree.[16] In practice, however, little differentiation is made between the two. Almost all master's programs accredited by the NLNAC require the applicant to have at least a 3.0 grade point average (GPA) and to demonstrate academic proficiency by achieving a satisfactory score on the Graduate Record Examination (GRE) or the Miller's Analogy Test before admission. The GRE is also used to recommend remedial coursework needed to correct deficiencies before the master's program is undertaken.

> *In the evolution of the various levels of education, the baccalaureate degree is a generalist's degree, the master's degree is a specialist's degree, and the doctoral degree is a generalist's degree, although at a much higher academic level than the baccalaureate degree.*

What Do You Think?

Have you ever been to an advanced practice nurse for care? How would you rate the quality of that care? If you have not been to an advanced practice nurse, would you consider going to one for care? Why or why not?

Doctoral Programs

In the evolution of the various levels of education, the baccalaureate degree is a generalist's degree, the master's degree is a specialist's degree, and the doctoral degree is a generalist's degree, although at a much higher academic level than the baccalaureate degree. The major purpose of early doctoral degrees was to prepare the individual to conduct advanced research in a particular area of interest.

A Wide Range of Choices

Currently there is a wide range of available doctoral degrees for nurses. The doctor of philosophy (PhD) degree is the most accepted academic degree and is designed to prepare individuals to conduct research. The doctor of education (EdD) degree is considered to be a professional degree, although in many programs there is little difference between the courses of study taken by the EdD and PhD candidates. In other programs, the PhD focuses primarily on research, whereas the EdD focuses more on administration in the educational setting. The classes and research credits differ somewhat between the two degrees.

Since the 1970s, other doctoral programs for nurses have been developed that stress the clinical rather than the academic nature of nursing.[17] These include the doctor of nursing science (DNSc) and the doctor of science in nursing (DSN), which is a clinically oriented nursing degree. The doctor of nursing (DN or ND) degree is for the person with a BS or MS in a field other than nursing who wants to pursue nursing as a career. It is a generalist's degree at a basic level of education.

In recent years, there has been some discussion of making these degrees the basic entry degree into the profession of nursing. An additional degree for nurses who wish to pursue a career in higher education, the doctor of nursing education (DNEd) degree, is available.

Few Programs, Tough Requirements

Despite the wide range of doctoral degrees in nursing, there are relatively few programs across the United States that offer these degrees. Many nurses who seek them may obtain them in fields such as higher education, psychology, college teaching, and adult education. Fewer than 2 percent of nurses hold doctoral degrees.

The requirements for all doctoral education degrees are similar, even though the specific degrees being sought may be different. The student must have attained a master's degree and must have achieved a satisfactory score on the GRE. Often there is an admission interview and preprogram examination that must be passed before the candidate can be formally admitted to the program. Doctoral programs are at least 60 college credit hours in length, require many statistics and research courses, and often have a residency requirement. Before the doctoral degree can be granted, the student must successfully complete both oral and written comprehensive examinations, as well as write a doctoral dissertation explaining the conduct of a major research project.

Some individuals pursuing doctoral degrees do so on a part-time basis while they are working full-time, whereas others attend classes full-time while working full-time, often completing the program in 3 to 4 years. Many programs require that the individual complete all the requirements within a 10-year time period. Although this may seem like a long time, it is not unusual for the dissertation process itself to take 2 to 3 years.

Leaders in the Profession

Nurses with master's or doctoral degrees are regarded as leaders in the profession of nursing. Many of the larger hospitals in the United States require their unit managers and supervisors to have master's degrees and their directors of nursing or vice presidents of nursing to have doctorates. Of course, in baccalaureate programs, the minimal requirement for teaching is the master's degree, and the doctorate is preferred. Nurses with these advanced degrees provide direction and leadership for the profession through their publications, research, and theory development. As health-care delivery becomes more complicated, larger numbers of nurses with advanced degrees will be required.

EDUCATION FOR ADVANCED PRACTICE

Advanced practice is one of those often misused terms in nursing that add to the public's confusion about educational levels of those in the profession. It is sometimes referred to as **expanded role** or **expanded practice.** Nurses who obtain certification are allowed to practice at a higher and more independent level depending on the nurse practice act of their individual state. Advanced practitioners diagnose illnesses, prescribe medications, conduct physical examinations, and refer clients to specialists for more intensive follow-up care. These nurses practice nursing under their own licenses as **independent practitioners** but often work closely with a physician so they can quickly refer clients who have medical problems that lie outside their scope of practice.

The Nurse Practitioner

The nurse practitioner levels of nursing are most widely accepted as advanced practice areas for nursing. These include the pediatric nurse practitioner (PNP), the neonatal nurse practitioner (NNP), the geriatric nurse practitioner (GNP), the obstetrics-gynecology (OB-GYN) nurse practitioner, the family nurse practitioner (FNP), the rehabilitation nurse practitioner (RNP), the psychiatric nurse practitioner, and the nurse midwife.

The certified registered nurse anesthetist (CRNA) and nurse midwife are the oldest of the advanced practice specialties for nurses and are already well accepted in the medical community. Other advanced practice nurses experience varying levels of acceptance from physicians, although the public in general likes the care they receive from advanced practice nurses. All states now have granted some type of **prescriptive authority** to nurse practitioners.

In the past, nurses with baccalaureate degrees (or even associate degrees in California as late as the 1990s) could attend highly concentrated courses of study for 1 to 2 years and become increasingly proficient in a particular specialty area without obtaining an MSN. They could then take the certification examination and become certified as nurse practitioners. Currently, most nurse practitioner programs are offered in major universities, requiring students to complete the master's degree before allowing them to take the certification examination.

The Clinical Nurse Specialist

One level of nursing that falls under the umbrella of advanced practice is the **nurse specialist,** or **clinical nurse specialist** (CNS). Although relatively few schools offer specific clinical nurse specialists curricula, these nurses are self-classified as clinical nurse specialists after completing a master's degree, or some additional education, in a particular clinical area. However, in a few states, such as Ohio, the clinical nurse specialist designation requires a master's degree and a special licensing examination. CNSs are usually hired by hospitals and often function as in-service educators for the hospital.

The Scope of Advanced Practice

In 1988, an amendment to the New York Nurse Practice Act established a separate scope of practice and title protection for nurse practitioners (NPs).

Subsequent to the NP amendment, there has been some confusion regarding which of the advanced nursing practice categories are included within the scope of practice, particularly clinical nurse specialists, nurse midwives, and certified nurse anesthetists. This confusion, especially in psychiatric mental health nursing and nurse anesthesia, is related to the legal interpretations of the NP amendment. The resultant debate about this issue has led to a clearer definition and understanding of the term *advanced practice nurse.*

The career opportunities for advanced practice nurses are numerous.[18] Many nurse practitioners work for county health departments, rural clinics, and on Native-American reservations; others work in hospitals, with physicians in private practice, and in rehabilitation centers. Some have even established their own independent clinics. They provide primary health-care services in areas where there is a lack of primary care physicians. Although many of these areas are traditionally rural, today inner-city areas also often need this type of health care.

In addition, a common element of several proposed national health-care plans is the requirement that a client seeking entry into the health-care system be evaluated by a primary health-care practitioner before referral to any specialized health-care practitioner. Although the family practice physician, or general practitioner, is the most common primary health-care provider to evaluate the client, the nurse practitioner can also function in this role. If any of these proposed health-care plans are adopted on a national level, the demand for nurse practitioners will increase tremendously.

Conclusion

In today's rapidly changing health-care environment, there is an ever-increasing need for health-care professionals who are educated to practice at the highest levels.[1] It is imperative that the schools that will be educating future nurses be responsive to the changes, challenges, and demands of an ever more sophisticated and technologically advanced health-care system. Nursing education is an important part of a much larger network of health-care systems, including the service and practice sector, government and regulatory agencies, and licensing and credentialing institutions. All of these interact with each other and together form what is called the health-care system.

The nursing profession has, over the years, developed a number of different types of education programs in an attempt to meet the demands of a growing health-care system. Some of the programs that were developed for specific needs that no longer exist should be examined for their usefulness and viability in today's advanced health-care atmosphere. Perhaps their resources could be rechanneled to programs that are more in tune with current needs. Students should carefully evaluate programs they might enter and decide which one best meets their care goals.

Meanwhile, nursing education continues to develop innovative approaches to help nurses meet the demands for more education, more technical skills, and more leadership ability. The ladder programs are a good example. By recognizing the dynamic state of nursing education, and implementing changes that respond to or even anticipate changes in the health-care system, the nursing profession will continue as one of the pillars of the health-care system.

Educators in nursing have begun to recognize that it is impossible to teach nursing students everything they need to know in the short time allowed for formal education. The demands of the changing health-care system will make that goal even more difficult. However, it may not be necessary to teach nursing students everything. It is more important to teach these students the thinking, decision-making, and management skills that will allow them to adjust to an ever-changing and developing health-care system.

Issues Now

What Nursing School Graduates Need to Know and Be Able to Do

It has always been a challenge for nursing educators to decide what needs to be taught to and learned by nursing students before they graduate. Some of the curricular content is dictated by the licensure examination, but high-quality nursing programs recognize that this test knowledge is the minimum required for safe practice at an entry level. The health-care marketplace demands more than the minimum. In this regard, the consumers of the products of nursing education, that is, the health care entities that hire nursing school graduates, have had an important if somewhat unstructured role in determining curricular content.

In an attempt to provide more structure to the input from the facilities, a study was conducted that asked administrators who worked at hospitals, home-health-care agencies and nursing homes to rank 45 skills or knowledge-based competencies they expected to see in the baccalaureate-level nursing school–graduate nurses they hired. The results showed a mix of skills and knowledge competencies that were most sought after. Those that ranked the highest included:

• Teaching clients health promotion and prevention
• Teaching clients about how life style affects health
• Effective supervision of less educated staff
• Effective delegation and monitoring of staff
• Efficient organization of routine daily tasks
• Safe administration of medications
• Competence in the use of computer databases and charting
• Ability to organize nursing care for 6 to 10 clients at the same time

Overall, the expectations for new graduates appear to be clustered around the ability to initiate and adapt to change, use critical thinking in problem solving, attain a basic level of skills, and be able to communicate with both clients and staff. It is interesting to note that the basic competencies have not changed much since Nightingale organized her first nursing school. Like her students, current students still need to master basic skills and learn to communicate effectively.

However, health care technology has advanced so rapidly in recent years that it has put a strain on both the faculty teaching nursing students and students attempting to master it. One advantage this study had over past studies that generally focused on hospital-based nursing practice was that it included home-based agencies and extended care facilities.

Sources: Utley-Smith, Q: 5 competencies needed by new baccalaureate graduates. Nursing Education Perspectives 25(4):166–170, 2004.
Manojlovich, M: Predictors of professional practice behaviors in hospital settings. Nursing Research 54(1):41–47, 2005.
Katz, T, et al.: Essential qualifications for nursing students. Nursing Outlook 52(6):277–289, 2004.

Critical Thinking Exercises

- Discuss why the current educational system for nurses leads to confusion over the role and scope of practice for nurses.
- The literature reports that there will be a nursing shortage well into the twenty-first century. What aspects of health-care reform are likely to produce changes in nursing education? Identify possible changes that may occur in nursing education because of the projected nursing shortage. Will these changes be beneficial or harmful to the profession of nursing?
- What historical factors had an important influence on the development of nursing education as it is currently conducted in the United States?
- What should the minimum level of education be for the professional nurse—ADN, BSN, or MSN? Defend your position.

References

1. Freeman, LH, et al.: New curriculum for a new century. Nursing Education 41(1):38–40, 2002.
2. Bellack, JP, and O'Neil, EH: Recreating nursing practice for a new century: Recommendations and implications of the Pew Health Professions Commission's Final Report. Nursing and Health Care Perspectives 21(1):14–21, 2002.
3. de Tornyay, R: Critical challenges for nurse educators. J Nurs Educ 35(4):146–147, 1996.
4. American Nurses Association: Position Paper on Education. ANA, Kansas City, MO, 1965.
5. Fitzpatrick, ML: Prologue to Professionalism. Robert J. Brady, Bowie, MD, 1983.
6. Jamieson, EM, et al.: Trends in Nursing History. WB Saunders, Philadelphia, 1968.
7. Hegner, BR, and Caldwell, E: Nursing Assistant: A Nursing Process Approach, ed. 6. Delmar Publishers, Albany, NY, 1995.
8. National League for Nursing: Trends in Education, 2002. Available at: www.nln.org.
9. Ketefian, S: Moving beyond traditional boundaries. J Prof Nurs 9:25–31, 1993.
10. Calhoun, J: The Nightingale pledge: A commitment that survives the passage of time. Nursing & Health Care 14:130–136, 1993.
11. National League for Nursing: Statistics on Education, 2002. Available at: www.nln.org.
12. Manthey, M: Continuing the case for the baccalaureate. J Prof Nurs 18(1):7, 2002.
13. Felton, G, et al.: How does NLNAC support the Pew Health Commission Competencies? Nursing and Health Care Perspectives 21(1):53, 2000.
14. Forni, PR: Nursing's diverse master's programs: The state of the art. Nursing & Health Care 8:770–775, 1987.
15. Lipman, TH, and Deatrick, JA: Enhancing specialist preparation for the next century. J Nurs Educ 33:53–58, 1994.
16. Kalisch, PA, and Kalisch, BJ: The Advance of American Nursing, ed. 3. JB Lippincott, Philadelphia, 1995.
17. American Association of Colleges of Nursing: Indicators of quality in doctoral programs in nursing. J Prof Nurs 3:72–74, 1987.
18. Lynch, MP, et al.: Advanced practice issues: Results of the ONS Advanced Practice Nursing Survey. Oncol Nurs Forum, 28(10):1521–1530, 2001.

Bibliography

Bosher, S: Linguistic bias in multiple-choice nursing exams. Nursing Education Perspectives 24(1):15–34, 2003.

Brady, M, et al.: A proposed framework for differentiating the 21 Pew competencies by level of nursing education. Nursing and Health Care Perspectives 22(1):30–35, 2002.

Callister, S, et al.: Inquiry in baccalaureate nursing education: Fostering evidence-based practice. Nursing Educator 44(2):59–65, 2005.

Emerson, R, and Records, K: Nursing profession in peril. J Prof Nurs, 21(1):5–9, 2005.

Katz, T, et al.: Essential qualifications for nursing students. Nursing Outlook 52(6):277–289, 2004.

Ferguson, L, and Day, R: Evidence-based nursing education: Myth or reality? Nursing Education 44(3):107–116, 2005.

Fondiller, SH: The advancement of baccalaureate and graduate nursing education 1952–1972. Nursing and Health Care Perspectives 21(1):10–13, 2002.

Freeman, LH, et al.: New curriculum for a new century. Nursing Education 41(1):38–40, 2002.

Hoffman, L, et al.: Outcomes of care managed by an acute care nurse practitioner vs attending physician team in a subacute medical intensive care unit. Am J Crit Care 14(2):121–130, 2005.

Jeffries, P: Technology trends in nursing education: Next steps. Nursing Education 44(1):3–5, 2005.

Long, K: Preparing nurses for the 21st century: Re-envisioning nursing education and practice. J Prof Nurs 20(2):1–4, 2004.

Manojlovich, M: Predictors of professional practice behaviors in hospital settings. Nursing Research 54(1):41–47, 2005.

Medley, C, and Home, C: Using simulation technology for undergraduate nursing education. Nursing Education (44):131–135, 2005.

Miller, J, et al.: A study of personal digital assistants to enhance undergraduate clinical nursing education. Nursing Education 44(1):19–27, 2005.

Rosenstein, A, and O'Daniel, M: Disruptive behavior & clinical outcomes. Nursing Management 36(1):18–28 2005.

Stewart, S, and Dempsey, L: A longitudinal study of baccalaureate nursing student's critical thinking dispositions. Nursing Education 44(2):81–85 2005.

Study looks at impact of nurses' education level. Am Nurse 35(6):5–6, 2005.

6

Critical Thinking

Joseph T. Catalano

Learning Objectives

After completing this chapter, the reader will be able to:

- Demonstrate logical, rational, and creative critical thinking.
- Describe the steps of the critical thinking process in resolving a client care issue.
- Apply critical thinking to client care.
- List five characteristics of critical thinking.

A DECISION PROCESS

The Art of Thinking

One of the most important responsibilities that nurses have is to make correct and safe decisions in a variety of client care situations. The decisions made by nurses affect the health status, recovery time, and even the survival or death of a client. For example, the critical care nurse must decide when to give certain medications on the basis of changes in the client's condition. The emergency room nurse must decide which clients to treat first based on the extent of their injuries. The hospital staff nurse must decide what PRN medication to give for which set of symptoms. The home health nurse must decide when to call the physician about a change in a client's condition.

The process by which these decisions are made involves the use of critical thinking. Critical thinking is based on reason and reflection, knowledge, and instinct derived from experience. It has also been defined as "the art of thinking about thinking." It is both an attitude about and an approach to solving problems. Critical thinking helps nurses make decisions about problems for which there are no simple solutions. Often nurses have to make these decisions with less than complete information.

Can We Define It?

Although critical thinking has always been used by nurses to some degree and is recognized as important in the provision of care, its status increased greatly when the National League for Nursing Accrediting Commission (NLNAC) designated critical thinking as one of its mandatory outcome objectives in 1992. It was removed as an outcome criterion in 1999 but remains an element that nursing schools must demonstrate as an essential part of the curriculum. Schools of nursing have been challenged to demonstrate where and how they teach and measure critical thinking in the curriculum. It is fairly easy to claim, "Yes, we teach our students how to think critically," but much more difficult to accurately define what critical thinking is and then demonstrate that the graduates of the program have attained and can use the skill.

A definition is a short statement that identifies and distinguishes something from all other things so that it can be recognized. Generally, things that are easy to define have one or a few definitions. Things that are more difficult to define tend to have many definitions that may or may not overlap. Critical thinking falls into the latter category. At least 10 primary definitions for critical thinking have been developed over the years by various experts on the subject. Perhaps a better approach to recognizing and developing critical thinking is to look at the characteristics that seem to be common to most of the definitions.

> *Creative thinkers are able to bring together bits of knowledge or information that may initially seem unrelated and formulate them into a plan that leads to effective decision making and solves the problem by finding connections between the thoughts and concepts.*

CHARACTERISTICS OF CRITICAL THINKING

Critical Thinking Is Creative

Nurses who think creatively explore new ideas and alternative ways of solving client care problems. Creative thinkers are able to bring together bits of knowledge or information that may initially seem unrelated and formulate them into a plan that leads to effective decision making and solves the problem by finding connections between the thoughts and concepts. This process is similar to the linear approach used in the nursing process. All the situational variables must be considered, and decision making becomes more complex as the number of variables increases.

Example of Creative Thinking

In a small hospital, a policy was instituted that required all postcesarean delivery clients to be monitored in the recovery room just like all other postoperative clients.

Because the operating room (OR) nurses were on call for the recovery room, they thought that they were being required to do more work with no additional staff. The circulating and scrub obstetric (OB) nurses could go home after the delivery. The OR nurses became very resentful of the extra call for the postdelivery clients and often called in sick the day after they were required to attend a postcesarean client. This practice left the OR short staffed during the day and led to increased tension and frequent unfriendly confrontations between the OR and the OB nurses.

The nurse managers of the OB and OR units resolved the problem by instituting a policy of "cross-training" with the OR and OB nurses. OB nurses were taught how to monitor the recovery of postoperative clients and were rotated through recovery for 1 week every 2 months to keep these skills current. The OR nurses were taught how to assist at cesarean deliveries and were rotated through the OB unit for 1 week every 2 months. This system kept the staffing levels constant and allowed the OB nurses to assist with the postcesarean delivery clients. As often happens with these types of decisions, not everyone was happy with the change, but it did reduce the resentment levels between the two units and gave the nurses a better appreciation of the other nurses' responsibilities.

What Do You Think?

Identify two situations that you have been involved with that required critical thinking. How did you resolve these situations? What elements of critical thinking did you use?

_____

_____

_____

_____

_____

_____

_____

_____

_____

_____

_____

_____

Critical Thinking Is Logical, Rational, and Reflective

Although the critical thinking process is often expanded beyond fundamental logical thinking, it must always be based on rationales and facts rather than emotions or egocentric impulses. Intuition can play a part in critical thinking when it is recognized as a rational thought process that brings together and processes a number of factors at the subconscious level rather than a simple "gut feeling."

If at all possible, critical thinkers must take the time to collect as much data as they can and examine them under the light of reason before making a decision or taking an action. Decisions must at times be made on a limited amount of information in situations where there is a high degree of risk and ambiguity. In these situations, the nurse's past experiences resolving similar situations as well as intuition can help. However, in most cases, merely jumping to conclusions often produces poor decisions and negative results. Logical reasoning is often divided into deductive and inductive reasoning.

Example of Deductive Reasoning

Deductive logic or reasoning is a process whereby the individual proceeds from the general to the particular. The conclusions reached by deductive reasoning based on a valid argument are certain and true:

Either John Smith or George Jones is to be given a dose of IV penicillin before surgery.

There was no order for IV penicillin for John Smith before surgery.

Therefore, George Jones is to be given IV penicillin before surgery.

The conclusion is valid. The rationale is that all of the information in the conclusion is found in the premises; therefore, the conclusion must logically follow if the premises are true.

Example of Inductive Reasoning

Inductive logic or reasoning involves proceeding from the particular to the general. The conclusions reached by inductive reasoning are probable or contingent. Inductive reasoning is more frequently used in health-care situations than deductive reasoning because of the wide range of variables involved in client care that almost always introduce a degree of uncertainty.

Mr. Jones has bacterial lobar pneumonia.

Antibiotics are usually used to treat this disease.

Therefore, Mr. Jones should probably be given an antibiotic.

The conclusion is valid. The rationale is that the conclusion is uncertain because the use of the word "usually" in the premise leaves room for alternative conclusions. For example, what if the cause of the lobar pneumonia was a viral infection? Then antibiotics would not be an appropriate treatment for the condition.

Errors in Reasoning

Keep in mind that all critical thinking, including both inductive and deductive reasoning, is open to fallacies. A fallacy is generally defined as an error in reasoning that leads to a conclusion that does not follow from its premises.[1] Some arguments are valid, sound, or cogent, whereas others are false, illogical, and invalid.

The Non Sequitur

The most common type of fallacy seen in nursing is the non sequitur, a fallacy in which the conclusion does not follow from the arguments or premise. For example, a 72-year-old male client who had a colon resection and colostomy 12 days ago and who is being prepared for discharge expresses fear about returning to his one-room apartment in the inner city. He also has a heart murmur. On these two factors alone, a nursing diagnosis of "severe dependency needs" is formulated.

Another common example of this fallacy is often seen when there are staffing shortages. It is not unusual for nursing supervisors to say to a staff nurse, "We need you to work this extra shift because everyone else called in. I know you take classes in the evening, but the clients always come first. Therefore, if you don't work, you might as well start looking for employment elsewhere." This situation also adds the element of irrelevant appeal to force.

How Fallacies Happen

People commit fallacies for various reasons. In some cases, individuals have such a strong ideological commitment to a religious, economic, or political belief that they refuse to listen to any ideas or opinions that contradict what they believe. Basically, their minds are closed to any alternative conclusions; thus, they stick to their own conclusions regardless of the reasoning process. Some individuals have difficulty acknowledging that they have made a mistake and will refuse to see the lack of logic in their reasoning and conclusions. Still others must "win" at all costs and will subvert the critical thinking process and logic by abuse, twisting the other person's words, and using personal attacks. Being able to recognize conclusions that are valid or invalid is an important part of critical thinking.

Practice Critical Thinking

For practice, analyze each of the following arguments, decide whether they are inductive or deductive, note whether they are valid or invalid, and give a rationale for the decision.

1. The largest city in a country is usually the capital of the country.
   New York City is the largest city in the United States.
   Therefore, New York City is the capital of the United States.
   Type of reasoning: _____
   Conclusion valid? Yes No
   Rationale: _____
   _____
   _____

2. All nurses are women.
   Pat is a nurse.
   Therefore, Pat is a woman.
   Type of reasoning: _____
   Conclusion valid? Yes No
   Rationale: _____
   _____
   _____

3. Nora is a premature infant who weighs 1 pound.
   Nora has two congenital abnormalities: myelomeningocele and ventricular septal defect.
   Premature infants with congenital abnormalities usually die within 2 weeks of birth.
   Therefore, Nora will die within the next 2 weeks.
   Type of reasoning: _____
   Conclusion valid? Yes No
   Rationale: _____
   _____
   _____

4. In prison, criminals perform hard labor.
   Tom is a prisoner performing hard labor.
   Therefore, Tom is a criminal.
   Type of reasoning: _____
   Conclusion valid? Yes No
   Rationale: _____
   _____
   _____

5. 96% of nurses are women.
   Terry is a nurse.
   Therefore, Terry is probably a woman.
   Type of reasoning: _____
   Conclusion valid? Yes No
   Rationale: _____
   _____
   _____

6. Mary is staggering around the room.
   Mary was just at a cocktail party.
   Therefore, Mary drank too much alcohol.
   Type of reasoning: _____
   Conclusion valid? Yes No
   Rationale: _____
   _____

7. Almost every identified carcinogen causes cancer in animals.

   Humans are animals.

   Therefore, almost every identified carcinogen causes cancer in humans.

   Type of reasoning: _____

   Conclusion valid? Yes No

   Rationale: _____

   _____

   _____

8. Bill owns a fishing boat.

   The bodies of Bill's dead wife and baby were found in the water.

   Therefore, Bill killed his wife and baby.

   Type of reasoning: _____

   Conclusion valid? Yes No

   Rationale: _____

   _____

   _____

9. Ada, Betty, and Clara are the staff nurse, the head nurse, and the supervisor (but not necessarily in that order).

   Ada was beaten by the head nurse in a bridge game.

   Betty is the supervisor's neighbor.

   Betty is unbeatable at bridge when playing the other two nurses.

   Clara wants to become a head nurse or supervisor.

   a. Who is the head nurse?

   b. Who is the supervisor?

   c. Who is the staff nurse?

   Type of reasoning: _____

   Rationale: _____

   _____

   _____

10. Smith, Jones, and Brown are a surgeon, a scrub nurse, and an OR tech (but not necessarily in that order).

    The OR tech, who is an only child, earns the least amount of money.

    Brown, who married Smith's sister, earns more than the scrub nurse.

    Who is the surgeon?

    Who is the scrub nurse?

    Who is the scrub tech?

    Type of reasoning: _____

    Rationale: _____

    _____

    _____

> *People commit fallacies for various reasons. In some cases, individuals have such a strong ideological commitment to a religious, economic, or political belief that they refuse to listen to any ideas or opinions that contradict what they believe.*

Keep in mind that these exercises are simplified examples of inductive and deductive reasoning and are presented as an introduction to logical reasoning. However, using simple reasoning processes alone in client care decisions can lead to serious fallacies and error in judgment. All the other characteristics of critical thinking discussed here must be included for sound clinical decision making.

Critical Thinking Is Independent

Nurses who think critically are not easily influenced by others with strong opinions. They demonstrate their autonomy by thinking for themselves and not passively succumbing to peer pressure or the belief system of the majority.

Example of Independent Thinking

An 82-year-old woman was brought into the emergency room (ER) by her family with complaints of "difficulty urinating." During the initial assessment, the RN noted that the client had 2+ pitting edema of her ankles and feet, congested lung sounds, and shortness of breath. The ER physician ordered a urinary catheter to be inserted, urinalysis, and a consultation with a urologist for the urinary complaint. The RN pointed out the client's history of congestive heart failure (CHF) and current symptoms and also the fact that only 10 mL of urine was obtained when the catheter was inserted. The ER physician insisted that the problem was urinary and refused to discuss the client's condition any more.

While waiting for the urinalysis results, the client became increasingly short of breath and restless. The RN called for a chest x-ray and measurement of arterial blood gases (ABG). The chest x-ray showed that 75 percent of the client's lung fields though the client had not requested it. The newly hired nurse felt uncomfortable making the call and refused on the grounds that it was a violation of client **confidentiality.** The experienced nurse became angry at the refusal and berated the new nurse with the statement, "We've been notifying the families of our clients for years and you're not going to change that practice."

The next day, the newly hired nurse had a conference with the OB unit nurse manager. The nurse manager decided that a series of in-service presentations on the right to privacy, and the code of ethics and requirements of the Health Insurance Portability and Accountability Act (HIPPA), should be attended by all members of the unit.[3]

> " *To use effective critical thinking, biases and stereotypes must be identified and eliminated.* "

were filled with fluid, and the ABGs showed respiratory acidosis with hypoxia. The nurse asked the physician to order furosemide (Lasix) for the client on the basis of these findings. The physician became angry, accused the nurse of practicing medicine, and refused to write the order. The nurse then called the client's attending physician, who decided to admit the client to the hospital and begin treatment with IV furosemide for the obvious CHF.

Critical Thinking Challenges Custom

A healthy, constructive questioning of long-used health-care practices prevents the nurse from mindlessly providing rote care. Improvement and advances in health-care practices occur only when nurses understand the rationale behind the practices, and then accept or reject them based on evidence that they either do or do not work as intended.[2]

Example of Challenging Custom

A newly hired nurse was beginning her first shift on the obstetric (OB) unit when a 28-year-old client in her sixth month of pregnancy was admitted with abdominal cramps and vaginal bleeding. A spontaneous abortion was suspected. Another nurse who had worked on the OB unit for 10 years knew the client and her family. She told the newly hired nurse to call the client's sister (her number was on the chart), even

Critical Thinking Is Free of Bias and Prejudice

Biases are unjustified personal opinions. When a bias, as well as **stereotype,** is taken as fact, it becomes a prejudice. A belief is not necessarily true just because it has been in existence for a long period of time or because many people believe it. To use effective critical thinking, biases and stereotypes must be identified and eliminated.

Analyzing and viewing a situation from all points of view before arriving at a conclusion prevents the nurse from making one-sided decisions. It also helps identify bias or prejudice on the part of physicians, nurses, and even clients and the backlash effect that it may produce on other decision makers.

Recognition of bias does not always eliminate it, but it helps the decision-maker compensate for it when making the final decision.

Example of Bias- and Prejudice-Free Thinking

A homosexual, HIV-positive client with full-blown symptoms of AIDS is admitted to a medical/surgical unit for care. The nurse assigned to care for the client has very strong religious beliefs about homosexuality. She believes that her obligation as a nurse requires her to care for this client despite his diagnosis and sexual preference, yet she also believes that caring for this client would tacitly condone his sexual preferences and lifestyle. She tries to place herself in the client's situation and recognizes that an ill client deserves high-quality care without consideration of his beliefs or background.

Critical Thinking Is Action Oriented
The goal of critical thinking in health care should always be the resolution of a problem or a method to improve client care. Critical thinking is used at all levels of the health-care system and is essential to the formulation and evaluation of policies and procedures, use of effective communication, and resolution of management and personnel conflicts.

Example of Action-Oriented Critical Thinking
A physician with a reputation for striking fear in the hearts of the nurses in the medical/surgical unit was in a particularly bad mood one day. After making his rounds, the physician loudly and publicly criticized the care that the nurses were giving to his clients and proceeded to announce numerous mistakes that the nurses had made over the past year. The unit manager took the physician aside and told him that if he was having problems with the nurses on the unit, he should follow correct channels to file complaints and not make a scene in the nurses' station where many of the clients could hear him.

The physician became even more irate and stormed out of the unit and went directly to the office of the vice president of nursing services (VPNS). He told the VPNS that he was filing an official **complaint** against the unit manager for unprofessional behavior, disrespect for a physician, and failure to follow medical orders. The VPNS told him that she would investigate the complaint and take appropriate action.

After talking with all the nurses on the medical/surgical unit and nurses on other units, as well as a number of physicians, the VPNS discovered that the physician who filed the complaint was well known for his capricious and obnoxious behavior toward nurses. He was referred to the hospital medical board, reprimanded for his behavior toward the nurses, and required to drop the complaint about the manager of the medical/surgical unit. In addition, a special meeting was called for all the physicians practicing in the hospital to discuss the problem and to better understand what was involved regarding professional behavior.

A healthy, constructive questioning of long-used health-care practices prevents the nurse from mindlessly providing rote care.

CRITICAL THINKING SKILLS

Although there are different approaches to developing critical thinking, certain concepts are common to the skill. Some individuals seem to have an innate ability to master these concepts, whereas others have difficulty with them. As with most skills, practice and repetition increase efficiency and the ability to make safe decisions in complex nursing situations where there are multiple variables that affect the client's health status.

Identify the Problem
The saying "It's hard to know when you have arrived if you don't know where you are going" applies particularly well to critical thinking. If the underlying problem has not been identified, then it is almost impossible to develop a plan to solve it. One way to identify the underlying problem is to try to restate the issue as a declarative statement. For example, a public health nurse may identify that "sexually transmitted diseases (STDs) among teenagers in our society are increasing at a rapid rate."

Gather Pertinent Data
It sometimes happens that when trying to apply critical thinking to the resolution of a problem, there is only a small amount of information that relates to the situation. On the other hand, in our information-oriented society, there may be an overabundance of data. It becomes necessary for the nurse to sort through the data, use the data that relate to the problem, and reject the data that are extraneous and perhaps misleading.

In the example of STDs in teenagers, the Internet can provide copious data, including general population statistics, racial and ethnic breakdowns, STD incidence by region, the most common STDs, treatment regimens, and even projections for the future.

Rational analysis and consideration of the data may produce a re-examination and refocusing of the problem. For example, after examining the abundance of information about teenage STD, the community health nurses may decide to focus their efforts on dealing with the problem in their community rather than the entire state.

What Do You Think?

What five values are most important to you? How do these influence the way you act? What happens when these values conflict?

_____

_____

_____

_____

_____

_____

_____

_____

_____

_____

_____

Your Values in Conext

Contextual Awareness

The Influence of Belief
Developing a contextual awareness requires primarily the use of deductive reasoning. Contextual awareness is a very broad concept that is not merely limited to values but includes everything that may affect the client, such as physical symptoms and environment. Everyone, including nurses, has feelings and beliefs about all issues. Some of these beliefs are personal; some are cultural; some are stated overtly, whereas others remain deeply rooted but hidden in the subconscious. In any case, these beliefs influence how situations are perceived and what decisions are made.

Values Clarification
To make solid decisions based on critical thinking, nurses must examine their own philosophy, beliefs, and value systems. **Values clarification** is an important element in critical thinking. At some point, preferably early in their careers, nurses should make

Box 6.1
Personal Values

Listed below are a number of values that almost everyone has. Circle the ones that are important to you, adding additional values as necessary. Then rank the values according to priority.

family	competency
education	empathy
career	flexibility
honesty	trust
good health	teamwork
respect	dependability
leisure time	punctuality
nonjudgmental	accountability
attitude	self-determination
cooperative work	independence
relationships	veracity
professional	justice
integrity	commitment

a list of all the things they consider valuable. It should also be recognized that values are not static and that values will be added or deleted or will change in priority with time.

In addition, nurses must examine their own philosophy of nursing and health care as it relates to that of the agency for which they are working. Then, they need to compare how societal values relate to their personal philosophy and that of the agency. Do societal values reflect or contradict the philosophy? How do the standards of care, the nurse practice act of the state, facility **protocols,** and even the code of ethics affect the care being provided?

Challenging Assumptions and Rituals

Does the Old Approach Really Work?
Challenging assumptions and rituals of care requires use of inductive reasoning. The nurse needs to ask whether there are any assumptions about the care provided, what they are, how they affect care, and whether any of these assumptions can be challenged.

In much the same way, rituals about care should also be identified and challenged. What are the rituals that are done routinely without much thought? Are they beneficial or can they be changed or eliminated?

The community health nurse, for example, may have the philosophy that STDs among teenagers represent a dangerous and serious threat to the health of the community. On the other hand, the community may have an underlying philosophy that teenage STD is to be expected and is one of the rites of passage that must be experienced. Where such a major difference in philosophy exists, it would be extremely difficult for the nurse to implement any action that would resolve the problem.

What Really Caused the Problem?
Some assumptions that could be challenged might revolve around the cause of the problem. An increase in STDs among teenagers may be caused by (1) a lack of sexual education in school, (2) a lack of morals in our society, or (3) an atmosphere of permissiveness and egocentrism that is projected in the media.

A nurse using critical thinking will often be able to identify more than one solution to a problem.

One health department philosophy about teenagers that may need to be challenged might be that all teenagers are rebellious, uncooperative, and promiscuous, when in reality, many teenagers work well with others, are highly productive, and have high moral standards.

Nurses also need to learn about and evaluate the value systems of those with whom they are working. Even though they may not agree with those values, it is important to recognize them and work with them when attempting to affect health. For example, when teaching a group of high-school students about STDs, it would be essential to know what their attitudes toward sex and health are. In all likelihood, these attitudes would be different from those of the nurse. An education program organized around only the nurse's belief and value system would be doomed to failure. Presenting the information from the students' viewpoint would help them better understand and perhaps be more willing to accept it.

Nurses also need to learn about and evaluate the value systems of those with whom they are working. Even though they may not agree with those values, it is important to recognize them and work with them when attempting to affect health.

Imagine and Explore Alternatives Creatively

Once the nurse has identified the problem and explored the assumptions and rituals, he or she needs to consider the possible alternatives to care delivery. However, the nurse does not need to do this alone.

This information can be obtained from a variety of sources, such as written reports, surveys, and published articles. Information may also be obtained informally from others, such as in discussions with individuals who work in the field or have dealt with a similar problem before, or via feedback from the clients who are receiving the care. No matter what the source of information, it needs to be evaluated critically for accuracy, consistency, cause and effect, and biases.[4]

A nurse using critical thinking will often be able to identify more than one solution to a problem. For example, possible solutions to the teenage STD problem may include providing condoms for all high-school students, performing tubal ligations on sexually active girls, or establishing strict nighttime curfews.

Although all these solutions may be effective, the nurse would have to evaluate the cause-and-effect relationship, value, and consequences of each of these courses of action. A nurse who is a critical thinker would consider each one of these before implementing a course of action.

CRITICAL THINKING IN DECISION MAKING

Although critical thinking is used in all aspects of decision making, it is particularly important in the nursing process. It is important to remember that although the nursing process and critical thinking are interrelated and interdependent, they are not identical.

As a way of looking at the world, critical thinking allows the nurse to consider new ideas and then evaluate those ideas in light of accepted information as well as client and personal value systems. Nurses are constantly making decisions in both their professional and personal lives. By viewing critical thinking as a purposeful mental activity in which ideas are evaluated and decisions reached, nurses will be able to make ethical, creative, rational, and independent decisions related to client care.[5]

Critical thinking, when applied to the nursing process, makes it a powerful client problem-solving tool. Critical thinking expands the usual linear nursing process into a gestalt that allows the nurse to sort through the multiple variables that are often encountered in client care. Effective use of critical thinking within the nursing process is evident when the nurse successfully applies knowledge from other disciplines in the resolution of client problems, deals with stressful environments, and creatively resolves unique nursing care problems.

> *Critical thinking, when applied to the nursing process, makes it a powerful client problem-solving tool.*

Conclusion

Nurses practicing in today's health-care system are required to master many skills. Critical thinking underlies many of these skills. By examining assumptions, beliefs, propositions, and meanings, nurses are able to make sound and valid decisions about client care. Critical thinking both underlies and expands the nursing process in the practical provision of nursing care. When students and nurses master critical thinking concepts and skills, they open their perspectives on client care. An important transformation occurs when students are taught how to think rather than what to think.

The profession of nursing is in an active state of change, continually developing new theories, redefining its practice, and adapting to changing public policy and social mandates. Nurses who use critical thinking in making nursing judgments tend to consider the client's human rights and be effective client advocates. These nurses will also be able to adapt the rules of the nursing process to meet a wide range of client needs.

Issues in Practice

Long Shifts = More Mistakes

Working Past The Limit

It would seem that any person with some common sense and the basic ability to reason logically would conclude that if nurses work longer and/or more frequent shifts, their chance for making errors in client care would increase. However, in an age when "evidence-based practice" is the buzz phrase, and nobody seems to rely much on common sense, there has to be scientific proof that there is a cause and effect relationship between the two elements.

Aiken and associates[1] demonstrated in a longitudinal study over 6 years that the death rate of postoperative clients increases when nurses' client loads exceed four surgical clients (along with increases in nurse dissatisfaction and turnover rates). In much the same way, a recent study by researchers in Pennsylvania concluded that there is a threefold increase in the incidence of errors among nurses who work for more than 12.5 hours in any given shift.

Ann Rogers, the study's lead author, in conjunction with her colleagues at the University of Pennsylvania, followed and analyzed the work habits of 393 hospital nurses over a 4-week period. The research was funded by the federal Agency for Healthcare Research and Quality and the Robert Wood Johnson Foundation, a philanthropy devoted to health issues.

The "Longest Shift" Prize

The researchers looked at data from 5317 shifts worked by the nurses they studied. The nurse who took home the "Longest Shift" prize worked a shift that lasted an amazing 23 hours and 40 minutes. During the study period, they found that over all, the nurses in the study worked shifts longer than 12.5 hours more than 40 percent of the time. Usually the overtime was not scheduled in advance and the nurses in the study worked an average of 55 minutes longer than was scheduled. One-third of the nurses worked overtime every day they worked during the four week study period.

Although there have been approximately 50 studies on the effects of long shifts and sleep deprivation among medical students and physicians, very few studies have centered on how long nursing shifts affect nurses, who compose the largest single group of health care professionals. In addition to hiring less qualified workers to fill in the gap left by the RN shortage, hospitals and other health-care facilities have been extending the lengths of nurses' shifts and having nurses working more shifts per week.

With health care's current focus on understanding why medication errors occur and how to prevent them, the data from the study found that the nurses in the study made 199 medical errors. The researchers also found 213 near medication errors in which nurses caught themselves before they administered the wrong medication. The researchers concluded that all the nurses in the study had an increased probability of making at least one medication error whenever they worked past the scheduled 12-hour limit.

(continued)

Issues in Practice <small>continued</small>

The researchers also concluded that there should be limited use of 12-hour shifts and that overtime associated with 12-hour shifts be eliminated completely. Similarly, the Institute of Medicine, an independent organization that advises the federal government on medical matters, also has recommended reducing the length of nurses' shifts, including limiting their workday to 12 hours.

Source: Reuters, CNN.Com Wednesday, July 7, 2004.

Critical Thinking Exercises

se the steps in the nursing process to provide a plan of care, including at least two nursing diagnoses, for the following client situation:

Mr. Y is 49 years old and has been complaining of chest pain starting in the center of his chest and radiating to his left arm and hand for 2 hours. He is having trouble breathing, is very pale, and has cool and moist skin. His pulse is 134 beats per minute and irregular; his blood pressure is 92/50 mm Hg, and his respiratory rate is 24 breaths per minute. He is very anxious and expresses concern about having to leave his job as an accountant because of these symptoms. He is diagnosed as having an acute anterior myocardial infarction and is admitted to the intensive care unit.

- What key assessment does the nurse need to identify as essential to this client's problem?
- What problems does this client have that a nurse can treat independently? Write nursing diagnoses for these problems.
- What can be accomplished in the nursing treatment of this client's problems (goals)?
- What type of activities can the nurse undertake to achieve the goals (intervention)?
- What does the nurse need to look for to see whether the interventions have worked (evaluation)?

References

1. Rogers, A: The working hours of hospital staff nurses and patient safety: Both errors and near errors are more likely to occur when hospital staff nurses work twelve or more hours at a stretch. Health Affiliates 23(4):202–212, 2004.
2. Allen, G, et al.: Reliability of assessment of critical thinking. J Prof Nurs 20(1):15–23, 2004.
3. Tanner, C: What have we learned about critical thinking in nursing? Nursing Education 44(2):47–49, 2005.
4. Erickson, P: Privacy measures cause headaches. The Oklahoman. April 4, 2004, 8D.
5. Stewart, S, and Dempsey, L: A longitudinal study of baccalaureate nursing students' critical thinking dispositions. Nursing Education 44(2):81–85, 2005.

Bibliography

Ali, N, et al.: Validaiton of critical thinking skills in online responses. Nursing Education 44(2):90–95, 2005.
Anderson, K: Teaching cultural competencies using an exemplar from literal journalism. Nursing Education 43(6):254–260, 2004.
Case, J, et al.: A qualitative tool for critical thinking skill development. Nurse Educator 29(4):147–152, 2004.
Daily, WM: The development of an alternative method in the assessment of critical thinking as an outcome of nursing education. J Adv Nurs 36(1):120–130, 2001.
Giddens, J, and Gloeckner, G: The relationship of critical thinking to performance on NCLEX. Nursing Education 44(2):85–90, 2005.
Martin, C: The theory of critical thinking of nursing. Nursing Education Perspectives 23(5):243–247, 2002.
Maslow, AH: Motivation and Personality. Harper & Row, New York, 1971.
Nokes, K, et al.: Does service-learning increase cultural competency, critical thinking and civil engagement? Nursing Education 44(2):65–71, 2005.
Smith, Q: 5 competencies needed by new baccalaureate graduates. Nursing Education Perspectives 25(4):166–175, 2004.
Twibeil, R, et al.: Faculty perceptions of critical thinking in student clinical experience. Nursing Education 44(2):271–281, 2005.
Winningham, ML, and Preusser, BA: Critical Thinking in Medical-Surgical Settings. Mosby, St. Louis, 2001.

2
Making the Transition to Professional

10 Ways to Take Care of Yourself

1. Know the symptoms of burnout, including chronic exhaustion, sleep changes, depression, loss of concern and empathy, feelings of anger and resentment.
2. Keep healthful, easy-to-fix meals and snacks on hand so you can re-energize yourself with good nutrition.
3. Know your limits and respect them.
4. Identify the things you have control over and tackle them. Find ways to let go of the things you can't control.
5. Learn to manage stress in healthful ways: use exercise, stretching, laughter, hobbies, and other positive strategies.
6. Every workday brings triumphs and failures. Savor the triumphs and move beyond the failures.
7. Watch your back! Back injuries are the #1 occupational hazard nurses face.
8. Look for ways to continue growing professionally and building confidence in your skills.
9. Make time for your family and loved ones. When you look back on your life, those moments will be the ones you treasure.
10. Apply to yourself the good advice you give others every day!

7

Ethics in Nursing

Joseph T. Catalano

Learning Objectives

After completing this chapter, the reader will be able to:

- Discuss and analyze the difference between law and ethics.
- Define the key terms used in ethics.
- Discuss the important ethical concepts.
- Distinguish between the two most commonly used systems of ethical decision making.
- Apply the steps in the ethical decision-making process.

A LEARNED SKILL

Nurses who practice in today's health-care system soon realize that making ethical decisions is a common part of daily nursing care. However, experience shows that in the full curricula of many schools of nursing, the teaching of ethical principles and ethical decision making gets less attention than the topics of nursing skills, pathophysiology, and nursing care plans. As health-care technology continues to advance at a rapid pace, nurses will find it more and more difficult to make sound ethical decisions. Many nurses feel the need to be better prepared to understand and deal with the complex ethical problems that keep evolving as they attempt to provide care for their clients.

Ethical decision making is a skill that can be learned. The ability to make sensible ethical decisions is based on an understanding of underlying ethical principles, ethical theories or systems, a decision-making model, and the profession's Code of Ethics. This skill, like others, involves mastery of the theoretical material and practice of the skill itself. This chapter presents the basic information required to understand ethics, the code of ethics, and ethical decision making. It also highlights some of the important bioethical issues that confront nurses in the current health-care system.

IMPORTANT DEFINITIONS

In Western cultures, the study of ethics is a specialized area of philosophy, the origins of which can be traced to ancient Greece. In fact, certain ethical principles articulated by Hippocrates still serve as the basis of many of the current debates. Like most specialized areas of study, ethics has its own language and uses terminology in precise ways. The following are some key terms that are encountered in studies of health-care ethics.

Values

Values are ideals or concepts that give meaning to the individual's life. Values are derived most commonly from societal norms, religion, and family orientation and serve as the framework for making decisions and taking action in daily life. People's values tend to change as their life situations change, as they grow older, and as they encounter situations that cause value conflicts. For example, prior to the 1950s, pregnancy outside of marriage was unacceptable, and unmarried women who were pregnant were shunned and generally separated from society. Today, it is much more accepted, and it is not uncommon to see pregnant high-school students attending classes.

> *A moral person is generally someone who responds to another person in need by providing care and who maintains a level of responsibility in all relationships.*

Values are usually not written down; however, at some time in their professional careers, it may be important for nurses to make lists of their values. This value clarification process requires that the nurse assess, evaluate, and then determine a set of personal values and prioritize them. This will help the nurse make decisions when confronted with situations in which the client's values differ from the nurse's own values.

Value conflicts that often occur in daily life can force an individual to select a higher priority value over a lower priority one. For example, a nurse who values both career and family may be forced to decide between going to work and staying home with a sick child.

> *Values are usually not written down; however, at some time in their professional careers, it may be important for nurses to make lists of their values.*

What Do You Think?

What type of value conflicts have you experienced in the past week? How did you resolve them? Were you satisfied with the resolution, or did it make you feel uncomfortable?

Morals

Morals are the fundamental standards of right and wrong that an individual learns and internalizes, usually in the early stages of childhood development. An individual's moral orientation is often based on religious beliefs, although societal influence plays an important part in this development. The word *moral* comes from the Latin word *mores,* which means customs or values.

Moral behavior is often manifested as behavior in accordance with a group's norms, customs, or traditions. A moral person is generally someone who responds to another person in need by providing care and who maintains a level of responsibility in all relationships.[1] In many situations in which moral convictions differ, it is difficult to find a rational basis for proving one side right over the other. For example, animal rights activists believe that killing animals for sport, their fur, or even food is morally wrong. Most hunters do not even think of the killing of animals as a moral issue at all.

Laws

Laws can generally be defined as rules of social conduct made by humans to protect society, and these laws are based on concerns about fairness and justice. The goals of laws are to preserve the species and promote peaceful and productive interactions between individuals and groups of individuals by preventing the actions of one citizen from infringing on the rights of another. Two important aspects of laws are that they are enforceable through some type of police force and that they should be applied equally to all persons.

Ethics

A System of Morals

Ethics are declarations of what is right or wrong and of what ought to be. Ethics are usually presented as systems of value behaviors and beliefs; they serve the purpose of governing conduct to ensure the protection of an individual's rights. Ethics exist on several levels, ranging from the individual or a small group to the society as a whole. The concept of ethics is closely associated with the concept of morals in both the development and purposes of both. In one sense, ethics can be considered a system of morals for a particular group. There are usually no systems of enforcement for those who violate ethical principles.

A **code of ethics** is a written list of a profession's values and standards of conduct. The code of ethics provides a framework for decision making for the profession and should be oriented toward the daily decisions made by members of the profession.

A Dilemma

An **ethical dilemma** is a situation that requires an individual to make a choice between two equally unfavorable alternatives. When ethical dilemmas are reduced to their elemental aspects, conflicts of one individual's rights with those of another, one individual's obligations with the rights of another, or a combination of one group's obligations and rights conflicting with those of another group usually form the basis of the dilemma.

Principles in Conflict

By the very nature of an ethical dilemma, there can be no simple correct solution, and the final decision must often be defended against those who disagree with it.

For example, a client went to surgery for a laparoscopic biopsy of an abdominal mass. After the laparoscope was inserted, the physician noted that the mass had metastasized to the liver, pancreas, and colon, and even before

the results of the tissue biopsy returned from the laboratory, the physician diagnosed metastatic cancer with a poor prognosis. When the client was returned to his room, the physician told the nurses about the diagnosis but warned them that under no circumstances were they to tell the client about the cancer.

When the client awoke, the first question that he asked the nurses was, "Do I have cancer?" This posed an ethical dilemma for the nurses. If they were to tell the client the truth, they would violate the principle of fidelity to the physician. If they lied to the client, they would violate the principle of veracity.

> *By the very nature of an ethical dilemma, there can be no simple correct solution, and the final decision must often be defended against those who disagree with it.*

KEY CONCEPTS IN ETHICS

In addition to the terminology used in the study and practice of ethics, several important principles often underlie ethical dilemmas. These principles include autonomy, justice, fidelity, beneficence, nonmaleficence, veracity, standard of best interest, and obligations.

Autonomy

Autonomy is the right of self-determination, independence, and freedom. Autonomy refers to the client's right to make health-care decisions for himself or herself, even if the health-care provider does not agree with those decisions.

Autonomy, as with most rights, is not absolute, and under certain conditions, limitations can be imposed on it. Generally these limitations occur when one individual's autonomy interferes with another individual's rights, health, or well-being. For example, a client generally can use his or her right to autonomy by refusing any or all treatments. In the case of contagious diseases, for example, tuberculosis (TB), that affect society, however, the individual can be forced by the health-care and legal systems to take medications to cure the disease. The individual can also be forced into isolation to prevent the disease from spreading. Consider the following situation:

June, who is the 28-year-old mother of two children, is brought into the emergency department after a tonic-clonic–type seizure at a shopping mall. June is known to the emergency room (ER) nurses because she has been treated several times for seizures after she did not take her antiseizure medications. She states that the medications make her feel "dopey" and tired all the time and she hates the way they make her feel.

Recently, June has started to drive one of her children and four other children to school in the neighborhood car pool 1 day a week. She also drives 62 miles one way on the interstate highway twice a week to visit her aging mother in a nursing home in a different city. The nurse who takes care of June this day in the ER knows that the state licensing laws require that an individual with uncontrolled seizures must report the fact to the Department of Motor Vehicles and is usually ineligible for a driver's license. When the nurse mentions that she is going to have to report the seizure, June begs her not to report it. She would have no means of taking her children to school or visiting her mother. She assures the nurse that she will take her medication no matter how it makes her feel.

Justice

Justice is the obligation to be fair to all people. The concept is often expanded to what is called distributive justice, which states that individuals have the right to be treated equally regardless of race, sex, marital status, medical diagnosis, social standing, economic level, or religious belief. The principle of justice underlies the first statement in the American Nurses Association (ANA) Code of Ethics for Nurses:

> The nurse provides services with respect for human dignity and the uniqueness of the client unrestricted by considerations of social or economic status, personal attributes, or the nature of health problems.[2]

What Do You Think?

Identify a situation in which a law is or may be unethical. Which system has higher authority? How do you resolve the conflict?

Distributive justice sometimes includes ideas such as equal access to health care for all. As with other rights, limits can be placed on justice when it interferes with the rights of others.

For example, a middle-aged homeless man who was diagnosed with type I, insulin-dependent diabetes mellitus demanded that

Medicaid pay for a pancreas transplant. His health record showed that he refused to follow the prescribed diabetic regimen, drank large quantities of wine, and rarely took his insulin. The transplant would cost $48,000, which is the total cost of immunizing all the children in the state for 1 year.

Fidelity

Fidelity is the obligation of an individual to be faithful to commitments made to himself or herself and to others. In health care, fidelity includes the professional's faithfulness or loyalty to agreements and responsibilities accepted as part of the practice of the profession. Fidelity is the main support for the concept of accountability, although conflicts in fidelity might arise from obligations owed to different individuals or groups.

For example, a nurse who was just finishing a very busy and tiring 12-hour shift may experience a conflict of fidelity when she is asked by a supervisor to work an additional shift because of the hospital's being short-staffed. The nurse has to weigh her fidelity to herself against fidelity to the employing institution and against the fidelity to the profession and clients to do the best job possible, particularly if she felt that her fatigue would interfere with the performance of those obligations.

> *Fidelity is the main support for the concept of accountability, although conflicts in fidelity might arise from obligations owed to different individuals or groups.*

Beneficence

Beneficence, one of the oldest requirements for health-care providers, views the primary goal of health care as doing good for clients under their care. In general, the term *good* includes more than providing technically competent care for clients. Good care requires that the health-care provider take a holistic approach to the client, including the client's beliefs, feelings, and wishes as well as those of the client's family and significant others. The difficulty in implementing the principle of beneficence is in determining what exactly is good for another and who can best make the decision about this good.

Consider the case of the man involved in an automobile accident who ran into a metal fence pole. The pole passed through his abdomen. Even after 6 hours of surgery, the surgeon was unable to repair all the damage. The man was not expected to live for more than 12 hours. When the man came back from surgery, he had a nasogastric tube inserted, so the physician ordered that the client should have nothing by mouth (NPO) to prevent depletion of electrolytes.

Although the man was somewhat confused when he awoke postoperatively, he begged the nurse for a drink of water. He had a fever of 105.7 F. The nurse believed the physician's orders to be absolute; thus she repeatedly refused the client water. He began to yell loudly that he needed a drink of water, but the nurse still refused his requests. At one point, the nurse caught the man attempting to drink water from the icepacks that were being used to lower his fever. This continued for the full 8-hour shift until the man died.

Nonmaleficence

Nonmaleficence is the requirement that health-care providers do no harm to their clients, either intentionally or unintentionally. In a sense, it is the opposite side of the concept of beneficence, and it is difficult to speak of one term without referring to the other. In current health-care practice, the principle of nonmaleficence is often violated in the short term to produce a greater good in the long-term treatment of the client. For example, a client may undergo painful and debilitating surgery to remove a cancerous growth to prolong his life.

By extension, the principle of nonmaleficence also requires that health-care providers protect from harm those who cannot protect themselves. This protection from harm is particularly evident in groups such as children, the mentally incompetent, the unconscious, and those who are too weak or debilitated to protect themselves. In fact, very strict regulations have developed around situations involving child abuse and the health-care provider's obligation to report suspected child abuse. (This issue is discussed in more detail in Chapter 8.)

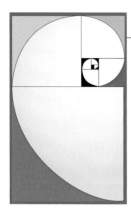

Issues in Practice

A Question of Distributive Justice

Jessica B was diagnosed with acute lymphocytic leukemia at age 4. She is now 7 years old and has been treated with chemotherapy for the past 3 years with varying degrees of success. She is currently in a state of relapse, and a bone marrow transplant seems to be the only treatment that might improve her condition and save her life. Her father is a day laborer who has no health insurance, so Jessica's health care is being paid for mainly by the Medicaid system of her small state in the Southwest.

The current cost of a bone marrow transplant at the state's central teaching hospital is $1.5 million, representing about half of the state's entire annual Medicaid budget. Although bone marrow transplants are an accepted treatment for leukemia, this therapy offers only a slim chance for a total cure of the disease. The procedure is risky, and there is a chance that it may cause death. The procedure will involve several months of post-transplant treatment and recovery in an intensive care unit far away from the family's home and will require the child to take costly antirejection medications for many years.

The family understands the risks and benefits. They ask the nurse caring for Jessica what they should do. How should the nurse respond? Does the nurse have any obligations toward the Medicaid system as a whole?

Veracity

A Right to Know

Veracity is the principle of truthfulness. It requires the health-care provider to tell the truth and not to deceive or mislead clients intentionally. As with other rights and obligations, limitations to this principle exist. The primary limitation is when telling the client the truth would seriously harm (principle of nonmaleficence) the client's ability to recover or would produce greater illness.

Health-care providers often feel uncomfortable giving a client bad news, and they tend to avoid answering these questions truthfully. An uncomfortable feeling is not a good enough reason to avoid telling clients the truth about their diagnosis, treatments, or prognosis. Clients have a right to know this information.

One common situation in which veracity is violated is in the use of placebo medications. At some point during their careers, most health-care providers will observe the placebo effect among some clients. Sometimes when a client is given a gel capsule filled with sugar powder and it seems to relieve the pain, this has the same effect as giving the person a narcotic, but without the side effects or potential for addiction. Of course, if the client was told that it was just a sugar pill (veracity), it would not have the same effect. How should nurses feel about this practice?

Costly Errors

Another issue that has come into the public eye in recent months is medical errors. Some studies indicate that the incidence of medical errors in the current health-care system is extremely high and accounts for as many as 44,000 deaths per year. Nurses are often involved in these incidents. What is the nurse's ethical obligation to reveal this information? Some believe that if there is no injury to clients, then the error need not be revealed.

Consider the following case study from the viewpoint of veracity:

Tisha S, a senior nursing student, was acting as the team leader during her final clinical experience. Jamie D, a close friend of Tisha's, was one of three junior nursing students on Tisha's team that day. Because of some personal problems, Jamie had been late and unprepared for several clinical experiences. She was informed by her instructor that she might fail unless she showed marked improvement during clinical training.

Claire B, a 64-year-old woman with diabetes and possible renal failure, was one of Jamie's clients. Mrs. B was having a 24-hour urine test to help determine her renal function. After the test was completed later that afternoon, she was to be discharged and treated through the renal clinic. Jamie understood the principles of the 24-hour urine test and realized that all the urine for the full 24 hours needed to be saved, but she became busy caring for another client and accidentally threw away the last specimen before the test ended. She took the specimen container to the laboratory anyway.

At the end of the shift, when Jamie was giving her report to Tisha, she confided that she had thrown away the last urine specimen but begged Tisha not to tell the instructor. This mistake would mean that the test would have to be started over again, and Mrs. B would have to spend an extra day in the hospital. Out of friendship, Tisha agreed not to tell the instructor, rationalizing that they had collected almost all the urine and she was going to be treated for renal failure anyway. When the instructor asked Tisha for her final report for the day, she specifically asked if there had been any problems with the 24-hour urine test. What would be the consequences of telling the truth and of not telling the truth?

Standard of Best Interest

The Client's Wishes

Standard of best interest describes a type of decision made about a client's health care when the client is unable to make the informed decision regarding his or her own care. The standard of best interest is on the basis of what health-care providers and the family decide is best for that individual. It is very important to consider the individual client's expressed wishes, either formally in a written declaration (e.g., a living will) or informally in conversation with family members.

A Designated Person

Individuals can also legally designate a specific person to make health-care decisions for them in case they become unable to make decisions for themselves. The designated person then has what is called durable power of attorney for health care (DPOAHC).

Issues in Practice

The nurse is caring for a critically ill client after a radical neck surgery in the surgical ICU. The client is connected to a ventilator and is on a sedation protocol with continuous IV infusion of midazolam HCl (Versed), a powerful sedative that requires constant monitoring and titration to maintain the required level of sedation. During the night shift, the nurse discovers that the medication bag is almost empty and the pharmacy, which is closed, did not send up another bag. She looks the medication up in a drug guide and proceeds to mix the drip herself. The night charge nurse was busy supervising a cardiac arrest situation out of the ICU and was unavailable to double-check how the medication was mixed.

Inadvertently, the nurse had mixed a double-strength dose of the medication. Thirty minutes after she hung the new drip, the client's blood pressure was 44/20. The client required a saline bolus and a dopamine drip to stabilize the blood pressure. The family was notified that the client had "taken a turn for the worse" and that they should come to the hospital immediately. In backtracking for the cause of the hypotension, the nurse realizes that she had mixed the sedative double-strength and reduces the rate by half.

When the family arrives, the client's blood pressure has started to return to normal. They ask the nurse what happened and why their mother was on the new IV medication. Should the family be told about the error? Who should tell them? The nurse? The physician? What approach should be used?

Source: McNutty, J: Disclosure of medical errors: An ethical dilemma. AACN News 19(3):4, 2002.

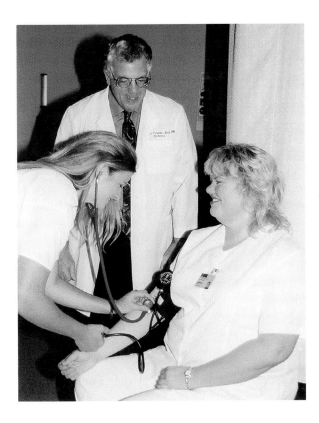

The Omnibus Budget Reconciliation Act (OBRA) of 1990 made it mandatory for all health-care facilities, such as hospitals, nursing homes, and home health-care agencies, to provide information to clients about the living will and DPOAHC.

The standard of best interest should be based on the principle of beneficence. Unfortunately, when clients are unable to make decisions for themselves and no DPOAHC has been designated, the resolution of the dilemma can be a unilateral decision made by health-care providers. Health-care providers' making a unilateral decision that disregards the client's wishes implies that the providers alone know what is best for the client; this is called paternalism.

Obligations

Obligations are demands made on an individual, a profession, a society, or a government to fulfill and honor the rights of others. Obligations are often divided into two categories.

Legal obligations. **Legal obligations** are those that have become formal statements of law and are enforceable under the law. For instance, a nurse has a legal obligation to provide safe and adequate care for clients assigned to him or her.

Moral obligations. **Moral obligations** are those based on moral or ethical principles but are not enforceable under the law. In most states, no legal obligation exists for a nurse on a vacation trip to stop and help an automobile accident victim.

> *Health-care providers' making a unilateral decision that disregards the client's wishes implies that the providers alone know what is best for the client; this is called paternalism.*

Rights

Rights are generally defined as something owed to an individual according to just claims, legal guarantees, or moral and ethical principles. Although the term right is frequently used in both the legal and ethical systems, its meaning is often blurred in daily usage. Individuals sometimes mistakenly claim things as rights that are really privileges, concessions, or freedoms. Several classification systems exist in which different types of rights are delineated. The following three types of rights include the range of definitions.

Welfare Rights

Welfare rights (also called **legal rights**) are based on a legal entitlement to some good or benefit. These rights are guaranteed by laws (e.g., the Bill of Rights of the U.S. Constitution), and violation of such rights can be punished under the legal system. For example, citizens of the United States have a right to equal access to housing regardless of race, sexual preference, or religion.

Ethical Rights

Ethical rights (also called **moral rights**) are based on a moral or ethical principle. Ethical rights usually do not need to have the power of law to be enforced. Ethical rights are, in reality, often privileges allotted to certain individuals or groups of individuals. Over time, popular acceptance of ethical rights can give them the force of a legal right.

An example of an ethical right in the United States is the belief in universal access to health care. In the United States, it is really a long-standing privilege, whereas in many other industrialized countries, such as Canada, Germany, Japan, and England, universal health care is a legal right.

> *Over time, popular acceptance of ethical rights can give them the force of a legal right. An example of an ethical right in the United States is the belief in universal access to health care. In the United States, it is really a long-standing privilege. . . .*

Option Rights

Option rights are rights that are based on a fundamental belief in the dignity and freedom of humans. These are **basic human rights** that are particularly evident in free and democratic countries such as the United States and much less evident in totalitarian and restrictive societies such as Iran. Option rights give individuals freedom of choice and the right to live their lives as they choose, but within a given set of prescribed boundaries. For example, people may wear whatever clothes they choose, as long as they wear some type of clothing.

ETHICS COMMITTEES

Physicians, nurses, and other staff members often encounter ethical conflicts they are unable to resolve on their own. In these cases, the interdisciplinary ethics committee can help the health-care provider resolve the dilemma. An increasing number of health-care facilities, particularly hospitals, have instituted ethics committees that make their consultation services available to health-care providers.

The people who belong to the ethics committee vary somewhat from one institution to another, but almost all include a physician, a member of administration, an RN, a clergy person, a philosopher with a background in ethics, a lawyer, and a person from the community. Members of

ethics committees should not have any personal agenda that they are promoting and should be able to make decisions without prejudice on the basis of the situation and ethical principles.

Depending on the institution, the scope of the ethics committee's duties can range widely, from very limited activity with infrequent meetings on an ad hoc basis to active promotion of ethical thinking and decision making through educational programs. Other common functions of ethics committees include evaluating institutional policies in the light of ethical considerations, making recommendations about complex ethical issues, and providing education programs for medical and nursing schools as well as the community. It is extremely important that nurses participate in these committees and that the ethical concerns of the nurses are recognized and addressed.

ETHICAL SYSTEMS

An ethical situation exists every time a nurse interacts with a client in a health-care setting. Nurses continually make ethical decisions in their daily practice, whether or not they recognize it. These are called normative decisions.

Normative ethics. **Normative ethics** deal with questions and dilemmas that require a choice of actions when there is a conflict of rights or obligations between the nurse and the client, the nurse and the client's family, or the nurse and the physician. In resolving these ethical questions, these nurses often use just one ethical system, or they may use a combination of several ethical systems.

The two systems that are most directly concerned with ethical decision making in the health-care professions are utilitarianism and deontology. Both apply to bioethical issues: the ethics of life (or, in some cases, death).

Bioethics. **Bioethics** and **bioethical issues** are terms that are in common use. These terms have become synonymous with health-care ethics and encompass not only questions concerning life and death but also questions of quality of life, life-sustaining and life-altering technologies, and biological science in general. It is in the context of bioethics that the following discussion of these two systems of ethics is undertaken.

Utilitarianism

Ethical Precepts

Utilitarianism (also called **teleology,** consequential-ism, or situation ethics) is referred to as the ethical system of utility. As a system of normative ethics, utilitarianism defines good as happiness or pleasure. It is associated with two underlying principles: "the greatest good for the greatest number" and "the end justifies the means." Because of these two principles, utilitarianism is sometimes subdivided into act utili-tarianism and rule utilitarianism.

Rule Utilitarianism

According to rule utilitarianism, the individual draws on past experiences to formulate internal rules that are useful in determining the greatest good. With act utilitarianism, the particular situation in which a nurse finds himself or herself determines the right-ness or wrongness of a particular act. In practice, the true follower of utilitarianism does not believe in the validity of any system of rules because the rules can change depending on the circumstances surrounding whatever decision needs to be made.

Act Utilitarianism

Situation ethics is probably the most publicized form of act utilitarianism. Joseph Fletcher, one of the best-known proponents of act utilitarianism, out-lines a method of ethical thinking in which the situa-tion itself determines whether the act is morally right or wrong. Fletcher views acts as good to the extent that they promote happiness and bad to the degree that they promote unhappiness. Happiness is defined as the happiness of the greatest number of people, yet the happiness of each person is to have equal weight.

Abortion, for example, is considered ethical in this system in a situation where an unwed mother on welfare with four other children becomes preg-nant with her fifth child. The greatest good and the greatest amount of happiness are produced by abort-ing this unwanted child.

Because utilitarianism is based on the con-cept that moral rules should not be arbitrary but should rather serve a purpose, ethical decisions derived from a utilitarian framework weigh the effect of alternative actions that influence the over-all welfare of present and future populations. As such, this system is oriented toward the good of the population in general and toward the individual in the sense that the individual participates in that population.

Advantages

The major advantage of the utilitarian system of ethical decision making is that many individuals find it easy to use in most situations. Utilitarianism is built around an individual's needs for happiness in which the individual has an immediate and vested interest. Another advantage is that utilitarianism fits well into a society that otherwise shuns rules and regulations.

A follower of utilitarianism can justify many decisions based on the happiness principle. Also, its utility orientation fits well into Western society's belief in the work ethic and a behavioristic approach to education, philosophy, and life.

Telling a Sad Truth?

The follower of utilitarianism will support a general prohibition against lying and deceiving because ulti-mately the results of telling the truth will lead to greater happiness than the results of lying. Yet truth telling is not an absolute requirement to the follower of utilitarianism. If telling the truth will produce widespread unhappiness for a great number of people and future generations, then it would be ethically bet-ter to tell a lie that will yield more happiness than to tell a truth that will lead to greater unhappiness.

Although such behavior might appear to be unethical at first glance, the strict follower of act util-itarianism would have little difficulty in arriving at this decision as a logical conclusion of utilitarian eth-ical thinking.

Disadvantages

Who Decides?

Some serious limitations exist when using utilitarian-ism as a system of health-care ethics or bioethics. An immediate question is whether happiness refers to the average happiness of all or the total happiness of a few. Because individual happiness is also important, one must consider how to make decisions when the individual's happiness is in conflict with that of the larger group.

More fundamental is the question of what constitutes happiness. Similarly, what constitutes the greatest good for the greatest number? Who determines what is good in the first place? Is it society in general, the government, governmental policy, or the individual? In health-care delivery and the formulation of health-care policy, the general guiding principle often seems to be the greatest good for the greatest number. Yet where do minority groups fit into this system?

Also, the tenet that the ends justify the means has been consistently rejected as a rationale for justifying actions. It is generally unacceptable to allow any type of action as long as the final goal or purpose is good. The Nazis in the 1930s and 1940s used this aphorism to justify many actions that may be viewed by others to be considerably less than good.

What is Good?

The other difficulty in determining what is good lies in the attempt to quantify such concepts as good, harm, benefits, and greatest. This problem becomes especially acute when dealing with health-care issues that involve individuals' lives. For example, an elderly family member has been sick for a long time, and that course of illness has placed great financial hardship on the family. It would be ethical under utilitarianism to allow this client to die or even to euthanize her to relieve the financial stress created by her illness.

Utilitarianism as an ethical system in the health-care decision-making process requires use of an additional principle of distributive justice as an ultimate guiding point. Unfortunately, whenever an unchanging principle is combined with this system, it negates the basic concept of pure utilitarianism.

Pure utilitarianism, although easy to use as a decision-making system, does not work well as an ethical system for decision making in health care because of its arbitrary, self-centered nature. In the everyday delivery of health care, utilitarianism is often combined with other types of ethical decision making in the resolution of ethical dilemmas.

> *Another advantage is that utilitarianism fits well into a society that otherwise shuns rules and regulations. A follower of utilitarianism can justify many decisions based on the happiness principle.*

Deontology

Ethical Precepts

Deontology is a system of ethical decision making based on moral rules and unchanging principles. This system is also termed the formalistic system, the principle system of ethics, or duty-based ethics. A follower of a pure form of the deontological system of ethical decision making believes in the ethical absoluteness of principles regardless of the consequences of the decision.

The categorical imperative. Strict adherence to an ethical theory, in which the moral rightness or wrongness of human actions is considered separately from the consequences, is based on a fundamental principle called the categorical imperative. It is not the results of the act that make it right or wrong, but the principles by reason of which the act is carried out. These fundamental principles are ultimately unchanging and absolute and derived from the universal values that underlie all major religions. Focusing on a concern for right and wrong in the moral sense is the basic premise of the system. Its goal is the survival of the species and social cooperation.

Unchanging Standards

Rule deontology is based on the belief that standards exist for the ethical choices and judgments made by individuals. These standards are fixed and do not change when the situation changes. Although the number of standards or rules is potentially unlimited, in reality—and particularly in dealing with bioethical issues—many of these principles can be grouped together into a few general principles.

These principles can also be arranged into a type of hierarchy of rules and include such maxims as the following: People should always be treated as ends and never as means; human life has value; one is always to tell the truth; above all in health care, do no harm; humans have a right to self-determination; and all people are of equal value. These principles echo such fundamental documents as the Bill of Rights and the American Hospital Association's Patient's Bill of Rights.

Advantages

The deontological system is useful in making ethical decisions in health care because it holds that an ethical judgment based on principles will be the same in a variety of given similar situations regardless of the time, location, or particular individuals involved. In addition, deontological terminology and concepts are similar to the terms and concepts used by the legal system.

The legal system emphasizes rights, duties, principles, and rules. Significant differences, however, exist between the two. Legal rights and duties are enforceable under the law, whereas ethical rights and duties are usually not. In general, ethical systems are much wider and more inclusive than the system of laws that they underlie. It is difficult to have an ethical perspective on law without having it lead to an interest in making laws that govern health care and nursing practice.

Disadvantages

The deontological system of ethical decision making is not free from imperfection. Some of the more troubling questions include the following: What do you do when the basic guiding principles conflict with each other? What is the source of the principles? Is there ever a situation where an exception to the rule will apply?

Although various approaches have been proposed to circumvent these limitations, it may be difficult for nurses to resolve situations in which duties and obligations conflict, particularly when the consequences of following a rule end in harm or hurt being done to a client. In reality, there are probably few pure followers of deontology, because most people will consider the consequences of their actions in the decision-making process.

> *Ethical theories do not provide recipes for resolution of ethical dilemmas. Instead, they provide a framework for decision making that the nurse can apply to a particular ethical situation.*

APPLICATION OF ETHICAL THEORIES

Ethical theories do not provide recipes for resolution of ethical dilemmas. Instead, they provide a framework for decision making that the nurse can apply to a particular ethical situation.

A Framework for Decisions

At times, ethical theories may seem too abstract or general to be of much use to specific ethical situations. Without them, however, ethical decisions may often be made without reasoning or forethought and may be based on emotions. Most nurses in attempting to make ethical decisions combine the two theories presented here.

What Do You Think?

Identify a situation in which you were faced with an ethical dilemma. Which system of ethical decision making did you use? Why did you select that system?

Nursing Code of Ethics

A code of ethics is generally defined as the ethical principles that govern a particular profession. Codes of ethics are presented as general statements and thus do not give specific answers to every possible ethical dilemma that might arise. These codes do, however, offer guidance to the individual practitioner in making decisions.

A Periodic Review

Ideally, codes of ethics should be reviewed periodically to reflect necessary changes in the profession and society as a whole. Although codes of ethics are not judicially enforceable as laws, consistent violations of the code of ethics by a professional in any field may indicate an unwillingness to act in a professional manner and will often result in disciplinary actions ranging from reprimands and fines to suspension of licensure.

Although similar, there are several different codes of ethics that nurses may adopt. In the United States, the American Nurses Association (ANA) Code of Ethics is the generally accepted code. After several years of work, the ANA revised the Code of Ethics in 2001 to be more reflective of the health-care challenges in the new century (Box 7.1). There is also a Canadian Nurses Association Code of Ethics.

Clearly Stated Principles

The ANA Code of Ethics has been acknowledged by other health-care professions as one of the most complete. It is sometimes used as the benchmark against which other codes of ethics are measured. Yet, a careful reading of this code of ethics reveals only a set of clearly stated principles that the nurse must apply to actual clinical situations.

For example, the nurse involved in resuscitation will find no specific mention of **no-code orders** in the ANA Code of Ethics. Rather, the nurse must be able to apply general statements to the particular situation. For example,

The nurse . . . practices with compassion and respect for the inherent dignity, worth and uniqueness of every individual, unrestricted by considerations of social or economic status, personal attributes or the nature of health care problems.

The nurse is responsible and accountable for individual nursing practice and determines the appropriate delegation of tasks consistent with the nurse's obligation to provide optimum patient care.

B o x   7 . 1

The American Nurses Association Code of Ethics

1. The nurse in all professional relationships practices with compassion and respect for the inherent dignity, worth, and uniqueness of every individual, unrestricted by considerations of social or economic status, personal attributes or the nature of health problems.
2. The nurse's primary commitment is to the patient, whether an individual, family, group, or community.
3. The nurse promotes, advocates for, and strives to protect the health, safety, and rights of the patient.
4. The nurse is responsible and accountable for individual nursing practice and determines the appropriate delegation of tasks consistent with the nurse's obligation to provide optimum patient care.
5. The nurse owes the same duties to self as to others including the responsibility to preserve integrity and safety, to maintain competence, and to continue personal and professional growth.
6. The nurse participates in establishing, maintaining, and improving health care environments and conditions of employment conducive to the provision of quality health care and consistent with the values of the profession through individual and collective action.
7. The nurse participates in the advancement of the profession through contributions to practice, education, administration, and knowledge development.
8. The nurse collaborates with other health professionals and the public in promoting community, national, and international efforts to meet health needs.
9. The profession of nursing, as represented by associations and their members, is responsible for articulating nursing values, for maintaining the integrity of the profession and its practice, and for shaping social policy.

Source: Code for Nurses with Interpretive Statements, 2001; p. 1. American Nurses Publishing, American Nurses Foundation/American Nurses Association, 600 Maryland Avenue, SW, Suite 100W, Washington, DC 20024-2571, with permission.

The ANA Code Revised

The revised Code of Ethics restates and reinforces the basic values and commitments that have been and remain essential to the profession of nursing. Traditional ethical principles such as veracity, justice, beneficence, and autonomy are re-emphasized. The nurse is still expected to practice with cooperation, wisdom, compassion, honesty, courage, and respect for the client's privacy. However, the revised code, in response to current health-care practices, defines new boundaries of duty and loyalty. Ethical challenges such as cost containment, delegation, and information technology require nurses to look at health care from new perspectives.

The revised code supports nurses in their attempts to upgrade their employment conditions and environment through measures such as collective bargaining. The revised code addresses and supports nurses who are involved in whistle-blowing when dealing with health-care team members who may be chemically impaired or otherwise incompetent in practice. It also supports nurses in their right to refuse to practice in treatments that violate their beliefs.

The revised code also expands nursing duties beyond individual nurse–client interactions. It recognizes that professional nurses now work in multiple practice areas and are responsible for developing and using the knowledge used in these expanded areas through research and collaborative practice. The 2001 Code for Nurses is an important document that nurses need to be familiar with, both to help ensure ethical practice and to shape an improved future for the profession of nursing.

THE DECISION-MAKING PROCESS

Nurses, by definition, are problem solvers, and one of the important tools that nurses use is the nursing process. The nursing process is a systematic step-by-step approach to resolving problems that deal with a client's health and well-being.

Although nurses deal with problems related to the physical or psychological needs of clients, many feel inadequate when dealing with ethical problems associated with client care. Nurses in any health-care setting can, however, develop the decision-making skills necessary to make sound ethical decisions if they learn and practice using an ethical decision-making process.

Modeling the Nursing Process

An ethical decision-making process provides a method for nurses to answer key questions about ethical dilemmas and to organize their thinking in a more logical and sequential manner. Although there are several ethical decision-making models, the problem-solving method presented here is based on the nursing process. It should be a relatively easy transition for the nurse to move from the nursing process used in the resolution of a client's physical problems to the ethical decision-making process for the resolution of problems with ethical ramifications.

The chief goal of the ethical decision-making process is to determine right and wrong in situations where clear demarcations are not readily apparent. This process presupposes that the nurse making the decision knows that a system of ethics exists, knows the content of that ethical system, and knows that the system applies to similar ethical decision-making problems despite multiple variables. In addition to identifying their own values, nurses also need an understanding of the possible ethical systems that may be used in making decisions about ethical dilemmas.

What Do You Think?

Identify a health care realted ethical situation that is currently in the news. What are the key elements of the dilemma? Discuss how to resolve it with your classmates.

The following ethical decision-making process is presented as a tool for resolving ethical dilemmas (Fig. 7.1).

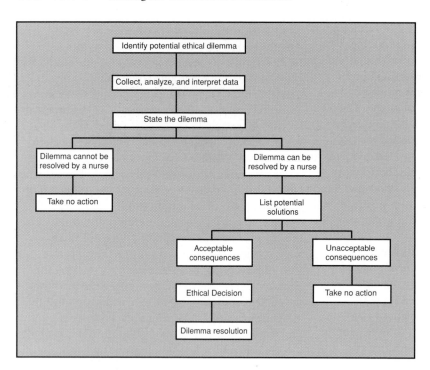

Figure 7.1 Ethical decision-making algorithm. (Adapted from Catalano, JT: Ethical decision making in the critical care patient. Crit Care Nurs Clin North Am 9(1):45–52, 1997.

Step 1: Collect, Analyze, and Interpret the Data

Obtain as much information as possible concerning the particular ethical dilemma. Unfortunately, such information is sometimes very limited. Among the important issues are the client's wishes, the client's family's wishes, the extent of the physical or emotional problems causing the dilemma, the physician's beliefs about health care, and the nurse's own orientation to issues concerning life and death.

Many nurses, for example, face the question of whether or not to initiate resuscitation efforts when a terminally ill client is admitted to the hospital. Physicians often leave instructions for the nursing staff indicating that the nurses should not resuscitate the client but should, instead, merely go through the motions to make the family feel better, which is sometimes referred to as a **slow-code order.** The nurse's dilemma is whether to make a serious attempt to revive the client or to let the client die quietly.

Important information that will help the nurse make the decision might include:

• The mental competency of the client to make a no-resuscitation decision

• The client's desires
• The family's feelings
• Whether the physician previously sought input from the client and the family
• Whether there is a living will or DPOAHC

Many institutions have policies concerning no-resuscitation orders, and it is wise to consider these during data collection. After collecting information, the nurse needs to bring the pieces of information together in a manner that will give the clearest and sharpest focus to the dilemma.

Step 2: State the Dilemma

After collecting and analyzing as much information as is available, the nurse needs to state the dilemma as clearly as possible. In this step, it is important to identify whether the problem is one that directly involves the nurse or is one that can be resolved only by the client, the client's family, the physician, or the DPOAHC.

Recognizing the key aspects of the dilemma helps focus attention on the important ethical principles. Most of the time, the dilemma can be reduced to a few statements that encompass the key ethical issues. Such ethical issues often involve a question of conflicting rights, obligations, or basic ethical principles.

In the case of a no-resuscitation order, the statement of the dilemma might be "The client's right to death with dignity versus the nurse's obligation to preserve life and do no harm." In general, the principle that the competent client's wishes must be followed is unequivocal. If the client has become unresponsive before expressing his or her wishes, then the family members' input must be given serious consideration. Additional questions can arise if the family's wishes conflict with those of the client.

> *Recognizing the key aspects of the dilemma helps focus attention on the important ethical principles. Most of the time, the dilemma can be reduced to a few statements that encompass the key ethical issues.*

Step 3: Consider the Choices of Action

After stating the dilemma as clearly as possible, the next step is to attempt to list, without consideration of their consequences, all possible courses of action that can be taken to resolve the dilemma. This brainstorming activity in which all possible courses of action are considered may require input from outside sources such as colleagues, supervisors, or even experts in the ethical field. The consequences of the different actions are considered later in this chapter.

Some possible courses of action for the nurse in the resuscitation scenario might include the following:

- Resuscitating the client to the nurse's fullest capabilities despite what the physician has requested
- Not resuscitating the client at all
- Only going through the motions without any real attempt to revive the client
- Seeking another assignment to avoid dealing with the situation
- Reporting the problem to a supervisor
- Attempting to clarify the question with the client

- Attempting to clarify the question with the family
- Confronting the physician about the question
- Consulting the institution's ethics committee

For nurses who are unsure about which issues can be referred to the ethics committee, the facility's policy and procedure manual can give direction.

Step 4: Analyze the Advantages and Disadvantages of Each Course of Action

Some of the courses of action developed during the previous step are more realistic than others. The identification of these actions becomes readily evident during this step in the decision-making process, when the advantages and the disadvantages of each action are considered in detail. Along with each option, the consequences of taking each course of action must be thoroughly evaluated.

Consider whether initiating a discussion might anger the physician or cause distrust of the nurse involved. Both these responses may reinforce the attitude of submission to the physician, and either could make continuing to practice nursing at that institution difficult. The same result might occur if the nurse successfully resuscitates a client despite orders to the contrary. Failure to resuscitate the client has the potential to produce a lawsuit unless a clear order for no resuscitation has been given. Presenting the situation to a supervisor may, if the supervisor supports the physician, cause the nurse to be considered a troublemaker and thus have a negative effect on future evaluations. The same process could be applied to the other courses of action.

When considering the advantages and disadvantages, the nurse should be able to narrow the realistic choices of action. Other relevant issues need to be examined when weighing the choices of action. A major factor would be choosing the appropriate code of ethics. The ANA Code of Ethics should be part of many client-care decisions affected by ethical dilemmas.

Step 5: Make the Decision and Act on It

The most difficult part of the process is actually making the decision, following through with action, and then living with the consequences. Decisions are often made with no follow-through, because nurses are fearful of the consequences of their decisions. By their nature, ethical dilemmas produce differences of opinion, and not everyone will be pleased with the decision.

In the attempt to solve any ethical dilemma, there will always be a question of the correct course of action. The client's wishes almost always supersede independent decisions on the part of health-care profes-sionals. A collaborative decision made by the client, physician, nurses, and family about resuscitation is the ideal situation and tends to produce fewer complica-tions in the long-term resolution of such questions.

Conclusion

Ethical dilemmas, by definition, are difficult to resolve. Rarely will a nurse find ethical dilemmas covered in policy, procedure, and protocol manuals, but nurses can develop the skills necessary to make appropriate ethical decisions. The key to developing these skills is the recognition and frequent use of an ethical decision-making model and application of the appropriate ethical theories to the dilemma. As an orderly approach in solving the often disorderly aspects of ethical questions encountered in nursing practice, the decision-making model presented in this chapter can be applied to almost every type of ethical dilemma. Although each situation is different, ethical decision making based on ethical theory can provide a potent tool for resolving dilemmas found in client-care situations.

Critical Thinking Exercises

1. Compare and contrast ethics with laws by delineating the purposes, scopes, and methods of enforcement of each.
2. Distinguish between the two types of obligations.
3. Compare the three categories of rights.
4. Analyze the following ethical dilemma case study using the ethical decision-making process:

- What are the important data in relation to this situation?
- State the ethical dilemma in a clear, simple statement.
- What are the choices of action and how do they relate to specific ethical principles?
- What are the consequences of these actions?
- What decision can be made?

Bill L, a veteran emergency room (ER) nurse, called the resident physician about a client just admitted to the ER after a fall from a ladder. The client, a 52-year-old man, had been fixing his roof when the accident occurred. He had suffered a minor head injury, a twisted ankle, and a badly bruised arm. He also had a long history of asthma and heavy smoking. Not long after his admission to the ER, the client became cyanotic, dyspneic, and semiconscious. By the time the resident physician arrived, the nurse had prepared the client for endotracheal intubation and had already notified the personnel in the medical intensive care unit (MICU) that they would be receiving this client.

After a hasty evaluation of the client, the resident decided to perform an emergency tracheostomy before transporting the client to the MICU. While performing the tracheostomy, the physician severed a major blood vessel and the client hemorrhaged profusely. After several tense minutes, the endotracheal tube was inserted, and the client was quickly transported to the MICU. The client remained cyanotic and had great difficulty breathing. Shortly after leaving the ER, the nurse realized that the oxygen tank that the client had been connected to was empty. The client never regained consciousness and died 3 days after admission. His death was due to respiratory failure and not to the injuries sustained in the fall.

When the client's wife came to the unit to collect the deceased's belongings, the nurse was torn between telling her about the mistakes that were made in the treatment of her husband and remaining silent. What are the key ethical principles involved in this situation? Are there any statements in the ANA Code of Ethics that may help resolve this dilemma? What would be the consequences of informing the client's wife of the truth? What are the consequences of not informing her?

References

1. Paul, R, and Elder, L: Ethical Reasoning. The Foundation for Critical Thinking, 2003 (www.crticalthinking.org).
2. Miracle, V: Rights of patients. Dimensions of Critical Care Nursing 23(3):129–130, 2004.

Bibliography

Bachrach, S: In the name of public health: Nazi racial hygiene. N Engl J Med 351(5):417–420, 2004.

Cook D, et al.: Withdrawal of mechanical ventilation in anticipation of death in the intensive care unit. N Engl J Med 329(1):123–132, 2003.

DePalo, V, et al.: Do-not-resusccitate and stratification-of-care forms in Rhode Island. Am J Crit Care 12(3):239–241, 2003.

Erlen, J: HIPAA: Clinical and ethical considerations for nurses. Orthopedic Nursing 23(6):410–413, 2004.

Engelhardt, HT, and Cherry, MJ: Allocating Scarce Resources. Georgetown University Press, Baltimore, 2002.

Irving, JA, and Sniper, J: Preserving professional ethics. J Prof Nurs 18(1):5, 2002.

Kennedy, W: Beneficence and autonomy in nursing: a moral dilemma. British Journal of Perioperative Nursing 14(11):500–506, 2004.

Mathes, M: Ethics, law, and policy: Ethical decision making and nursing. Medical Surgical Nursing 13(6):429–431, 2004.

Milton, C: Ethical issues: The ethics of respect in nursing. Nursing Science Quarterly18(1):20–23, 2005.

Oxtoby, K: Consent: Obtaining permission to care. Nursing Times 101(1):22–24, 2005.

Quinn, S: Health policy and ethics forum. Ethics in public health research: Protecting human subjects: The role of community advisory boards. Am J Public Health 94(6):918–922, 2004.

8

Bioethical Issues

Joseph T. Catalano

Learning Objectives

After completing this chapter, the reader will be able to:

- Discuss the key ethical principles involved in:

  Abortion

  Genetic research

  Fetal tissue research

  Organ transplantation

  Use of scarce resources

  Assisted suicide

  Acquired immunodeficiency syndrome (AIDS)

  Children

- Discuss the nurse's role in these ethical dilemmas.

- Analyze and make a thoughtful ethical decision in a complex situation.

THE CLIENT'S WELL-BEING

In the recent history of nursing, numerous biomedical and ethical dilemmas have arisen. Historically, nurses have been concerned with moral responsibility and ethical decision making. The nursing code of ethics and its frequent revisions demonstrate the profession's concern with providing ethical health care.

The earliest codes of ethics made obedience to the physician the nurse's primary responsibility. The present code of ethics recognizes that the primary responsibility of the nurse is the client's well-being. This change in emphasis reflects the profession's increased self-awareness, independence, and growing accountability for its actions. Unfortunately, this new attitude has also heralded an era of increased tension, self-doubt, and ethical confusion. By examining the issues and identifying the key moral and ethical conflicts, nurses will be able to accept their moral responsibilities and make good ethical decisions.

In the course of their careers, nurses are likely to encounter any number of ethical dilemmas. Although a complete analysis of every issue is beyond the scope of this book, some of the more common situations and their important ethical features are presented as examples of ways to analyze such dilemmas and to make informed decisions. The resolution of ethical dilemmas is never an easy task, and it is likely that someone may disagree with the decision.

ABORTION

A Polarizing Issue

Few issues evoke as strong an emotional reaction as abortion. Because of its religious, ethical, social, and legal implications, the abortion issue touches everyone in one way or another. There seems to be very little middle ground. People are either strongly in favor of abortion or oppose it completely. In a recent presidential election, abortion was once again a central issue, and the outcome of the election may very well have been decided by the candidates' positions on the law that supports the practice.

What Do You Think?

Do you support or reject elective abortion? On what ethical principles do you base your belief? What advice would you give to a pregnant teenager who wanted to have an abortion?

_____

_____

_____

_____

_____

_____

_____

_____

_____

_____

_____

A Matter of Convenience?

Elective abortion is the voluntary termination of a pregnancy before 24 weeks of gestation. An elective abortion may be either therapeutic or self-selected. Strictly speaking, a therapeutic abortion would be one performed in consultation with and on the recommendation of a physician or psychiatrist, based on the conclusion that the mother's health or psychological state would be damaged without the abortion.

Self-selected, or elective, abortions are those performed solely on the mother's own decision, without consultation with a physician or psychiatrist, usually for economic or convenience reasons. In the case of *Roe v. Wade* in 1973, the Supreme Court changed the legal status of elective abortion in the United States, but the ethical basis and moral status of this decision remain controversial.

A careful reading of the court's decision in *Roe v. Wade* reveals that the justices made no decision about the ethics or morality of elective abortion. Rather, the court said that, according to the U.S. Constitution, all people have a right to determine what they can do with their bodies (i.e., the right to self-determination) and that such a right includes termination of a pregnancy.

A Conflict of Rights?

The fundamental issues at the heart of the abortion debate center on the question of when life begins and the right of freedom of choice. Those who argue against abortion believe that life begins at the moment of conception and therefore hold that abortion is an act of killing. Proponents of abortion argue that the fetus is not really human until it reaches the point of development when it can live outside the mother's body (i.e., the age of viability, about 20 weeks). From a deontological standpoint, abortion represents a basic conflict of rights.

On one hand, a woman's rights to privacy, self-determination, and freedom of choice are at issue. In the United States, these rights are fiercely held and are considered to be issues of public policy and **constitutional law.** Indeed, these rights form the basis of the *Roe v. Wade* decision.

The conflicting right from the antiabortion side of the dilemma is the fetus's right to life. In most Western civilizations, particularly those that are based on Judeo-Christian beliefs, the casual and intentional taking of a human life is strongly prohibited. Life is the most basic good, because without it there can be no other rights. In general, the right to life is considered to be the most profound of the rights and is absolute in most situations.

When one is attempting to resolve the ethics and morality of abortion, these two conflicting rights need to be weighed against each other. Nurses are often placed in situations where they must help clients make decisions about abortion. Just as frequently, they are asked to participate in the procedure itself.

Where Your Values Fit In

In practice, ethical issues are always affected by the health-care provider's moral values. In the dilemma over abortion, nurses must analyze their own values and perceptions of their roles to make the best decisions. As a client **advocate,** should a nurse be for or against abortion? How can a nurse avoid influencing the woman's decision about abortion? Can a nurse ethically and legally refuse to assist at abortions? Should the client's reason for wanting an abortion or her stage of pregnancy (first or second trimester, or later, requiring a partial-birth procedure) have any influence on the nurse's decision?

These questions are not easily answered, but understanding the underlying principles involved in the issue may help defuse some of the emotional impact that often surrounds this topic. As in all complicated ethical dilemmas, the nurse needs to remember that the client must receive competent, high-quality care regardless of the nurse's own personal values or moral beliefs.

> *In practice, ethical issues are always affected by the health-care provider's moral values. In the dilemma over abortion, nurses must analyze their own values and perceptions of their roles to make the best decisions.*

GENETICS AND GENETIC RESEARCH

The ability to alter genetic material to produce organisms that differ greatly from their original form is now a reality. Scientific and popular literature is filled with reports of new ways to identify and change the genetic material of all types of living creatures.

The Future is Now

Currently, genetically altered bacteria (e.g., *Escherichia coli*) are used to produce various medications, including a purer form of insulin. Genetically altered corn is now growing in very hot, dry places and is resistant to most insects. Abnormal genes that indicate individuals who are at risk for various types of cancer, Alzheimer's disease, Parkinson's disease, and Down syndrome have been identified.

In the twentieth century, society became so accustomed to the idea that science should be allowed to do whatever it is capable of doing that very few questions have been asked about the ethics of genetic engineering and research. As with most scientific research and techniques, the techniques of genetic engineering are ethically neutral. Procedures such as refining recombinant DNA, gene therapy, altering germ cells, and cloning other cells are neither good nor bad in themselves. The potential for misuse of these procedures is so great, however, that it may permanently alter or even destroy the human species.

Ethics of Genetic Research

Several ethical issues need to be considered when genetic engineering and research are being conducted, including those involving the safety of genetic research, the legality and morality of genetic screening, and the proper use of genetic information. Recently proposed laws attempt to regulate genetic research to prevent the production of a supervirus or superbacterium that could exterminate the entire human population.[1]

Mandatory Screening

With current technology, it is possible to detect genetic patterns in newborn infants that are linked to breast and colon cancer, heart disease, Huntington's disease, and Parkinson's disease. The advantage to insurance companies, which could screen individuals as early as infancy for costly and potentially lethal diseases later in life, is obvious: these individuals could be excluded from health and life insurance coverage, thus saving the insurance companies a great deal of money.

Although this practice would most likely be unethical, the concept of mandatory genetic screening is not unrealistic. Because it requires just one blood sample from a person at some point during that person's life, it is possible that this type of screening could even be done without the individual's knowledge or consent.

Informed Consent

Informed consent is permission granted by a person based on full knowledge of the risks and benefits of what is being done. The basic question is, Do parents violate the right of informed consent if they give permission to have gene testing performed on their newborn and have the results released to an insurance company? Do insurance companies violate informed consent if they somehow obtain the information without the knowledge of the client? (Informed consent is discussed in detail in Chapter 9.)

Confidentiality

Similarly, confidentiality is at great risk of being violated by genetic screening. The confidentiality,

fidelity that exist between the health-care ...er and the client have been the basis of the ...rapeutic relationship. In some cases, individuals may be denied employment based on the results of genetic testing. In this time of the information super-highway and vast computerized databases, very little of a client's health history remains confidential.[2]

Emotional Impact

An important ethical implication for nurses is the emotional impact that genetic information may have on the client. Knowledge of the possible long-term outcome of one's health, particularly if that knowledge is negative, may cause a client **anxiety,** or the person may become depressed or suicidal. Nurses must further hone their teaching and counseling skills to assist clients in dealing with the implications of this type of information.

Obstetric nurses have been involved with genetic screening procedures for years. Some of the most important information obtained from amniocentesis deals with the genetic composition of the fetus. It is important that the mother understand the procedure and the type of information it may yield and that she give informed consent for this procedure.

Self-determination

Nurses have a strict ethical obligation to refuse to participate in mandatory, involuntary screening programs as well as a strict prohibition about revealing genetic test results to unauthorized individuals. Forcing clients to be tested who are strongly opposed to finding out information about their genetic status is clearly a breach of those clients' right to self-determination.

However, much as the current practice of routine screening for diseases such as tuberculosis, hepatitis, and blood lead levels promotes the general health of the population, so does the screening for genetic diseases. Clients who are strongly opposed to such genetic screening must be allowed the option to refuse it to maintain their right to self-determination.

Promise or Threat?

Now that the human genome has been decoded, a whole new world of possibilities—both positive and negative—has been opened for health-care providers. The impact of the Human Genome Project, cloning research, and other related genetic procedures is on par with the discovery of bacteria and antibiotics. The potential for the cure of almost all known diseases, ranging from viral infections to cancer to the regeneration of spinal cord nerves, is now possible.

On the other side of the issue, there is the potential for the development of superviruses that could wipe out the population of the earth. Nurses need to watch each development very closely and call their legal representatives when they believe science is moving into dangerous areas.[3]

USE OF FETAL TISSUE

Fetal tissue research has been conducted since at least the early 1990s. Traditional fetal tissue research has been generally limited to taking living cells from an aborted fetus and transplanting them into people who have chronic or severe diseases. The procedure has been found to be helpful to a limited extent in the treatment of Alzheimer's disease and Parkinson's disease.

Growing Tissue on Demand

Artificial Conception. During 1997 to 2000, the Human Genome Project added a new twist to this research. Rather than using tissue from aborted fetuses, scientists are now growing their own fetal tissue in the laboratory through **artificial insemination** and in vitro fertilization procedures. These test-tube fetuses are then dissected. Various fetal tissues are used for genetic and other types of research. The legal system has become aware of abuses of these procedures and has proposed legislation to control their use, including limiting the age of in vitro fetuses to 6 weeks. After 6 weeks, such fetuses will have to be destroyed.

Stem Cell Research. Stem cell research is a closely related issue. Stem cells are the very early cells present in the developing fetus that have not yet begun to differentiate; that is, all the cells are identical and contain all the genetic material needed to reproduce an identical individual. Stem cells can be separated and then placed in an environment where they will form more stem cells, or the genetic material from the stem cell can be removed and replaced, or the genetic material can be removed, manipulated, and then replaced. Recent federal administrative decisions permitted federal funding for stem cell research on a limited basis; however, there are no restrictions on privately funded stem cell research.

Like stem cells, fetal tissue is highly desirable for research and transplantation because it lacks some of the genetic material that makes more mature tissues and organs more likely to cause rejection in the host. These fetal tissues are also in a rapid growth mode and naturally develop more quickly than do tissues from other sources. Scientists involved in this research see fetal tissue as one of the most important means of curing diseases.

The Source of the Material

Even a superficial consideration of these procedures necessarily raises many important ethical issues. Basic to the ethics of this type of research is the source of the research material. In the past, most of the material came from elective abortions.

Potential for Abuse. Because of the immaturity and lack of differentiation of cells during the first trimester of pregnancy, the best fetal tissue comes from fetuses aborted during the second trimester. Most scientists agree that second-trimester fetuses have well-developed nervous, cardiovascular, gastrointestinal, and renal systems and are capable of feeling pain. Even though fetal tissue research has not led to an increase in abortions, the potential for abuse is tremendous.

Paying for Fetuses? It is also not definite whether the fetal tissue research scientists are paying others for these aborted fetuses. If payment is being made for aborted fetuses, it would seem to violate both the laws that prevent payment for organs used in transplantation and the moral respect for humanity. Questions also arise concerning who is giving permission for the use of fetuses in transplantation procedures. Does anyone really own them?

In Vitro Fertilization. Another important ethical issue concerns the use of in vitro fertilization as a source for fetal tissue. Many religious groups question the morality of the procedure itself. Even if in vitro fertilization is considered ethical for procedures such as surrogate motherhood, is it ethical to create fetuses that are going to be used only for research and transplantation? From whom are the ova and sperm coming? Have the people from whom these have been obtained given permission for such use of their tissues? What about the rights of a fetus that was created in a test tube without ever having a hope of a normal life?

The Nurse's Role

The 1988 directive, which was extended indefinitely in 1990, to prevent the Department of Health and Human Services from using federal money for fetal tissue research, was amended in 2001 to allow this type of research on a very limited basis with federal funding. Local biomedical ethical panels can make decisions about this type of research. Many of these panels, which consist mainly of research scientists, have ruled in favor of continuing research.

Nurses may have an important role to play in issues involving fetal tissue research. Although they will not likely be involved directly in research, nurses are often employed in facilities where elective abortions are performed. Nurses employed in such places must become aware of the issues involved in abortion. They also should know where the aborted fetuses are taken and how they are disposed of. Nurses should also remain informed about developing procedures and techniques regarding fetal tissue research; they should support legal and ethical efforts to control its abuses.

> *Whenever a human organ is transplanted, many people are involved, including the donor, the donor's family, medical and nursing personnel, and the recipient and his or her family.*

ORGAN TRANSPLANTATION

Despite widespread public and medical acceptance of organ transplantation as a highly beneficial procedure, ethical questions still remain. Whenever a human organ is transplanted, many people are involved, including the donor, the donor's family, medical and nursing personnel, and the recipient and his or her family. Society in general could also be added to this group because of the high cost of organ transplantation, which is usually paid from tax money directly or indirectly in the form of increased insurance premiums. Each of these persons or groups has rights that may conflict with the rights of others.

The Good of the Donor

Currently, the three primary sources for organ and tissue donations are living related donors, living unrelated donors, and **cadaver donors.** Most institutions that perform transplants or organizations that are involved in obtaining organs and tissues have developed complex procedures to help deal with the ethical and legal issues involved in transplantation. Despite these efforts, some ethical uncertainties remain whenever the issue of organ transplantation is raised.

When the Donor Is a Child

One particularly sensitive issue is exemplified when a child donates an organ, for example, a kidney transplant for a sibling, a procedure that poses some serious risk. Although parents are usually required to give consent for medical procedures for their children, by legal definition, a child younger than 18 years of age cannot give informed consent to such a procedure. It can be argued, however, that ethically the donor child, as a participant, should have input in making such a decision. At what age can a child have a say in the decision? Can a child be forced, for example, to donate a kidney even if he or she refuses? (See the discussion of children's ethics later in this chapter.)

One situation that illustrates this dilemma is that of a teenage girl who developed leukemia. The only way to save her life was to find a bone marrow donor who matched her genetic type. When no donor could be found, the parents decided to have another baby in the hope that the bone marrow of the second child would match that of the first child. After the baby was born, it was found that the bone marrow did indeed match, and when the child was old enough to donate safely, the bone marrow was taken and transplanted into the older child.

When Does Death Occur?

Despite the best efforts of the medical and legal community to establish criteria for death, some ethical questions still linger about what constitutes death. Because organs such as the heart, lungs, and liver need to come from a donor whose heart is still beating, some clinicians fear that there will be a tendency for physicians to declare that a person is dead before death actually occurs.

The most widely accepted criterion for death is **brain death.** Some researchers, however, question whether the death of the brain actually means that a person ceases to exist as a human. Are there some other criteria that ought to be examined in conjunction with brain death?

Selecting the Recipient

One of the most difficult ethical issues involved in organ transplantation is the selection of recipients. Because fewer organs are available than the numerous people who need them, the potential ethical dilemmas are great.

Legislating Donation

The **Uniform Anatomical Gift Act** was passed to increase the supply of organs for donation and attempt to reduce some of the confusion over organ donation. The national organ recipient list attempts to list and rank all people who need organs in a nondiscriminatory manner. Some important criteria for ranking include need, length of time on the list, potential for survival, prior organ transplantation, value to the community, and tissue compatibility.

Nurses can be, and often are, involved in some aspect of the organ donation process. Many states have passed laws that require health-care workers to ask the family members of potential organ donors whether they have ever thought about their dead or dying loved one being used for organ donation (Box 8.1).

The Nurse's Responsibility

Many nurses, particularly nurses who work in critical care units, provide care for clients who may potentially become organ donors. Nurses in operating rooms may help in the surgical procedures that remove organs from a cadaver and transplant them into a recipient's body. Other nurses provide the postoperative care for clients who have received a transplanted organ. Home-health-care nurses give the follow-up care to such clients at home.

Nurses working with organ transplantation need to be sensitive to the potential for manipulation. Most people who are seeking organ transplantations are desperately ill or near death. They and their families can be very easily manipulated or can themselves become very manipulative.

Obtain Permission Gently

On the other side, the families of potential organ donors are usually distraught about the sudden and traumatic loss of a loved one. They too are vulnerable to psychological manipulation. Because of the emotionally fragile state of the family of a trauma victim, they are vulnerable to guilt and grief. Health-care providers should avoid appealing to these emotions when obtaining permission to harvest organs for transplantation.

As a general rule, neither the donor nor his or her family should play any part in the selection of a recipient. Nurses need to avoid making statements or giving nonverbal indications of their approval or disapproval of potential recipients.

The traditional belief has been that life should be preserved at all costs and by any means available. Health-care providers feel uncomfortable when cost considerations are mentioned regarding treatments for terminally ill clients.

USE OF SCARCE RESOURCES IN PROLONGING LIFE

In these days of huge federal budget deficits and attempts to control them by shrinking the health-care budget, money for health care is becoming more difficult to obtain. It is recognized that most public money allocated for health care is spent during the last year of life for many elderly clients. Expensive procedures, therapies, technologies, and care are provided to terminally ill individuals to extend their lives by a few days or even a few hours. It is not unusual to spend as much as $5000 a day on a client receiving care in an intensive care unit.

Preserving Life at Any Cost

The traditional belief has been that life should be preserved at all costs and by any means available. Health-care providers feel uncomfortable when cost considerations are mentioned regarding treatments for terminally ill clients. Yet, in the context of current problems in society, such considerations are both economic and ethical realities. The necessity of conserving resources has forced society, through governmental action, to face this issue.

All the currently proposed health-care plans take into consideration some type of cost-control

Box 8.1

Organ Donation

Seven Questions That Families Often Ask About Organ Donation and How You Should Answer Them

Many families refuse to donate a loved one's organs simply because they do not fully understand organ donation. By being prepared to address their concerns, you can help them make a decision they are comfortable with.

Here are the most common questions families ask about organ donation. Review them along with the answers so that you are prepared the next time that you need to counsel a family on this sensitive issue.

1. *Whose consent is needed to allow organ donation?*

   Consent must come from the patient's legal next of kin, even if the patient has a signed donor card or an organ donation sticker on his or her driver's license.

2. *How can you ask us to make this decision at such a tragic time?*

   "I know that this is a very stressful time for you, but I need to ask that you think about organ donation. Is it what your loved one would have wanted?"

   "I understand that you may not be able to say yes right now, and that's okay. However, if you decide to donate, we need to know as soon as possible so that any tissues or organs may be removed in time to help another person."

3. *What does brain death mean?*

   Brain death is an irreversible condition that occurs when blood no longer flows to the brain and the brain tissue dies. Although the brain is dead, other organs and tissues can function if supported by artificial means. A doctor will pronounce brain death only after everything possible has been done for your loved one and there is no chance of survival.

4. *Is the body disfigured when the organs are removed?*

   Surgeons use as few incisions as possible to recover the donated organs or tissues. Donation shouldn't interfere with an open casket funeral, if that's what you have planned.

5. *Will we be charged for donation costs?*

   No. All costs related to removal of the organs are covered by the donor program. However, you'll still be responsible for the funeral, burial arrangements, and related costs.

6. *How are recipients chosen?*

   Recipients are chosen from the United Network of Organ Sharing, a national computer registry. They're selected according to degree of need, how long they've been on the waiting list, and certain medical criteria, such as blood type compatibility, tissue matching, and body size.

7. *We're not sure if our religion allows organ donation. What should we do?*

   Many religions support organ donation; but if you're concerned, speak with your religious leader.

Teresa M. Odell, RN
Coordinator, Nursing Staff Education
Cobb Hospital and Medical Center
Kennesaw, GA

Source: Odell, TM: Organ donation. What families need to know. Nursing 94 December 1994, p. 321, with permission.

measures related to restricting payment for client care. In addition, the **hospice care** movement and a growing number of physicians and other health-care professionals support **palliative** care for the terminally ill that provides pain relief and comfort measures but does not try to prolong the person's life.

In reality, the current health-care system is already rationing care to some degree. Many people who are not covered by health-care insurance do not seek health care. Groups such as the poor, who are covered by massive governmental programs, shy away from seeking health care because of the numerous restrictions placed on it. Individuals who are covered by insurance often have restrictions placed on them by the insurance companies.

The Ethics of Tube Feeding

The long-standing controversy over tube feedings has been given new life recently by the Schiavo case in Forida.[4] Tube feeding is a relatively simple procedure that is used in all areas of health care, from feeding premature infants in the neonatal intensive care unit to maintaining the elderly postoperative client at home under the supervision of home-health-care staff. Additionally, it is a way of maintaining nutrition and hydration, two of the most basic needs of life. Nurses who work with terminally ill clients often believe that once a feeding tube has been inserted, it cannot be removed for any reason because that would constitute active euthanasia, or mercy killing. But is that belief justified in all circumstances? Consider the following scenario:

> Her large family—consisting of her husband of many years, three sons, and two daughters—were very upset. Mrs. Ada Floral, 82 years old, had just suffered a massive stroke that rendered her unresponsive. Although she was breathing on her own, she had no voluntary movements and seemed to be completely paralyzed. Magnetic resonance imaging (MRI) showed a large area of bleeding around the midbrain and brain stem. Her pupils were constricted and unresponsive. The physician explained that the prognosis was extremely grave, and the likelihood of Mrs. Floral's survival was minimal.
>
> However, the family members all agreed that "everything" should be done, so the physician reluctantly initiated aggressive medical therapy with IV glucocorticoids, osmotic diuretics, antihypertensives, and physical therapy. After a week, there was no change. The family wondered whether Mrs. Floral might be "starving to death" and asked the physician to have a feeding tube inserted and feedings started.
>
> One month later, the still-unresponsive Mrs. Floral is being cared for at home by her family with the supervision of the local hospice/home-health-care program. She is off all IV medications; however, she is receiving some medications, a commercially prepared feeding, and water through the feeding tube. Some of the family members are beginning to question whether they did the right thing by insisting that everything be done and wish to remove the feeding tube so that Mrs. Floral can die a peaceful and dignified death rather than just hanging on for months. Other family members feel that if they give permission for the tube's removal, they would be killing their mother and could not live with the guilt.
>
> The hospice nurse in charge of the case had discussed the issue with the family. She too believes that once a feeding tube has been placed, it should not be removed, even if all the family agrees on its removal. She feels that it's not an issue a family can "just change their minds about." Although she is in frequent contact with Mrs. Floral's physician, she has not mentioned that the family is thinking about removing the feeding tube in fear that the physician might agree.

Is the hospice nurse correct in her belief about the removal of the feeding tube? When do tube feedings stop being beneficial to clients? Is there a right to death with dignity? What ethical rationales could be used for removal of the feeding tube in this case?

Should Care Be Restricted?

The use of public funds for health care is an ethical issue that revolves around the principle of distributive justice. In this context, distributive justice requires that all citizens have equal access to all types of health care, regardless of their income levels, race, sex, religious beliefs, or diagnosis. Many complex issues are involved in this dilemma.

These issues go far beyond the questions of who gets what type of care and where and how the care takes place. Some type of **universal health-care coverage** is likely to be mandated for all Americans sometime in the future. Is it fair that some individuals (taxpayers) pay for the health care of others? Should individuals who contribute to their own poor state of health by smoking, drinking, taking illicit drugs, or overeating be provided with the same type of care as those who do not put themselves at risk? Who is going to make the decisions about who gets expensive treatment such as organ transplantations, experimental medications, placement in intensive care units, or life-extending technologies?

The use of criteria such as age, potential for a high-quality life, and availability of resources for determining who receives life-extending technologies is gaining wider acceptance, but is this a valid ethical position? Nurses are often involved in situations in which terminally ill clients are brought to the hospital for end-of-life care. Nurses need to play an active role in helping formulate policies concerning the issues they face daily.

What Do You Think?

Are you for or against universal health-care insurance for all U.S. citizens? Discuss your rationale for your position.

THE RIGHT TO DIE

The right-to-die issue is an extension of the right to self-determination issue discussed in Chapter 9. It also overlaps with the dilemma of **euthanasia** and assisted suicide. Health-care providers often become involved in the decision-making process when clients are irreversibly comatose, vegetative, or suffering from a terminal disease. The choices that the families of such clients often face are death or the extension of life using painful and expensive treatments.[5]

What Is Extraordinary?

One of the difficulties in resolving right-to-die issues is understanding the terminology used. Often a client who has a living will states that he or she wants no extraordinary treatments if he or she should become comatose or unable to make decisions involving health care. But what constitutes extraordinary treatments? A general definition of ordinary treatments includes any medications, procedures, surgeries, or technologies that offer the client some hope of benefit without causing excessive pain or suffering.

Using this definition, extraordinary treatments (sometimes called heroic measures) are those treatments, medications, surgeries, and technologies that offer little hope for curing or improving the client's condition. Although these general definitions provide some guidelines for making decisions about ordinary and extraordinary treatments, discerning the nature of the specific modalities remains difficult.

Ventilation

For example, a ventilator is a machine that assists a client's breathing. In intensive care units (ICUs), it is a common mode of treatment for many types of clients, including postoperative clients, clients with cardiac and respiratory diseases, and victims of trauma. Does its widespread and frequent use make the ventilator an ordinary mode of treatment? Many would say yes, whereas others would say it is still extraordinary because of its invasive nature and complicated technology.

Cardiopulmonary Resuscitation

Another issue often included in the right-to-die debate is that of codes and "do-not-resuscitate" (DNR or no code) orders. Cardiopulmonary resuscitation (CPR) is

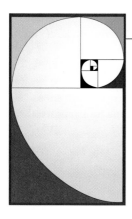

Issues in Practice

An Issue of Distributive Justice

The Numbers of Americans Without Health Insurance Continue
to Rise

The Centers for Disease Control (CDC) have been collecting data on the percentage of adults and children who do not have health insurance in the United States beginning in 1997. In 1997, the rate of uninsured adults in the United States was 12.8 percent. By 2002 the rate had risen to 19.1 percent, and in 2003, the last year for which data is available, the rate had risen to 20.1 percent. Although no specific reasons were cited for this increase, the increased numbers of uninsured occurred during a time period when the U.S. economy took a downturn with a rise in unemployment.

On the positive side, the United States improved in its health care coverage for children. The rate of children without health insurance coverage decreased from 13.9 percent in 1997 to 10.1 percent in 2003. Officials at the CDC's National Center for Health Statistics cite efforts by states to increase coverage for children living at or near the poverty line as the single most significant factor in this increase.

The rate of Americans of all ages who had no health insurance in 2003 was 15.2 percent, which increased from 14.7 percent in 2002. These percentages translate into approximately 43.6 million Americans without health care insurance. However, the distribution by race is unequal. Hispanics have an uninsured rate three times higher than whites and almost twice as high as blacks.

The United States does not offer universal health insurance coverage to its citizens as Canada and many European nations do. Most Americans receive coverage through their employers or purchase it from private insurance companies. Despite efforts over the years by the Democratic party to institute universal health insurance for all Americans, the health insurance lobby has managed to block the legislation with backing from the Republicans. The lack of health insurance coverage was one of the major themes of Democratic presidential nominee John Kerry's campaign for the White House.

The Institute of Medicine estimates that over 18,000 Americans die each year because they lack health insurance. Even with health insurance coverage, approximately 14 percent of families in the United States have accumulated enough debt from medical expenses to place a significant strain on their financial resources.

Source: Reuters, CNN.Com Wednesday, July 1, 2004.

widely taught to both health-care providers and the general public. It is often used to treat clients who have suffered heart attacks and have gone into cardiac arrest as well as clients suffering from electrical shock, drowning, and traumatic injuries.

In the hospital setting, the nursing staff is obligated to perform CPR on all clients who do not have a specific DNR order. This leads to situations in which terminally ill clients may be subjected to CPR efforts several times before they die.[6]

> *The expressed desires about future medical care are known as advance directives. They are the best means to guarantee that a client's wishes will be honored.*

Advance Directives

As an issue of self-determination, it is essential that the client's wishes about health care be followed. All client communication to the nurse about desires for future care should be documented. If at all possible, the client should be encouraged to designate an individual to act as a moral surrogate—a designated decision maker—should the client become unable to make his or her own decisions. The expressed desires about future medical care are known as advance directives. They are the best means to guarantee that a client's wishes will be honored.

A Formal Document

Advance directives, in the form of a living will or durable power of attorney, can and should specify which extraordinary procedures, surgeries, medications, or treatments can or cannot be used. These directives are often in the form of formal documents that need to be witnessed by two individuals who are not related to the client (Box 8.2).

As useful as advance directives are in helping the client decide on future care, clients often are unable to anticipate all the possible types of treatments used. For example, an elderly client with a long history of cardiovascular disease specified in his living will that he did not want CPR performed and did not want a ventilator. When his heart developed

Box 8.2

Checklist for Evaluating a Patient's Living Will Document

1. Statement of intention states the document was written freely when the patient was competent.
2. Statement of when the document goes into effect. This is usually when the patient is no longer able to make decisions for himself or herself.
3. A section specifies general health-care measure to be excluded from care.
4. Open section for specific measures (ventilators, pacemakers, etc.) and any other specific instructions concerning care.
5. Proxy statement (sometimes called durable power of attorney), which is optional but a strong addition. Allows another person to make decisions in situations that may not have been anticipated in the living will. (Check your state law concerning details of proxy selection.)
6. Substitute proxy. This section is optional. Specifies who can make decisions, if first choice proxy is not available.
7. Legal statement that the proxy(s) may make decisions.
8. Witness selection statement. Many states require that witnesses not be related or members of the health-care team.
9. Signature and date. Must be signed and dated by the patient. Some states have very specific regulations concerning how long the will is valid. It may range from a few months to 5 years.
10. Legal signatures of witnesses are required.
11. Notary seal, if required by state law. State laws differ on notary seal requirement. It is usually required if a proxy is selected.

a potentially lethal dysrhythmia that rendered him unresponsive, his physician made the decision to cardiovert* the client using the electric cardioverter because this mode of treatment was not specifically forbidden by the client's living will. Strictly speaking, the physician did not violate the letter of the living will, but did he violate its spirit?

A Legal Requirement

Advance directives, which include living wills, are now a required part of the health care of all clients. The Omnibus Budget Reconciliation Act of 1990 requires that all hospitals, nursing-care facilities, home-health-care agencies, and caregivers ask clients about advance directives and provide information concerning living wills and durable power of attorney (DPOA) to help clients make informed health-care decisions. However, the federal law mandates only the requirements and not the directives to implement the law. The actual implementation of the law is left to the individual states. Because of the vagueness of the law, a great deal of confusion exists, particularly with regard to living wills.

Nurses play an important role in ensuring that clients understand the implications of their choices pertaining to decisions that may prolong their lives during medical emergencies. Because of their "frontline" position as caregivers within the health-care system, nurses must understand this role, specifically as it pertains to living wills.

Ethical Difficulties of Living Wills

What Did the Client Know?

Although a living will seems to be a simple solution to a complex care situation, there are some ethical difficulties inherent in their use that nurses need to know about. Primary among these ethical difficulties is the question of the person's level of knowledge of potential and future health-care problems at the time the will was formulated. Because living wills are often formulated long before they are to be used, there may later be serious questions about how informed the person was about the disease states and treatment modalities that might later affect care. If

there is any indication that the person did not understand the full implications of future therapies or potential medical problems, then the validity of the living will is in question.

A Moral Conflict

A second ethical difficulty for nurses encompasses the principles of beneficence and nonmaleficence. The principle of beneficence states that a health-care professional's primary duty is to benefit or do good for the client. The principle of nonmaleficence states that health-care providers should protect the client from harm. It is sometimes difficult to determine whether the primary duty is to produce benefit or prevent harm.

Generally, most health-care providers think that the duty to avoid harming the client outweighs the concerns for providing benefit. When evaluated from the beneficence and nonmaleficence viewpoints, living wills seem to violate the principle of providing benefit to the client. This perception makes many health-care providers ethically uncomfortable. In some situations, the implementation of a living will might actually involve the termination of some modes of treatments already in use. Termination seems to constitute harm to the client.

In either case, respecting a living will might often appear to health-care providers to be a violation of their duty to help clients and preserve life. Nurses, as well as other health-care providers, often experience a sense of frustration when they are not allowed to use all the skills they have learned to preserve life.

Lack of Clarity

A third difficulty nurses and other health-care workers may have with living wills is their formulation and legal enforcement. In general, the language used in the standard living will document is broad and vague. Living wills are often not specific enough to include all the forms of treatments that are possible for the many types of illnesses that might render a person incompetent to make decisions. Health-care providers may have little direction as to the care they are to give if the circumstances at the time the living will was formulated are significantly different from the declared wishes of the client.

Furthermore, unless the particular state has enacted into law a special type of living will called a

---

*Cardioverting is a procedure in which electrical shock is used to change the heart rhythm from ventricular tachycardia or other rhythms to normal sinus rhythms.

Issues in Practice

In the current health-care environment, nurses may encounter elderly clients who function independently at home and have not officially or legally been declared incompetent, but whose behavior might indicate that they are unable to make rational decisions about their care. Consider the following situation:

A 74-year-old client, Buster Mack, had been a long-haul truck driver for most of his life and was still driving his big rig into his 60s. He had been in relatively good health until 5 years ago, when he was diagnosed with lung cancer. A lobectomy was performed at that time, and he was treated with follow-up radiation and chemotherapy, but the cancer had slowly metastasized to the bone. His current hospitalization was because of a syncopal episode witnessed by a neighbor in the front yard of Mr. Mack's home, where he lives by himself.

During the admission assessment, the nurse observed that Mr. Mack had trouble focusing on the questions, and often the answer was unrelated to the question or in the form of a long rambling account of something that happened many years ago. Although he knew he was in a hospital (he could not remember the name), he had no idea where it was or what the date was. His demeanor was cooperative and pleasant, and he laughed easily when the nurse joked with him. He could not remember whether he had any family left living, although the name and address of a son in a distant city were listed on the old records.

Mr. Mack signed all the admission papers and consent forms placed in front of him for a number of neurological tests. His physician was fearful that the cancer might have spread to his brain and wanted to do a magnetic resonance imaging (MRI) test, spinal tap, and brain scan. The MRI and brain scan showed a small tumor in an area of the brain where it could be removed rather easily. Mr. Mack's physician, in consultation with a neurosurgeon, felt that an immediate craniotomy with removal of the tumor was required. After explaining the procedure to Mr. Mack, the physicians placed the consent to operate form on his overbed table and gave him a pen. He promptly signed it and gave it back.

Later on that day during her shift assessment, the nurse checked on Mr. Mack. The neighbor who had found him unconscious was visiting at the time. When the nurse asked Mr. Mack whether he was ready for the surgery scheduled for the next morning, he had a blank look on his face. On further questioning, the nurse concluded that Mr. Mack had no idea about what was going to happen to him the next day. The neighbor, who helped Mr. Mack with his bills and other paper work at home, stated: "He'll pretty much sign anything that you put in front of him." At this point the nurse felt that Mr. Mack was incapable of making an informed decision about the craniotomy.

The nurse called both the primary physician and the neurosurgeon about her observations. She was told bluntly that the consent had been signed and that they were going to operate on Mr. Mack the next day for his own good. If she wanted what was best for the client, she would just drop the issue.

Should the nurse just drop the issue? Is there anything she could do to resolve the problem? What ethical principles are involved with this situation?

natural death act, the living will has no mechanism of legal enforcement. Also, when a client travels from one state to another, the legal effect of the living will may be in question. Does the nonresident state have an obligation to honor it?

In some states, a living will is considered only advisory, and the physician has the right to comply with the living will or treat the client as the physician deems most appropriate. There is no protection for nurses or other health-care practitioners against criminal or civil liability in the execution of living wills in states without a natural death act. Once a valid living will exists, it only becomes effective when the person who formulated it meets the qualifications for the natural death act. In most states, the individual must be diagnosed as having a terminal condition where the continuation of treatment and life support would only prolong the client's dying process, but there is no clear consensus on the definition of *terminal condition*.

A Guide for the Care Provider

Despite all these difficulties, living wills are still a good way for a client to make health-care wishes known to health-care providers. Documents that are specific about treatment modalities, are written in a "legal" format, and are signed by two or more witnesses tend to be treated with an increased level of respect by health-care providers (Fig. 8.1).

Nurses can help clients plan ahead for their care should they become unable to make decisions for themselves. Although the nurse should not make the decisions for the client, the nurse can provide important information about the various treatment modalities that the client is considering. The nurse can also help clients clarify their wishes and guide them through the process of formulating an advance directive.

EUTHANASIA AND ASSISTED SUICIDE

Although the term *euthanasia* simply means a "good" or peaceful death, it has taken on the connotation of some type of action that produces death. A distinction needs to be made between passive and active euthanasia. Passive euthanasia usually refers to the practice of allowing an individual to die without any extraordinary intervention. This umbrella definition includes practices such as DNR orders, living wills, and withdrawal of ventilators or other life support.

Active Euthanasia

Active euthanasia usually describes the practice of hastening an individual's death through some act or procedure. This practice is also sometimes referred to as mercy killing and takes many forms ranging from use of large amounts of pain medication for terminal cancer clients to use of poison, a gun, or a knife to end a person's life.

The Case of Dr. Kevorkian

Assisted suicide—brought to public attention by Dr. Jack Kevorkian, a Michigan physician who publicly practiced it for many years—can be considered a type of active euthanasia or mercy killing. The central issue that Dr. Kevorkian demonstrated was whether it is ever ethically permissible for health-care personnel to assist in taking a life. In most states the practice is illegal. The legal definition of homicide—bringing about a person's death or assisting in doing so—seems to fit the act of assisted suicide. In the past, there has been a great deal of hesitation on the part of the legal system to prosecute persons who are involved in assisted suicide or juries to convict physicians who participate in the activity.

> " *The central issue that Dr. Kevorkian demonstrated was whether it is ever ethically permissible for health-care personnel to assist in taking a life.* "

A Killing on TV

In the fall of 1998, Dr. Kevorkian raised the legal and ethical stakes. On a nationally broadcast network news show, *60 Minutes,* he not only admitted to administering a lethal medication to a client without the client's assistance, but he also played a videotape that showed the whole episode.

The client, who had Lou Gehrig's disease (amyotrophic lateral sclerosis), had requested that Dr. Kevorkian help him end his life. The client had signed a **consent** form and release and was even given an extra 2 weeks to "think about it." The client waited only for 3 days before making his final request for the lethal medication.

INSTRUCTIONS	**PENNSYLVANIA DECLARATION**
PRINT YOUR NAME	I, _____, being of sound mind, willfully and voluntarily make this declaration to be followed if I become incompetent. This declaration reflects my firm and settled commitment to refuse life-sustaining treatment under the circumstances indicated below.

I direct my attending physician to withhold or withdraw life-sustaining treatment that serves only to prolong the process of my dying, if I should be in a terminal condition or in a state of permanent unconsciousness.

I direct that treatment be limited to measures to keep me comfortable and to relieve pain, including any pain that might occur by withholding or withdrawing life-sustaining treatment. |
| **CHECK THE OPTIONS WHICH REFLECT YOUR WISHES** | In addition, if I am in the condition described above, I feel especially strongly about the following forms of treatment:

I ( ) do ( ) do not want cardiac resuscitation.
I ( ) do ( ) do not want mechanical respiration.
I ( ) do ( ) do not want tube feeding or any other artificial or invasive form of nutrition (food) or hydration (water).
I ( ) do ( ) do not want blood or blood products.
I ( ) do ( ) do not want any form of surgery or invasive diagnostic tests.
I ( ) do ( ) do not want kidney dialysis.
I ( ) do ( ) do not want antibiotics.

I realize that if I do not specifically indicate my preference regarding any of the forms of treatment listed above, I may receive that form of treatment. |
| **ADD PERSONAL INSTRUCTIONS (IF ANY)** | Other instructions: |
| © 2000 PARTNERSHIP FOR CARING, INC. | |

Figure 8.1 Sample advance directive. Because the laws on advance directives vary widely from state to state, there is no standard advance directive whose language conforms exactly with all states' laws. (Reprinted with permission of Partnership for Caring, formerly Choice in Dying, 200 Varick Street, New York. For more information visit www.partnershipforcaring.org.)

Under Michigan law, Dr. Kevorkian could have been charged with **manslaughter** or even first-degree murder. Dr. Kevorkian admitted that his **motivation** for the act was to be tried under these laws as a test case for active euthanasia. He was arrested 2 weeks later on a charge of first-degree murder; however, he felt very strongly that a jury would not convict him. The trial verdict was guilt of second-degree murder, and he is currently serving a term of 25 years to life in prison. This verdict reinforced the belief of most health-care professionals that mercy killing or assisted suicide is always ethically wrong.

The unfortunate fallout from Dr. Kevorkian's conviction is that many physicians have become even more reluctant to write DNR orders or comply with clients' and/or families' wishes to allow clients to be removed from life support. Clearly they do not understand the distinctions between active and passive euthanasia.

APPOINTING A SURROGATE	**PENNSYLVANIA DECLARATION PAGE 2 OF 2**

Surrogate decisionmaking:

I ( ) do ( ) do not want to designate another person as my surogate to make medical treatment decisions for me if I should be incompetent and in a terminal condition or in a state of permanent unconsciousness.

PRINT THE NAME, ADDRESS AND PHONE NUMBER OF YOUR SURROGATE

Name: _____
Address : _____
Phone: _____

PRINT THE NAME, ADDRESS AND PHONE NUMBER OF YOUR ALTERNATE SURROGATE

Name and address of substitute (if surrogate designated above is unable to serve):

Name: _____
Address: _____
Phone: _____

PRINT THE DATE

I made this declaration on the _____ day of _____ .
                                          (day)   (month, year)

SIGN THE DOCUMENT AND PRINT YOUR ADDRESS

Declarant's signature: _____
Declarant's address: _____

WITNESSING PROCEDURE

The declarant, or the person on behalf of and at the direction of the declarant, knowingly and voluntarily signed this writing by signature or mark in my presence.

YOUR TWO WITNESSES MUST SIGN AND PRINT THEIR ADDRESSES

Witness's signature: _____
Witness's address: _____

Witness's signature: _____
Witness's address: _____

© 2000
PARTNERSHIP
FOR CARING, INC.

Courtesy of **Partnership for Caring, Inc.**   6/96
1620 Eye Street, NW. Suite 202, Washington, DC 20006 800-989-9455

F i g u r e 8 . 1 (*Continued*)

An Issue of Self-Determination

A Last Act of Control?

The fundamental ethical issue in these situations is the right to self-determination. In almost every other health-care situation, a client who is mentally competent can make decisions about what care to accept and what care to refuse. Yet, when it comes to the termination of life, this right becomes controversial. Supporters of the practice of assisted suicide believe that the right to self-determination remains intact, even with regard to the decision to end one's life. It is the last act of a very sick individual to control his or her own fate. Many believe that medical personnel should be allowed to assist clients in this procedure, just as they are allowed to assist clients in other medical and nursing procedures.

An Unacceptable Practice?

Those who oppose assisted suicide find these arguments unconvincing. Legally, ethically, and morally, suicide in U.S. society has never been an accepted practice. Health-care staff go to great lengths to prevent suicidal clients from injuring themselves. In addition, it would seem that individuals in the terminal stages of a disease, who are overwhelmed by pain and depressed by the thought of prolonged suffering, might not be able to think clearly enough to give informed consent for assisted suicide. Also, because the termination of life is final, it does not allow for spontaneous cures or for the development of new treatments or medications.

Nonmaleficence is the term that describes the obligation to do no harm to clients. Whether assisting in or causing the death of a client is a violation of this principle is most likely to be an issue that will continue to be debated for some time. Several states have passed laws permitting assisted suicide, but these states have very strict guidelines. The American Nurses Association (ANA) and other nurses' organizations oppose assisted suicide as a policy and believe that nurses who participate in it are violating the code of ethics.

> *Most acute care facilities will make some exceptions for the treatment of clients with AIDS, for example if the nurse is pregnant, is receiving chemotherapy, or has had other immunity problems. In most situations, however, the nurse is obligated to provide the best nursing care possible for all clients, including those with AIDS.*

HUMAN IMMUNODEFICIENCY VIRUS AND ACQUIRED IMMUNODEFICIENCY SYNDROME

The number of human immunodeficiency virus (HIV) and acquired immunodeficiency syndrome (AIDS) cases continues to rise again in the United States despite educational efforts on its prevention and spread. Several Asian countries are also seeing a recent dramatic increase in cases of HIV/AIDS. In some parts of Africa, it is estimated that as much as 60 percent of the population is infected with the virus.

An Emotional Issue
HIV and AIDS have evoked strong emotions both in the public and in the medical community. Nurses, who for years held strongly to the ethical principle that all clients regardless of race, sex, religion, age, or disease process should be cared for equally, are

questioning their obligation to take care of clients who have AIDS.

The Right to Privacy
Several ethical issues underlie the AIDS controversy. One of the most important is the right to privacy. Although there is a general requirement to report infection with HIV/AIDS to the Centers for Disease Control and Prevention (CDC), many states have strict laws regarding the confidentiality of the diagnosis. Unauthorized revelation of the diagnosis of HIV/AIDS brings the possibility of a lawsuit against the health-care provider or institution. However, the right to privacy is not absolute. Diseases such as tuberculosis, gonorrhea, syphilis, and hepatitis, which are highly contagious and sometimes fatal, must be reported to public health officials.

If the right to privacy can be violated when the public welfare is at stake, does AIDS represent this type of threat? Is it unjust to ask health-care providers to care for clients with this disease without knowing that the client has it? Is it just to violate a client's privacy when the disease carries with it a potential for social stigma and isolation? Does the client have a right to know that a health-care provider is infected with HIV/AIDS?

The Right to Care
Another important ethical issue is the right to care. Can a nurse refuse to care for a client with AIDS? Obviously, a fundamental right of a client is to receive care, and a fundamental obligation of a nurse is to provide care.

The Nurse's Own Interest
The first statement of the ANA Code of Ethics for Nurses is that a nurse must provide care unrestricted by any considerations. Most acute care facilities will make some exceptions for the treatment of clients with AIDS, for example if the nurse is pregnant, is receiving chemotherapy, or has had other immunity problems. In most situations, however, the nurse is obligated to provide the best nursing care possible for all clients, including those with AIDS.

What Cost to Society?
What about the tremendous cost involved in treating individuals who have AIDS? Studies estimate that the medical cost of treating a client with AIDS from the time of diagnosis to the time of death is approximately $900,000.[4] In the face of this crisis, governmental

agencies, which bear the brunt of paying for AIDS treatment, will have to make some difficult decisions concerning this issue. With more than 2 million people already infected with this disease, the cost to society is astronomical.

Nurses have the obligation to care for all clients, including those with AIDS, but ought physicians, hospitals, or governmental agencies also be held to this same precept? Should our society regard health care as a right or a privilege?

ETHICS INVOLVING CHILDREN

Although children are universally acknowledged as the hope of the future, many children remain poorly fed, clothed, housed, and educated and are in dire need of all types of health care, even in affluent countries such as the United States. In the past few years, there has been a marked increase in the reporting of incidents of child neglect and abuse by parents.

The Power of Parents

Our society generally acknowledges the tremendous decision-making power that parents have on behalf of their children; however, there are limits to how parents may decide to act. These limits are sometimes obvious, such as in cases of physical abuse and cruelty to children; however, they may also be less conspicuous, such as in cases of neglect or decisions about withholding medical care for religious reasons. Health-care professionals often find themselves trying to make decisions about the appropriateness of a parent's actions toward a child.

The legal and ethical factors surrounding the decisions that health-care providers must make about child health issues are complicated and sometimes contradictory, ranging from laws about reporting suspected abuse to obtaining permission for treatment. This section focuses on child abuse and the ethical issues that it creates for nurses and the issues of informed consent as it pertains to children.

Issues involving children have always been an important consideration in our society. Whereas the political attention seems to focus on education, drug and alcohol abuse, and child health-care issues, ethical concerns in **pediatrics** are never forgotten and often serve as the unspoken basis for the more visible issues.

Child health ethical issues are numerous and diverse, ranging from mass screening for diseases to withholding permission for treatment.

Child Abuse

Case Study

Emily, who is 8 months old, is brought to the hospital by her 17-year-old unemployed mother, who stated that the baby refused to eat at home and vomited a lot. Emily was very small for her age and was below the growth curve for weight. She was also neurologically introverted and showed little interest in her surroundings. She slept a great deal of time. She was admitted to the hospital with a diagnosis of nonorganic failure to thrive.

During her stay in the hospital, Emily ate well and gained a significant amount of weight. Her neurological status also improved.

One nurse suspected that this was a case of neglect (a form of child abuse) and suggested to the physician that child protective services be notified to evaluate the case. The physician resisted because there was not enough evidence to make a definitive case and thought that it was unfair to the parents to make such a claim. The other nurses felt that by reporting the case they would lose the trust of the mother and cause her to avoid health care for Emily in the future. They also cited a case in which nurses and the hospital were sued when they reported a teenage mother for neglect; the accusation later proved to be false.

Emily was sent home after 3 weeks but was re-admitted 1 month later with the same complaints of poor feeding. She had lost weight since her discharge from the hospital, and she was again neurologically withdrawn. The physician still refused to notify child protective services because of the lack of hard evidence. He thought that an investigation and possible removal of the child from the home was too extreme based on the data available. The nurse still believed that the mother should be reported on the basis of suspicions that could be substantiated legally.

Ethics Regarding Child Abuse

There is a general legal requirement in most states that suspected child abuse must be reported by health-care providers as well as by anyone who suspects that child abuse has occurred. Abuse is more obvious when the child has physical injuries that do not fit the medical history or are atypical for the age group. However, in cases of neglect, the evidence may be very minimal or even nonexistent. Often nurses and physicians who specialize in the care of children rely on their experience in making decisions about reporting or not reporting suspected abuse.

A conflicting ethical principle that is sometimes forgotten in the reporting of suspected child abuse is the family's right to privacy and self-determination. It is an equally fundamental right that Emily's parents be allowed to live their lives according to their own values, free from intrusions.

Decisions about reporting suspected child abuse or neglect rest on the underlying ethical principles of beneficence and protection of the best interests of the child. It is always difficult to decide how far ranging these concerns for "best interest" should be. Physicians tend to focus on solving the immediate problem. Nurses have a more holistic viewpoint and tend to see children in relationship to their environments as well as the environments of the parents. Nurses also tend to think of themselves as saviors, protecting the unfortunate or disadvantaged from a malignant social system and often making value judgments about the lifestyles of others from their middle-class vantage point.

A conflicting ethical principle that is sometimes forgotten in the reporting of suspected child abuse is the family's right to privacy and self-determination. However, when the child is a client in the hospital, beneficence usually outweighs fidelity and veracity.

Resolving The Dilemma

How is the nurse going to resolve this dilemma? Should she report the case and go against the physician's decision? Should she just agree with the physician and defer to his greater experience and better judgment? Should she submit the problem to the hospital ethics committee? Are there any other possible options for action in this case?

It is likely that the physician was correct in his decision about this case, although his ethical reasoning may leave something to be desired. Legally, it is unlikely that there would be sufficient proof to remove the infant from the mother because home monitoring could achieve the same results. Therefore, how can the ethical obligations for the best interest of the child be met?

One very plausible solution is to monitor the child closely through frequent follow-up either at the physician's office or at the local health department. In addition, a follow-up and home evaluation

could be arranged through a home-health-care agency, which could also make available other community resources to help in Emily's care. If the infant continued to fail to gain weight, or if it was later determined that Emily's mother was indeed unable to care adequately for her, the case could then be referred to child protective services.

The role of the nurse who cares for the very young or abused child is one of client advocate. These children need help and protection, and at times, for their very survival, must be taken out of an abusive home setting. Nurses need to be aware of and use all the assets available in these situations, including the police, child protective services, welfare, and home-health-care agencies.

Informed Consent and Children

Case Study

Peter, one of a pair of 7-year-old identical twins, developed a severe bilateral glomerulonephritis after a strep throat infection. The renal involvement was so severe that it did not respond to any medical treatment, and both of his kidneys had to be removed. Paul, Peter's identical twin, was evaluated for kidney donation and, as expected, matched on all six antigens as well as blood type and size. Paul seemed to understand what had happened to his brother and agreed to donate one of his kidneys to keep his brother alive.

However, the children's parents were having some trouble agreeing on whether Paul should donate a kidney to Peter. The twins' mother felt that the donation and transplant should be permitted because it would indeed help keep Peter alive and would also make Paul feel that he was an important part of the process. She argued that if Peter ever did die, Paul would be overcome with guilt knowing that he could have saved his brother but did not.

The twins' father was not as certain about the transplant procedure. He thought that Paul was too young to make a truly free decision of that type and that he did not really understand the serious nature of a kidney removal operation. He thought that Paul, because he was so young, might have been unduly influenced by subtle, yet powerful pressures from his family. No one had directly told Paul that he *must* donate one of his kidneys, yet the fact that his brother's survival may well depend on his decision could have had a major effect on his willingness to donate. Because Peter was being maintained on dialysis and seemed to be doing fairly well, the twins' father thought that he should be put on the transplant list to see whether a suitable nonrelated donor could be found.

The nurses on the unit where Peter was being cared for were equally divided about whether the transplant should be performed. At various times during Peter's lengthy stay in the hospital, they had all been asked by the parents, usually one parent at a time, whether or not they should go ahead with the transplant.

Case Study Analysis
The question, as related to the case study, is, "Does a 7-year-old child have sufficient rational decision-making ability to decide to donate a kidney to his brother?" If, after assessing the child carefully, the answer is "yes," then under the rights-in-trust doctrine, the right to self-determination can be turned over to the child and he can make his own decision. If the answer is "no," then the child should not be permitted to donate the kidney.

There are other ethical principles that can be brought to bear on this decision. From a utilitarian viewpoint, the child should be allowed to donate the kidney, because it would provide the greatest good or happiness for the greatest number of people. Similarly, love-based ethics, or the Golden Rule system of ethical decision making, would also support the donation on the grounds that Paul identifies closely with his brother and appears to understand the issues involved in donation. However, from an egoistic or beneficent viewpoint, because the transplant has little benefit for the donor and will surely cause pain and place him at risk for postoperative complications, the operation should not be permitted.

As with many ethical dilemmas, there is no perfect answer to this situation. The best that can be done is to ensure that the parents and children have as much of the necessary information as possible and support their decisions.

By recognizing the rights of children as individuals, their importance to society is also recognized. However, parents and health-care professionals also have the duty to nurture, support, and guide children

Box 8.3
Determining the Greatest Good

Sherry is an RN who works for a rehabilitation center that deals mainly with developmentally delayed children. For several years, Sherry has been following the case of Margie N, who is now 8 years old and has Down syndrome and moderate retardation. Margie has made steady, if slow, progress in achieving basic motor and cognitive skills but still requires close supervision of all activities and care for all basic hygiene needs. Margie is still not advanced enough to participate in group activities at the center's day clinic.

Mrs. N, Margie's mother, a 42-year-old widow, has been providing a high level of care for Margie at home as well as meeting the child's demands for love and attention. Recently, Mrs. N has been diagnosed with systemic lupus erythematosus (SLE), which has displayed as its primary symptoms severe joint pain and stiffness. During the past several months, Mrs. N has been finding it increasingly difficult to care for Margie because of the progressive nature of the SLE.

Mrs. N is trying to make a decision about long-term care for Margie. She trusts Sherry's judgment completely and often relies on the information and teaching given by the nurse to make changes in Margie's care. Sherry is uncertain about what advice she should give. She recognizes that the high level of care and comfort provided by Mrs. N have been an essential part in the advances Margie has made up to this point, but she also recognizes that Mrs. N may soon reach a point at which that care can no longer be provided. It seems that to do what is good for Mrs. N (i.e., placing Margie in an institution) would be harmful to Margie, whereas doing what is good for Margie (i.e., leaving her at home) would be harmful to Mrs. N. What is the best course of action in this situation? Are there any alternative solutions to this dilemma?

as they grow into adolescence and adulthood. Nurses who work with children are challenged to support their independence by encouraging them to be responsible for and participate in their own health care.

> *Whenever there is an ethical dilemma involving child health-care issues, a three-way relationship develops involving the child, the health-care professional, and the parents.*

Ethical Principles Regarding Child Health Care

One important difference between adults and children that always needs to be included in ethical decisions about child health issues is that children are dependents. As dependents, they generally are not attributed the right to self-determination that is fundamental to adult decision making.

A Three-Way Relationship

Whenever there is an ethical dilemma involving child health-care issues, a three-way relationship develops involving the child, the health-care professional, and the parents. Generally, the parents have the primary role in deciding health-care issues for their under-aged, dependent children based on what they consider to be in the child's best interests.

Current routine child health practices reinforce this principle. Young children are given immunizations and medications, have blood drawn for tests, and even have operations such as tonsillectomies or myringotomies, all without asking for their permission. This exemption to the principle of self-determination in children is based on the belief that young children do not yet have the capacity to make fully rational decisions. Yet, the final expectation for children is that at some point in their lives they develop the capacity to make informed, correct decisions. The primary questions then become, When do they develop this capacity for rational decision making? and How should they be treated until they develop this capacity?

What Do You Think?

If you were the nurse, what would you suggest to the twins' parents? What ethical issues would be involved in your suggestions?

_____

_____

_____

_____

_____

_____

_____

_____

_____

_____

_____

_____

Safeguarding the Child's Rights

The legal system has fixed the age for rational decision making at age 18. Children who are younger than 18 years of age, with a few exceptions, require the permission of the parent for any and all medical procedures. Children older than 18 years of age can make their own decisions about health care.

The difficulty with fixing an age is that it is arbitrary and does not reflect the reality of the individual child's development. From experience it can be observed that many children who are 9 or 10 years old exhibit rather advanced and adult-like decision-making skills, whereas other children who may be 18 or 19 years of age display a marked lack of this ability.

The more serious question, however, is, How should underaged children be treated? One solution is to deny, because of their age, that they have rights and then treat them as being incompetent by bringing to bear paternalistic, best-interest interventions. Another approach is to say that children do have the same rights as adults except that these rights are temporarily suspended until the child is sufficiently mature to exercise them. This is called rights-in-trust, and the rights are turned over to the child at the appropriate time. The question then becomes, When is the appropriate time?

One approach is to turn over all the rights to the child at the same time, for example, when he or she reaches 18 years of age. Another approach is to gradually release individual rights as the child grows older and is prepared to exercise them. In either case, appropriate adults, including nurses, have the role of safeguarding the child's rights and act as guardians, protectors, and advocates of the children under their care.

Conclusion

Ethical issues are a factor in the daily practice of all nurses. Any time a nurse comes in contact with a client, a potential ethical situation exists. In today's world, with rapidly advancing technology and unusual health-care situations, ethical dilemmas are proliferating. Nurses can be prepared to deal with most of these dilemmas if they keep current with the issues and are able to follow a systematic process for making ethical decisions. At some point, difficult decisions must be made, and we should not avoid making them. One of the worst elements of ethical decision making is that it is very unlikely that everyone involved in the dilemma will be happy with the decision. However, if the decision is made after the situation has been analyzed and if it is on the basis of sound ethical principles, it can usually be defended.

Issues in Practice

Case Study in Ethics

Analyze the following case study using the ethical decision-making process:

Ms. Sally Jones, RN, a public health nurse for a rural health department, was preparing to visit Mr. Weems, a 58-year-old client who was recently diagnosed with chronic bronchitis and emphysema. Mr. Weems was unemployed as a result of a farming accident and had been previously diagnosed with hypertension and extreme obesity. Ms. Jones was making this visit to see why Mr. Weems had missed his last appointment at the clinic and whether he was taking his prescribed antibiotics and antihypertensive medications.

As Ms. Jones pulled up in the driveway of his house, she noticed Mr. Weems sitting on the front porch smoking a cigarette. She felt a surge of anger, which she quickly suppressed, as she wondered why she spent so much of her limited time teaching him about the health consequences of smoking.

During the visit, Ms. Jones determined that Mr. Weems had stopped taking both his antihypertensive and antibiotic medications and rarely took his expectorants and bronchodilators. He coughed continuously, had a blood pressure of 196/122, and had severely congested lung sounds. Mr. Weems listened politely as Ms. Jones explained again about the need to stop smoking and the importance of taking his medications as prescribed. She also scheduled another appointment at the clinic in 1 week for follow-up.

As she drove away to her next visit, Ms. Jones wondered about the ethical responsibilities of nurses who must provide care for clients who do not seem to care about their own health. Mr. Weems took little responsibility for his health, refused to even try to stop smoking or lose weight, and did not take his medications. She wondered whether there was a limit to the amount of nursing care a noncompliant client should expect from a community health agency. She reflected that the time spent with Mr. Weems would have been spent much more productively screening children at a local grade school or working with mothers of newborn infants.

Critical Thinking Exercises

- What data are important in relation to this situation?
- State the ethical dilemma in a clear, simple statement.
- What are the choices of action and how do they relate to specific ethical principles?
- What are the consequences of these actions?
- What decisions can be made?

References

1. Hook, C: Primer on medical genomics part XIII: Ethical and regulatory issues. Mayo Clinic Practice 79(5): 645–650, 2004.
2. Terzioglu, F: Nurses' views on their role in genetics. JOGNN, 33(6):756–764, 2004.
3. Heller, BR, et al.: 10 Trends to watch. Nursing and Health Care Perspectives 24(1):9–14, 2002.
4. Goode, A: Schiavo case should prompt discussin about health care wishes. Oklahoma City Nursing Times 43(4):15, 2003.
5. Stinson, C, et al.: Ethical dilemma: Voluntary stoppping of eating and drinking. Dimensions of Critical Care Nursing 23(1):38–43, 2004.
6. Pieknik, R: DNR: The ethics of resuscitation. Surgical Technology 36(4):12–22, 2004.

Bibliography

Berger, J: Ethical challenges of partial do-not-resuscitate (DNR) orders: Placing DNR orders in the context of a life-threatening conditions care plan. Arch Intern Med 163(19):2270–2275, 2003.

Clendinen, D: "My father wasn't there" The care of Terri Schiavo has universal and personal resonance. The New York Times, October 26, 2003, 12.

Conway A: Ethical issues in the neonatal intensive care unit. Critical Care Nursing Clinics of North America 16(2):271–278, 2004.

Engelhardt, HT, and Cherry, MJ: Allocating Scarce Resources. Georgetown University Press, Baltimore, 2002.

Ewing, A, and Catlin, A: Pediatric ethics, issues, & commentary. Pediatric Nursing 30(6):471–472, 2004.

Fontanarosa, P: Controversies: Surrogate consent for living related organ donation. JAMA 291(6):728–731, 2004.

Grace, P: Patient safety and the limits of confidentiality. AJN 104(11):33–37, 2004.

Jenkins, J: Ethical implications of genetic information. Online Journal of Issues in Nursing February 9, 2001.

Horner, S. Ethics and genetics: Implications for CNS practice. Clinical Nurse Specialist 18(5):228–231, 2004.

Husted, G: When is a health care system not an ethical health care system? Suspending the do-not-resuscitate order in the operating room. Critical Care Nursing Clinics of North America 12(2): 157–163, 2004.

Koppelman, E: The dead donor rule and the concept of death: Severing the ties that bind them. American Journal of Bioethics 3(1):1–9, 2003.

McNeil, D: Vegetative or minimally conscious? The New York Times, October 26, 2003.

Offit, K, and Gostin, L: Health law and ethics: The "duty to warn" a patient's family members about hereditary disease risks. JAMA 292(12):146914–73, 2004.

Paul, R, and Elder, L: Ethical Reasoning. The Foundation for Critical Thinking, 2003 (www.crticalthinking.org).

Rushton, C, and Ferrell, B: Ethics and palliative care in pediatrics: When should parents agree to withdraw life-sustaining therapy for children? AJN 104(4):54–64, 2004.

9

Nursing Law and Liability

Mary Evans and Tonia Aiken

Learning Objectives

After completing this chapter, the reader will be able to:

- Distinguish between statutory law and common law.
- Differentiate civil law from criminal law.
- Explain the legal principles involved in:

  Unintentional torts

  Intentional torts

  Quasi-intentional torts

  Informed consent

  Do-not-resuscitate (DNR) orders
- Describe the trial process.
- List methods to prevent litigation.
- Identify the elements in delegation.

THE LEGAL SYSTEM

For many nurses, the mere mention of the word *lawsuit* provokes a high level of anxiety. At first glance, the legal system often seems to be a large and confusing entity whose intricacies are designed to entrap the uninitiated. Many nurses feel that even a minor error in client care will lead to huge settlements against them and loss of their nursing license. In reality, even though the number of lawsuits against nurses has been increasing since the early 1990s, the number of nurses who are actually sued remains relatively small.

It is important to remember that the legal system is just one element of the health-care system. Laws are rules to help protect people and to keep society functioning. The ultimate goal of all laws is to promote peaceful and productive interactions between and among the people of that society.

An understanding of basic legal principles will augment the quality of care that the nurse delivers. In our litigious society, it is important to comprehend how the law affects the profession of nursing and the individual nurse's daily practice.

SOURCES OF LAW

There are two major sources of laws in the United States: statutory law and common law (Box 9.1). Most laws that govern nursing are state-level statutory laws because licensure is a function of the state's authority.

Statutory Law

Statutory law consists of laws written and enacted by the U.S. Congress, the state legislatures, and other governmental entities such as cities, counties, and townships. Legislated laws enacted by the U.S.

Box 9.1
Division and Types of Law

I. Statutory Law
A. Criminal Law
   1. Misdemeanor
   2. Felony
B. Civil Law
   1. Tort Law
      a. Unintentional tort
      b. Intentional tort
      c. Quasi-intentional tort
   2. Contract Law
   3. Treaty Law
   4. Tax Law
   5. Other

II. Common Law
A. Criminal Law
   1. Misdemeanor
   2. Felony
B. Civil Law
   1. Tort Law
      a. Unintentional tort
      b. Intentional tort
      c. Quasi-intentional tort
   2. Contract Law
   3. Treaty Law
   4. Tax Law
   5. Other

Congress are called federal **statutes.** State-drafted laws are called state statutes. Individual cities and municipalities have legislative bodies that draft **ordinances,** codes, and regulations at their respective levels.

The laws that govern the profession of nursing are statutory laws. Most of these laws are written at the state level, because licensure is a responsibility of the individual states. These laws include the nurse practice act, which establishes the state board of nursing, individual licensure procedures, and schedule of fees for the state.

Common Law

Common law is different from statutory law in that it has evolved from the decisions of previous legal cases that form a **precedent.** These laws represent the accumulated results of the judgments and decrees that have been handed down by courts of the United States and Great Britain through the years.

Common law often extends beyond the scope of statutory law. For example, no statutes require a person who is negligent and causes injury to another to compensate that person for the injury. Court decisions that have addressed the same legal issues over and over, such as negligence, however, have repeatedly ruled that the injured person should receive compensation. The way in which each case is resolved creates a precedent, or pattern, for dealing with the same legal issue in the future. The common laws involving negligence or malpractice are most frequently encountered by the nurse.

Common law or case law is law that has developed over a long period. The principle of *stare decisis* requires a judge to make decisions similar to those that have been handed down in previous cases if the facts of the cases are identical. Common law decisions are published in bound legal reports. Generally speaking, common law deals with matters outside the scope of laws enacted by the legislature.

DIVISIONS OF LAW

In the U.S. legal system, there are many divisions in the law. A major example of such a division is the difference between criminal law and civil law, either of which may be statutory or common in origin.

Criminal Law

A System of Protection
Criminal laws are concerned with providing protection for all members of society. When someone is accused of violating a criminal law, the government at the county, city, state, or federal level imposes punishments appropriate to the type of **crime.** Criminal law involves a wide range of **malfeasance,** from minor traffic violations to murder.

Although most criminal law is created and regulated by the government through the enactment of statutes, a small portion falls under the common law. Statutes are developed and enacted by the legislature (state or federal) and approved by the executive branch, such as a governor or the president. Criminal law is further classified into two types of offenses: (1) **misdemeanors,** which are minor criminal offenses, and (2) **felonies,** which are major criminal offenses.

In the criminal law system, an individual accused of a crime is called the defendant. The prosecuting attorney represents the people of the city, county, state, or federal jurisdiction who are accusing the individual of a crime. A **criminal action** is rendered when the person charged with the crime is brought to trial and convicted. Penalties or sanctions are imposed on the violators of criminal law and are based on the scope of the crime. They can involve a range of punishment from community service work and fines to imprisonment and death.

> *The most common violation by nurses of the criminal law is through failure to renew nursing licenses. In this situation, the nurse is in effect practicing nursing without a license, which is a crime in all states.*

What Do You Think?

Do you know anyone who has filed a malpractice suit or a health-care provider who was the defendant in a malpractice suit? What was the situation that caused the case? How was it resolved? If you have never been involved with a malpractice suit or do not know anyone who has, how would you feel if a lawsuit were to be brought against you?

_____

_____

_____

_____

_____

_____

_____

_____

_____

_____

_____

_____

_____

_____

The Nurse's Involvement

Nurses can become involved with the criminal system in their nursing practice in several ways. The most common violation by nurses of the criminal law is through failure to renew nursing licenses. In this situation, the nurse is in effect practicing nursing without a license, which is a crime in all states.

Nurses also become involved with the illegal diversion of drugs, particularly narcotics, from the hospital. This is a more serious crime, which may lead to imprisonment. Recent cases involving intentional or unintentional deaths of clients and assisted suicide cases have also led to criminal action against nurses.

Civil Law

Nurses are much more likely to become involved in civil lawsuits than in criminal violations. **Civil laws** generally deal with the violation of one individual's rights by another individual. The court provides the forum that enables these individuals to have their disputes resolved by an independent third party, such as a judge or a jury of the defendant's peers.

The individual who brings the dispute to the court is called the **plaintiff.** The formal written document that describes the dispute and the resolution sought is called the complaint. The individual against whom the complaint is filed is called the **defendant,** who, in conjunction with his attorney, prepares the **answer** to the complaint. In civil cases, the **burden of proof** rests with the plaintiff.

Civil law has many branches, including contract law, treaty law, tax law, and tort law. It is under the tort law that most nurses become involved with the legal system.

Tort Law

A **tort** is generally defined as a wrongful act committed against a person or his or her property independent of a contract. A person who commits a tort is called the **tort-feasor** and is **liable** for **damages** to those who are affected by the person's actions. The word *tort,* derived from the Latin *tortus* (twisted), is a French word for injury or wrong. Torts can involve several different types of actions, including a direct violation of a person's legal rights or a violation of a standard of care that causes injury to a person. Torts are classified as unintentional, intentional, or quasi-intentional.

Unintentional Torts

Negligence

Negligence is the primary form of **unintentional tort. Negligence** is generally defined as the **omission** of an act that a reasonable and prudent person would perform in a similar situation or the commission of something a reasonable person would not do in that situation. **Nonfeasance** is a type of negligence that occurs when a person fails to perform a legally required duty.[1]

Malpractice

Malpractice is a type of negligence for which professionals can be sued (professional negligence). Because of their professional status, nurses are held to a higher standard of conduct than the ordinary layperson. The standard for nurses is what a reasonable and prudent nurse would do in the same situation: "A registered nurse is charged with utilizing the degree and skill and judgment commensurate with his or her education, experience, and position."[2]

For instance, it is reasonable and prudent that the nurse put the side rails up on the bed of a client who had just received an injection of a narcotic pain medication, because the drug causes drowsiness and sometimes confusion. If the nurse gave an injection of a narcotic medication but forgot to put the side rails up, and the client fell out of bed and fractured his hip, the nurse can be sued for the negligent act of forgetting to put the side rail up.

> *Because of their professional status, nurses are held to a higher standard of conduct than the ordinary layperson.*

Four elements are required for a person to make a claim of negligence:

1. A duty was owed to the client (professional relationship).
2. The professional violated the **duty** and failed to conform to the standard of care (breach of duty).
3. The failure to act by the professional was the **proximate cause** of the resulting injuries (causality).

4. Actual injuries resulted from the breach of duty (damages).

If any of these elements are missing from the case, the client will probably not be able to win the lawsuit (Box 9.2).

Case Study

Consider the following situation:

Mr. Fagin, a 78-year-old client, was admitted from a nursing home for the treatment of a fractured tibia after he fell out of bed. After the fracture was reduced, a fiberglass cast was applied, and Mr. Fagin was sent to the orthopedic unit for follow-up care. While making her 0400 rounds, the night charge nurse (a registered nurse [RN]) discovered that Mr. Fagin's foot on the casted leg was cold to touch, looked bluish-purple, and was swollen approximately $1\frac{1}{2}$ times normal size. The nurse noted these findings in the client's chart and relayed the information to the day shift nurses during the 0630 shift report.

The charge nurse on the day shift promptly called and relayed the findings to Mr. Fagin's physician. The physician, however, did not seem to be concerned and only told the nurse to "Keep a close eye on him, and don't bother me again unless it is an absolute emergency." A short time later, Mr. Fagin became agitated, complained of severe pain in the affected foot, and eventually began yelling uncontrollably. The charge nurse called the emergency room (ER) physician to come to check on the client. The ER physician immediately removed the cast and noted an extensive circulatory impairment that would not respond to treatment. A few days later, Mr. Fagin's leg was amputated. His family filed a malpractice lawsuit against the hospital, the physician, and both the night and day charge nurses.

Are all the elements present in this case for a bona fide lawsuit? What could have been done to prevent this situation from happening? How should nurses deal with reluctant or hostile physicians?

Professional Misconduct

Malpractice is more serious than mere negligence because it indicates professional misconduct or

Box 9.2

Malpractice Considerations

Nursing malpractice is based on the legal premise that a nurse can be held legally responsible for the personal injury of another individual if it can be proven that the injury was the result of negligence.[2] Nursing malpractice is based on four elements: (1) duty, (2) breach of duty, (3) causation (the "but for" test), and (4) damage or injury.

Inappropriate work assignment and inadequate supervision are a breach of duty and could be the basis for finding a nurse's actions to be negligent. Failure or breach of duty to delegate is established by proving that a reasonably prudent nurse would not have made a particular assignment or delegated a certain responsibility or that supervision was inadequate under the circumstances.

The act of improper delegation of tasks or inadequate supervision must be evaluated in light of the "but for" test related to the injury. If the person who performed the injurious act had not been assigned or delegated to perform the task, or had been adequately supervised, the injury could have been avoided. Consequently, the nurse is not being held liable for the negligent act of her subordinate, *but for the lack of competence in performing the independent duties of delegation and supervision.*

Off-site Consideration

Registered nurses who practice in public health, community, or home care settings must rely frequently on written or telephone communication when delegating patient care duties to assistive personnel. The nurse who must supervise from off site has a particular duty to assess the knowledge, skills, and judgment of the assistive personnel before assignments are made. Regular supervisory visits and impeccable documentation will help the registered nurse ensure that care provided by assistive personnel is adequate.

Source: Aiken, TD: Legal, Ethical, and Political Issues in Nursing. FA Davis, Philadelphia, 1994.

unreasonable lack of skill in performing professional duties. Malpractice suggests the existence of a professional standard of care and a deviation from that standard of care. A professional **expert witness** is often asked to testify in a malpractice case to help establish the standard of care to which the professional should be held accountable.

A 1988 case in South Dakota presents an example of nursing malpractice. The nurse failed to question the physician's order to discharge a client when she discovered that the client had a fever. In this case, a supervisory nurse provided expert testimony and reported to the judge that the general standard of care for nurses is to report a significant change in a client's condition, such as an elevated temperature. It is the nurse's responsibility to question the physician's order as to appropriateness of discharge.

The records on this case indicated that the client's elevated temperature was charted after the physician had completed his rounds. The nurse did not notify the physician of the client's fever, and the client was subsequently discharged. The client was

readmitted a short time after discharge and died in the hospital. The nurse was found negligent. The court held that negligence can be determined by failure to act as well as by the commission of an act.

Many other types of actions by nurses can produce malpractice lawsuits. Some of the more common actions include:

- Leaving foreign objects inside a client during surgery
- Failing to follow a hospital standard or protocol
- Not using equipment in accordance with the manufacturer's recommendations
- Failing to listen to and respond to client's complaints
- Not properly documenting phone conversations and orders from physicians
- Failure to question physician orders when indicated (e.g., too large medication dosages, inappropriate diets, etc.)
- Failing to clarify poorly written or illegible physician orders
- Failing to assess and observe a client as directed
- Failing to obtain a proper informed consent
- Failing to report a change in a client's condition, such as vital signs, circulatory status, and level of consciousness
- Failing to report another health-care provider's **incompetency** or negligence
- Failing to take actions to provide for a client's safety, such as not cleaning up a liquid spill on the floor that causes a client to fall
- Failing to provide a client with sufficient and appropriate education before discharge

If the Nurse Is Liable

If a nurse is found guilty of malpractice, several types of actions may be taken against the nurse. The nurse may be required to provide monetary compensation to the client for general damages that were a direct result of the injury, including pain, suffering, disability, and disfigurement. In addition, the nurse is often required to pay for special damages that resulted from the injury, such as all involved medical expenses, **out-of-pocket expenses,** and wages lost by the client while he or she was in the hospital.

Optional damages, including those for emotional distress, mental suffering, and counseling expenses that were an outgrowth of the initial injury, may be added to the total settlement. If the client is able to prove that the nurse acted with conscious disregard for the client's safety or acted in a malicious,

willful, or wanton manner that produced injury, then an additional assessment of punitive or exemplary damages may be added to the award.

Intentional Torts

An **intentional tort** is generally defined as a willful act that violates another person's rights or property. Intentional torts can be distinguished from malpractice and acts of negligence by the following three requirements: (1) the nurse must intend to bring about the consequences of the act, (2) the nurse's act must be intended to interfere with the client or the client's property, and (3) the act must be a substantial factor in bringing about the injury or consequences.

The most frequently encountered intentional torts are assault, battery, false imprisonment, abandonment, and intentional infliction of emotional distress. With intentional torts, the injured person does not have to prove that an injury has occurred, nor is the opinion of an expert witness required for adjudication. Punitive damages are more likely to be assessed against the nurse in intentional tort cases, and some intentional torts may fall under the criminal law if there is gross violation of the standards of care.

Assault and Battery

Assault is the unjustifiable attempt to touch another person or the threat of doing so. **Battery** is actual harmful or unwarranted contact with another person without his or her consent. Battery is the most common intentional tort seen in the practice of nursing.

For a nurse to commit assault and battery, there must be an absence of consent on the part of the client. Before any procedure can be performed on a competent, alert, and normally oriented client, the client must agree or consent to the procedure being done. Negligence does not have to be proved for a person to be successful in a claim for assault and battery.

A common example of an assault and battery occurs when a nurse physically restrains a client against the client's will and administers an injection against the client's wishes.

False Imprisonment

False imprisonment occurs when a competent client is confined or restrained with intent to prevent him or her from leaving the hospital. The use of restraints alone does not constitute false imprisonment when they are used to maintain the safety of a confused, disoriented, or otherwise incompetent client. In general, mentally impaired clients can be detained against their will only if they are a threat to injure themselves or others. The use of threats or medications that interfere with the client's ability to leave the facility can also be considered false imprisonment.

Intentional Infliction of Emotional Distress

Intentional infliction of emotional distress is another common intentional tort encountered by the nurse. To prove this intentional tort, the following three elements are necessary: (1) conduct exceeds what is usually accepted by society, (2) the health-care provider's conduct is intended to cause mental distress, and (3) the conduct actually does produce mental distress (causation). Any nurse who is charged with assault, battery, or false imprisonment is also at risk for being charged with infliction of emotional distress.

A 1975 case is an example of infliction of emotional distress. In *Johnson v. Women's Hospital,* a mother wished to view the body of her baby who had died during birth. After she made the request, she was handed the baby's body floating in a gallon jar of formaldehyde.[1] The Johnson case demonstrates a clear lack of respect shown to the mother. If the mother in this delicate situation had been treated with dignity and respect, the situation would have been avoided.

Client Abandonment

Because of the ongoing nursing shortage, **abandonment** of clients has become an important legal and ethical issue for health-care providers. Abandonment occurs when there is a unilateral severance of the professional relationship with the client without adequate notice and while the requirement for care still exists. The nurse–client relationship continues until it is terminated by mutual consent of both parties.

From an ethical standpoint, the issue of abandonment falls under the umbrella of beneficence. From the legal view, client abandonment can be considered an intentional tort, breach of contract, or in some cases where injury occurs, malpractice. The key phrase to keep in mind when discussing client abandonment is "without adequate notice." If the client knows that the nurse's shift is scheduled to end at 7:00 P.M., then the client as well as the hospital both have adequate notice.

It is not uncommon for nurses in today's health-care system to be approached by nursing supervisors with the statement, "Everyone else called in, so you will have to work a double shift or you could be charged with client abandonment." In this case, the abandonment becomes the hospital's responsibility, not the nurse's. Nurses sometimes feel uncomfortable about going on strike because it seems to imply client abandonment; however, if there is adequate notice about the strike and the facility has had time to make arrangements for care or discharge of clients, then there is no client abandonment. The growing practice of emergency client diversion that occurs when facilities can no longer safely care for emergency clients as the result of lack of space or staffing has the potential to fall under the legal definitions of abandonment.

Quasi-Intentional Torts

A **quasi-intentional tort** is a mixture of unintentional and intentional torts. It is defined as a voluntary act that directly causes injury or distress without intent to injure or to cause distress. A quasi-intentional tort does have the elements of volition and causation without the element of intent. Quasi-intentional torts usually involve situations of communication and often violate a person's reputation, personal privacy, or civil rights.

Defamation of Character

Defamation of character, which is the most common of the quasi-intentional torts, is harmful to a person's reputation. Defamation injures a person's reputation by diminishing the esteem, respect, good will, or confidence that others have for the person. It can be especially damaging when false statements are made about a criminal act or an immoral act or when there are false allegations about a client's having a contagious disease. In *Schessler v. Keck* (1954), a nurse was found liable for defamation of character when she told a friend that a caterer for whom she was caring was being treated for syphilis. Even though the statement was false, when the information became public, it destroyed his catering business.[1]

Defamation includes **slander,** which is spoken communication in which one person discusses another in terms that harm that person's reputation. **Libel** is a written communication in which a person makes statements or uses language that harms another person's reputation. To win a defamation lawsuit

Box 9.3

Registered Nurse Licensure

The legislature of each state enacts laws that govern the practice of nursing. The purpose of licensing law is to ensure that the public is protected from unqualified practitioners by developing and enforcing regulations that define who may practice in the profession, the scope of that practice, and the level of education for the profession.

A fundamental premise of nursing practice is that a professional nurse is personally responsible for all acts or omissions undertaken within the scope of practice. The American Nurses Association defines delegation as "the transfer of responsibility for the performance of an activity from one person to another while retaining accountability for the outcome."[1] Additionally, the nurse is responsible for the adequate supervision of a delegated task to a subordinate. If the nurse fails to delegate appropriately or supervise adequately, any injuries resulting from the acts of the subordinate may result in licensure ramifications. The state licensing board may take disciplinary actions.

against the nurse, the client must prove that the nurse acted maliciously, abused the principle of **privileged communication,** and wrote or spoke a lie.

Medical record documentation is a primary source of defamation of character. Through the years, the client's chart has been the basis of many defamation lawsuits. Discussion about a client in the elevators, cafeteria, and other public areas can also lead to lawsuits for defamation if negative comments are overheard.

Invasion of Privacy

Invasion of privacy is a violation of a person's right to protection against unreasonable and unwarranted interference with one's personal life. To prove that invasion of privacy has occurred, the client must show that (1) the nurse intruded on the client's seclusion and privacy, (2) the intrusion is objectionable to a reasonable and prudent person, (3) the act committed intrudes on private or published facts or pictures of a private nature, and (4) public disclosure of private information was made.[3] Examples of invasion of privacy include using the client's name or picture for the sole advantage of the health-care provider, intruding into the client's private affairs without permission, giving out private client information over the telephone, and publishing information that misrepresents the client's condition. The Health Insurance Portability and Accountability Act (HIPAA) of 1996, which is now fully implemented, has added some additional confusion to the issue of confidentiality in the health-care setting.

Breach of Confidentiality

Privileged Communication

Confidentiality of information concerning the client must be honored. A breach of confidentiality results when a client's trust and confidence are violated by public revelation of confidential or privileged communications without the client's consent. Privileged communication is protected by law and exists in certain well-defined professional relationships, for example physician–client, psychiatrist–client, priest–penitent, and lawyer–client.

Privileged communication ensures that the professional who obtains any information from the client cannot be forced to reveal that information, even in a court of law under oath. Nurses do not have privileged communication with clients. However, they can be bound, by extension, under the seal of privileged communication if they are in a room with a physician when the client reveals personal information.

Most breach of confidentiality cases involve a physician's revelation of privileged communications shared by a client. Nurses who overhear privileged communication or information, however, are held to the same standards as a physician with regard to that information.

Privileged client information can only be disclosed if it is authorized by the client. In accord with the recently enacted HIPAA regulations, all health-care facilities must have specific guidelines dealing with client information disclosure. Disclosure of information to family members violates

HIPAA regulations unless the client is under 18 years of age or gives permission to do so. For instance, a client may not wish to disclose to a family member a specific diagnosis, such as cancer. If this is the case, the nurse should honor this request; otherwise, it is considered a violation of HIPAA regulations.

Electronic Pitfalls

Use of computerized documentation and telemedicine have led to several lawsuits based on breach of confidentiality and malpractice. (See Chapter 18 for examples.) The HIPAA regulations are the government's attempts to force the legal system to keep pace with the use of computers and electronic record keeping. Cases exist in which medical records have been lost because of computer failure.

Other issues, such as correction of errors in **charting,** are complicated by use of computers. On paper charts, health-care providers had to draw a line through the erroneous entry, initial the entry, and date it. With computerized charting, simply hitting the delete button will completely erase all evidence of an incorrect entry.

FACING A LAWSUIT

Because of the rapid proliferation of lawsuits since the 1990s, there is now a higher probability that a nurse, at some time in his or her career, will be involved either as a witness or as a party to a nursing malpractice action. Knowledge of the litigation process increases nurses' understanding of the way in which their conduct is evaluated before the courts.

Knowledge of the litigation process increases nurses' understanding of the way in which their conduct is evaluated before the courts.

The Statute of Limitations

A malpractice suit against a nurse for negligence must be filed within a specified time. This period, called the **statute of limitations,** generally begins at the time of the injury or when the injury is discovered and lasts until some specified future time. In most states, the limitation period lasts from 1 to 6 years, with the most common duration being 2 years. However, in cases involving children, the statute of limitations extends until the person reaches 21 years of age. If the client fails to file the suit within the prescribed time, the lawsuit will be barred.

The Complaint

Filing the suit (also called the complaint) with the court begins the litigation process. The written complaint describes the incident that initiated the claim of negligence against the nurse. Specific allegations, including the amount of money sought for damages, are also stated in the **legal complaint.** The plaintiff, who is usually a client or a family member of a client, is the alleged injured party, and the defendant (i.e., the nurse, physician, or hospital) is the person or entity being sued. The first notice of a lawsuit occurs when the defendant (nurse) is officially notified or served with the complaint. All defendants are accorded the right of **due process** under constitutional law.

The Answer

The defendant must respond to the allegations stated in the complaint within a specific time frame. This written response by the defendant is called the answer. If the nurse had liability insurance in force at the time of the negligent act, the insurer will assign a lawyer to represent the defendant nurse. In the answer, the nurse can outline specific defenses to the claims against him or her.

The Discovery

After the complaint and answer are filed with the court, the discovery phase of the litigation begins. The purpose of discovery is to uncover all information relevant to the malpractice suit and the incident in question. The nurse may be required to answer a series of questions that relate to the nurse's educational background and emotional state, the incident that led to the lawsuit, and any other information the plaintiff's lawyer deems important. These written questions are called **interrogatories.**

In addition, the plaintiff's lawyer may seek requests for production of documents. These are documents related to the lawsuit, including the plaintiff's medical records, **incident reports, card file,** the institution's policy and procedure manual concerning the specific situation, and the nurse's job description. The plaintiff is also required to disclose information as part of the discovery process that includes the plaintiff's past medical history.

The Deposition

The next step in the process is the taking of a deposition from each party to the lawsuit, as well as any potential witnesses, to assist the lawyers in the trial preparation. A **deposition** is a formal legal process that involves the taking of testimony under oath and is recorded by a court reporter. These are usually wide-ranging in scope and often include information not allowed in a trial, such as **hearsay** testimony. In some cases, videotaped depositions may be used. Nurses can prepare for a deposition by keeping some key points in mind (Box 9.4).

The deposition **testimony** is reduced to a written document called an **affidavit** for use at trial. If a witness during the trial changes testimony from that given at the deposition, the deposition can be used to contradict the testimony. This process is called impeaching the witness. Impeaching a witness

on a specific issue can create doubt about that witness's credibility and can thus weaken other areas in the witness's testimony. In some situations, witnesses can later be charged with **perjury** if it is proved that they gave false testimony under oath.

The Trial

The **trial** often takes place years after the complaint was filed. Once **jurisdiction** is determined, the *voir dire* process, more commonly called jury selection, begins. After jury selection, each attorney presents opening statements. The plaintiff's side is presented first. Witnesses may be served with **subpoenas** that require them to appear and provide testimony.

Each witness or party is subject to direct examination, cross-examination, and redirect examination. Direct examination involves open-ended questions by the attorney. Cross-examination is performed by the opposing lawyer, and questions are asked in such a way as to elicit short, specific

Box 9.4

Giving a Deposition

1. Do not volunteer information.
2. Be familiar with the client's medical record and nurse's notes.
3. Remain calm throughout the process and do not be intimidated by the lawyers.
4. Clarify all questions before answering; ask the lawyer to explain the question if you do not understand.
5. Do not make assumptions about the questions.
6. Do not exaggerate answers.
7. Wait at least 5 seconds after a question is asked before answering it to allow objections from other lawyers.
8. Tell the truth.
9. Do not speculate about answers.
10. Speak slowly and clearly, using professional language as much as possible.
11. Look the questioning lawyer in the eye as much as possible.
12. If unable to remember an answer, simply state "I don't remember" or "I don't know."
13. Think before answering any question.
14. Bring a resume or curriculum vitae to the deposition in case it is requested.
15. Request a break if you are tired or confused.
16. Avoid becoming angry with the lawyers or using sarcastic language.
17. Avoid using absolutes in the answers.
18. If a question is asked more than once, ask the court recorder to read the answer given previously.
19. Be sure to read over the deposition just before the trial.

Source: Aiken, TJ, and Catalano, JT: Legal, Ethical, and Political Issues in Nursing. FA Davis, Philadelphia, 1994.

responses. The redirect examination consists of follow-up questions to address issues that were raised during the cross-examination.

After both parties have presented their case, the lawyers deliver their closing arguments. The case then goes to a jury or a judge for deliberation. If the facts are not in dispute, the judge may render a **summary judgment.** The decision or ruling made about the case can be appealed if either party is not satisfied. The party appealing the decision is called the **appellant.**

POSSIBLE DEFENSES TO A MALPRACTICE SUIT

Contributory Negligence

Damages awarded vary from one state to another and also with the types of injuries sustained. In a state with contributory negligence laws, clients are not allowed to receive money for injuries if they contributed to that injury in any manner. For example, the nurse forgot to raise the bed rail after administering an injection of a narcotic pain medication to a client who had an operation but instructed the client to turn on the call light if he wanted to get out of bed. The client fell while attempting to go to the bathroom; because he did not use the call light, he contributed to his own injuries and thus could not receive compensation.

Comparative Negligence

In a state with comparative negligence laws, the awards are based on the determination of the percentage of fault by both parties. For example, in the afore-

mentioned case, if $100,000 was awarded by the jury, it may be determined that the nurse was 75 percent at fault and the client was 25 percent at fault. In that case, the client would receive $75,000. In general, if the client is 50 percent or more at fault, no award will be made. As can be seen, determination of these types of awards is highly subjective, and an **appeal** about the decision is often made to a higher court.

Case Study

Consider the following case:

Ms. Gouge, a 44-year-old client who weighs 307 lb, was admitted to a large university medical center ER with complaints of chest pain and disorientation and a blood pressure of 208/154. She also displayed aphasia, hemiplegia, and loss of sensation and movement on her right side.

After a magnetic resonance imaging (MRI) scan of the head, it was discovered that she had a nonoperative cerebral aneurysm. In addition to appropriate medical treatment for blood pressure and circulation, her family physician told her that she had to lose a significant amount of weight. The nurse in the physician's office instituted a weight loss teaching plan for Ms. Gouge, planned out a calorie-restricted low-fat diet, and gave her a large amount of information about healthy diet and a videotape of low-impact aerobic exercises. At a follow-up visit 1 month later, Ms. Gouge weighed 315 lb.

Six months later, Ms. Gouge's aneurysm ruptured, leaving her in a vegetative state.

Ms. Gouge's family filed a lawsuit against the physician and his office nurse claiming that they had failed to institute proper and appropriate preventive measures and that they had failed to inform the client of the seriousness of her condition.

Did the nurse's decisions or actions contribute to the filing of this suit? Is there any contributory negligence? What is the nurse's role in defending against this suit? What might the nurse have done to prevent the suit in the first place?

Assumption of Risk

When the client signs the informed consent form for a particular treatment, procedure, or surgery, it is implied that he or she is aware of the possible complications of that treatment, procedure, or surgery. Under the assumption-of-risk defense, if one of those listed or named complications occurs, the client has no grounds to sue the health-care provider. For example, a common complication from hip replacement surgery is some loss of mobility and range of motion of the affected leg. Even if a client, after having a hip replaced, is able to walk only using a walker, he or she still does not have any grounds for a lawsuit.

> *Health-care providers are sometimes hesitant to provide care at the scene of accidents, in emergency situations, or during disasters because they fear lawsuits. The Good Samaritan Act is designed specifically to protect health-care providers in these situations.*

Good Samaritan Act

Health-care providers are sometimes hesitant to provide care at the scene of accidents, in emergency situations, or during disasters because they fear lawsuits. The **Good Samaritan Act** is designed specifically to protect health-care providers in these situations. A health-care professional who provides care in an emergency situation cannot be sued for injuries that may be sustained by the client if that care was given according to established guidelines and was within the scope of the professional's education.

For example, a nurse who finds a person in cardiac arrest administers cardiopulmonary resuscita-

tion (CPR) to revive the person. In the process, she fractures several of the client's ribs. The client would not be able to sue the nurse for the fractured ribs if the CPR was administered according to established standards.

Good Samaritan laws do, however, have some limitations. They do not cover nurses for grossly negligent acts in the provision of care or for acts outside the nurse's level of education. For example, in the case of a person choking on a piece of meat, the nurse initially attempts the Heimlich maneuver but without success. As the person loses consciousness, the nurse decides to perform a tracheostomy. The client survives but can sue the nurse for injuries from the tracheostomy, because this is not a normal part of a nurse's education.

Unavoidable Accident

Sometimes accidents happen without any contributing causes from the nurse, hospital, or physician. For example, a client is walking in the hall and trips over her own bathrobe. She breaks an ankle. There were no puddles on the floor or obstacles in the hall, and the client was alert and oriented. Because no one is at fault, there are no grounds for a lawsuit.

Defense of the Fact

Defense of the fact is based on the claim that the actions of the nurse followed the standards of care, or that even if the actions were in violation of the standard of care, the actions themselves were not the direct cause of the injury. For example, a nurse wraps a dressing too tightly on a client's foot after surgery. Later, the client loses his eyesight and blames the loss of vision on the nurse's improper dressing of his foot.[4]

Going through the litigation process can produce high levels of anxiety. Placing every aspect of the nurse's conduct under scrutiny in a trial is very stressful. All aspects of the alleged negligent act will be examined and re-examined. Often events that happened years before can be brought in to establish a "pattern of behavior." Every word of the nurse's notes and the medical record will be closely analyzed and questioned. Nurses can survive the litigation process with the help of good attorneys and by being honest and demonstrating that they were acting in the best interests of the clients. From this viewpoint, it is easy to see the importance of carrying nursing liability insurance.

ALTERNATIVE DISPUTE FORUMS

Although most lawsuits against nurses are settled through the court system, there are other methods of settling them. Because of the large number of cases and the resultant overload of the judicial system, other methods of resolving disputes have become increasingly popular. These alternative forums of dispute resolution are being used for many types of conflicts and are seen more frequently in the area of torts, contracts, employment, and family law matters. Mediation and arbitration are the most commonly used alternatives to trial.

Mediation

Mediation is a process that allows each party to present his or her case before a mediator, who is an independent third party trained in dispute resolution. The mediator listens to each side individually. This one-sided session is called a caucus. The mediator's role is to find common ground between the parties and encourage resolution of the disputed matters by compromise and negotiation. The mediator aids the parties in arriving at a mutually acceptable outcome. The mediator does not act as a decision maker, but rather encourages the parties to come to a "meeting of the minds."

Arbitration

Arbitration, in contrast, allows a neutral third party to hear both parties' positions and then make a decision or ruling on the basis of the facts and evidence presented. Arbitration, by agreement or by statutory definition, can be binding or nonbinding. **Arbitrators** or mediators can be, and frequently are, retired judges who work on an hourly-fee basis or practicing attorneys. In the family law area, they are frequently social workers or specially trained mediators. Negligence and malpractice issues are frequently resolved through arbitration and mediation.

COMMON ISSUES IN HEALTH-CARE LITIGATION

Informed Consent

Informed consent is both a legal and an ethical issue. Informed consent is the voluntary permission by a client, or by the client's designated proxy, to carry out a procedure on the client. Clients' claims that they did not grant informed consent prior to a surgery or invasive procedure can and do form the basis of a small percentage of lawsuits.

Although these lawsuits are most often directed against physicians and hospitals, nurses can become involved when they provide the information but are not performing the procedure. The person who is performing the procedure has the responsibility to obtain the informed consent. However, some physicians have gotten into the habit of giving nurses the consent forms and saying, "Get the client to sign this." Informed consent can only be given by a client after the client receives sufficient information on:

- Treatment proposed
- Material risk involved (potential complications)
- Acceptable alternative treatments
- Outcome hoped for
- Consequences of not having treatment

The physician should provide most of this information. Nurses can reinforce the physician teaching and even supplement the information but should not be the primary or only source of information for the informed consent. It is often difficult to draw a clear distinction between where the physician's responsibility ends and that of the nurse begins.

What Do You Think?

Have you ever had a surgical procedure where you signed an informed consent form? Did it meet all five criteria listed? Which ones were missing?

> *Nurses can reinforce the physician teaching and even supplement the information but should not be the primary or only source of information for the informed consent. It is often difficult to draw a clear distinction between where the physician's responsibility ends and that of the nurse begins.*

Exceptions to Informed Consent

There are two exceptions to informed consent:

1. Emergency situations when the client is unconscious, incompetent, or otherwise unable to give consent.
2. Situations where the health-care provider feels that it may be medically contraindicated to disclose the risk and hazards because it may result in illness, severe emotional distress, serious psychological damage, or failure on the part of the client to receive lifesaving treatment.

Patient Self-Determination Act

The Patient Self-Determination Act of 1990, sponsored by Senator John Danforth, is a federal law that requires that all federally funded institutions inform clients of their right to prepare advance directives. The advance directives are meant to encourage people to discuss and document their wishes concerning the type of treatment and care that they want (i.e., life-sustaining treatment) in advance, so that it will ease the burden on their families and providers when it comes time to make such a decision.

There are two types of advance directives: the living will and medical durable power of attorney (Box 9.5). The **living will** is a document stating what health care a client will accept or refuse after the client is no longer competent or able to make that decision. The medical durable power of attorney, or health-care proxy, designates another person to make health-care decisions for a person if the client becomes incompetent or unable to make such decisions.

Each state outlines its own requirements for executing and revoking the medical durable power of attorney and living wills.

Incompetent Client's Right to Self-Determination

The courts are protective of incompetent clients and require high standards of proof before allowing a physician to terminate any life-sustaining treatment for that client.

Nancy Cruzan was 30 years old and in a persistent vegetative state. She had a gastrostomy feeding and hydration tube inserted to assist with feedings, which her husband consented to. Her parents, however, petitioned the court for removal of the tube. In the Cruzan case, the court held that the state had the right to err on the side of life. The U.S. Supreme Court recognized that a living will would have been sufficient evidence of Cruzan's wishes to sustain or to remove her feeding tube.

The issue before the U.S. Supreme Court was whether the state of Missouri could use its own standard of clear and convincing proof for removal of the tube or whether there was a 14th Amendment due process guarantee of a "right to die" that would override the state statute. It was decided that the constitutional right would not be extended and the state procedural requirement would be allowed, at which time the burden of proof was put on Cruzan's family to show that she would not have wanted to continue living in this manner.

Many aspects of the recent Terri Shiavo case in Florida parallel the Cruzan case. In the Shiavo case, after the feeding tube was removed by order of a Florida judge, the U.S. Congress became involved and passed a bill that was signed by George W. Bush that required the case be heard by the U.S. Supreme Court. The goal was to have the tube reinserted until the high court could rule on the case. It is interesting to note that not much progress has been made in developing legal solutions for this type of case during the almost 20 years since the Cruzan case.

The Nurse's Role in Advance Directives

Because laws vary from state to state, it is important that nurses know the laws of the state in which they practice that pertain to advance directives, clients' rights, and the policies and procedures of the institution in which they work. Nurses must

B o x   9 . 5

Common Questions about Advance Directives

Q. Which is better—a living will or a medical durable power of attorney for health care or health-care proxy?

A. The documents are different and allow the nurse to do two different things. The living will states what health-care procedures a client will accept or refuse after the client is no longer competent or able to make that decision. The medical durable power of attorney or health-care proxy allows a client to designate another person to make health-care choices for him or her.

Q. If I change my mind and have a living will, can I cancel the living will or durable medical power of attorney?

A. Yes, each state has ways that your advance directives can be cancelled or negated. Most states require an oral or written statement, destruction of the document itself, or notification to certain individuals, such as the physician. Again, each state's statute should be checked for the specific details required.

Q. If I have a living will in one state, is it good in all states?

A. It may or may not be, depending on the requirements for the living will. It is important that you have your living will checked by an attorney to determine whether or not it may be effective in the states in which you are traveling or working.

Q. If I have a living will and have medical durable power of attorney who should get copies?

A. Copies should be given to your next of kin, your physician, and your attorney so that more than one person has a copy and knows what your intentions are. Some states will allow you to register your living will with certain state agencies such as the Secretary of State. There are also national groups that will allow you to register your living will with them so that there is access to it.

Nurses must also teach about advance directives and document all critical decisions, discussions with the client and client's family about such decisions, and the basis for the decision-making process.

---

inform clients of their right to formulate advance directives and must realize that not all clients can make such decisions.

It is important for the nurse to establish trust and rapport with a client and the client's family so the nurse can assist them in making decisions that are in the client's best interests. Nurses must also teach about advance directives and document all critical decisions, discussions with the client and client's family about such decisions, and the basis for the decision-making process. Discrimination must also be prevented against clients and their families on the basis of their decisions regarding their advance directives.

It is important that nurses determine whether or not clients have been coerced into making advance directive decisions against their will. Nurses need to become involved in ethics committees at hospitals or nursing specialty groups at local, state, or national levels to better help clients make decisions about advance directives.

Because laws vary from state to state, it is important that nurses know the laws of the state in which they practice that pertain to advance directives, clients' rights, and the policies and procedures of the institution in which they work.

Do-Not-Resuscitate Orders

Protection for the Nurse

Although a do-not-resuscitate (DNR) instruction may be included in an advance directive, DNR orders are legally separate from advance directives. For the health-care professional to be legally protected, there should be a written order for a "no code" or a DNR order in the client's chart.

Each hospital should have a policy and procedure that outlines what is required with regard to a client's condition for a DNR order. The DNR order should be reviewed, evaluated, and reordered. Different facilities have established different time periods for these reviews. Nurses must also know whether there is any law that regulates who should authorize a DNR order for an incompetent client who is no longer able to make this decision. Hospitals often have policies and procedures describing what must be done and which clients fit the requirements for a DNR order. The American Nurses Association (ANA) has published a position statement on nursing care and DNR decisions.

Nurses face many legal dilemmas when dealing with confusing or conflicting DNR orders. For example, it may be difficult to interpret a DNR order when it has been restricted: for instance, "do not resuscitate except for medications and defibrillation" or "no CPR or intubation." Often a lack of proper documentation in the medical records indicating how the DNR decision was reached can be an important and crucial issue if a medical malpractice case is involved and it is disputed whether or not the client or family actually gave consent for a DNR order.

Many facilities have developed DNR decision sheets for recording information about DNR discussions or the sheets are dated and signed by the client and those family members who took part in the discussion. It then becomes a permanent part of the medical record.

Protection for the Client

It is very important that nurses not stigmatize clients by the use of indicators for DNR orders, such as dots on the wristband or dots over the bed. Health-care providers' attitudes often change because they feel that the client is "going to die anyway." This abandonment can jeopardize the care of a client designated with a DNR order. However, it is also important for the nurses and staff to know whether an order is to be honored and what the policies and procedures are with regard to transfer clients and DNR orders that accompany the incoming client.

Information about the DNR status of a client should be obtained during shift reports. If there has not been a periodic review, is the order still in effect? If a client is transferred from one facility to another and has a DNR order that is time-limited and has not been reordered, what should a nurse do?

> *Nurses are encountering an increasing number of incidents where conflicts occur between institutional and professional standards, for example in staffing ratios.*

Standards of Care

A Measure of Action

Standards of care are the yardstick that the legal system uses to measure the actions of a nurse involved in a malpractice suit. The underlying principle used to establish standards of care are on the basis of the actions that would likely be taken by a reasonable person (nurse) placed in the same or similar circumstances.

The standard usually includes both objective factors (e.g., the actions to be performed) and subjective factors, including the nurse's emotional and mental state. Specifically, a nurse is judged against the standards that are established within the profession and specialty area of practice. The ANA and specialty groups within the nursing profession, such as the American Association of Critical-Care Nurses (AACN), publish standards of care that are updated continually as health-care technology and practices change.

External Standards. Both external and internal standards govern the conduct of nurses. External standards include nursing standards developed by the ANA, the state nurse practice act of each jurisdiction, criteria from accrediting agencies such as the Joint Commission on Accreditation of Healthcare Organizations, guidelines developed by various nursing specialty practice groups, and federal agency regulations. Nurses are encountering an increasing number of incidents where conflicts occur between institutional and professional standards, for example in staffing ratios. These conflicts are difficult to resolve and may require deliberation and decisions from institutional committees. As a general rule, when a conflict exists, it is safer legally to follow professional standards.

Internal Standards. Internal standards include nursing standards defined in specific hospital policy and procedure manuals that relate to the nurse in the particular institution. The nurse's job description and employment contract are examples of internal nursing standards that define the duty of the nurse.

Criteria for Good Care

The rationale for advancing standards of care for the nurse is to ensure proper, consistent, and high-quality nursing care to all members of society. When nurses violate their duty of care to the client as established by the profession's standards of care, they leave themselves open to charges of negligence and malpractice. Until recently, nurses were held to the standards of the local community. National criteria have now replaced most **locality rule standards of care.** Individual nurses are held accountable not only to acceptable standards within the local community but also to national standards as well.

Although standards of care may appear to be specific, they are merely guidelines for nursing practice. Because every client's situation is different, the appropriate standard of care may be difficult to identify in a specific case. More than one course of nursing action may be considered appropriate under a proper standard of care. The final decision must be guided by the nurse's judgment and understanding of the client's needs.

The Nurse Practice Act

The nurse practice act defines nursing practice and establishes standards for nurses in each state. It is the most definitive legal statute or legislative act regulating nursing practice. Although nurse practice acts vary in scope from one state to another, they tend to have similar wording based loosely on the ANA model published in 1988. The nurse practice act provides a framework for the court on which to base decisions when determining whether a nurse has breached a standard of care.

Most state nurse practice acts define scope of practice, establish requirements for licensure and entry into practice, and create and empower a board of nursing to oversee the practice of nurses. In addition, nurse practice acts identify grounds for disciplinary actions such as suspension and revocation of a nursing license.[4]

The judicial interpretation of the nurse practice act and its relationship to a specific case provide guidance for decisions about future cases. Many state legislatures have responded to the expanded role of the nurse by broadening the scope of their nurse practice acts. For example, the addition of the term *nursing diagnosis* to many states' nurse practice acts reflects the legislature's recognition of the expansion of the nurse's role.

In addition, occupational roles such as nurse practitioner, **nurse clinician,** and clinical nurse specialist are beginning to be included in nurse practice acts. It is important to remember that as the nurse's role expands, so does the legal accountability of the role itself.

PREVENTION OF LAWSUITS

What can the nurse do to avoid having to go through the stressful, sometimes financially and professionally devastating, process of litigation? The following guidelines provide some ways to avoid a lawsuit.

> *The medical record is the single most frequently used piece of objective evidence in a malpractice suit. In preparation for the trial, the lawyers attempt to reconstruct the events surrounding the incident in a minute-by-minute time line.*

Medical Record

The medical record is the single most frequently used piece of objective evidence in a malpractice suit. In preparation for the trial, the lawyers attempt to reconstruct the events surrounding the incident in a minute-by-minute time line. The client's **chart** is the most important source for this time line. Maintaining an accurate and complete medical record is an absolute requirement (Box 9.6).

The old adage "if it isn't written, it didn't happen" remains true in most situations; however, recent court trials have recognized some exceptions. Some judges and juries have begun to recognize that charting by exception is a valid form of health-care record keeping. Charting by exception, very closely related to problem-oriented charting, was developed initially to save busy nurses time

Box 9.6

Some Documentation Guidelines

Medications
- Always chart the time, route, dose, and response.
- Always chart PRN medications and the client response.
- Always chart when a medication was not given, the reason (client in x-ray, physical therapy, etc.; do not chart that the medication was not on the floor), and the nursing intervention.
- Chart all medication refusals and report them to the appropriate source.

Physician Communication
- Document each time a call is made to a physician even if he or she is not reached. Include the exact time of the call. If the physician is reached, document the details of the message and the physician response.
- Read verbal orders back to the physician and confirm the client's identity as written on the chart. Chart only verbal orders that you have heard from the source, not those told to you by another nurse or unit personnel.

Formal Issues in Charting
- Before writing on the chart, check to be sure you have the correct client record.
- Check to make sure each page has the client's name and the current date stamped in the appropriate area.
- If you forgot to make an entry, chart "late entry" and place the date and time at the entry.
- Correct all charting mistakes according to the policy and procedures of your institution.
- Chart in an organized fashion following the nursing process.
- Write legibly and concisely and avoid subjective statements.
- Write specific and accurate descriptions.
- When charting a symptom or situation, chart the interventions taken and the client response.
- Document your own observations and not those that were told to you by another party.
- Chart frequently to demonstrate ongoing care and chart routine activities.
- Chart client and family teaching and the response.

Source: From Tappen, RM, et al.: Essentials of Nursing Leadership and Management, ed. 2. FA Davis, Philadelphia, 2001, p 169, with permission.

and to save the facility money by reducing the volume of documents created and stored. In institutions where charting by exception is used, the nurse charts only those elements of client care that are abnormal or unusual or that constitute a health-care problem. If the client is stable and recovering as expected, there may be very little written in the chart about his or her physical or mental assessments.

Trying to recall specific events from 2 to 6 years ago without the benefit of written notes is almost impossible. In general, the client record should *not* contain personal opinion, should be legible, should be in chronological order, and should be written and signed by the nurse. Although opinions have a relatively low value in legal proceedings, the documentation should indicate the nursing judgments made. An entry should never be obliterated or destroyed. If a nurse questions a physician's order, a record must be made that the physician was contacted and the order clarified.

Rapport With Clients

Establishing a rapport with the client through honest, open communication goes a long way in avoiding lawsuits. Treating clients and their families with respect and letting them know that the nurse really cares about them may well prevent a lawsuit. Many

What Do You Think?

Think about being involved in a legal or courtroom activity, either as a defendant, complainant, witness, or juror. What would your role be in each situation?

people are willing to forgive a nurse's error if they have good rapport and a trusting relationship with a nurse who they believe is interested in their well-being.

Current Nursing Skills

Keeping one's nursing knowledge and skills current is vital to preventing errors that may lead to lawsuits. It is better to refuse to perform an unfamiliar procedure than to attempt it without the necessary knowledge and skills. Taking advantage of in-service training, workshops, and continuing nursing education classes is an important part of maintaining the nurse's skill level. Nurses must practice within their level of competence and scope of practice.

Knowledge of the Client

Recognizing the client who is lawsuit-prone can help reduce the risk of litigation. Some common characteristics of this type of client include constant dissatisfaction with the care given, constant complaints about all aspects of care, and negative comments about other nurses. This client often complains about the poor care given by nurses on the previous shift. This client may also have a history of lawsuits against nurses.

Being direct, solving problems with the client, and helping the client become involved in his

or her care are helpful to diffuse this negative behavior. Also, even more careful documentation of the care provided and the client's responses to the care can be helpful if a lawsuit is later filed.

> *Being direct, solving problems with the client, and helping the client become involved in his or her care are helpful to diffuse this negative behavior.*

LIABILITY INSURANCE

Maintenance of proper liability insurance is a necessity. Nurses who do not carry liability insurance place themselves at high risk. The nurse's personal assets as well as the nurse's wages may be subject to a judgment awarded in a malpractice action. Even if the client does not win at the trial, the litigation process, including hiring a lawyer and paying the costs of experts, can be financially devastating.

Claims-Made and Occurrence Policies. A professional liability insurance policy is a contract with an insurer who promises to assume the costs paid to the injured party in exchange for payment of a premium (Box 9.7). There are two types of malpractice poli-

B o x 9 . 7

What to Look for in an Insurance Policy

The following factors should be reviewed to determine what is the best policy for your type of nursing practice:

1. Type of insurance policy (claims-made or occurrence basis)
2. Insuring agreement

The insurance company's promise to pay in exchange for premiums is called the insuring agreement. The insurance company agrees to pay a money award to a plaintiff who is injured by an act of omission or commission by a health-care provider who is insured by the company.

3. Types of injuries covered

The language must be scrutinized to determine whether it is broad or limiting. Some companies will agree to pay only if the insured nurse is sued for damages, which means the nurse must be sued for a money amount or award. If the nurse is sued for a specific performance lawsuit or an injunctive relief action, which means that the nurse will either have to perform something or discontinue doing something, that particular insurance policy may not be adequate. Also, most insurance policies do not cover the nurse for disciplinary actions.

4. Exclusions

Items that are not covered by a policy are called exclusions. It is important to review the exclusions. Some of the more common exclusions include sexual abuse of a client, injury caused while under the influence of drugs or alcohol, criminal activity, and punitive damages. Punitive damages are used to punish the defendant for egregious acts or omissions.

Who Is Covered Under the Policy
The purchaser is the named insured and can be an individual, institution, or group. Others who may be covered by the policy are nurses, employees, agents, and volunteers, among others.

Limitations and Deductions
In exchange for payment of the premium, the insurance company agrees to pay up to a certain amount on behalf of the insured. This amount is called the limit of liability. It is usually expressed in two ways: the amount that can be paid per incident (per occurrence), and the amount that will be paid for the entire policy year. For example, if you have a policy that states $1,000,000/$3,000,000, it means that the company will pay up to $1 million per incident and a total of $3 million per policy year.

The insurance industry relies on the A. M. Best Company to evaluate both the financial size and relative strengths of insurance companies. An A. M. Best rating of A or better should be a prerequisite for purchase of any policy.

The Right to Select Counsel
Some insurance companies allow nurses to select their own attorneys to represent them in a medical negligence claim. Others retain attorneys or law firms, and the nurse does not have the opportunity to make that selection.

The Right to Consent to Settlement
Some policies allow the nurse to decide whether or not a case should be settled or go to trial, whereas others do not.

cies: claims-made and occurrence. **Claims-made policies** protect only against claims made during the time the policy is in effect. **Occurrence policies** protect against all claims that occurred during the policy period, regardless of when the claim is made. Generally, the occurrence type of liability insurance offers more protection. Claims-made policy coverage can be broadened by purchasing a tail that is a separate policy that extends the time of coverage.

Some hospitals have liability insurance policies for the nurse as a part of the nurse's employment package with the institution. This hospital policy may be limited to claims arising from the nurse's employment and might not apply in a situation in which a nurse renders care outside the institution, for instance, at an automobile accident site. It is preferable to have liability insurance coverage that includes all situations in which the nurse may be involved.

Individual indemnity insurance coverage independent of the facility's policy is recommended for all nurses. With passage of the **Federal Tort Claims Act,** and similar state laws, nurses who were formerly protected from lawsuits by working at federal or state health-care facilities can now be sued for malpractice like nurses at any other facility.

REVOCATION OF LICENSE

Self-Enforced Standards

One of the most severe punishments that a nurse can experience is revocation of the license to practice nursing. The nursing profession is responsible for monitoring and enforcing its own standards through the state licensing board. These actions may or may not be related to tort law, contract law, or criminal charges. Each state's licensing board is charged with the responsibility to oversee the professional nurse's competence.

The state's nursing board receives its authority to grant and revoke licenses from specific statutory laws. The underlying rationale for establishment of a licensing

board is to protect the public from uneducated, unsafe, or unethical practitioners. If nurses fail to adhere to the standards of safe practice and exhibit unprofessional behavior, they can be disciplined by the state nursing licensing board. One of the remedies that these boards can use is suspension or revocation of a nurse's license.

The Disciplinary Hearing

A disciplinary hearing is held to review the charges of the nurse's unprofessional conduct. This hearing is less formal than the trial process, and the nurse is allowed to present evidence and be represented by legal counsel at the hearing. Due process requires that the nurse be notified in advance of the specific charges being made. The question of what constitutes unprofessional conduct is an issue frequently dealt with at the disciplinary hearing. Each respective state's nurse practice act provides guidance with regard to the specifics of unprofessional conduct.

> *The nursing profession is responsible for monitoring and enforcing its own standards through the state licensing board.*

Unprofessional conduct can be reported by a nursing peer, supervisor, client, or a client's family. Many cases are dismissed before the hearing takes place if the board finds there is no support for the allegation being made against the nurse. If a hearing is necessary, it is in the best interest of the nurse to seek legal counsel because of the potential risk of license revocation.

License revocation is a serious consequence for the nurse because it removes the nurse's right to practice. Drug abuse, administering medication without a prescription, practicing without a valid license, and any singular act of unprofessional or unethical conduct can constitute grounds for losing a nursing license.

Conclusion

The legal system and its effects on the practice of nursing are ever-present realities in today's health-care system. Nurses need to be aware of the implications of their actions but should not be so overwhelmed by fear that it reduces their ability to care for the client. The more advanced and specialized the

nurse's practice becomes, the higher the standards to which the nurse is held. Nurses will be challenged throughout their careers to apply legal principles in the daily practice of nursing. An awareness of what constitutes malpractice and negligence will aid in the prevention of litigation.

Issues in Practice

HIPAA Has Unintended Side Effects

Much like new medications, new laws have long-term side effects that sometimes do not become evident until they have been in use for a period of time. The Health Insurance Portability and Accountability Act (HIPAA) of 1996 is now in the full implementation stage, and some unintended results have occurred. The initial focus of the law was aimed at concerns about the rapidly growing area of medical informatics[1] and the risks of violation of client privacy posed by electronically transmitted medical information. However, the rules and standards were expanded to limit how all health-care providers, including nurses, physicians, pharmacists, insurance companies, hospitals, nursing homes, home-health-care agencies, and even schools of nursing, are permitted to use and release medical information.

Extreme Compliance

Because violation of HIPAA rules is a federal offense with extensive fines, all health-care facilities and providers are going to great lengths to comply with the many standards. Many new policies and procedures have been developed and implemented by health-care facilities to protect the privacy of clients, reflecting the high premium the law puts on medical privacy.

Some of the required policies include the practice of offering clients written notices explaining how the physician or facility uses the client's medical information and how it can be released to other health-care providers. Clients also receive information concerning their right to see their medical records and the ability to make corrections. They have the right to obtain a list of business associates of the physician or facility that have access to medical information. Clients must sign a form acknowledging that they received the information. Many times, however, clients sign the form but do not read it because they are in a hurry, too ill, or too anxious to really care what it says.

The law requires that health-care institutions build fire walls into their computer networks that severely limit the amount of information that different departments are able to access. In some cases, the fire wall has a positive effect. For example, billing clerks are able to see that a test was run on a client, but no longer are able to see the test's results. In other cases, the same fire wall can create problems. For example, a dietitian attempting to adjust the diet of a client in renal failure may not be able to access important lab test results such as potassium, calcium, and phosphate that may be critical to the client's survival.

Are These Laws Necessary?

Initially there was delay in the transfer of information from physician to hospital, hospital to physician, and even physician to physician. Some of the confusion arose because of modifications in the initial version of the law by the Bush administration. Under the modified law, physicians are **not** required to obtain a client's consent before releasing information for medical purposes.

Privacy of information has always been an element in the provision of health care, and many health-care providers believe the HIPAA laws are unnecessary

(continued)

Issues in Practice   continued

and an added burden to the provision of care. The codes of ethics of the American Medical Association (AMA) and the American Nurses Association (ANA) have clear statements concerning the requirement that their respective health care professionals keep information private. The requirement for privacy can be traced to the very early stages in the development of professional health care as elements in the Hippocratic Oath and the Nightingale Pledge. As nurses and physicians are socialized into the profession, they clearly understand the requirements of client privacy.

Health-care facilities are in the process of retraining employees and volunteers to become obsessive/compulsive about privacy. They are being required to turn charts over so that clients' names cannot be seen, remove chart holders from areas that are visible to the public, double check FAX numbers and e-mail addresses before sending medical information, and are forbidden from discussing clients in any area where the public may overhear the exchange of information. Almost all facilities have been required to renegotiate contracts, or at minimum send out addendums to contracts to be signed, with anyone who does business with the facility, such as lawyers, insurance companies, nursing schools, and transport services. Large institutions may have as many as 500 agencies that may have access to some part of the medical record and need a new contract with each one.

One area of the law that has created additional confusion is public access to the hospital's main directory. Under a strict interpretation of the HIPAA rules, facilities cannot even acknowledge that a client is receiving care in that facility without the client's consent. There have been a number of documented cases where clients have been admitted unconscious or in a condition where they could not sign the release for inclusion in the hospital's directory. In facilities where the interpretation of the law implies that clients are excluded in the directory unless they chose to be included, relatives, and even physicians, had difficulty finding them.

The Effect on the Student

Nursing students can expect a renewed and vigorous emphasis on client privacy issues as a result of HIPAA. Because of the policies that have evolved from the HIPAA rules, some nursing schools are finding it difficult for students to obtain information for the traditional nursing care plans they are required to submit after clinical experiences. Elaborate measures are being initiated to remove all identifying information about the client, including basic information such as age and sex. Also, an essential element in many leadership/management courses for nursing students is chart audits for quality control issues. Because of restrictions on access to medical records, students may no longer be able to conduct chart audits.

Although many consumer groups still consider HIPAA as an important piece of legislation, the long-term side effects, some of which are yet to be acknowledged, have created unforeseen problems in health care delivery. The law's goal of protecting the privacy of clients is heroic; however, implementation has proved somewhat less than ideal. But get ready—if it hasn't already, HIPAA is coming your way, soon!

(See Catalano, J. Nursing Now: Today's Issues, Tomorrow's Trends, FA Davis, 2006, Chapter 18, p 323 for more detail on informatics.)

(Source: NYTimes.com, Health: Tarkan, L: A Privacy Law's Unintended Results, 6/4/2003.

Critical Thinking Exercises

Consider the following case: *Thomas v. Corso* (Md. 1982):

The client was brought to the hospital emergency room (ER) after being involved in an automobile accident. The ER nurse assessed and recorded the client's vital signs and a complaint of numbness in his right anterior thigh. The client was able to move the right leg, and there was no discoloration or deformity. After he was given meperidine (Demerol) for his pain, his blood pressure (B/P) dropped to 90/60, and the nurse notified the ER physician of the change. The physician ordered the nurse to arrange for admission to the hospital, which she did.

The client was transferred to a medical/surgical unit, but he could not be placed in a room because of an influenza epidemic. Rather, the client was placed in the hall next to the nurses' station for close observation. A nurse checked the client's vital signs about 20 minutes after the transfer and noted that the B/P was now 70/50, respiratory rate 40, and pulse 120. His skin was cool and diaphoretic, his breathing was deep and rapid, and he was asking for a drink of water. The client also complained of pain in his leg, but the nurse did not give him more pain medication because of his blood pressure.

The nurse assessed him about 30 minutes later and found his skin warmer, although he still complained of pain and thirst. The nurse also noted a strong odor of alcohol on the client's breath. An assistant supervisor also assessed the client's condition but refused to give him any water because he had obviously been drinking alcohol. She had been told about the low blood pressure by the client's nurse but attributed it to the alcohol and pain medication combination. The nurse checked his vital signs again and found a B/P of 100/89. Thirty minutes later it was 94/70, pulse 100, and respirations 28. When the nurse next assessed the client an hour later, he had a Cheyne-Stokes respiratory pattern, no pulse, and no blood pressure. She started cardiopulmonary resuscitation (CPR) and called a "code blue," but after a lengthy attempt at resuscitation, the client died.

An autopsy was performed and showed that the client had a lacerated liver and a severe fracture of the femur with bleeding into the tissues. The coroner determined that traumatic shock, secondary to the fractured femur and lacerated liver, was the cause of death. His family sued the nurses for poor judgment and the hospital for malpractice and won.

- What mistakes were made by the nurses in this case?
- What legal liability did the nurses incur by their actions?
- How can the nurses best prepare for trial in this case?
- What actions could the nurses have taken with this client to prevent a lawsuit?
- What are your feelings toward inebriated clients? Did the nurses' attitudes about inebriation affect their judgments?
- Why are clients who are drunk at higher risk for injury and poor medical outcomes than other clients?

References

1. Guido, G: Legal Issues in Nursing: A Source Book for Practice, ed. 2. Appleton & Lange, E. Norwalk, CT, 1997.
2. Menikoff, J: Law and Bioethics. Georgetown University Press, Baltimore, 2001.
3. Fiesta, J: Legal update, 1995, Part 2. Nursing Management 27(6):24–25, 1996.
4. Aiken, TD: Legal, Ethical, and Political Issues in Nursing. FA Davis, Philadelphia, 1994.

Bibliography

Austin, S: Legal checkpoints: Respect the scope of your license and practice. Nurse Manager 35(12):18, 20, 2004.

Berntsen, K: Looking beyond tort reform toward safer healthcare systems. Journal of Nursing Care Quality 20(1):9–12, 2005.

Brown, P: Not documented! Not done! New focus on healthcare quality makes documentation critical. ASBN UPDATE 8(1):7, 27, 2004.

Cogar, S: The legal nurse consultant's role in defending law enforcement officers. Journal of Legal Nurse Consultant 15(1):3–6, 2004.

Croke, E: Nurses, negligence and malpractice. AJN 103(9):54–63, 2003.

Future looks bleak as malpractice premiums continue upward spiral. Healthcare Risk Management 24(1):1–4, 2002.

Goode, A: Schiavo case should prompt discussion about health-care wishes. Oklahoma City Nursing Times 43(4):15, 2003.

Gosciminski, L: Point of view: How to avoid a lawsuit. Nursing Spectrum 16(15):3, 2004.

Griffith, R: Living wills, duty of care and the right to treatment. British Journal of Community Nursing 9(11):488–91, 2004.

Grace, P: Patient safety and the limits of confidentiality. AJN 104(11):33–37 2004.

Klein, C: Legal file: The great malpractice debate. Nurse Practitioner 29(9):53, 2004.

Salladay, S: Ethical problems. Confidentiality: disguised as a family member. Nursing 2004 34(12):28, 2004.

Skyrocketing malpractice premiums hamper access to care. OR Manager 20(7):16, 2004.

Sullivan, E: Issues of informed consent in the geriatric population. Journal of Perianethesia Nursing 19(6): 430-32, 2004.

Yeo, T, and Edmunds, M: Advocacy in practice: What to expect from medical liability tort reform. Nurse Practitioner 29(5):7, 2004.

10

Taking and Passing Tests

Joseph T. Catalano

Learning Objectives

After completing this chapter, the reader will be able to:

- Discuss the importance of a positive attitude when taking examinations.
- Recognize the importance of careful reading of questions and answers.
- Use critical thinking in identifying the key information sought in the question stem.
- Apply key test-taking strategies to help improve examination grades where the student's knowledge may be lacking.

TEST-TAKING STRATEGIES

Knowledge First

The multiple-choice question test format is one of the most commonly used. Of course the best way to get a good grade on any exam is to know the material. There is no substitute for knowledge. However, some individuals seem always to do well on multiple-choice question tests, whereas others seem to have problems with that test format. The individuals who always do well are not necessarily more intelligent than you; rather, they may have intuitively mastered some of the strategies or "tricks" necessary to do well on multiple-choice tests. Fortunately, once you become aware of these strategies and master them, you also will be able to improve your scores on this type of examination format.

Knowing the material is the most important determinant of your grade on an exam. However, knowing how to take a multiple-choice examination and optimizing the selection of the correct answers is a skill that will help you score higher than you might otherwise have.

> *The best way to get a good grade on any exam is to know the material. There is no substitute for knowledge.*

Strategy in Action

When mastery of test taking skills is combined with knowledge of the key material, the probability of passing any exam, including the National Council Licensure Examination (NCLEX), increases greatly. The following section lists and describes these important test-taking strategies that can be used when taking classroom exams, the NCLEX, or certification exams. Strategies 1 to 11 work best when you know the material pretty well and you are fairly confident about the correct answer. Strategies 12 to 34 can be used when you are unsure of the material or do not have a clue about what the question is asking.

A number of sample questions throughout the chapter demonstrate how the particular test taking strategy might help you answer the question. Try to answer the question the best you can before checking the answer at the end of the chapter.

STRATEGY 1. Think positive and avoid test anxiety. The night and morning before the exam, sit back, relax, and say the following to yourself: "I am intelligent and I will pass." "I'll show the instructor that I can do it." "I can do well on this exam." Avoid negative people; don't even talk to them!

STRATEGY 2. Cover up the answers and read the question carefully, trying to formulate your own answer. Looking at the answers right away pulls your attention away from the question. As you read the question and answers, try to understand what knowledge the question is asking for.

Clarify the Question. Look for and make a mental note of any key words, qualifiers, or statements that may help select the correct answer or eliminate the incorrect ones. Ask yourself: "What is this question really asking?" Rephrase it in your own words. It will usually be about a disease process, client problem or nursing action, or a symptom. Look at the details. Is it asking for a nursing action? A client response? A family response? Every word counts. If the question provides information about client age, gender, or marital status, it is probably important in selecting the correct answer, especially on the NCLEX.

Restate the Question. Ask yourself, "What information do I need to have to answer this question?" "Is there information in the client situation I can use to answer the question? What type of information is the question stem asking me for?" Restate the question in your own words to see if you really understand it. Create a mental pool of answers before you look at the answers given to the question. Then see

if any of your answers are similar to those that are provided.

One Question at a Time. Treat each question individually. Use only the information that is provided for that particular question in answering. Even though there may be client situations somewhere else in the examination that are similar to the one you are currently working on, avoid returning mentally to these previous items for help. You should also be careful about reading into a question information that is not actually provided. Avoid making clients in the questions sicker than they already are. Avoid recalling exceptions or unusual clients that you may have encountered in your clinical rotations when trying to answer questions.

> " *Avoid making clients in the questions sicker than they already are. Avoid recalling exceptions or unusual clients that you may have encountered in your clinical rotations when trying to answer questions.* "

Remember that there are no staffing shortages or lack of equipment in the NCLEX hospital. If the question mentions a piece of equipment, you can use it in the answer. By and large, questions on the NCLEX ask for "textbook" levels of knowledge of the material. Instructors will often give you study guides that outline the type of material they will include on their tests.

Let's practice restating the question and figuring out what knowledge is required:

1. A client is admitted with sudden acute respiratory syndrome (SARS). Which statement made by the client indicates that additional teaching is required?
2. A postpartum client is being sent home with a prescription for methylergonovine (Methergine) 0.4 mg. What should the nurse include in the discharge teaching plan?

STRATEGY 3. Uncover the answers one by one and ask yourself, "Does it answer the question?" Eliminate the incorrect answers and then leave them alone. Read *all* the answers carefully. Priority-type questions may have more than one correct answer. Many mistakes are made on this type of examination because the person taking the test did not read all parts of the question carefully. Look for the most specific answer to the question.

Restate this question, figure out what knowledge is needed, and then make a mental pool of answers before looking at the answers given:

3. Identify the nursing action that is most effective in preventing autonomic dysreflexia in a client with a spinal cord injury.
   a. Give the client a PRN dose of oxazepam (Serax) before PT (possible)
   b. Keep the client in the sitting position as much as possible (no)
   c. Encourage a fluid intake of at least 1000 mL per day (no)
   d. Maintain the patency of the urinary catheter (possible)
4. A 22-year-old woman is brought into the ER for a fractured radius by her boyfriend who said she fell off the sofa when napping. The nurse finds new injuries on top of old injures upon exam. How should the nurse chart these findings?
   a. Three new and four old ecchymotic areas located on right and left arms (possible)
   b. Many injuries on arms from physical abuse (no)
   c. Ecchymotic areas on both arms from unknown reasons (possible)
   d. Several injuries on arms from what looks like a baseball bat (no)

STRATEGY 4. Make sure you are actually "seeing" the words in the question and the answers. Picture what the words are saying about the question and examine the root words, suffixes and prefixes. A large percentage of mistakes are made because test takers misread the question.

Sample question for strategy 4:

5. A client who was in an automobile accident has been in skeletal traction for 10 days. Identify the complication the nurse will anticipate for this client.
   a. Orthostatic hypotension
   b. Diarrhea
   c. Muscular hypertrophy
   d. Decreased level of consciousness

STRATEGY 5. Take the time to do the test well the first time. After you select an answer, go back and reread the question to make sure they match. On your class tests, do *not* go back at the end and reread all the questions and answers. Mark the ones you are unsure of as you go through the first time and then go back and look only at those. You cannot do this on the NCLEX because once an answer is selected, the question cannot be accessed again.

Sample question for strategy 5:

6. Select the nursing action that is most helpful in relieving the pain from an episiotomy in a 1 day postpartum client.
   a. Increase fluid intake to 2000 to 3000 mL per day.
   b. Encourage the client to breast-feed the infant every 3 hours or on demand.
   c. Apply cold compresses to the perineum every 2 hours.
   d. Administer methylergonovine (Methergine) as prescribed PRN.

STRATEGY 6. Don't spend a lot of time on questions you don't know. Manage your time wisely, but don't rush—use all the available time. Generally allow 1 minute per question. If you are spending more than 2 minutes on any question, put an answer down and move on to the next question if you are taking the NCLEX or, on classroom tests, put a mark by the question and come back to it later on.

Although the NCLEX examination, strictly speaking, is not timed, the graduate is never sure how many questions will need to be answered. If you plan on taking all 265 questions in 6 hours, you will need approximately 80 seconds per question. Actually, most individuals who take this type of test average approximately 45 seconds per question; thus, it is likely that you will be finished well before the time limit is reached. Take a watch along to the examination. Theoretically, you could sit in front of the computer screen for 6 hours with the same question. There is a mandatory 10-minute break at 2½ hours and another optional break at 4 hours. Of course, breaks can be taken any time during the exam, but that time is lost from the total allowed time.

STRATEGY 7. Don't change your answers! Trust your intuition. When a question and the answers are read for the first time, an intuitive connection is made between the right and left hemispheres of the brain. The end result is that the first answer selected is usually the best choice. Educational psychologists have shown that test takers change the wrong answer to the correct answer only around 1% of the time. Most of the time they change the correct answer to the wrong answer or one wrong answer to another wrong answer.

> *Don't change your answers! Trust your intuition.*

When you read a question too many times, you may start to read into it elements that are really not there. On the NCLEX, once an answer is selected, it cannot be changed, but on class tests, change answers only when you are 100 percent sure that the answer you are changing to is correct. If there is any doubt at all, don't change your answer.

STRATEGY 8. Pay attention to where the client is in the recovery/disease process. One day postoperative clients have different needs than 4 day post op clients. The assessments of clients who have been on antibiotics for a week will be different from clients who were just started on antibiotics. A client newly diagnosed with diabetes will require different care than a 10-year diabetic.

Sample question for strategy 8:

7. Identify the assessment of a client who had a neuroblastoma removed 3 hours ago that would require immediate intervention by the nurse.
   a. Diminished appetite
   b. Pinkish tinged urine
   c. Temperature of 99.8°F
   d. Dressing saturated with bright red blood

STRATEGY 9. Look for priority or qualifying words in the question stem. Some important words can help determine what type of information is being elicited in the answer. Some of these words are:

First	Better
Best	Fastest
Most	Highest priority
Initial	

When words like these appear in the question stem, it is an indication that more than one of the choices are correct and perhaps all four of them are correct. The task then becomes selecting the one answer that should be first or the answer that ought to receive the highest priority. Remember Maslow's hierarchy of needs (physiological and safety have highest priority), the ABCs (airway, breathing, circulation) of cardiopulmonary resuscitation (CPR), and nursing process. The first step in the nursing process is always assessment, so if you have a question asking about what the nurse should do first, look for the answer with an assessment in it. Remember to always assess the client before the equipment.

Sample questions for strategy 9:

8. A client is admitted with the symptoms of anthrax infection, including fever of 102°F, severe dyspnea, tachypnea, and chest pain. Which nursing diagnosis has highest priority?
   a. Anxiety related to fear of death
   b. Pain related to pressure on the sternum
   c. Hyperthermia related to bacterial infection
   d. Ineffective airway clearance related to retained respiratory secretions

9. A 62-year-old client who has a history of coronary artery disease is brought into the emergency room

(ER) complaining of chest pain. What action should the nurse take first?

a. Give the client nitroglycerin gr 1/150 sublingual now.

b. Call the client's cardiologist about his admission.

c. Check his blood pressure and note the location and degree of chest pain.

d. Place the client in an elevated Fowler's position after loosening his shirt collar.

10. A client diagnosed with sickle cell disease is admitted in acute crisis. Which action by the nurse has highest priority?

a. Open the airway and begin high-flow oxygen therapy.

b. Administer prescribed narcotic pain medications

c. Establish a strong therapeutic relationship

d. Begin prescribed rehydration with IV fluids

STRATEGY 10. For delegation questions, match the activity with the person.

Know the person's skill level and education.

Know the job description.

Evaluate the client's status (acute = not appropriate vs. chronic = OK to assign; unstable = not appropriate vs. stable = OK to assign.

LPNs can do most skills but for the NCLEX:

• **Cannot** do admission assessments
• **Cannot** give IV push medications
• **Cannot** write nursing diagnoses
• **Cannot** do most teaching
• **Cannot** do complex skills
• **Cannot** take care of clients with acute conditions
• **Cannot** take care of unstable clients

UAPs/CNAs/Aides on the NCLEX:

• Look for the lowest level of skill required for the task.
• Look for the most uncomplicated task.
• Look for the most stable client.
• Look for the client with the chronic illness.

In the real world of health care, these individuals often perform functions beyond their legal scope of practice, but for the NCLEX, these are the general limitations.

Sample questions for strategy 10:

11. Identify the task that the RN may delegate to an LPN if all of the clients are stable

a. Adding potassium (KCL) to a bag of D5W that is already hanging

b. Developing a nursing diagnosis for a newly admitted client with diarrhea

c. Teaching a newly diagnosed diabetic client how to self-administer insulin

d. Turning a comatose client with a head injury side to side every 2 hours

12. Which client would be most appropriate for the charge RN to assign to an LPN?

a. A ventilator-dependent client with COPD

b. A client with dementia who is clutching her chest

c. A client with a history of head trauma transferred from the ICU 1 hr ago

d. A newly admitted client who is vomiting bright red blood

13. The medical unit is staffed today with three RNs and one LPN. To which client would it be appropriate to assign the LPN?

a. A man with TB who is being discharged today

b. A woman who fell and is now in skeletal traction

c. A woman who is scheduled for an EGD

d. A man newly diagnosed with gout

14. Select the task that is most appropriate for the RN to delegate to a CNA.

a. Suction a client with a new tracheostomy

b. Change a sterile dressing on a 60-year-old man with fresh skin grafts

c. Complete the initial postoperative assessment on a client just returned from the RR.

d. Obtain the temperature of a 29-year-old woman who is receiving the final 30 minutes of a whole blood transfusion.

STRATEGY 11. Once you realize something is seriously wrong with the client, do NOT delay care! Serious conditions require immediate treatment. Delaying action only allows the client to die slowly rather than quickly.

Sample question for strategy 11:

15. While the labor and delivery nurse is administering IV oxytocin (Pitocin) to augment labor, he or she notices that the fetal monitor is showing late decelerations and loss of beat-to-beat variability. What is the initial action the nurse should take?

a. Re-assess the FHT in 15 min.

b. Call the physician immediately.

c. Increase the rate of the primary IV.

d. Turn off the medication.

What if you are unfamiliar with the material and really don't know the answer? Don't panic! Use the rest of these strategies to help you figure out the answer or at least increase your odds of answering it correctly.

> *What if you are unfamiliar with the material and really don't know the answer? Don't panic! Use the strategies in the book to help you figure out the answer or at least increase your odds of answering it correctly.*

STRATEGY 12. An educated guess is better than no answer at all. There is no penalty for guessing on the NCLEX, and you have to put an answer down to move on to the next question. On both the NCLEX and classroom tests, if you are unable to make any decision at all about the correct answer, you should just select one and move on. There is at least a one-in-four chance of choosing the correct answer. However, studies have shown that answer 3 (c) has the highest probability (30%), answer 2 (b) the next highest, answer 4 (d) the third highest, and answer 1 (a) the lowest probability of being the correct answer. Wild guessing for large numbers of questions, of course, will have a negative effect on the total score.

STRATEGY 13. If you know the other three answers are wrong, then the one that is left is correct. Use the process of elimination to select the correct answer. Usually there are one or more of the answers that can easily be identified as being incorrect. By eliminating these from the possible choices, you will be better able to focus attention on the answers that have been identified as having some chance of being correct. Go back and read the stem question over again to try to determine exactly what type of information is being asked. If you are still unable to decide which of the remaining two answers is correct, select one and move on. Using this method increases the probability of choosing the correct answer to 50-50.

Sample question for strategy 13:

16. What action should the nurse take for a client who is developing Stevens-Johnson syndrome?
    a. Place tight tourniquets in the antecubital spaces of both arms.
    b. Give all medications through the client's arterial line.
    c. Hold the client's next dose of Bactrim and notify the physician.
    d. Inform the family that the client will die within 24 hours.

STRATEGY 14. If part of the answer is incorrect, the whole answer is incorrect. One incorrect part of a multipart answer makes the whole answer incorrect.

Sample question for strategy 14:

17. Identify the side effects a nurse should evaluate for a client who is receiving oral prednisone (Deltasone).
    a. Edema, hypotension, mood swings
    b. Dehydration, hyperglycemia, hirsutism
    c. Unstable moods, moon face, hypoglycemia
    d. Euphoria, hyperglycemia, hypertension

STRATEGY 15. Look for the answer that has the broader focus. Another method that may be used when the choices have been narrowed down to two is to examine the answers and try to determine whether one answer may include the other. The answer that is broader, more inclusive, or that includes the other answer, is usually the correct one. The answer that is most complete leaves the least room for error.

Sample questions for strategy 15:

18. Select the finding by the nurse that best identifies when a 10-year-old child with acting-out behavior requires help.
    a. Frequent fights with peers
    b. Multiple aspects of the child's life are affected
    c. Grades start to decline
    d. Stressful relationships with siblings and parents
19. Identify the best instructions for the RN to give to the C.N.A. for ambulating a client who has been on bed rest for 3 days.
    a. Put non-skid shoes on the client before ambulating.
    b. Ambulate the client 50 feet and notify me if there are any problems.
    c. Ambulate the client only as far as she can go without becoming tired.
    d. Ambulate the client to the nurses station and back and return her to bed if she becomes tired.

STRATEGY 16. Watch for similarities in the content of the options. When answers are grouped by similar concepts, activities, or situations, select the one that is different. If three of the four choices have some common element that makes them similar, and the fourth answer lacks this element, the different answer is probably correct.

Sample questions for strategy 16:

20. How can the nurse best help a 7-year-old boy diagnosed with acute lymphoblastic leukemia cope with the fear of dying?
    a. Instruct the parents to avoid bringing up the subject of death.
    b. Redirect the child's questions to safe topics when he mentions death.
    c. Answer the child's questions at the level of his understanding.
    d. Emphasize that nurses are not allowed to make prognosis about death.
21. A woman has been treated for severe chronic emphysema for several years using bronchodilators and relatively high doses of prednisone (Deltasone). Select the activity that would pose the least risk for this client in relation to the side effects of prednisone therapy.
    a. Shopping at the mall on Saturday afternoon.
    b. Spring-cleaning her two-story house.
    c. Attending Sunday morning church services.
    d. Serving refreshments at her 6-year-old son's school play party.

STRATEGY 17. Look for negatives in the question stem. Although there are very few negative questions on the NCLEX, negative words or prefixes in the question stem change how the correct answer is selected. Some common negatives include:

Least	Except
Unlikely	Inconsistent
Inappropriate	Untoward
Unrealistic	All but
Lowest priority	Atypical
Contraindicated	Incorrect
False	Not

In general, when a negative question is asked, it indicates that three of the choices are correct and one is incorrect. The incorrect choice is the answer. When a negative question appears, the test taker needs to ask: "What is it they don't want me to do in this situation?" or "What is the wrong statement?" On the NCLEX, negative questions are often disguised so that you have to read them carefully to figure out what they are asking. Phrases such as "What indicates the need for more teaching," are really telling you that one of these statements the client made is incorrect—which is it? The negative word is often at the end of the question like a hook on a fishing line. If you don't read the whole question, you'll miss it!

In general, when a negative question is asked, it indicates that three of the choices are correct and one is incorrect. The incorrect choice is the answer.

Sample questions for strategy 17:

22. Identify the client statement about taking aspirin at home for arthritis that requires further discharge instructions.
    a. "I need to take it with food or milk."
    b. "A small amount of blood in my urine is normal."
    c. "I should call the clinic if I develop large black-and-blue areas on my body."
    d. "Ringing in my ears may mean that I am taking too much medication."
23. Identify a side effect of a benzodiazepine-class medication that would be considered atypical.
    a. Syncope
    b. Depression
    c. Tremor
    d. Excitement

STRATEGY 18. Do not panic if a totally unfamiliar question is encountered. Some standardized diagnostic examinations and the NCLEX are designed so that no one gets a 100%. As a result, there are questions that are very complex, which deal with disease processes, medications, and laboratory tests that may be unfamiliar to the test taker. Questions like this may be encountered no matter how much review or study has been done. Often the "A+" students have the most difficulty with this type of test because they are not used to seeing questions they don't have a clue about answering.

Remember, nobody knows everything! When encountering these types of questions, it is important to not panic. Take a few deep breaths and think to yourself, "I can answer this question!" It is just one question out of many. Use some of the strategies already discussed in this chapter to select the best answer. Remember that nursing care is very similar in many situations even though the disease processes may be quite different. Select the answer that seems logical and involves good general nursing care. Common sense can go a long way in dealing with these types of questions.

Sample question for strategy 18:

24. What is the best action for the nurse to take when she or he discovers that a 9-year-old girl has a positive Rovsing's sign?
    a. Have the child rest quietly and assess the vital signs.
    b. Call a code blue and begin CPR.
    c. Inform the child's parents that she only has 3 months to live.
    d. Confront the child about which adult member of the family had been sexually molesting her recently.

STRATEGY 19. Remember, if you have never heard of it, probably no one else ever has either! Don't select answers that are totally unfamiliar. Stick with the things you know.

Sample question for strategy 19:

25. The nurse is caring for a client diagnosed with Smith-Strang disease. Identify the lab test the nurse would consider most significant for this client.
    a. ∀-5 ST 1
    b. CA 155 Antigen
    c. ICD
    d. UA

STRATEGY 20. If you can't figure out the answer any other way, look at the length of the answers. This is not a very reliable method, but it might work sometimes. The average length answer is most often correct. The NCLEX is difficult because the material itself is difficult, but the examination is not designed to be tricky or difficult for the sake of confusing the test taker. On the other hand, the test question writers are not going to make the correct answer obvious. Therefore, if one answer is much longer or shorter than the other three, it is probably not the correct choice.

Be wary of answers that sound like they are trying to rationalize the correct choice by using a lot of explanation, particularly when the other answers do not have lengthy explanations. Such answers are probably incorrect. You should also avoid answers that are different from the other three because of measurements or the way in which they are presented.

> *The NCLEX is difficult because the material itself is difficult, but the examination is not designed to be tricky or difficult for the sake of confusing the test taker.*

Sample question for strategy 20:

26. How can the nurse best administer tetracycline oral liquid suspension to an 8-year-old child?
    a. Quickly
    b. Through a drinking straw

c. With milk or antacid to prevent stomach irritation and vomiting
d. Hidden in the child's food so that the bitter taste will be disguised and the child will complete the full course of treatment

STRATEGY 21. If there is a lengthy client situation or case study, read the stem question before reading the case study. Reading the question first will help you focus on the information you will need to obtain from the case study. This is a way to save a little time. On the NCLEX, the amount of space for the client situation is limited to half the computer screen, so this will not be a problem.

STRATEGY 22. Avoid automatically passing the decision or intervention to the physician. Class tests as well as the NCLEX are for nurses and deal with conditions and problems that nurses should be able to resolve independently. Often a nursing action can and should be taken prior to notifying the physician. However, it is an important element of nursing knowledge and judgment to know when notifying the physician is appropriate, but do so only when there is nothing else the nurse can do to help the client.

Sample question for strategy 22:

27. A postlobectomy client pulls out his chest tube while going to the rest room. What is the appropriate initial nursing action?
    a. Call the physician immediately.
    b. Position the client on the operative side.
    c. Insert a new sterile chest tube and reconnect it to underwater seal drainage.
    d. Cover the insertion site with an occlusive dressing.

STRATEGY 23. Avoid answers that focus on medical knowledge or are a medical action. It is unlikely that questions on class tests or the NCLEX would require a medical action as an answer. The NCLEX in particular focuses on information to measure competency as a nurse. Remember that nurses cannot legally initiate medical actions independently. There are two exceptions to this rule. One exception is where standing protocols exist, but unless the question tells you there are standing orders or protocols, do NOT assume they exist. The second exception is when a treatment or medication is causing immediate harm to the client. These should be stopped immediately and the physician notified.

Sample question for strategy 23:

28. What is the most appropriate action to take when the nurse notes late fetal heart rate decelerations in a pregnant client who is in labor?
    a. Insert a urinary catheter to relieve pressure on the fetus.
    b. Begin oxygen by non-rebreather mask at 10 L/min to decrease fetal hypoxia.
    c. Initiate a magnesium sulfate IV drip at 1 gram/hour.
    d. Position the client on her left side.

STRATEGY 24. Avoid selecting answers that have absolutes in them. Answers that have absolutes in them are almost always incorrect choices. Some absolute words to be aware of include:

Always	All
Every	Never
Only	None

Humans are very complex biochemical entities. Every person is different and almost every rule will have an exception.

Sample question for strategy 24:

29. Which factor should the nurse include in the teaching plan of a client with a home prescription for reserpine (Serpalan)?
    a. Walk 2 miles every day.
    b. Never eat any candy or ice cream.
    c. The physician is the only one who can cut your toenails to prevent bleeding.
    d. Try to take the medication at the same time each day.

STRATEGY 25. Avoid answers that make the client seem inferior, immoral, unworthy, or ignorant. Nurses are obligated by the code of ethics to treat all clients equally, regardless of race, sex, lifestyle preferences, disease process, or economic status. Be careful of cultural differences and biases that can color the way the nurse interacts with a client. Also be particularly cautious in situations that are emotionally charged, such as child abuse, drug or alcohol addiction, spousal abuse, teen pregnancy, HIV, sexually transmitted disease (STD), or homosexuality.

Sample question for strategy 25:

30. Identify the most therapeutic statement by the nurse to a 14-year-old girl who admits she is

sexually active and has just been informed that she has gonorrhea and is 3 months pregnant.
a. "You obviously lack the intelligence to understand how to use the birth control pills and condoms you were given at the clinic at your last visit."
b. "Tell me how you think your pregnancy will affect your life."
c. "I hope you now understand the consequences of your lack of moral standards."
d. "Tell me how you feel when your classmates call you a slut behind your back."

STRATEGY 26. Look for answers that have words identical or similar to those in the question stem. If there is no other way to determine the correct answer, similarities to the stem may act as a clue to the correct answer, but this will require careful reading of both the stem and answers. With therapeutic communication questions, look for the answer that reflects or restates the emotions the client is expressing and ask open ended questions.
Sample questions for strategy 26:

31. Which assessments indicate to the nurse that a client was developing steal syndrome after the insertion of an AV graft in the left forearm?
a. Hypotension and irregular pulse
b. Weak radial pulses and mottled fingers of the left hand
c. Elevated temperature and purulent urinary drainage
d. Bruit and thrill over the surgical site
32. Select the most therapeutic response when a client says to the nurse, "That stupid doctor of mine makes me so mad I could spit nails! I want to leave this dump now!"
a. "You seem very angry. Tell me why you want to leave."
b. "If you sign the AMA sheet, you can go home now."
c. "It is your right to change to a new physician if you are not satisfied with your care."
d. "If there is no one to care for you at home, legally the hospital cannot release you."

STRATEGY 27. Watch for grammatical clues that may be a tip-off to the correct answer. All the options should be grammatically consistent with the question stem; however, question writers tend to pay more

attention to this detail with the correct answer. Answers that grammatically do not match the stem or disagree in number (singular/plural) are usually incorrect. When the stem is an incomplete statement, the options should complete the sentence in a grammatically correct manner.
Sample questions for strategy 27:

33. Identify the assessments that would lead the nurse to suspect that a newly admitted client was developing Kugelberg-Welander disease.
a. Compression fracture of L4
b. Blood-tinged urine
c. Muscle atrophy and twitching of the extremities
d. Grade 3 pansystolic murmur over the PMI
34. An important therapeutic measure for the nurse to take when treating a client with a *Dracunculus medinensis* is to:
a. Maintain a steady traction by winding around a small object like a pencil
b. Keeping the client on strict bed rest throughout the treatment period
c. Soaking the affected area in warm bath water several times a day
d. Active and passive range of motion every 4 hours

STRATEGY 28. Look for qualifiers in the answers. The answer that includes a qualifying word when the others do not is often the correct answer. Qualifying words include:

Generally	Might
Tends to	About
Usually	Approximately
Often	Most
May	Many

Sample question for strategy 28:

35. What is the most accurate information for the nurse to provide to the parents of an infant with gray syndrome?
a. Gray syndrome is always caused by a genetic defect.
b. You can take the baby home after 2 weeks' treatment with antibiotics.
c. The baby will require open heart surgery to live past age 3.
d. Approximately 40% of newborns with gray syndrome die by the fifth day of life.

STRATEGY 29. When two of the answers are opposites, one of them is usually correct. Look for answers that, when considered, cover all the possibilities of action. One of the answers must be correct and you have improved your odds to 50-50.

      Sample question for strategy 29:

36. What should the nurse conclude when she or he finds a positive Scarf sign while assessing a newborn infant?
   a. The infant was born after 30 weeks' gestation.
   b. The mother of the infant used cocaine during her pregnancy.
   c. There is a genetic predisposition for sickle cell disease.
   d. The infant was born before 30 weeks' gestation.

STRATEGY 30. When asked about numerical values or dates, the one in the middle range is more often correct. Numerical ranges can be from large to small or small to large. Dates can range from present to past or past to present. Extremes in numerical values or dates are usually incorrect.

      Sample question for strategy 30:

37. Identify the serum medication level that indicates to the nurse that a client with seizure disorder was taking his or her clonazepam (Klonopin) as prescribed.
   a. 142 ng/mL
   b. 112 ng/mL
   c. 72 ng/mL
   d. 12 ng/mL

STRATEGY 31. Avoid looking for a pattern in the selection of answers. Although you may be able to detect a pattern in your teacher-made exams, the questions and answers on the NCLEX are arranged by the computer in a random fashion without any particular pattern.

      If something appears to be in a pattern, ignore it. Any pattern is just coincidental. For example, if question 6 had answer 1, question 7 had answer 2, question 8 had answer 3, question 9 had answer 4, question 10 had answer 1, and question 11 had answer 2, you might expect that question 12 would require answer 3. This is probably not the case.

      Here is another example of a pattern-type situation that sometimes occurs with answers on this type of test. Questions 22 to 29 all have 3 as their correct answers. The answer to question 30 also seems to be 3, but the tendency may be not to select it because

of all the other choice 3 answers on the previous questions. The correct answer may very well be 3, and if that is the best choice, go ahead and select it. It is important that each question be treated individually.

STRATEGY 32. If you don't have a clue about what the question is asking, select the answer that has the most serious or worst client outcome if no action were to be taken by the nurse.

      Sample question for strategy 32:

38. Which complications can the nurse anticipate a client diagnosed with antiphospholipid antibody syndrome (AAS) to develop?
   a. Ecchymotic areas on the trunk and back
   b. Osteoporosis and hirsutism
   c. Weakness of the legs
   d. Cerebrovascular accident and pulmonary emboli

STRATEGY 33. Avoid answers that leave the client or family alone. Only on very rare occasions should clients or family be left alone. To have effective therapeutic communication, the nurse must interact with the client and family.

> *Be positive about the examination. Motivational research has shown that people who have a positive attitude about an examination score higher than people who are negative about it.*

      Sample question for strategy 33:

39. Select the best action for the nurse to take when a client in the ICU dies and his distraught family is present.
   a. Allow the family grieving time alone with their deceased loved one.
   b. Contact the client's religious leader by phone.
   c. Provide a quiet space apart from the unit for grieving.
   d. Stay at the bedside to answer questions.

Strategy 34. Be positive about the examination. Motivational research has shown that people who have a positive attitude about an examination score higher than people who are negative about it. Believe in yourself. Think positive thoughts all the time. Not only will you do better on tests, but you will be a happier and friendlier person too!

Box 10.1

ABCs for Success in Nursing School

A: Apply yourself to the task at hand. Learn all that you can about everything. This is the profession that you have chosen. To be successful, you must give it all that you've got.

B: Be organized. Set up a three-ring binder or notebook with a calendar and dividers for each subject.

C: Children do NOT belong in the classroom. If you have children, make care arrangements with a back-up plan for unexpected illnesses or babysitter call-ins.

D: Dress for success. Make sure you follow the dress code policy for the clinical rotations. Prepare for your clinical days the night before by washing and ironing your uniform.

E: Exercise regularly. It is a great stress reducer. Start it before you need it.

F: Front of the class is where it's at! Students who sit up front can see better, hear better and are less distracted.

G: Group study. It helps reinforce learning. Follow the rules for group study.

H: Healthy habits will keep you physically and mentally fit for nursing school. Eat right: stay away from fatty foods and eat lots of fruits and vegetables. Rest. Nursing school is physically and mentally demanding.

I: Introduce yourself to the course instructors and your advisor early on. They are there to help you.

J: Journal your experiences in nursing school. You will be surprised by how much you have learned from month to month.

K: Keep all your books and notes until you pass the NCLEX. They make good references and you may need them in other classes later on.

L: Look up procedures and skills in designated books prior to doing the skill with the instructor in lab or clinic.

M: Make your own flash cards from index cards to study while waiting at stop lights or other places.

N: Network with students that have gone before you. The information they give you about courses and instructors will be helpful.

O: Ooze enthusiasm! Look forward to each new leaning experience; volunteer for activities; join your student nursing association and encourage other students. Strive to be the kind of nurse that you would want caring for your family members.

P: Practice test taking. The more test questions you practice answering, the less test anxiety you will experience.

Q: Question things you don't understand or think are incorrect. Don't administer a medication if you have any question about it.

R: Research, used correctly, is an important tool. Learn how to look things up before you do them. Help in research projects if asked.

S: Study skills are essential for success. Develop some. Find out what works for you. Repetition is the best teacher: listen, read, write, and talk about it.

T: Teach others what you have learned. You will really have to know and understand a topic to teach it and you will remember it forever.

U: Unwind after a day in class or clinical. Find things to do that will take your mind off school and clinicals for a while. Meditate, listen to music, exercise, take a hot bath, dance, take up a hobby, play a computer game, an so on.

V: Vent your emotions. Have a designated sounding board (friend, spouse, parent) who is willing to listen to you with out criticizing or trying to solve the problem. Keeping emotions inside can lead to high blood pressure and ulcers.

W: Watch out for information on the Internet when doing papers. Not all of the information is high quality.

Box 10.1

ABCs for Success in Nursing School (Continued)

X: Excuses don't cut it in nursing school. Your instructors have heard them all before. It is better to just say "I don't know" than trying to bluff your way through.

Y: You can if you think you can! Think positive all the time. What you truly believe, you can achieve.

Z: Zap negative thoughts! Think positive all the time. Stay away from negative people; they will bring you down and add to your stress level. Seek out positive people who want you to be successful in school and your career.

GENERAL STUDY TIPS

STUDY USING IMAGES. Most people remember pictures better than words. Outline the pictures in your books with magic marker, highlighter, crayon, lipstick, whatever. Color in the pictures in the book or draw your own pictures. Try to visualize what is being taught. If you can see it in a picture, you understand it and are more likely to remember it.

Act out situations (role play) when you group study. The more senses involved, the better the learning; connect it with an emotion—humor, anger, fear. Your best teachers will often tell a funny story to demonstrate a point. They are connecting the learning with an emotion so you can remember it better. You can do this yourself.

DON'T CRAM! DON'T CRAM! DON'T CRAM! DON'T CRAM! DON'T CRAM! If you always do what you've always done, you will always get what you always got! The day before the next class, review the notes from the last class at a rate of 15 min per hour of class; it increases memory by 30 to 50 percent. Ask questions during class; it reinforces memory. **Play "stump the professor"** by trying to find a question in the book you are pretty sure the teacher doesn't know the answer to. You'll remember it forever.

GROUP STUDY RULES. These few simple rules will make the study session much more effective:

1. Be selective of the members—4 to 6 max; too many people makes the group hard to control and lessens learning. Be selective of the members. Study with people you like and get along with. Don't ask the

class clown or gossip to participate in the group. Avoid negative classmates like the plague.

2. Prepare before the group meets: assign topics or content to prevent the "what are we going to study tonight" syndrome. The goal of group study is for the members of the group to help each other learn. If someone doesn't know anything, they are not going to be much use to the group.

3. Limit the length of the session to 60 to 90 minutes maximum. Sessions that go longer start to get off track and people will start to get negative.

4. Use role playing to reinforce information. It adds a visual and/or emotional (usually humor) element that reinforces memory.

5. Remain positive. You can never be too positive.

6. Relax; have fun, but don't turn it into a party. It's OK to have some light snacks and drinks, but don't over do it. You can party AFTER you pass the test.

PRACTICE DOING QUESTIONS LIKE THE ONES THE PROFESSOR ASKS ON EXAMS. After the first test, try to formulate your own questions about the material you study. Get a review book that has a lot of questions in it and practice taking those questions. When you do test reviews in class, try to understand why you missed the questions you missed. Was it due to lack of knowledge? Failure to critically think? Not reading the question carefully? Changing the answer?

MAKE NOTES ABOUT KEY CONCEPTS WHEN YOU READ OR ARE IN CLASS. Create your own flash cards (e.g., med name on front, side effects on back or disease on the front, symptoms on the back). Summarize what you have read and **think, think, think about it.** Don't just memorize. Try to become interested in the material. If you find a topic boring try to relate it to something that interests you.

OVER-LEARN THE MATERIAL. Everyone forgets stuff. You can improve the chance of remembering if you continue to review and relearn material. Go back over material you are unsure of or have questions about.

NEVER LEAVE A CLASS IF YOU DO NOT CLEARLY UNDERSTAND THE CONTENT THAT WAS COVERED. The teacher is getting paid to explain the material so you can understand it. If you don't understand it, the teacher is not earning his or her salary. Keep asking questions until it's explained in a way that is clear to you. Especially ask WHY questions. Some teachers don't like these questions, but your best teachers will ask you "why questions" during the presentation of material. This is important because when you understand "why" you are using critical thinking. Then you won't have to memorize the material, because you understand it.

If you are still having problems after class, make an appointment with the teacher to see if it can be explained more clearly.

GET RID OF NEGATIVE THOUGHTS. If you think any of the following, you are guilty of negative thoughts:

• "I have to get a perfect score."
• "I'm always anxious during a test."
• "I'm a loser because I didn't remember that answer."
• "If he/she asks about _____, I'm dead."
• "I don't know what I'll do if I fail the exam."
• "My family will think I'm stupid if I fail."
• "My classmates will think I'm stupid if I fail."
• "I'll think I'm stupid if I fail."
• "No one ever understands what this teacher is talking about."
• "I just know I won't know the answers during the exam."
• "Everyone knows I can't get an A, so why even try?"
• "I'm not smart enough to be a nurse."
• "The teacher asks such tricky questions, so it doesn't matter if I study or not."
• "I'll be happy if I can make a C minus."
• "The information just flies out of my head when I sit down to take an exam."

THINK POSITIVE! THINK POSITIVE! THINK POSITIVE! Oh, and if you are having a really bad time on a test, THINK POSITIVE some more!

Conclusion

Mastering test taking and study skills is like mastering any other sills. It takes some concentration and practice. The test-taking and study skills outlined above can be used both for preparation for class room exams as well as preparing for the NCLEX.

Although nothing is as effective for passing an examination as paying attention in class, good note taking and thorough study, mastering these test-taking skills may improve your scores.

ANSWERS TO THE QUESTIONS IN CHAPTER 10

1. What type of disease is SARS? Which statement is incorrect (wrong) about SARS?

2. What is Methergine? Which statement about Methergine is **correct? Correct answer:**

3. What is autonomic dysreflexia? What triggers it? What can the nurse do to prevent autonomic dysreflexia? **Correct answer: d.** Autonomic dysreflexia is a condition found in clients with spinal cord injuries where a localized stimulus, like a distended bladder or impaction, causes a systemic response.

4. What information should the nurse include when charting? What is good charting? **Correct answer: a.** Good charting is specific, detailed, and descriptive. It should never include judgments, opinions, or suppositions.

5. Correct answer: a. If you selected answer *c,* you probably were thinking "atrophy," which is the decrease in size of a muscle when it isn't used for a long period of time. The word "hypertrophy" means the enlargement of something, which would not occur in this client.

6. Correct answer: c. Although the other answers may be appropriate nursing measures, they do not address the problem of pain relief.

7. Correct answer: d. The client is fresh postoperative, and one of the important assessments the nurse must make is the condition of the dressing. A dressing saturated with blood indicates a problem that needs attention. The other assessments are to be expected in a recent postoperative client.

8. Correct answer: d. Airway-related nursing diagnoses have highest priority (ABCs of CPR).

9. Correct answer: d. The first step in the nursing process is assessment. Always look for an assessment type answer when asked what to do first.

10. Correct answer: d. Rehydration dilutes the blood cells and prevents the clumping and clot formation that causes permanent damage from sickle cell crisis. Answer *a* may seem correct except for the fact that high flow oxygen will make the crisis worse. Also, a closed airway is not a problem in sickle cell.

11. Correct answer: d. *a.* IV med: no; *b.* nursing Dx: no; *c.* teaching: no. The client in *d* is stable and chronic and this is a procedure an LPN is qualified to do.

12. Correct answer: a. A ventilator-dependent client with COPD is stable with a chronic disease process. Client *b* is unstable/chronic; client *c* is unstable/chronic; client *d* is unstable/acute.

13. Correct answer: b. This client is stable and does not require any teaching at this point. Situations *a, c,* and *d* require teaching.

14. Correct answer: d. This client is stable and the procedure is uncomplicated. *a.* Client is unstable with a complicated procedure; *b.* client is stable but procedure is complicated; *c.* client is unstable and procedure is complicated.

15. Correct answer: d. Late decelerations and loss of variability indicate fetal distress likely caused by excessively strong contractions from the medication. Stopping it is the only way to save the fetus.

16. Correct answer: c. Stevens-Johnson syndrome is a type of erythemic edema that is commonly seen in clients who are taking Bactrim for urinary tract infections. The other three answers are things that the nurse should never do.

17. Correct answer: d. Prednisone causes fluid retention, resulting in hypertension and edema; raises the blood sugar, resulting in hyperglycemia; affects the mood, causing instability; and causes abnormal fat distribution, resulting in moon face and buffalo hump.

18. Correct answer: b. It includes all of the other answers.

19. Correct answer: d. It includes all the other measures when ambulating a client and therefore offers the most complete instructions.

20. Correct answer: d. All the other answers try to avoid talking about death with the child.

21. Correct answer: b. All the other answers place the client at risk for infection by exposure to large groups of people in open public areas.

22. Correct answer: b. The other three answers would be considered correct for a client taking aspirin. There should never be any blood in the urine.

23. Correct answer: d. The negative or "hook" word is atypical. It means unexpected. Benzodiazipine class medications are used as antianxiety agents and sedatives. You wouldn't expect them to cause excitement.

24. Correct answer: a. Rovsing's sign is an indication of appendicitis. The child should rest quietly until she can go to surgery.

25. Correct answer: d. Smith-Strang disease is a metabolic disease that produces methionine malabsorption syndrome leading to abnormal urine with a very strong smell. A UA will show these abnormalities. The other tests are made-up.

26. Correct answer: b. Tetracycline liquid stains the teeth and is best given to children through a straw. Note that answer *a* is very short, and answers *c* and *d* have long rationales.

27. Correct answer: d. Covering the site quickly is an acceptable nursing action and will prevent the pneumothorax from becoming larger. The physician can be called later.

28. Correct answer: d. Late decelerations are often caused by pressure on the umbilical cord, and changing position is a simple and effective way to relieve the pressure that is an independent nursing action. The other three measures are medical in nature and would require an order.

29. Correct answer: d. The other three choices all have absolute words in them.

30. Correct answer: b. Good therapeutic communication answers reflect or explore the client's feelings. The other three answers all make judgments about the girl's moral character or intelligence.

31. Correct answer: b. Steal syndrome occurs when too much of the arterial blood is shunted away from the hand. Note that answer *b* is the only one with the word *left* in it, matching the stem question that has the word *left*.

32. Correct answer: a. Good therapeutic responses reflect the emotions and content of the client's statements.

33. Correct answer: c. Kugelburg-Welander disease is a neuromuscular disorder that affects primarily teenagers, leading to loss of coordination and paralysis starting in the legs. Note that answer *c* is the only

plural answer matching grammatically the question that asks for "assessments."

34. Correct answer: a. A *Dracunculus medinesis* is a type of parasitic worm that infects the upper part of the leg. It can be removed by maintaining a slow steady traction force on it over a period of time. Note that answer *a* is the only one of the answers that grammatically completes the open-ended statement of the stem question.

35. Correct answer: d. Gray syndrome occurs in infants who were treated with chloramphenicol during the newborn period and is highly lethal. Note that answer 4 is the only one with a qualifying word, *approximately.*

36. Correct answer: d. Scarf sign is elicited when the elbow of the infant can be drawn across the chest without resistance. It is a sign of prematurity. Note that answers *a* and *d* cover all the possible options for age.

37. Correct answer: c. The therapeutic range for clonazepam is 20 to 80 ng/mL. Throw out the high and low, and the answer that is most in the middle of the extremes is answer *c.*

38. Correct answer: d. AAS is a disease process that causes blood clot formation. CVA and PE are caused by blood clots and are the most serious of the conditions listed in the answers.

39. Correct answer: d. Staying at the bedside and answering questions is the best method to use therpeutic communications. All the other answers take the nurse away from the family.

Bibliography

Christiaens, G: Strategies for coping with test anxiety. Imprint 51(4):68–69, 2004.

King, N: How to prepare for the certification examination. Insight 29(2):26, 2004.

Ludwig, C: Preparing for certification: Test-taking strategies. MedicalSurgical Nursing 13(2):127–128, 2004.

McDonald, M: NLN Assessment and Evaluation Division. Review guide to RN pre-entrance exam, ed. 2. Jones and Bartlett Publishers, Boston, 2004.

Nugent, P: Test Success: Test-Taking Techniques for Beginning Nursing Students, ed. 4. F.A. Davis Company, Philadelphia, 2004.

Smith, K: Lifelong learning, professional development, and informatics certification. Computer Informatics Nursing 22(3):172–178, 2004.

11

NCLEX: What You Need to Know

Joseph T. Catalano

Learning Objectives

After completing this chapter, the reader will be able to:

- Describe the NCLEX-RN, CAT test plan.
- Discuss the NCLEX-RN, CAT test format.
- Analyze and identify the different types of questions used on the NCLEX-RN, CAT.
- Select the most appropriate means for preparing for the NCLEX-RN, CAT.

I DON'T WANT TO TAKE THIS EXAM!

The primary purpose of licensure examinations is to protect the public from unsafe or uneducated practitioners of a profession. When you pass the National Council Licensure Examination (NCLEX), it indicates that you have the minimal level of knowledge or competency deemed necessary by the state to practice nursing without injury to clients. Licensure is a legal requirement for all professions that deal with public health, welfare, or safety.

Most people have varying levels of anxiety before taking an exam. The more important the examination, the higher the anxiety levels. Anxiety is sometimes defined as fear of the unknown. This chapter presents key information about the NCLEX test plan to better help you understand and anticipate what you are going to encounter when you take the exam. It also includes some suggestions for study for the NCLEX and do's and don'ts for the exam itself. It is hoped that this information will help lower your anxiety levels about the NCLEX. Sample practice questions throughout the chapter give you an idea of how the NCLEX asks about different types of nursing information. Try to answer these questions as you read the chapter. The answers and rationales are found at the end of the chapter.

NCLEX TEST PLAN

The NCLEX is a computerized, **criterion-referenced examination** that you take after you graduate from a school of nursing. Unlike a **norm-referenced examination,** which bases a passing score on the scores of others who took the exam, criterion-referenced examinations

Issues Now

Handling Your Anxiety

First, it is perfectly reasonable to be slightly anxious about taking the NCLEX. You have expended plenty of blood, sweat, and tears to come to this point. As one diploma grad told me, "I was in debt up to my ears and running out of money fast when I took the NCLEX. Passing was literally my meal ticket." Even if you're not in such dire financial straits, it's no small thing to be tested on years of accumulated knowledge. You would have to be comatose not to feel butterflies in your stomach at this point. Do not be anxious about being anxious.

Because you cannot go back and change answers, treat each question as an exam in itself; once you hit the enter key the second time, immediately turn your attention to the next question. Tell yourself not to be surprised by anything. You are at a psychological disadvantage if you expect the computer to turn off at a certain number and it doesn't. So if you can, avoid looking at the question number as you answer each question.

If you are distracted by the clicking of other people's computers or other such annoying sounds, you can ask for earplugs. The testing service provides them; they are disposable and not entirely unattractive.

Finally, there are going to be other people close to you or next to you who may sit down at the computer at the same time as you do. They may get up before you, but ignore them. The testing centers administer many different tests, so you can realistically tell yourself that the person next to you who finished in 45 minutes was not even taking the NCLEX. Even if they were taking the NCLEX, you do not need to think about it. A little denial in this situation can go a long way.

Source: Dunham, KS: How to Survive and Maybe Even Love Nursing School. FA Davis, Philadelphia, 2001, pp. 180–181, with permission.

compare your knowledge to a pre-established standard. If you meet or exceed the standard, you pass. The NCLEX measures nursing knowledge of a wide range of material, but mostly measures your ability to think critically and make good sound judgments about nursing care. With computerized adaptive tests such as the NCLEX, the computer selects questions in accordance with the examination plan and how you answered the previous questions.

Changes in the Test Plan

Over the years since its institution, several substantive changes were made in the NCLEX Computerized Adaptive Testing for Registered Nurses (NCLEX-RN, CAT) test plan. The changes included reorganization of the test plan into three primary components: (1) client needs, (2) level of cognitive ability, and (3) integrated concepts and processes. The third component was expanded to include nursing process, caring, communication, cultural awareness, documentation, self-care, and teaching and learning.

Additional changes were made in October 2001 and October 2002 to the format and examination test vendor. The percentages of questions in the various needs categories were redistributed in 2003 to their current levels. In 2004, alternative format questions were added (discussed below). In 2005, the length of time allowed to complete the exam was increased from 5 hours to 6 hours. There was also an increase in the number of pharmacology questions (up to 19 percent), and the difficulty level was increased by 0.078 logits (about 7 percent), discussed below.

Client Health Needs

The NCLEX asks questions about four general groups of material called client health needs:

- Safe and effective care environment
- Physiological integrity
- Psychosocial integrity
- Health promotion and maintenance needs

Safe and Effective Care Environment (21 to 33 Percent)

a. Management of care: 13 to 19 percent of NCLEX questions
b. Safety and infection control: 8 to 14 percent of NCLEX questions

The questions in this category make up between 21 and 33 percent of the total questions on the NCLEX. These questions deal with overt safety issues in client care, such as use of restraints, medication administration, safety measures to prevent injuries (such as putting up side rails), prevention of infections, isolation precautions, safety measures with pediatric clients, and special safety needs of clients with psychiatric problems.

This needs category also includes questions about laboratory tests, their results, and any special nursing measures associated with them; legal and ethical issues in nursing; a small amount of nursing management; and quality assurance issues. Questions on these issues are interspersed with other questions throughout the examination.

Physiological Integrity (43 to 67 Percent)

a. Basic care and comfort: 6 to 12 percent of NCLEX questions
b. Pharmacological and parenteral therapies: 13 to 19 percent of NCLEX questions
c. Reduction of risk potential: 13 to 19 percent of NCLEX questions
d. Physiological adaptation: 11 to 17 percent of NCLEX questions

The physiological integrity needs are concerned with adult medical and surgical nursing care, pediatrics, and **gerontology.** This category comprises the largest groups of questions, with about 43 to 67 percent of the total number of questions on the NCLEX. The more common health-care problems, both acute and chronic conditions, that nurses deal with on a daily basis include:

- Diabetes
- Cardiovascular disorders
- Neurological disorders
- Renal diseases
- Respiratory diseases
- Traumatic injuries
- Immunological disorders
- Skin and infective diseases

There are also questions about nursing care of the pediatric client, including such topics as:

- Growth and development
- Congenital abnormalities
- Child abuse
- Burn injury

- Fractures and cast and traction care
- Common infective diseases in children
- Common childhood trauma such as eye injuries

Psychosocial Integrity (6 to 12 Percent)

a. Coping and adaptation: 5 to 11 percent of NCLEX questions

b. Psychosocial adaptation: 5 to 11 percent of NCLEX questions

Psychosocial integrity needs are health-care issues that revolve around the client with psychiatric problems. This material also deals with coping mechanisms for high-stress situations such as acute illness and life-threatening diseases or trauma. These clients do not necessarily have any psychiatric disorders. This category constitutes at most 12 percent of the examination and includes questions about the care of clients with eating disorders, personality disorders, anxiety disorders, depression, schizophrenia, and organic mental disease. Also included in the psychosocial needs section are questions about therapeutic communication, crisis intervention, and substance abuse.

> *Being able to remember and understand information is the most basic way of learning. Although this type of knowledge is important and underlies the other levels of knowledge, it is not sufficient to ensure safe nursing care.*

Health Promotion and Maintenance (6 to 12 Percent)

a. Life span growth and development: 7 to 12 percent of NCLEX questions

b. Prevention and early detection of disease: 5 to 11 percent of NCLEX questions

Health promotion and maintenance needs deal with birth control measures, pregnancy, labor and delivery, the care of the newborn infant, growth and development, and contagious diseases, particularly sexually transmitted diseases. This section constitutes approximately 12 percent of the total examination. Teaching and counseling are important parts of the nurse's care during pregnancy, and knowledge of

"These are my Health Promotion tutors."

diet, signs and symptoms of complications, fetal development, and testing used during pregnancy is necessary.

Levels of Cognitive Ability

The level of cognitive ability is a component of the NCLEX that measures how information has been learned and how it can be used by the nurse. For the NCLEX, knowledge is tested at three different levels.

Level 1

Level 1 consists of knowledge and comprehension questions. Fewer than 10 percent of the questions are at this level; however, there is a good chance that you may not see any level 1 question.. These questions involve recalling specific facts and the ability to understand those facts in relationship to a pathophysiological condition; they cover knowledge of specific anatomy and physiology, medication dosage and side effects, signs and symptoms of diseases, laboratory test results, and the elements of certain treatments and interventions.

Being able to remember and understand information is the most basic way of learning. Although this type of knowledge is important and underlies the other levels of knowledge, it is not sufficient to ensure safe nursing care. An example of a level 1 question is:

1. A client is admitted to the medical unit with respiratory failure. Identify the normal range for the PO_2.
   a. 10–30 mm Hg
   b. 35–55 mm Hg
   c. 10–20 cm H_2O
   d. 70–100 mm Hg

Level 2

Level 2 questions add an additional step to the answering process. These questions presume that you have the basic information memorized and then ask you to analyze, interpret, and apply information to specific situations. Analysis and application questions are more difficult to answer because they require you to do more than simply repeat the information you have read or heard in class. Analysis requires the ability to separate information into its basic parts, decide which of those parts are important, and then make a decision about what the information is telling you. Application requires that you be able to use that information in client care decisions.

Some examples of this type of question involve interpreting electrocardiographic (ECG) strips, interpreting blood gas values, making a nursing diagnosis based on a set of symptoms, or deciding on a treatment plan. These questions provide a better indication of your ability to safely care for clients. An example of a level 2 question is:

2. A client is becoming progressively short of breath. The results of his arterial blood gas (ABG) tests are pH, 7.13; PO_2, 48; PCO_2, 53; and HCO_3, 26. What do these values indicate?
   a. Metabolic acidosis
   b. Respiratory alkalosis
   c. Respiratory acidosis
   d. Metabolic alkalosis

Level 3

Level 3—synthesis, judgment, and evaluation—takes the process a step further. Over 90 percent of the questions on the NCLEX are at either level 2 or level 3. Questions at the synthesis and judgment level ask you to process information on more than one fact; apply rules, methods, principles or theories to a situation; *and* make judgments and decisions about

client care. The way you can identify these higher-level questions is by recognizing that they require you be able to *process two or more* facts, concepts, theories, rules, or principles of care before you can answer the question.

One factor that adds to the difficulty of answering level 3–type questions is that there is often more than one correct answer. You may be asked to choose the best, or highest priority, answer from among several correct answers. Questions at this level often ask about the priority of care to be given, the priority of nursing diagnosis formulated, how to best evaluate the effectiveness of care you are giving, and the most appropriate nursing action to be taken. Your ability to make decisions about nursing care at these higher levels is the best indication of your critical thinking ability and best demonstrates the ability to provide safe nursing care. Three examples of level 3 questions are:

3. A client is becoming progressively short of breath. The results of his arterial blood gas (ABG) tests are pH, 7.13; PO_2, 48; PCO_2, 53; and HCO_3, 26. What action should the nurse take first?
   a. Call a code blue and begin cardiopulmonary resuscitation.
   b. Call the physician and report the condition.
   c. Make sure the client's airway is open and begin supplemental oxygen.
   d. Give the ordered dose of 200 mg aminophylline intravenous piggyback (IVPB) now.

4. After receiving shift report at 0645, identify the client the nurse should assess first.
   a. 65-year-old man with stable angina
   b. 37-year-old woman with possible GI bleeding; vital signs stable
   c. 56-year-old woman with COPD and an oxygen saturation of 89%
   d. 19-year-old man with Type I diabetes and a fasting blood sugar of 55 mg/dL

5. The nurse assesses a 7-month-old hospitalized girl and finds that the infant has a positive tonic neck reflex. What intervention would be most important for the nurse to include in the child's nursing care plan?
   a. Daily head circumference measurements
   b. Measure intake and weigh all diapers
   c. Position the infant on her back for naps
   d. Assess neuro/developmental levels each shift

Integrated Concepts and Processes

The integrated concepts and processes component includes the following:

- Nursing process
- Concepts of caring
- Therapeutic communication
- Cultural awareness
- Documentation
- Self-care
- Teaching and learning

These concepts are integrated throughout the examination and are included as elements in the four needs categories.

Nursing Process

The nursing process has traditionally been a very important part of the NCLEX. The NCLEX-RN, CAT uses the five-step nursing process: assessment, analysis, planning, intervention and implementation, and evaluation. Each of the questions you will be asked on the NCLEX falls into one of these five categories.

It is important that you keep in mind the steps of the nursing process when answering questions. Often questions that ask, "What should the nurse do first?" are looking for an assessment-type answer because that is the first step in the nursing process. Questions on the nursing process are no longer equally divided on the examination. Recent analysis has shown a higher percentage of questions in the implementation phase of the nursing process.

ASSESSMENT. The **assessment** phase primarily establishes the database on which the rest of the nursing process is built. Some components of the assessment phase include both subjective and objective data about the client, significant history, history of the present illness, signs and symptoms, environmental elements, laboratory values, and vital signs. Often the examination will ask you to distinguish between appropriate and inappropriate assessment factors. An example of an assessment phase question is:

6. What would be the most important information for the nurse to obtain when a client is admitted for evaluation of recurrent episodes of Stokes-Adams syndrome?
   a. Ability to perform aerobic exercises for 15 minutes

b. Bradycardia and increases in blood pressure
c. Changes in level of consciousness
d. Ability to discuss fat and sodium diet restrictions

ANALYSIS. The analysis phase of the nursing process involves developing and using nursing diagnosis for the care of the client. The NCLEX uses the North American Nursing Diagnosis Association (NANDA) nursing diagnosis system. Questions concerning nursing diagnosis will often ask you to prioritize the diagnoses. (See Chapter 10 for information about prioritization). An example of an analysis phase question is:

7. A client is admitted to the unit with a diagnosis of bronchitis, congestive heart failure, and fever. The nurse assesses him as having a temperature of 101.8°F, peripheral edema, dyspnea, and rhonchi. The following nursing diagnoses are all appropriate, but which one has the highest priority?
   a. Anxiety related to fear of hospitalization
   b. Ineffective airway clearance related to retained secretions
   c. Fluid volume excess related to third spacing of fluid (edema)
   d. Ineffective thermoregulation related to fever

PLANNING. The planning phase of the nursing process primarily involves setting goals for the client. Included in the planning phase are such factors as determining expected outcomes, setting priorities for goals, and anticipating client needs based on the assessment. These questions may ask you to identify the most appropriate goal or may ask you to identify the highest-priority goal from several appropriate goals. You can prioritize goals the same way you did the nursing diagnosis. Remember that a good goal is measurable, client centered, time limited, and realistic. An example of a planning phase question is:

8. A client is found to be in respiratory failure and is placed on oxygen. Which goal has the highest priority for this client?
   a. Walk the length of the hall twice during a nurse's shift.
   b. Complete his bath and morning care before breakfast.

c. Maintain an oxygen saturation of 90% throughout the shift.
d. Keep the head of the bed elevated to promote proper ventilation.

INTERVENTION AND IMPLEMENTATION. The **intervention** and **implementation** phase of the nursing process involves identifying nursing actions that are required to meet the goals stated in the planning phase. Some of the material in the intervention and implementation phase includes:

• Provision of nursing care based on the client's goals
• Prevention of injury or spread of disease
• Therapy with medications and their administration
• Giving treatments
• Carrying out procedures
• Charting and record keeping
• Teaching about health care
• Monitoring changes in condition

An example of an intervention and implementation phase question is:

9. When the nurse ambulates a client who has been on bed rest for 3 days, he suddenly becomes very restless, displays extreme dyspnea, and complains of chest pain. Select the most appropriate nursing action.
   a. Call a code blue.
   b. Continue to help the client walk, but at a slower pace.
   c. Give the client an injection of his ordered pain medication.
   d. Return the client to bed and evaluate his vital signs and lung sounds.

EVALUATION. The **evaluation** phase of the nursing process determines whether or not the goals stated in the planning phase have been met through the interventions. The evaluation phase also ties the nursing process together and makes it cyclic. If the goals have been achieved, it is an indication that the plan and implementation were effective, and new goals need to be established. If the goals were not met, then you have to go back and find the difficulty. Were the assessment data inadequate? Were the goals defective? Was there a deficiency in the implementation?

> *Contrary to rumor, no graduates are randomly selected to take all 265 questions.*

Evaluation is a continual process. Material in the evaluation phase includes comparison of actual outcomes with expected outcomes, verification of assessment data, evaluation of nursing actions and client responses, and evaluation of the client's level of knowledge and understanding. Evaluation questions are often worded very similarly and are relatively easy to identify after you have experienced a few of them. An example of an evaluation question is:

10. A client is being prepared for discharge. He is to take theophylline by mouth at home for his lung disease. Which statement by the client indicates to the nurse that her teaching concerning theophylline medications has been effective?
    a. "I can stop taking this medication when I feel better."
    b. "If I have difficulty swallowing the time-released capsules, I can crush them or chew them."
    c. "If I have a lot of nausea and vomiting or become restless and can't sleep, I need to call my physician."
    d. "I need to drink more coffee and cola while I am on these medications."

NCLEX FORMAT

You will take the NCLEX examination on a personal computer at a Pearson Professional Center (Box 11.1). The majority of the questions are in a multiple-choice format and are constructed similarly. They include a client situation, a stem or stem question, and four answers, or distractors, like the sample questions you have seen so far in this chapter.

All the multiple-choice questions on the NCLEX stand alone, although a similar situation may be repeated. Occasionally a single question may be included without a case situation.

Choosing the Right Answer

For the multiple-choice questions, you are asked to select the best answer from among the four possible

Box 11.1
Example of Computer Examination Question

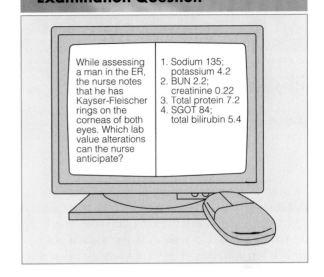

While assessing a man in the ER, the nurse notes that he has Kayser-Fleischer rings on the corneas of both eyes. Which lab value alterations can the nurse anticipate?

1. Sodium 135; potassium 4.2
2. BUN 2.2; creatinine 0.22
3. Total protein 7.2
4. SGOT 84; total bilirubin 5.4

choices. No partial credit is given for a "close" answer; there is only one correct answer for any particular question. The questions are totally integrated from the content areas that were previously discussed along with the approximate percentages that were identified. Each question carries an equal weight or value toward the final score.

When the question appears on the screen, read the question and answers. When you decide what the correct answer is, place the cursor in the circle in front of the answer, and click (Fig. 11.1). This selects the answer. If you decide to change the answer (not a good idea; see Chapter 10), place the cursor on the answer you selected and click again. It will remove the indicator and you can move the cursor to another answer. When you are sure you have selected the correct answer, click the "N" next button on the button bar at the bottom of the screen. That question will disappear and a new one will appear. You cannot go back and change an answer after you click the "N" next button.

Alternative Format Questions
In 2004, alternative format questions were added to the exam. The latest information on these questions is that between 2 and 10 percent of the total number of questions will be alternative format and that each graduate will have at least one of them on the exam. After the initial trial period in 2004, these questions began counting toward the final score on the exam.

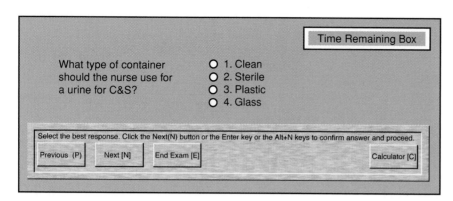

Figure 11.1 Sample multiple-choice question. Select the answer by placing the cursor in the circle and click or type in the answer. Change the answer by placing the cursor in a new circle and click. Move to the next question by clicking on the "Next (N)" button at the bottom of the screen.

There are several types of these questions. They are scored like the multiple-choice questions in that there is only one correct answer. They are also given a difficulty rating based on the same criteria as the multiple-choice questions. If you want to practice these types of questions, go to www.ncsb.org/testing, where you will find several examples.

Fill in the Blank
These alternative format questions may ask for a range of information. They may be calculation questions or ask for knowledge. After you read the questions, you need to type the answer in the box provided (Fig. 11.2). If it is a calculation question, you may use the pop-up calculator that is accessible by clicking the cursor on the "C" calculator button on the button bar (Fig. 11.3). After you have typed in your answer, you can go back and change it. Once you have decided that it is correct, click on the "N" next button and a new question will appear.

Multiple Answers
With the multiple-answer format questions, you are given a list of options or answers to a question and must select all that are correct. You need to get them all correct in order to get credit for the question. To select the options you think are correct, place the cursor in the circle or box before the option and click (Fig. 11.4). If you decide that one of the options is not really the one you want, you can click on the circle again and it will be removed. When you decide you have the options you want, click on the "N" next button and the next question will appear on the screen.

Sequencing Items
Sequencing format questions provide you with a question and then four or more options (items) that are related to the question. Your task with this type of question is to place them in the proper sequence (Fig. 11.5). You do this by selecting the circle or box in front of the option you think is number one and

Figure 11.2 Alternative format question. Fill in the blank by clicking on the "Calculator (0)" button at the lower right corner of the bar.

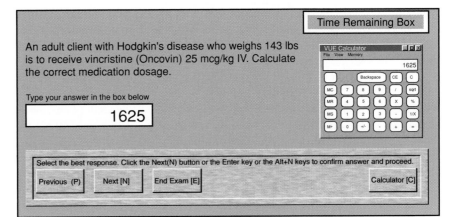

Time Remaining Box

An adult client with Hodgkin's disease who weighs 143 lbs is to receive vincristine (Oncovin) 25 mcg/kg IV. Calculate the correct medication dosage.

Type your answer in the box below

1625

Select the best response. Click the Next(N) button or the Enter key or the Alt+N keys to confirm answer and proceed.

Previous (P)   Next [N]   End Exam [E]   Calculator [C]

Figure 11.3 Alternative format question. Fill in the blank by using the calculator to click on number buttons. Then type in the answer box. Do *not* use spaces or commas in the answer. Close the calculator by clicking on the "X" button on the calculator screen.

Time Remaining Box

The nurse is caring for a client who has a draining wound infected with MRSA. Which infection control precautions should be used? Select all that apply.
- ○ wear a protective gown when entering the room
- ○ put on a particulate respirator mask when giving meds
- ○ wear gloves when delivering the meal tray
- ○ have visitors wear a mask when entering the room
- ○ wear sterile gloves when removing the dressing
- ○ put on a face shield before irrigating the wound

Select the best response. Click the Next(N) button or the Enter key or the Alt+N keys to confirm answer and proceed.

Previous (P)   Next [N]   End Exam [E]   Calculator [C]

Figure 11.4 Alternative format question—multiple answer.

Time Remaining Box

Identify the proper sequence for assessment of the abdomen starting with the number 1 for the first assessment. Type the number in the box before the statement.
- 3 Percussion
- 1 Inspection
- 4 Palpation
- 2 Auscultation

Select the best response. Click the Next(N) button or the Enter key or the Alt+N keys to confirm answer and proceed.

Previous (P)   Next [N]   End Exam [E]   Calculator [C]

Figure 11.5 Alternative format question—sequencing items.

typing in "1." Then move to the option you believe is number two and type that number in, and so forth. You can change the numbering by clicking on the boxes to remove the numbers.

A variation on this type of question uses the "drag and drop" format. With drag and drop, you will be given a series of items in a box on the left side of the screen. You will be asked to sequence them by clicking on them one at a time and putting them in the proper order in a box on the right hand side of the screen. When you have the options sequenced the way you think they should be, click on the "N" next button on the button bar and a new question will appear on the screen.

Identify the Area (or Hot Spot)
These types of questions provide you with a picture or diagram and then ask you to identify an area or a structure on the picture (Fig. 11.6). You place the cursor on the area that you think is correct and click. An "X" will appear. If you decide that is not where you really want the "X" you can click on the "X" again to remove it and then place the cursor in a new spot and click again. Once you decide that you have it where you want it, click on the "N" next button and the next question will appear on the screen.

Chart/Exhibit Items
A chart or exhibit item will present you with a chart, graph, or some other picture or graphic item or with a series of charts, graphs, or other pictures. You will need to be able to read the chart, graph, or picture to obtain the information to answer the question. Then you will be asked to select the correct answer from four or more options by using the information you gleaned from the chart, graph, or picture.

How Many Questions?
You may take between 75 and 265 questions, depending on how you answer. Of the first 75 questions, only 60 count. The other 15 are "trial" questions that will be used on future examinations, but you do not know which ones do not count, so you need to do the best you can on all of them. The NCSBN is attempting to establish reliability and validity data on these questions.

If you seem to be getting a lot of questions in a particular category, for example pediatrics, it may mean one of two things. The NCSBN may be testing pediatric questions on your exam so you are receiving a lot of them, or it may mean that you are having some problems answering pediatric questions correctly. The computer will continue to give you questions in a particular content area until you meet the goals of the test plan. The computer randomly draws the questions you are seeing from a pool of over 4,000 questions.

Contrary to rumor, no graduates are randomly selected by the computer to take all 265 questions. You can pass or fail the test with either 75 or 265 questions or any number in between. The average number of questions taken over the past 5 years is 119, and the average time is just over 2 hours.

How Long It Takes
There is a maximum time limit of 6 hours for the entire examination, although there is no minimum

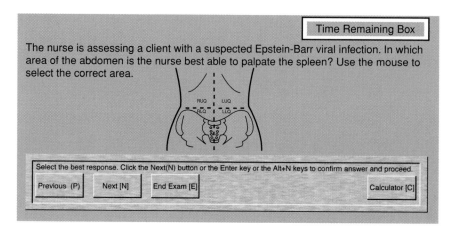

Figure 11.6 Alternative format question—identify area. With this type of question, you are given a diagram or picture and asked to locate a structure or area. Place the cursor on the area you think is correct and click. An "X" will appear in that area. To deselect the answer, click on the "X" and move the cursor to the new area. When finished, click on "Next (N)."

time limit. There is a mandatory break where the computer "locks up" about $2^1/_2$ hours into the test. For 10 minutes, you will not be able to answer any questions. There is another optional break at about 4 hours into the test, although the computer will not lock up at this time. You can take breaks at any time during the exam if you need to use the rest room, but remember that you will lose this time off of your total time for the exam.

The exam is not really a timed exam except for the overall time limit. Theoretically you could sit at the computer for the full 6 hours with question number 1 on the screen. The computer does not make you take questions at any particular rate. Most people can answer a multiple-choice question in about 45 seconds. As a rule of thumb, if you are spending more than 2 minutes on any single question, put an answer down and move on to the next question.

If you calculate that you are going to take 265 questions in 6 hours, it comes out to about 80 seconds per question. Some of the alternative format questions may take a little longer to answer, although some may take less time than the multiple-choice questions. Take a watch along and keep an eye on the "Time Remaining" box at the top of the screen.

How It's Graded

The test is graded on a statistical model that compares your responses with a pre-established standard. If you can demonstrate a knowledge level consistently above the standard, you will pass the examination.

Because the NCLEX-RN examination is given by computerized adaptive testing (CAT), increases in the passing standard do not necessarily require a higher number of items to be answered correctly by the graduate. However, it does require that you answer questions correctly at a slightly higher difficulty level than last year's graduates. Questions are assigned a difficulty value on a seven-logit (unit) scale called the NCLEX-RN logistic scale, ranging from the easiest (–3), which all graduates should answer correctly, to the most difficult (3), which almost all graduates would be expected to miss (Box 11.2).

Level of Difficulty

The difficulty level of the questions is determined by the question writers and question reviewers and is

Box 11.2

NCLEX-RN Logistic Scale

Logits
3 Most difficult
2
1

0 Approximate pass level
–1
–2
–3 Least difficult

based on factors such as when the material is usually presented in nursing programs (material presented earlier is considered less difficult) and the complexity of the material. To you, the test taker, difficulty level is somewhat relative. If you know the answer to a question, then it will seem relatively easy to you even if it is classified by the test writers as a higher difficulty-level question. Similarly, if you do not know the answer, then that question will be difficult for you even if it is determined to be at a relatively low difficulty level.

No Happy Questions. Keep in mind also that there are no "happy" questions on the NCLEX. There is always something wrong, and if there is a problem in the question, you need to worry about it. Also, as a general guiding principle, anything you know really well from your classes will NOT be on the NCLEX, so anticipate difficult questions.

After you finish the mandatory tutorial on the use of the computer, the first real question you will see will be at a medium difficulty level, probably a little above or a little below the pass criteria. If you answer it correctly, the next question will be a little more difficult. If you answer that one correctly, the next question will also increase in difficulty and so forth until you start missing questions. Then the computer will give you slightly less difficult questions. The computer is trying to establish your "zone of knowledge." If that zone is above the pass standard, then you will pass the exam.

Your Zone of Knowledge. If you miss the first question, and many graduates do because of anxiety, the computer will give you a slightly easier question for number 2. If you answer that one correctly, then the next one will increase in difficulty level, and so forth until you start missing questions. If the computer can clearly determine your zone of knowledge within the first 75 questions, then it will stop the test and ask you complete a short survey.

     The reason many graduates take more than 75 questions is because the computer is having difficulty establishing a clear zone of knowledge above or below the pass standard. It will keep giving questions until a clear determination is made. Graduates who take all 265 questions have answered questions above and below the pass standard throughout the whole exam. If you do have to take all 265 questions, it does not necessarily mean you failed.

> *Keep in mind that the NCLEX is designed so that no one can answer all the questions correctly. Even your most knowledgeable nursing instructor would not be able to answer some of the questions on the exam.*

EXAMPLE: LOW DIFFICULTY LEVEL

11. What blood test does the nurse evaluate as the best measure of a client's long-term control of diabetes mellitus?
    a. Fasting blood sugar
    b. Arterial blood gases
    c. Glucose tolerance test (GTT)
    d. Glycosylated hemoglobin (Hgb A_{1C})

EXAMPLE: MID-DIFFICULTY LEVEL (PASS CRITERIA)

12. While evaluating the results of a pulmonary function test, the nurse notes that an adult man who is short of breath has a vital capacity of 2800 mL, a tidal volume of 375 mL, and a residual volume of 2200 mL. Select the action the nurse should avoid implementing for this client.
    a. Position the client with the head of the bed elevated 45 degrees.
    b. Encourage fluid intake of 2 to 3 liters per 24 hours.

c. Begin oxygen by non-rebreather mask.
d. Encouraging the client to cough and to breathe deeply every hour during the shift.

EXAMPLE: HIGH DIFFICULTY LEVEL

13. While monitoring a client with a pulmonary artery catheter, the nurse notes catheter fling artifact on the pressure tracing. Identify the nursing measure that best compensates for this problem.
    a. Record only mean pressures.
    b. Ask the physician to reposition the catheter.
    c. Irrigate the catheter forcefully with heparinized saline solution.
    d. Level and zero the transducer before taking readings.

Remember that it is probably a good sign that you are getting difficult questions. It means that you are answering questions above the pass standard. You do not want a lot of easy questions on the NCLEX. Also keep in mind that the NCLEX is designed so that no one can answer all the questions correctly. Even your most knowledgeable nursing instructor would not be able to answer some of the questions on the exam.

     However, the NCLEX asks "entry-level" type questions that tend to be very "text-bookish." When you are answering NCLEX questions, look for the expected textbook-type knowledge. Don't look for exceptions. Each examination is different and unique to the person taking it because future questions depend on how you answered previous questions.

NCLEX BACKGROUND INFORMATION

Revisions in the Passing Standard

Passing standards are established by a nine-nurse panel of National Council members that includes diverse representation (regional, nursing specialty, minority, educator, new RNs). Their efforts combine with a survey of nursing professionals such as nursing administrators of all types of facilities and directors of nursing. After consideration of all the data, including current trends in health care, the National

Council Board of Directors may determine that safe entry-level practice for RNs requires a higher level of knowledge, skills, and abilities than was required in previous years.

The passing standard and test content is generally evaluated on a 3-year cycle, but revisions are not made every cycle. The National Council last revised the passing standard of the NCLEX-RN, CAT in 2005. It was raised 0.078 logit. Generally the national average pass rate drops by about 4 percent whenever there is an increase in the difficulty level.

Test Vendor and Logistics

The test vendor for the NCLEX is VUE, a subsidiary of NCS Pearson Professional Centers. The tests are given at Pearson Professional Centers. The test items and the format of the examination always stay the same even if vendors should change because the exam is owned by the National Council of State Boards of Nursing (NCSBN), which contracts with vendors to administer the examination.

After graduates have completed their nursing program, they apply to the state board of nursing. Appointments at the examination sites are made on a first-come, first-served basis. The centers are required to schedule the examination within 30 days from the time you apply. Each state establishes its own time interval for application after graduation, generally within 1 year.

There are both morning and afternoon sessions of 6-hour duration. Depending on the size of the center, between 8 and 15 graduates may be taking the test at the same time. There may be other people at the center taking examinations in other disciplines at the same time as the nursing graduates.

Testing by Computer

The computer skills required are minimal. The mouse is used for the majority of the examination, with minimal typing required. A digital picture is taken at the time you enter the examination room, and that picture, along with your information, appears on one of the computer screens in the room. A digital thumb print and signature are also obtained when you enter the exam center.

You sit at the computer with your picture on it and complete a three-question tutorial on the use of the mouse and computer. You have two attempts at completing the tutorial successfully. If you are unable to do so after the second try, a person who is working

at the testing center will come and help you. After the examination is completed, you will be asked to complete a short computerized personal data questionnaire and an evaluation of the examination site.

Questions appear one at a time on the computer screen, with a button bar on the bottom of the screen and a "time remaining" box in the upper corner. After you select an answer, the question is replaced with another question and answers. No question is ever repeated, nor are you able to change the answer once you have clicked on the "N" next button.

An on-screen pop-up calculator is available for answering dosage and other questions that require calculations. Because of the increased emphasis on pharmacology and the concern about mediation errors, it is probably safe to assume that the difficulty level of future calculation questions will increase markedly.

Security

Security is very tight at the examination sites. All exam sessions are video taped and there is a proctor in the room monitoring all the test-takers. Although cheating on the NCLEX is virtually impossible—every examination is different—it is important not to even look like you are attempting to cheat. Do not talk to the person next to you. Keep your eyes on your own computer. Do not take out any papers or electronic devices during the exam. Magic slates are generally provided for use as "scrap paper," so you will not need any paper or pens during the exam. Lockers are provided and you must leave all your personal belongings at the door, so do not bring a lot of things with you to the examination site.

How the Test Is Graded

The NCLEX is graded on a pass-fail basis. If the graduate has failed the examination, the entire examination must be taken again. The National Council of State Boards of Nursing (NCSBN) requires a 45-day waiting period before repeating the examination, and first-time takers are given preference over those who are repeating the examination. A number of states have restricted the number of times the graduate can retake the test, usually to three. Check with your state board of nursing for the particular regulations.

When the computer shuts off, it knows if you passed or failed, but it will not give you that information at that time. At the end of the day, after the last testing session, results are downloaded electronically to NCSBN in Chicago. The next business day, they notify the state board of nursing electronically and send hard copy; then it is up to the state board of nursing to notify you.

The exam results may be sent to you by mail, usually within 7 to 10 days after the examination has been completed, although this time frame varies from state to state. Most states now offer online results within 72 hours after the exam. Check with your state board of nursing to make sure they offer this service and how to access the site. The NCSBN offers a service that allows you to obtain unofficial results by telephone 3 days after taking the examination. The telephone number is 900-225-6000; the cost for the call is $7.95. You can also access the NCSBN on the Web at www.nclex.com/store.asp. Not all states participate in the service, and your employment agency may or may not accept the results.

NCLEX STUDY STRATEGIES

There are several ways to prepare for examinations, including the NCLEX. To attempt to take the examination with an attitude of "If I don't know it by now, I never will" is to court failure. Carefully directed study and preparation will considerably increase the chances of passing the examination. Review Chapter 10 for general tips on how to study for and take exams. Below is some specific information for preparation for the NCLEX.

The NCSBN Web Site
You can access the NCBSN Web site at www.ncsbn.org. This Web site can provide significant help as you prepare to take the NCLEX. It provides the most recent information on any changes in the test, has a sample tutorial about the exam, and even has some sample questions. The more you can learn about the exam before you have to take it, the lower your anxiety and the better you will do.

Review Books
The material covered by review books is the key material found on the NCLEX. These books usually follow the NCLEX Test Plan very closely. A review book is, however, just that; it reviews the material that you should already know. Reviewing is important to reinforce learning and recall of information you may not have used in a year or more.

What Do You Think?

When was the last time you sat in on a group study session? List three of the problems you encountered at the session. How could they be solved?

Review books are not really designed to present any new information about key material. If you are totally unfamiliar with the material in a particular section of the review book, then reading a more complete textbook on that particular subject area will be necessary.

Another important function of a review book is to point out areas of weakness. If you find sections that seem to contain "new" material, it is important to investigate that section in more detail. If you find most of the material familiar and easy to grasp, then you are probably well on your way to success on the NCLEX.

Group Study
Group study can be an effective method of preparation for an examination such as the NCLEX. To optimize the results of group study sessions, several rules should be followed.

RULE 1. *Be very selective when choosing the members of the study group.* They should have a similar frame of mind and orientation toward studying. They should be graduates who are also going to be taking the NCLEX. The ideal size for a study group is between four and six people. Groups larger than six become difficult to organize and handle. After the group has been formed and has begun its study sessions, it may be necessary to ask an individual to leave the group for not participating or for being disruptive to the study process or displaying negative attitudes about the examination.

RULE 2. *Have each individual prepare a particular section for each group study session.* Study groups generally meet once or twice a week. For example, if next week the group is going to study the endocrine system, assign group member 1 the anatomy and physiology of the system, member 2 the pathological conditions, member 3 the medications used for treatment, and member 4 the key elements of nursing care. When the group comes together, have each individual present his or her prepared section. This type of preparation prevents the "What are we going to study tonight?" syndrome that often plagues group study sessions.

> *No matter what other study and preparation methods are used, individual preparation for the NCLEX is a necessity.*

Following this process organizes the study group and allows for more in-depth coverage of the topic. It also permits the members of the group to ask questions of the other members, thereby reinforcing the information being discussed.

RULE 3. *Limit the length of the study session.* No single study session should be longer than between 60 and 90 minutes. Sessions that go longer tend to get off the topic and foster a negative attitude about the examination. Try to avoid making group study sessions into party time. A few snacks and refreshments may be helpful to maintain the group's energy level, but a real party atmosphere will detract significantly from the effectiveness of the study session.

RULE 4. *Use role playing to reinforce information.* The more senses you can involve in the learning process, the better the learning.

RULE 5. *Remain positive.* Although group study times should not be party times, relax and have some fun with the study.

> *Experts recommend that you take between 3000 and 5000 practice questions before you take the NCLEX. Obviously starting early in this process is important along with some planning and time management.*

Individual Study Tips

No matter what other study and preparation methods are used, individual preparation for the NCLEX is a necessity. This preparation can take several forms.

TIP 1. As previously discussed, use of a review book is valuable to indicate areas of deficient knowledge. Reading and studying the appropriate textbooks and study guides can be helpful if it is approached correctly. It is important that the graduate mentally organize the information being read into a format similar to that found in the NCLEX. After reading each page of a textbook or study guide, the graduate should be able to ask three or four multiple-choice questions about that information. These questions can be asked silently or written out and should answer the question "How might the NCLEX test my knowledge of this material?"

TIP 2. Practice answering questions similar to those found on the exam you are going to take or the NCLEX itself. Take practice exams on the computer. Most of the review books come with a CD that has practice questions on it. It will help alleviate some of the unknowns, particularly if you have not had a lot of experience with computer-based exams.

Learning the Format. Experts recommend that you take between 3000 and 5000 practice questions before you take the NCLEX. Obviously starting early in this process is important along with some planning and time management. When practice questions are answered, several important mental processes occur.

Getting Comfortable. First, you are becoming more familiar with and therefore more comfortable with the format of the examination. In research, this process is termed the practice effect; it must be accounted for when analyzing the results from pretest/post-test-type research projects. Individuals will have better results after a test even without any type of intervention because of having practiced answering questions on the pretest. Similarly, your score on the NCLEX may increase by as much as 10 percent through answering practice questions.

Reinforcing Information. A second result of answering practice questions is that it reinforces the information already studied. Although it is unlikely that a question on the NCLEX examination will be identical to a practice question, there are many similarities. Realistically, only a limited number of questions can be asked about any given subject. After a while, the questions will begin to sound very similar.

Identifying Weak Spots. A third advantage of answering practice questions is that it quickly reveals subject areas that you will need to study. It is relatively easy to say, "I understand the renal system pretty well." It is quite another to answer correctly 10 or 15 questions about that system. If you answer the questions correctly, then you can move on to the next topic. If you miss the majority of the questions, however, then further review is required.

In order to obtain the optimal benefit from working practice questions, it is probably best to spend 30 to 45 minutes each day working 20 to 100 questions rather than trying to do 1000 questions on one day during the week-end.

After you have answered the questions, you need to review them and compare your answers with the answers provided in the study book. You should also look at the rationales and the categories into which the questions fall. Try to understand why you missed the questions you did. Was it lack of knowledge? Didn't read the question carefully? Didn't use critical thinking?

TIP 3. Complete a 265-item test in one sitting in 6 hours. Many Web sites provide testing materials and sample examinations. One is http://passneclex.mcphu.eduwww.sjsu.edu/depts/itl/graphics/main.html.

TIP 4. Take the NCLEX as soon as possible after you graduate. The NCSBN has done some studies that show the following:

• The NCLEX taken less than 26 days after graduation has an 89 percent average pass rate.
• The NCLEX taken between 27 and 39 days after graduation has an 80 percent average pass rate.
• The NCLEX taken between 40 and 62 days after graduation has a 72 percent average pass rate.

• The NCLEX taken more than 62 days after graduation has a 45 percent average pass rate.

Formal NCLEX Reviews

The NCSBN does not endorse or sponsor any review courses for the NCLEX directly, but many companies offer reviews shortly after graduation. An on-line comprehensive review course for the NCLEX-RN examination on the NCSBN Web site is offered by an independent company (http://www.nclex.com). These review courses range from 2 to 5 days and basically cover the information found in review books. They are rather expensive, and the quality of NCLEX reviews varies. In general they are only as good as the people who are presenting the material. Also, look at the reported pass rate of the graduates after they take the review. Those with higher pass rates are probably better.

PREPARING FOR THE BIG DAY

Several Months to A Week Before the Exam

1. Get mentally and physically prepared. Eat a good healthy diet. Exercise regularly. Drink lots of water (64 ounces per day) to rid your body of accumulated toxins. Avoid alcohol, street drugs, and even over-the-counter medications like antihistamines that can affect your ability to concentrate and think. Ease off on the caffeine and stop smoking.
2. Practice doing NCLEX type questions—lots of them!

The Night Before the Exam

1. If you are unfamiliar with the area where the test center is located, drive to the test site. Note parking facilities and places where you can get a meal. This will save you from getting lost the next day and help you be on time.
2. Review formulas, common medications, information that can be summarized in tables, or on cards and lists. It is probably not a good time to pull out all your old text books and notes and try to read them. Concentrate on things that are visual and may have caused you some problems in the past, like the list of cranial nerves or the glands and hormones in the endocrine system. Don't try to

study everything. The "If I don't know it now, I never will" attitude is a negative thought process. You can always learn something.

3. Avoid strange or exotic foods that you have never eaten before. This can be a real temptation if you have to travel away from home and stay in a hotel the night before the exam. Stick to your usual diet. New or unusual foods may cause some gastrointestinal consequences that can be very distracting during the exam.

4. Go to bed at a reasonable hour. It is probably best to stick to your normal schedule. Staying up all night trying to study is going to be counterproductive. You will be nervous and may have some problems sleeping, but stay away from sleep aids. They will interfere with your decision-making ability on the exam. Even if you are not sound asleep, the fact that you are resting will be helpful.

The Day of the Exam

1. Stick to your regular schedule and routine as much as possible. Avoid drinking excessive amounts of caffeine beverages to try to "stay awake." They will only make you nervous and may increase the amount of time you need to spend on breaks in the rest room.

2. Eat breakfast, especially if you are scheduled for the morning session. Eat something with some glucose for a quick start (bread with jelly) and eat something with protein to get you through the morning (cereal and milk; egg and bacon). If you are taking the exam in the afternoon, eat some lunch but avoid a large meal with a lot of greasy food. It will make you sleepy and sit in your stomach like a lump.

3. Don't let the security at the site fluster you. They will take a digital picture, thumb print, and signature. They make you leave all your belongings at the door. There will be someone walking around the room during the exam. Just concentrate on your computer and answer the questions and you will do fine.

4. Wear comfortable clothes. You don't get extra points on the NCLEX for looking like a fashion model. Dress appropriately for the season but keep in mind that some buildings are very cool in the summer because of air conditioning and very hot in the winter because of heating systems. Wear something you have worn before. Sweat clothes are a good choice, particularly because you can dress in layers. If it is too warm, you can take a jacket off; if it is cold, you can leave it on.

5. Think positive! If you truly believe you will do well, you will do well. If you go into the exam with an "I'm never going to pass this—I'm too dumb" attitude, you probably are not going to do as well.

Conclusion

Taking and passing the NCLEX-RN, CAT is a necessary step in the process of becoming a professional registered nurse. Like all licensure examinations, its purpose is to protect the public from undereducated or unsafe practitioners. The examination is comprehensive and includes material from all areas of the graduate's nursing education. Although most graduates have some anxiety about taking this examination, knowledge about its format and content and strategies for taking the examination can lower anxiety to an acceptable level.

Critical Thinking Exercises

- Obtain an NCLEX-RN, CAT review book. Analyze the questions in the practice examination for type, cognitive level, and level of difficulty.
- Identify three to five other students in your class with whom you would feel comfortable working in a study group. Organize a study group session before the next major course examination.
- When you get the results of your next course examination, identify why you missed the questions you missed and what strategies might have been used to answer those questions correctly.

ANSWERS TO QUESTIONS IN CHAPTER 11

1. Correct answer: d. You either have or do not have the knowledge for this particular laboratory test.

2. Correct answer: c. Not only do you need to know the normal values for each of the blood gas components given, you must also be able to use that information in determining the underlying condition.

3. Best answer: c. Choices b and d are also actions that should be carried out, but at this time, opening the airway and oxygenating the client must receive highest priority. Not only does this question require that you know the normal values and be able to interpret them, but it also requires that a decision be made about the seriousness of the condition (analysis) and a selection of the type of care to be given from several correct options (judgment).

4. Correct answer: d. This question measures critical thinking and decision-making ability by asking you which of these clients is the sickest or least stable. Type I diabetics may have symptoms of hypoglycemia even when their blood glucoses are normal. This one is below normal and all the other clients are stable.

5. Correct answer: d. This question requires you to know what a tonic neck reflex is and its significance. It is present in the newborn because of immaturity of the CNS and usually is gone by 1 month. If a child at 7 months still has it, it indicates a delay in neurological development.

6. Correct answer: c. Stokes-Adams syndrome is a suddenly occurring episode of asystole. The client becomes unconscious quickly.

7. Correct answer: b. Nursing diagnoses that deal with the airway always have highest priority.

8. Correct answer: c. Choice a is unrealistic for this client; choice b is not client-centered; choice d is a nursing intervention, not a goal. Maintaining an oxygen saturation of 90 percent is realistic, measurable and within normal limits.

9. Correct answer: d. These are symptoms of a pulmonary embolism, which is a common complication of prolonged bed rest.

10. Correct answer: c. Answer c lists some side effects of theophylline medications that may indicate the onset of toxicity. The physician needs to know about these so that the theophylline level can be

determined and the dosage adjusted accordingly. Other instructions that the client could be given when taking theophylline medications include to avoid excessive amounts of caffeine, never to suddenly stop taking the medication, to take it with a full glass of water and a small amount of food, and to watch for interactions with over-the-counter (OTC) medications.

11. Correct answer: d. Laboratory tests and their significance are considered basic knowledge and are taught in the early part of most nursing programs.

12. Correct answer: c. The PFT indicates that the client has COPD. High levels of oxygen that can be delivered by a non-rebreather mask can put the client into respiratory arrest.

13. Correct answer: a. The question asks about how to compensate for the problem, not correct it. Invasive hemodynamic monitoring is considered advanced medical/surgical nursing and is usually presented during the last year of nursing school.

Computer Screen Box 11.2. Correct answer: 4. Kayser-Fleischer rings are caused by the deposition of a golden brown pigment from an increased copper level secondary to hepatolenticular disease, a familial disorder of abnormal copper metabolism. The liver is damaged, and the tests related to the liver are abnormally high. Other symptoms include dysphasia, dysarthria, rigidity, and coarse resting tremors (wing-beating tremors).

Bibliography

Crow, C: Requirements and interventions used by BSN programs to promote and predict NCLEX-RN success: A national study. J Prof Nurs 20(3):174–186, 2004.

Cunningham, H: Strategies to promote success on the NCLEX-RN for students with English as a second language. Nurse Educ 29(1):15–19, 2004.

Haas, R: The use of discriminant function analysis to predict student success on the NCLEX-RN. Journal of Nursing Education 43(10):440–446, 2004.

Miller, J: Tips on taking the NCLEX-RN. Imprint 52(1): 28–30, 32, 2005.

NCLEX-RN Passing standard raised for public safety. ASBN Update, Winter, 2004, p 9.

Seldomridge, L: Can success and failure be predicted for baccalaureate graduates on the computerized NCLEX-RN? J Prof Nurs 20(6):361–368, 2004.

Waterhouse, J, and Beeman, P: Predicting NCLEX-RN success. Can it be simplified? Nursing Education Perspectives 24(1):35–39, 2003.

Wendt, A: The NCLEX-RN examination: charting the course of nursing practice. Nurse Educ 28(6):276–280, 2003.

12

Reality Shock in the Workplace

Kristy Baker

Learning Objectives

After completing this chapter, the reader will be able to:

- Describe the concept of reality shock.
- Describe appropriate documents and procedures for job interviews.
- List evidential artifacts used to develop professional nursing portfolios.
- Define burnout and list its major symptoms.
- Discuss the key factors that produce burnout.
- List the important elements in personal time management.
- Analyze how the nurse's humanity affects nursing practice.
- List at least four health-care practices nurses can use to prevent burnout and to improve their professional performance.

WHAT IS REALITY SHOCK?

That is not how we do it in the real world. How many times do new graduate nurses hear that sentence? In many ways, that sentence is correct in identifying the fact that in nursing school, students are instructed in the ideal theoretical, research-based, and instructor-supervised practice. Although demanding physically, mentally, and emotionally, nursing school shelters students from the realities of the real world, where nursing practice consists of not only theory and research, but heuristic practice, human emotion and response, policies, regulations, and the push and pull of life responsibilities. Things are different in the real world. The transition from nursing student to registered nurse is referred to as **transition shock,** or **reality shock.**

MAKING THE TRANSITION FROM STUDENT TO NURSE

At any point in their lives, most people fulfill several different roles simultaneously. Sometimes, **role conflict** occurs. Role conflict exists when a person is unable to integrate the three distinct aspects of a given role: *ideal, perceived,* and *performed role images.* For a nursing student, a significant role conflict may be when they transition from the role of student to registered nurse.

Ideal Role
In the academic setting, the student is generally presented with the ideal of what a nurse should be. The ideal role projects society's expectations of a nurse. It clearly delineates obligations and responsibilities as well as the rights and privileges that those in the role can claim. Although the ideal role presents a clear image of what is

"So...when do we go to lunch?"

expected, it is often somewhat unrealistic to believe that everyone in this role will follow this pattern of behaviors.

An Angel of Mercy. The ideal role of the nurse might require someone with superhuman physical strength and ability with unlimited stamina who possesses superior intelligence and decision-making ability, yet remains kind, gentle, caring and altruistic, not caring about money. This perfect nurse can communicate with any client at any time and is able to function independently and know more than even the physician. This angel of mercy is able to prevent grievous errors in client care while continuing to always be responsive to clients' needs and requests while carrying out the physicians orders with accuracy and absolute obedience. Perceptive students soon begin to suspect that this ideal role of nurse does not exist anywhere in the real world.

Perceived Role

The perceived role is an individual's own definition of the role that is often more realistic than the ideal role. When individuals define their own roles, they may reject or modify some of the norms and expectations of society that were used to establish the ideal role. Intentionally or unintentionally, though, the ideal role is often used as the intellectual yardstick against which the perceived role is measured.

After a minimal amount of clinical experience, nursing students may realize that nurses do not possess extraordinary physical strength or intellectual ability but may continue to accept unconditionally, as part of their perceived role, that nurses must be kind, gentle, and understanding at all times with all clients and other health-care staff. The perceived role is the role with which the nursing student often graduates.

Performed Role

The performed role is defined as what the practitioner of the role actually does. Reality shock occurs when the ideal or perceived role comes into conflict with the performed role. Many new graduate nurses soon realize that the accomplishment of role expectations depends on many factors other than their perception and beliefs about how nursing should be performed. The environment has a great deal to do with how the obligations of the role are met.

In nursing school, where students are assigned to care for one or two clients at a time, there is plenty of time to practice therapeutic communication techniques; to provide completely for the physical, mental, educational, emotional, and spiritual needs of the client; and to develop an insightful care plan. The realities of the workplace may dictate that a nurse be assigned to care for six to eight clients at a time. In this situation, the perceived role of the nurse may have to be set aside for the more realistic performed role, from communicator to task organizer. Meeting all of the client's physical, psychological, social, and spiritual needs becomes less possible, and the care plan becomes more brief and to the point.

Cognitive Dissonance. Such situations can produce what is called **cognitive dissonance** in many new graduate nurses; that is, they know what they should do and they know how they should do it, yet the circumstances do not allow them to carry it out. The end result is increased anxiety. High levels of anxiety, left unrecognized or unresolved, can lead to various physical and emotional symptoms. When these symptoms become severe enough, a condition called burnout may result. In today's health-care climate and with the current nursing shortage, it is important that health-care agencies retain high-quality nurses and that nursing schools prepare graduates for their transition from student to nurse.

> *The Department of Health and Human Services currently projects a shortfall of up to 800,000 registered nurses by the year 2020.*

A NURSING SHORTAGE

A lack of qualified nurses has been present in the health-care system for so long that the term *nursing shortage* has become a truism. However, as recent history has demonstrated, the demand for nurses increases and decreases with changes in the health-care system. In addition, the demand for nurses is to some extent regional. Some areas of the country have a higher demand for registered nurses, and others may have fewer available jobs. However, studies about employment opportunities project that there will continue to be a shortage of nurses well into this century.[1]

What Do You Think?

Is there a nursing shortage in your region? Does it affect the health care that you can obtain at your local hospital? How can the nursing shortage be "fixed?"

_____

_____

_____

_____

_____

_____

_____

_____

_____

_____

_____

_____

Nurses in Demand

The demand for nurses is finally being recognized by high school counselors and employment agencies.

They are now encouraging young people to enter nursing schools, and enrollment is up. After several years of declines in nursing school enrollments that reduced the number of graduates by almost 30 percent nationally, nursing schools are starting to see dramatic increases in enrollment. Drops in enrollment tend to occur when the economy is strong.

In short, when the economy is strong, there are more opportunities outside of the traditional female employment areas for young women to pursue. Also, overall enrollment in higher education also decreases during periods of strong economic growth and increases when the economy takes a downturn.

There are several reasons for the increased demand for registered nurses. One of the primary reasons is the ever-increasing demand for health care. As the population of the United States continues to age, and there is a recognition that an older population has increased health-care needs, the demand for well-educated, highly skilled nurses will continue to increase. It is also important to note that a high percentage of the currently working registered nurses are in this group that will retire within the next 10 years and therefore will not be an active part of the workforce. The Department of Health and Human Services currently projects a shortfall of up to 800,000 registered nurses by the year 2020.[2]

Over the past several years, some facilities have tried to cut costs by reducing the number of their most expensive personnel, the registered nurses. Most of these facilities have recognized that although a reduction in registered nurse positions may reduce the costs in the short term, the long-term effects to the quality of health care are devastating. It is obvious that exchanging qualified nurses for lower-paid unlicensed technicians will eventually have an effect on the quality of client care. Hospitals and other health-care facilities are experiencing the results of personnel cutting practices in reduction in the number of clients seeking care at these facilities as well as closing units and losing revenue.

Decentralized Care

Certain groups of nurses are in higher demand than ever; these include nurses who can practice independently in several different settings, multiskilled practitioners, home care nurses, community nurses, and hospice nurses.[3] A major trend in health care today is to move the care out of the hospital and into the community and home settings. Provision of nursing services in these settings often requires that a nurse have at least a bachelor's degree or even higher education. Fewer than 50 percent of all new graduate nurses today are graduating from bachelor's degree programs.[4]

Although most nurse practitioners are currently based in community clinics, there is an ever-expanding opportunity for them to become involved in the care of hospitalized clients. A key element in many of the proposed health-care reform plans is that clients would be required to be evaluated by a primary health-care provider before they could be referred to secondary health-care providers or specialists. The advanced-practice education of nurse practitioners would make them eminently qualified to fill this role of primary health-care provider.

Certain specialty areas (e.g., intensive care units, neonatal units, and burn units) are always seeking nurses. As with community nurses, nurses who provide care in specialty units must be able to work independently and to draw from a large base of theoretical knowledge.

The nursing profession and nursing educators need to increase their vigilance when there are nursing shortages to maintain the high standards of the profession, to recruit high-quality students, and to retain professional nurses.

Preceptorships allow students to experience a more realistic employment situation before they graduate.

A POSITIVE TRANSITION TO PROFESSIONAL NURSING

The reality shock that new graduates often experience can be reduced to some extent. Some schools of nursing have instituted preceptor clinical experiences during the last semester of the senior year. The main goal of this type of clinical experience, which occurs just before graduation, is to help the student feel more comfortable in the role of registered nurse. Preceptorships allow students to experience a more realistic employment situation before they graduate.

A student who works with a preceptor is assigned to one registered nurse for supervision for

most of the semester. The student experiences the role of the registered nurse by working the same hours and on the same unit as the nurse to whom he or she is assigned. As the role expectations of the workplace are absorbed by the student during the preceptor experience, the student's perceived role expectations also change, allowing movement from the student role to that of practicing professional with less anxiety and stress.

Another experience that lessens role transition shock may be called an internship or externship depending on the name used by the hospital. Internships or externships are available to students between the junior and senior years at some hospitals. These experiences allow students to work in a hospital setting as nurses' aides, while permitting them to practice, with a few restrictions, at their level of nursing education. These experiences are invaluable for gaining practice in skills and for becoming socialized into the professional role.

Employment in Today's Job Market

Although the health-care industry is in dire need of registered nurses, employers are still looking for the best of the best for the positions they have available.

What Do You Think?

Have you ever been on a job interview? What were some of the mistakes you made? How can you correct these mistakes in the future?

Initial Strategies

Employers are looking for graduates who can function independently, require little retraining or orientation, and can supervise a variety of less-educated and unlicensed employees. The ability to use critical thinking skills in making sound clinical judgments is a must in today's fast-paced, complicated, and highly technical health-care systems.

Although these requirements may seem daunting, some strategies can be used to increase the chance of being hired. Students should take advantage of preceptor and intern or extern experiences in their junior and seniors year and attempt to meet their clinical obligations in the institution where they desire employment. In this way, the student can evaluate the hospital closely and observe its working conditions and the type of care provided to clients.

The hospital, on its part, has the opportunity to examine closely the student's knowledge, skills, personality, and ability to relate with clients and staff. The hospital benefits by getting **employees** that are familiar with the hospital before employment starts, thus decreasing the overall time of paid adjustment (referred to as "orientation").

> *First impressions are important. Preparing a neat, thorough, and professional-looking resume is worth the time and effort.*

The Resume

In today's job market, the **resume** is often the institution's first contact with the nurse seeking employment, and it has a substantial effect on the whole hiring process (Box 12.1). First impressions are important. Preparing a neat, thorough, and professional-looking resume is worth the time and effort. If you have access to a computer, a good-looking resume can be prepared at almost no cost. If a computer is not available, it is a good idea to spend a few dollars to have the resume professionally prepared and reproduced.

A Complete Picture

The goal of a resume is to provide the hospital with a complete picture of the prospective employee in as little space as possible. It should be easy to read and visually appealing and have flawless grammar and spelling. Although various formats may be used, all resumes should contain the same information. Each area of information should have a separate heading (see Box 12.1).

Many books are available in local bookstores that can serve as a guide in organizing the information in a resume. Many new computers now come from the factory loaded with software for the preparation of resumes in different formats. Keep an electronic copy of the resume for future use or reference. The required information includes the following:

• Full name, current address (or address where the person can always be reached), and a telephone number (including area code) and e-mail address.
• Educational background (all degrees), starting with the most recent, naming institution, location, dates of attendance, and degrees awarded. Usually high school graduation information is not necessary.
• Former employers, again starting with the most recent. Give dates of employment, title of position, name of immediate supervisor, supervisor's telephone number, and a short description of the job responsibilities. Should non–health-care-related work be included? Very basic jobs, for example, cooking hamburgers at Big Bob's Burgers, could probably be omitted unless it fills in a large gap in your employment history. However, if the job required supervision of other employees or demonstrated some higher degree of responsibility such as developing budgets, handling money, or preparing work schedules, it should be included and described.
• Describe any scholarships, achievements, awards, honors, or activities that have been received, starting with the most recent.
• List professional memberships, offices held, and date of memberships.
• List any publications. If both books and journal articles were published, list the books separately, starting with the most recent.
• Include an "Other" category to describe any unpublished materials produced (e.g., an internal hospital booklet for use by clients), research projects, **fellowships,** grants, and so forth.
• Provide professional license number and annual number for all states where licensed, along with the date of license and expiration date.

Box 12.1

Sample Resume

Mary P. Oak
100 Wood Lane, Nicetown, PA 22222 Telephone (333) 555-1234 (H) e-mail: moak@aol.com

Objectives

Obtain an entry-level position as a Registered Nurse; deliver high-quality nursing care; continue my professional development.

Skills

- Good organizational and time management skills
- Communication and supervisory ability
- Sensitivity to cultural diversity

Education

Mountain University, Nicetown, PA
Bachelor of Science in Nursing, May, 2006

Experience

Supercare Hospital, Hilltown, PA
Nursing Assistant, 2004 to present

    Responsibilities: Direct client care, including bathing, ambulation, daily activities, feeding paralyzed clients, assisting nurses with procedures, charting vital signs, and entering orders on the computer.
Big Bob's Burgers, Hilltown, PA
Assistant Manager, 1999–2004

    Responsibilities: Supervised work of six employees; counted cash-register receipts at end of shift; inventoried and ordered supplies.

Awards

Nursing Student of the Year, 2005
Mountain University, Nicetown, PA
Pine Tree Festival Queen, 1999
Hilltown High School, Hilltown, PA

Professional Membership

National Student Nurses Association, 2005 to present
Mountain University, Nicetown, PA

References

References should be included on a separate sheet of paper. Most institutions require three references. After obtaining permission from the individuals listed as references, the nurse preparing the resume should make sure to have current and accurate titles, addresses, e-mail addresses, and telephone numbers.

    An individual selected for a reference must know the applicant well in either a professional or a personal capacity, have something positive to say about the applicant, and be in some type of position of authority. The director of the nursing program, esteemed nursing faculty, supervisory-level personnel at a health-care facility, and even a physician make good references. It is best not to list relatives, unless the hospital is asking specifically for a personal reference.

    Do not obtain letters of reference until the facility asks for them. Many facilities are now using e-mail or phone references in place of letters as a time saving method.

The Cover Letter

A cover letter should be sent with every resume (Box 12.2). Like the resume, it should be neatly typed without errors and should be short and to the point. Although a friendly, rambling letter might provide insight into a prospective employee's underlying personality, most personnel directors or directors of nursing are too busy to read through the whole document. The letter should be written in a business letter format, centered on the page and should include the name and title of the person who will receive the letter. Letters beginning "To Whom It May Concern" do not make as favorable an impression.

Organizing the Letter

The statement of interest and name of the position should constitute the opening paragraph of the letter. The prospective employee should mention where he or she heard about the position. This information should be included in the first paragraph as well as a date when the applicant would be able to begin working.

The second paragraph should give a brief summary of any work experience or education that qualifies the applicant for this position. Newly graduated nurses will have some difficulty with this part, but they should include their graduation date, the name of the school they graduated from, the prospective date for taking the NCLEX, and the name of the director of the program. This paragraph should also state which shifts the applicant is willing to work.

The third paragraph should be very short. It should express thanks for consideration of the nurse's resume, a telephone number, and an e-mail address. Both the letter and resume should be sent by first-class mail in a 9-by-12-inch envelope so that the resume will remain unfolded, thus making it easier to handle and read.

Box 12.2

Sample Cover Letter

Mary P. Oak
100 Wood Lane
Nicetown, PA 22222

May 25, 2006

Mr. Robert L. Pine
Director of Personnel
Doctors Hospital
Gully City, PA 44444

Dear Mr. Pine:

I am interested in applying for the Registered Nurse position in the General Medical/Surgical Unit. I have five years of experience in providing care for a variety of clients with medical/surgical health-care problems as a nursing assistant. I completed my baccalaureate degree in nursing on May 9, and am scheduled to take the NCLEX examination on June 3. Enclosed find my resume.

I believe that my organizational and time management skills will be a great asset to your fine health-care facility. I work well with all types of staff personnel, and having been a nursing assistant for the past five years, I can appreciate the problems involved in their supervision.

Thank you very much for consideration of my resume and application. I will call you within the next few days to arrange a date and time for an interview. Feel free to call me at home anytime (333) 555-1234 or contact me by e-mail: moak@ol.com.

Sincerely,

Mary P. Oak

Will They Ever Answer?

Waiting for a reply can be the most difficult part of the process. Resist the urge to call the hospital too soon. Because most health-care institutions recognize the high anxiety levels of new graduates, they attempt to return calls within 1 to 2 weeks after receipt of the application. If no response is given after 3 weeks, the nurse should call the hospital to see whether or not the application was received. Mail does get lost. If the application has been received, the applicant should make no further telephone calls. Harassing the personnel director or director of nursing about a job is not usually an effective employment strategy.

> *Harassing the personnel director or director of nursing about a job is not usually an effective employment strategy.*

The Portfolio

Today's current work climate requires recruiters to interview, screen, and hire the most qualified person for the job in a short amount of time. The nursing shortage and a work force that embraces career portability has created the need to often recruit and hire nurses on a moment's notice.

Evidence of Positive Outcomes

Professional portfolios are being looked at closely by many non-artist professions to document skill qualifications, continued competency, accountability for professional development, and credible evidence to support employment claims during an interview. Nursing is one of the professions embracing this concept, and if the trend continues, student nurses of today will become the next generation of the 2.6 million registered nurses in the United States who use portfolios instead of resumes to interview for jobs, become certified, maintain certifications, and demonstrate competency.

Health-care employers today are looking for nurses who believe that high-quality performance on the job is more important than just having a job. Professional nurses can apply the nursing process to their own personal development, and evidence of positive outcomes is placed in the portfolio.

Constructing a portfolio requires looking at a career as a collection of experiences, which can be grouped and re-ordered to match the changing direction of one's career journey.[6] A portfolio also offers an opportunity for nurses to evaluate their experiences, create new goals, create and implement a plan, and then evaluate it. The portfolio supports the lifelong process of self- and career development.[7]

Assembling a Portfolio

Once a student has decided to initiate a portfolio as a professional vehicle for showcasing his or her experiences, education, skill-set, accomplishments, and what they have the potential to achieve, it will require time and effort commitment to create it. The effort, however, is well worth it in the long run.

The initial development of a portfolio may be somewhat time-consuming, but once developed, keeping it current should become part of a professional's routine activities. Many books are available that describe the format and organization of a portfolio; however, an example is discussed here.

Use a Binder. One format that many experts agree on is a three ring binder. This should include a table of contents, and the various sections should be separated by dividers.

Ask Yourself Questions. Questions to ask you prepare to gather materials for your portfolio include, What do I want to do next in my career? Why do I think I am qualified for this job? What do I want to tell the employer about myself? Why should my employer promote me?

> *Portfolios are an excellent way to impress potential employers, reach a larger employment pool, and put the Internet to work for a prospective employee.*

Interview a Professional. Once a decision has been made on an employment area of interest, it is helpful to discuss the needed skills and education with someone who is currently employed in that work setting. Personal interviews can provide information about what skills or education is required. It is a good idea to show the nurse being interviewed a draft of the portfolio to see if any of the information it contains is reflective of the required information or if there is a need to pursue further education or skill development before attempting to move into this field of nursing.

Showcase Your Education. Box 12.3 lists work samples that can be included in the portfolio. Box 12.4 lists basic categories for organizing the portfolio. Remember, these are just examples, and each nurse needs to use a format that will best showcase his or her education, work experience, skill-set, and accomplishments.

Use the Internet. Consider creating a Web version of the portfolio. Links can be created to digitized versions of portfolio information, examples of presentations the nurse has created, or photos of accomplishments or events. Portfolios are only limited by

Box 12.3

Examples to Collect for a Professional Portfolio

1. Education and training examples
2. General work performance examples
3. Examples regarding using data or nursing informatics
4. Examples pertaining to people skills
5. Examples demonstrating skills with equipment

Items that may be collected to support these areas include, but are not limited to the following:

Articles	Awards
Brochures	College transcripts and degrees
Drawings and designs	Grants
Flyers	Forms
Letters of commendation	Letters of reference
Manuals and handbooks	Merit reviews
Photographs	PowerPoint presentations
Presentations	Professional memberships
Proposals	Research
Resumes	Scholarships
Technical bulletins	Training certificates
Videos	Military service and awards

the nurse's imagination and access to space on the Web. Portfolios are an excellent way to impress potential employers, reach a larger employment pool, and put the Internet to work for a prospective employee. Even if the nurse has a Web version, it is a good idea to bring the portfolio to an interview.

As discussed in the previous section, a resume is an excellent tool for allowing the prospective health-care recruiter or employer to receive a concise overview of a potential employee in as little space as possible, and it will serve as a frame of reference once the interview process is complete. A nurse who offers to share a portfolio during the interview process provides tangible evidence of skills, accomplishments, and future potential. Showing a well-prepared portfolio leaves a positive lasting impression with the interviewer and provides a foundation to build upon as the nurse's career develops into the future.

> *The interview starts the moment the applicant enters the office. Conservative business clothes that are clean, neat, and well pressed are an absolute necessity.*

Interviews

The next important step in the process is the interview. The interview allows the institution to obtain a firsthand look at the applicant, as well as providing an opportunity for the applicant to obtain important information about the institution and position requirements. The interview often produces high levels of anxiety in new graduates who are interviewing for what might be their first real job.

Make a Good Impression

Again, first impressions are important (Box 12.5). The interview starts the moment the applicant enters the office. Conservative business clothes that are clean, neat, and well pressed are an absolute necessity. Similarly, a conservative hairstyle and a limited amount of accessories, jewelry, and makeup produce the best impression. Smoking, chewing gum, biting fingernails, or pacing nervously do not make good first impressions. The interviewer recognizes that interviews are stress producing and will make

Box 12.4

Categories to Organize Your Professional Portfolio

1. **Career Goals:** Where do you see yourself in 2–5 years?
2. **Professional Philosophy/Mission Statement:** What are your guiding principles?
3. **Traditional Resume:** Concise summary of education, work experience, achievements.
4. **Skills, Abilities, and Marketable Qualities:** Examples that support skill area, performance, knowledge or personal traits that contribute to your success and ability to apply that skill.
5. **List of Accomplishments:** Examples that highlight the major accomplishments in your career to date.
6. **Samples of Your Work:** See Box 11.2; you can also include CD-ROMs.
7. **Research, Publications, Reports:** Include examples of your written communication abilities.
8. **Letters of Recommendation:** A collection of any kudos you have received including clients, past employers, professors, etc.
9. **Awards and Honors:** Certificates of award, honor, or scholarship.
10. **Continuing Education:** Certificates from conferences, seminars, workshops, etc.
11. **Formal Education:** Transcripts, degrees, licenses, and certifications.
12. **Professional Development Activities:** Professional associations, professional conferences, offices held.
13. **Military Records, Awards, and Badges:** Evidence of military service, if applicable.
14. **Community/Volunteer Service:** Examples of volunteer work, especially as it may relate to your career.
15. **References:** A list of three to five people who are willing to speak about your strengths, abilities, and experience; prepared letters from same.

allowances for certain stress-related behaviors, but do try to avoid the mistakes listed in Box 12.6.

Arriving a few minutes early allows time for last-minute touch-ups of hair and clothes and gives the applicant a chance to calm down. Carrying a small briefcase with a copy of the resume, cover letter, references, and information about the hospital also makes a favorable impression.

Come Prepared

Mental preparation is as important to a successful interview as physical preparation. Most interviewers will start with some "small-talk" to attempt to put the interviewee at ease. Resist the temptation to launch into a long and rambling account of personal experiences. Next, the interviewer will usually ask about the resume or portfolio, if one is used. A quick review just before the interview is helpful so that the person being interviewed can avoid appearing ignorant about what information that is contained in the resume or portfolio.

Expect questions about positions held for only a short time (less than 1 year), gaps in the employment record (longer than 6 months), employment outside the field of nursing (e.g., waitress, clerk), educational experiences outside the nursing program, or unusual activities outside the employment setting. Answer the questions honestly but briefly. Most personnel directors or directors of nursing are busy and do not appreciate long, detailed, chatty answers. Applicants can anticipate being asked:

- Why do you want this position?
- Why have you selected this particular facility?
- Why do you think that you are qualified for the position?
- What unique qualifications do you bring to the job to make you more desirable than other applicants?
- Where do you see yourself five years from now? Ten years from now?

Using the portfolio will help answer some of these questions. By showing tangible examples of qualifications and accomplishments, the interviewee can help the busy interviewer discern between actual performance and mere rehearsed answers.

Box 12.5

Fashion Do's and Don'ts of Interviews

The Do List

Men

1. Do shave or trim facial hair closely.
2. Do use after-shave and/or cologne sparingly (a little goes a long way).
3. Do carry a money clip or leather wallet, and a small, plain functional briefcase.
4. Do wear leather shoes that are polished and in good repair. Lace-up or slip-on shoes are best.
5. Do wear calf-length dark socks.
6. Do wear a tailored suit (blue, gray, beige are best) with a dress shirt (lighter in color than the suit). Do wear a conservative tie.
7. Do shut off your cell phone or beeper.

Women

1. Do apply perfume or cologne sparingly (a little goes a long way).
2. Do invest in a good haircut/perm. Clean, neat, and conservative is best.
3. Do wear shoes that are polished and in good repair. Plain pumps with medium heels are best.
4. Do carry a briefcase or simple (small) handbag that matches your shoes.
5. Do wear hose that coordinate in color, style, and texture with your shoes and outfit. Do take an extra pair for emergencies.
6. Do apply makeup lightly and carefully.
7. Do apply conservatively colored nail polish carefully.
8. Do dress conservatively.
9. Do wear colors that make a strong statement, such as shades of gray in medium to charcoal, or blue in a medium to navy.
10. Do wear small, conservative earrings.
11. Do shut off your cell phone and beeper.

The Don't List

Men

1. Don't overstuff wallet, money clip, or briefcase.
2. Don't carry a can of smokeless tobacco in your back pocket or pack of cigarettes in a shirt pocket.
3. Don't wear sandals, running shoes, or cowboy boots.
4. Don't wear socks that are a lighter color than your trousers.
5. Don't wear green or flashy colors.

Women

1. Don't wear sneakers, sandals, cowboy boots, or heels more than 1-1/2 inches high.
2. Don't overstuff your handbag or briefcase.
3. Don't apply makeup so that it looks artificial and heavy.
4. Don't use black or bright or dramatic colored nail polish.
5. Don't wear skimpy or low-cut outfits, leather, or fringed apparel.
6. Don't wear large, dangling earrings or have other body piercing such as nose rings, lip rings, tongue rings, multiple earrings.

Sources: Iacono, M: The selection process: interview tips for nurse managers. Journal of Perianesthesia Nursing 19(5):345–347, 2004.
Puetz, B: The winning job interview: do your homework. AJN 2005 Career Guide: 30–32, 34–35, 2005.

Box 12.6

20 Worst Job Interview Mistakes

1. Arriving late
2. Arriving too early (10–15 minutes is OK)
3. Dressing wrong (see Box 12.5)
4. Having your cell phone or beeper go off during the interview (and answering it)
5. Drinking alcohol or smoking prior to the interview
6. Chewing gum and/or blowing bubbles
7. Bringing along a friend, relative, or children
8. Not being prepared—not having an interview "dress rehearsal"
9. Calling the interviewer by his or her first name
10. Not knowing your strengths and weaknesses
11. Asking too many questions of the interviewer (a few are OK)
12. Not asking any questions at all
13. Asking about pay and vacation as the first questions
14. Accusing the interviewer of discrimination
15. Bad-mouthing your present or former boss or employer
16. Name-dropping to impress the interviewer
17. Appearing lethargic and unenthusiastic
18. Weak, "dead fish," or bone-crusher handshake
19. Looking at your watch during the interview
20. Losing your cool or arguing with the interviewer

Sources: Littlewood, S: Making your job application stand out. Nursing Times 14–20; 100(37):50–51, 2004.
Cole, M: Interview game: pass the torch of knowledge. Nursing Spectrum 16(10):17, 2004.
Formichelli, L: What should you expect from employers? Diversity In Allied Health Careers Spring 2003, 31–33.
World, H: Nurses must use detective skills to unearth clues to lead them to their dream job. Nurse Week 5(4):21–22, 2004.

Forbidden Topics

Because of the emphasis placed on political correctness and discrimination issues in recent years, there are a number of areas that prospective employers are not supposed to discuss, but sometimes do anyway. These include questions about sexual preferences or habits, age, race, plans for a family, personal living arrangements, **significant others,** and religious or political beliefs.

If these questions are asked, the applicant needs to consider the implications of not answering them. Although there is no legal obligation for the applicant to answer, refusal to do so or pointing out that the question should not have been asked in the first place may be unwise. If these personal questions that violate an individual's right to privacy or seem discriminatory are answered by the graduate and then the graduate is not hired for the position, there may be grounds for some type of legal action based on discrimination.

Ask Your Own Questions

At some point in the interview, usually toward the end, applicants are asked whether they have any questions. Although most do have questions, many applicants are afraid to ask. In fact, asking questions can be seen as a demonstration of independence, initiative, and intellectual curiosity—all traits that are highly valued by health-care providers. It is important that the first questions are not about salary, vacations, and other benefits. Questions that indicate interest in the institution are included in Box 12.7.

After these questions have been answered, the applicant may want to ask about salary, raises, vacations, and other benefits. It would also be wise to inform the interviewer of the dates scheduled for the National Council Licensure Examination (NCLEX) so that arrangements can be made for time off. The applicant should also ask for written material on the

Box 12.7

Questions Interviewees Should Ask

- What are the responsibilities involved in the position?
- Who are the other staff or personnel working on this unit?
- What is the typical client-to-staff ratio for the unit?
- Are their any mandatory rotating shifts, weekend obligations, overtime, or floating?
- Does the hospital offer opportunities for continuing education, clinical ladder, advancement, or movement to other departments?
- Please describe the facility's policies for employee health and safety.

nurse's contract with the agency, including benefits and job descriptions. Often the interviewer will provide this information without being asked in the course of answering some of the other questions.

It is appropriate to close the interview by asking for a tour of the facility. A tour allows first-hand evaluation of the workplace and a chance to observe the staff and clients in a real work setting. The interviewer may not be able to provide a tour at that time and so may ask another individual (e.g., a secretary) to take the applicant on the tour.

Follow Up

As with the resume, making frequent calls about the results of the interview is unwise. It is, however, appropriate for the applicant to send a letter within 1 week after the interview to thank the interviewer for his or her time and express appreciation for being considered for the position (Box 12.8). The applicant should also acknowledge how much it would mean to him or her to become a member of the staff at such a high-quality agency or hospital, but avoid overdoing the complements.

If the position is offered, a formal letter of acceptance or refusal should be sent to the institution. Health-care facilities will not hold positions indefinitely, and failure to accept the position formally in a timely manner may result in them offering the position to someone else.

> *Health-care employers today are looking for nurses who believe that high-quality performance on the job is more important than just having a job. Professional nurses can apply the nursing process to their own personal development, and the evidence of positive outcomes is placed in the portfolio.*

WHEN NURSES BURN OUT

The **burnout syndrome** has existed for many years and has been recognized as a problem that can be

---

B o x   1 2 . 8

Sample Follow-up Letter

Mary P. Oak
100 Wood Lane
Nicetown, PA 22222

June 20, 2006

Mr. Robert L. Pine
Director of Personnel
Doctors Hospital
Gully City, PA 44444

Dear Mr. Pine:

Thank you very much for considering my resume and for the interview on June 3, 2006. I learned a great deal from the interview and from my tour of the hospital after the interview.

I am writing to let you know that I am still interested in the position and was wondering about the status of my application. If at all possible, I would appreciate it if you could either call me or write a note relating to my potential employment at your facility.

Feel free to call me at home any time (333) 555-1234, or contact me by e-mail: moak@aol.com.

Sincerely,

Mary P. Oak

reduced or even prevented. A widely accepted definition of burnout is a state of emotional exhaustion that results from the accumulative **stress** of an individual's life, including work, personal, and family responsibilities. Although the term is not often applied to students, many of the symptoms of burnout can be observed in these aspiring nurses.[8]

Who Burns Out?

The people who are most likely to experience burnout tend to be more intelligent than average, hard-working, idealistic, and perfectionist. There are certain categories of jobs and careers that tend to produce a higher incidence of burnout: situations and positions in which there is a demand for consistently high-quality performance, unclear or unrealistic expectations, little control over the work situation, and inadequate financial rewards. These jobs or careers tend to be very demanding and stressful, with little recognition or appreciation of what is being done. Also, jobs in which there is constant contact with people (customers, clients, students, or criminals) rank high on the burnout list.

Even with the most superficial knowledge of nursing, it is easy to see that many of these elements are present in the nurse's work situation. It is possible to recognize nurses who are in the early stages of burnout by identifying some classic behaviors (Box 12.9).

B o x   1 2 . 9

Symptoms of Burnout

- Extreme fatigue
- Exhaustion
- Frequent illness
- Overeating
- Headaches
- Sleeping problems
- Physical complaints
- Alcohol abuse
- Mood swings
- Emotional displays
- Anxiety
- Poor-quality work
- Anger
- Guilt
- Depression

How It Starts

One of the earliest indications of burnout is the attitude that work is something to be tolerated, rather than eagerly anticipated. Nurses in the early stages of burnout often are irritable, impatient, cynical, pessimistic, whiny, or callous toward coworkers and clients. These preburnout nurses take frequent sick days, are chronically late for their shifts, drink too much, eat too much, and often are not able to sleep.

Eventually, as their idealism erodes, their work suffers. They become careless in the performance of their duties, uncooperative with their colleagues, and unable to concentrate on what they are doing, and they display a general attitude of boredom and **apathy.** If allowed to continue, burnout may lead to feelings of helplessness, powerlessness, purposelessness, and guilt.[9]

Avoiding Burnout

Despite this bleak picture, nurses do not have to fall victim to the burnout syndrome. Many nurses practice their profession for many years, manage to deal with the stress, and find great personal satisfaction in what they do. These satisfied and motivated nurses have developed ways to deal with the stress of their careers while maintaining their goals and purpose as nurses.

The first step in dealing with burnout is to be able to recognize its signs. Many nurses who are burning out use denial and rationalization to block recognition of burnout, because it is just too painful for them to think they put so much time, money, and effort into preparing for a career they no longer want or enjoy. It is important to realize that it is not the career that is producing the burnout, but rather the difficulty in coping with the stresses the career is producing. Although it may not be possible to change the requirements of the profession significantly, it is possible to learn how to cope more effectively with stress.

Manage Stress and Time

Although there are many schools of thought about stress and time-management techniques, several common threads run through many of these theories. These views include setting personal goals, identifying problems, and using strategies for problem solving.

Issues in Practice

Critical Incident Stress Debriefing Teams

Responding to Major Stressful Events

Nurses are familiar with the stresses routinely found in their daily work and usually develop skills that are successful to some degree in dealing with it. Most nurses believe that traumatic events in their work setting are a part of the job and that they should be able to handle them without difficulty. However, as recent history has shown, major and overwhelming stressful events, such as the devastation of the World Trade Center, can strike without warning. As individuals and a nation, we experience a sense of horror, helplessness, and powerlessness in addition to the normal stress responses of shock, disbelief, anger, and grief. The end result may well be a complex of symptoms similar to burnout syndrome, including physical symptoms, depression, and chronic anxiety.

In response to major tragedies that have occurred over the past decade, the critical incident stress debriefing (CISD) process was developed to help people deal with major acts of violence and traumatic disasters. The American Red Cross has been instrumental in training and providing resources for local CISD teams that are made up of mental health professionals specially trained in crisis intervention, stress management, and post-traumatic stress disorder (PTSD). After a major incident, employers often call for the formation of the teams to support their workers though the immediate post-trauma period.

To be most effective, the CISD teams need to be on site within 2 to 3 days after serious events ranging from the death of coworkers, natural disasters such as tornados, or acts of terrorism. The goal of the team is to encourage the participants to verbalize their feelings and thoughts, identify and develop their coping skills, and generally lower overall grief and anxiety levels.

Post-Traumatic Stress Disorder

One of the keys when working with nurses is to have them recognize that they are not expected to be able to handle all situations and that it is appropriate to ask for help. Although nurses study the stress response and grieving process in nursing school, it is sometimes hard for them to apply the information about normal stress reactions to themselves. When nurses do not recognize that they are having difficulty in responding to traumatic stress, they increase their risk for developing long-term stress reactions. When they do not seek help, they can develop the symptoms of PTSD anywhere from a few days to as long as 6 months after the event.

Warning signs of PTSD include:

1. Recurring nightmares and inability to sleep
2. Intrusive and vivid flashbacks
3. Prolonged depression
4. High levels of anxiety
5. Maladaptive coping behaviors such as drug and alcohol abuse

The CISD session generally requires up to 3 hours. Sessions can be longer or shorter depending on the nature of the event and number of people affected.

(continued)

Issues in Practice _{continued}

In addition to the opportunity to express emotions and feeling, the participants are educated in some ways to reduce anxiety and promote mental and physical health that include:

1. Not watching televised replay of the event over and over
2. Staying with friends as much as possible
3. Avoiding unhealthy, high-fat diets
4. Engaging in regular aerobic exercise as much as possible
5. Avoiding excessive dependence on alcohol and drugs for sleep
6. Getting back to a comfortable routine as soon as possible
7. Feeling comfortable seeking professional help when needed

During the CISD sessions, nurses are asked for their input about the process. If the team feels it is necessary, additional referrals for long-term treatment may be recommended.

Although they do have a number of skills that help them deal with traumatic events in their workplace, nurses are not super-people and should not expect that they can handle all stressful events without help. The CISD process was developed to allow individuals, including nurses, to obtain help soon after the event to promote coping and resolution of major traumatic events.

Sources: Antai-Otong, D: Overwhelming stressful events: Proactive response key to coping. American Nurse 34(1):9, 2002.
McGown, B: Self-reported stress and its effects on nurses. Nursing Standard 15(42):33–38, 2001.

Set Personal Goals

Goals and goal setting are an important part of client care. Nursing students—and by extension, practicing nurses—are highly proficient in the planning stage of the nursing process, in which goal setting is the primary task. They know that a good set of goals should be client centered, time oriented, and measurable and that they should write these goals with every care plan they prepare.

In their personal lives, however, these nurses may rush full-tilt into one erratic day after another, subordinating their own needs to the needs of others and working long, hard hours, but without accomplishing very much and feeling frustrated about it. What is the problem here? Very simply, nurses can prepare realistic, beneficial goals for their clients, but they seem to be unable to do the same for themselves.

Long-Term Goals
Personal goals should include both long-term and short-term goals. Typically, personal long-term goals

look into the future at least 10 years and include a statement about what the nurse wants to achieve during his or her lifetime. Some examples are going back to school to obtain an advanced degree, becoming a director of nursing, or even writing a book about nursing.

Practicing nurses who are caught up in the whirlwind of everyday life find it difficult to formulate statements about the future. One other important characteristic of long-term goals is that they need to be flexible. As life circumstances change, modifications are required.

Short-Term Goals
Short-term goals are those that the nurse expects to accomplish in 6 months to 2 years. These goals should be aimed primarily at making the nurse's professional or personal life more satisfying and fulfilling. Like long-term goals, they do not need to be related to work. Perhaps visiting a foreign country, going on a skiing trip in the mountains, and even learning how to paint a picture or play the piano may

be achievable in a relatively short time. In the professional realm, joining a professional organization, becoming a head nurse, or changing an outdated hospital policy are goals that can be achieved in a short time. The fact that everyone ages over time cannot be altered, but that time can also be used to achieve personal satisfaction in life and increase knowledge and accomplishments.

> *It is important to realize that it is not the career that is producing the burnout, but rather the difficulty in coping with the stresses the career is producing.*

An End Achieved
Although goal setting is an important first step in dealing with the stress that leads to burnout, any good nurse recognizes that a plan without implementation is useless. As difficult as goal setting may be for nurses, carrying it out may be even more difficult. Although goal achievement requires a degree of hard work and personal sacrifice, when people are working toward something they really want, the effort that it takes to achieve the end actually becomes enjoyable. At first glance, this process may seem like a lot of work (and it is), but it becomes an exciting adventure in its own right.

Identifying Problems
Another important step in dealing with burnout is to identify the problems that are producing the stress. Again, nurses are taught as students that they need to identify client problems so they can work toward solving them.

Self-Diagnosis
Formulation of a nursing diagnosis is nothing more than precisely stating a client's problem. One thing nurses realize early in the learning process is that what may appear to be an obvious problem may in reality not be a problem at all. Conversely, something that a client only mentions in passing may turn out to be the real source of the client's nursing needs. Perhaps nurses should look at their own lives and attempt to formulate nursing diagnoses

What Do You Think?

List three tasks that you have put off today. Why did you avoid doing these? How can you get them done sooner?

that deal with their stress-related problems (setting the North American Nursing Diagnosis Association list aside).

For example, a new graduate has just completed a shift during which he was assigned to eight complete-care clients. He has had to supervise two badly prepared nurses' aides and has put in 55 minutes of overtime (for which he will not be paid) to complete the charting. This nurse is feeling tired, frustrated, and even a little bit guilty because of an inability to provide the type of care that he was taught in nursing school.

What is the problem? A possible nursing diagnosis might be: Alterations in personal satisfaction related to excessive workload, evidenced by sore feet, headache, shaky hands, feelings of guilt, frustration, and small paycheck.

Goals and Interventions
Now that the problem has been identified, goals and interventions can be introduced to solve the problem. The goals may range from organizing time better to refusing to take care of so many complete-care clients. Interventions, depending on the goals, can include activities such as attending a time-management

seminar, talking to the head nurse, or changing a policy in the policy and procedure book.

STRATEGIES FOR PROBLEM SOLVING

Nurses already know the nursing process as a client problem-solving technique. Why not apply the same knowledge and skills to personal problems? The stress level only increases if problems are left unsolved.

Although specific problems may require specific solutions, several widely accepted methods exist to deal with the general stresses produced by everyday work and personal life. Included in these methods are activities such as recognizing that nurses are only human, improving time-management skills, practicing what is preached, and decompression.

Time-Management Skills
In modern life there is often not enough time to do everything that needs to be done. The key to time management is setting priorities. In the world of nursing and client care, nurses are often required to do many tasks. Multitasking, the process of doing several tasks at the same time, tends to fragment the nurse's attention and concentration.

Nurses need to recognize that only some nursing activities are essential to the safety and well-being of clients. These include thorough assessment and ensuring that the clients get their medications on time, that their comfort needs are met, and that accidental injuries are prevented. Beyond these actions, nurses really have a great deal of discretion in what they can do when providing care to clients.

Make Room for Fulfillment
Burnout results mainly from personal and professional dissatisfaction. If nurses feel fulfilled in what they are doing, burnout is much less likely to occur. Activities that may increase nurses' satisfaction include spending time talking with clients, learning new skills, and decreasing the anxiety of families through teaching and listening. After such activities have been identified, time should be set aside for them during the shift. The real secret in using time management to prevent burnout is for the nurse to use the time left for those nursing activities that bring the most professional and personal satisfaction.

Several skills need to be developed to be able to allow time during a shift for these preferred activities. First, the nurse must learn to delegate by letting the licensed practical nurses (LPNs) or aides do those tasks they are supposed to be able to do. Many nurses graduate from nursing school with the attitude that if you want it done right, you need to do it yourself. After becoming familiar with the LPN and nurse's aide job descriptions, nurses need to give others a chance to prove themselves.[10]

Overcome Procrastination
Another necessary skill is overcoming procrastination. Most people have a natural tendency toward procrastination, particularly when unpleasant or difficult tasks are involved. The primary reasons that people postpone or delay doing something is because they either do not want to begin or do not know where to begin the task. More time and energy are expended in inventing excuses for putting off tasks than would be taken in doing the task.

The Most Distasteful Task. The best way to overcome procrastination is by starting the task, even if it is only a small step. An effective method is to select the most distasteful task to be done that day and to commit just 5 minutes to it. After 5 minutes are over, the task can be either set aside or continued. It is very likely that once the task is started and momentum builds, the task will be carried out to completion.

Tasks can be prioritized by listing them in three categories. Category A tasks (e.g., assessments, passing out medications, treatments, and dressing changes) are important and need to be completed on time. Category B tasks (bath, linen change, lunch break, charting) are important, but can be postponed until later in the shift. Category C tasks (cleaning up, organizing the supply room) are tasks that can either be delegated or wait until the next day.

Problems Don't Solve Themselves. For daily tasks, both pleasant and unpleasant, the best time to do them is immediately. If achievement of the plan requires delegation, then it needs to be done at the beginning of the shift, not at the middle or end of the shift. Often nurses have a built-in fear of taking chances. As a result, they avoid doing things if there is a chance of failure, in the hope that somehow the problem will resolve itself.

Any time an important decision is made, there is a chance that someone will disagree or that the decision will be incorrect. These types of situations need to be viewed as a challenge or an opportunity rather than a life-altering risk to be avoided. Although mistakes in health care do have the potential to be fatal, learning from mistakes is one of the most fundamental ways of increasing knowledge.

Time management, like other skills, requires some practice. Once a nurse masters this skill, his or her life becomes more satisfying.

Practicing What You Preach

Because nursing is oriented toward keeping people healthy as well as curing illness, nurses spend a large amount of their time teaching clients about eating well; getting enough sleep; going for regular dental, eye, and physical examinations; avoiding too much drinking and smoking; and exercising regularly. It might make an interesting student research project to have nurses rank themselves on how well they have incorporated these health maintenance activities in their own lives. The results would probably indicate a low overall score on the "practice what you preach" scale.

Nurses know all about the food pyramid, but they do not translate that knowledge into feeding themselves properly. In reality, there are going to be some busy days when it is impossible to eat right,

but it should be possible, on a regular basis, to follow a diet that will promote health and reduce the buildup of fat plaques in the arteries.

It is important to get enough sleep to avoid chronic fatigue. People can adjust to a state of fatigue, but it tends to decrease the enjoyment that they find in life, as well as make them irritable, careless, and inefficient. Most people need between 5 and 8 hours of good sleep each night. It also probably would not hurt for nurses to take a short nap during the afternoon on their days off.

The Right Kind of Exercise

Many nurses feel they get enough exercise during their busy shifts, and, in truth, the average staff nurse walks between 2 and 5 miles during each 8-hour shift. Unfortunately, this type of walking does not qualify as the type of aerobic exercise recommended for an improved cardiovascular condition. Exercise, in order to be beneficial, must be done consistently and must raise the heart rate above the normal range for an extended period. The short sprint-type walking involved in client care does not accomplish this goal.

Walking 1 to 2 miles a day outside of work is a beneficial, simple exercise that will improve health. Nurses can also use a wide variety of exercise equipment for those days when walking outside is undesirable. The important requirement is that the exercise be done consistently and frequently. Regular exercise not only improves the cardiovascular system but also helps improve stamina, raise self-image, and promote a general sense of well-being.

Decompression Time

The profession of nursing is stressful, even under ideal circumstances. Nurses are required to deal with other people constantly and to carry out numerous tasks that are potentially dangerous. At the end of any shift, even the most skilled and best-organized nurse has a sense of internal tension. This tension must be released or it will eventually cause a major explosion or (if turned inward) produce anxiety.

Establish a Daily Decompression Routine

It may take a little time to discover, through trial and error, what works to reduce the tension built up during the shift. Some effective techniques include setting aside approximately 30 minutes of private, quiet time to dream and reflect about the day's activities. Perhaps relaxing in a tub of hot soapy water or

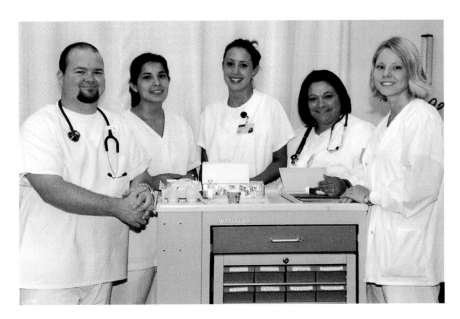

sitting in a favorite reclining chair might meet the need for decompression. Relaxation activities, such as swimming, shopping, or even going for a drive, can help reduce tension and act as a time for decompression. Of course, stress-management techniques learned at seminars (e.g., self-hypnosis or meditation) can be used by those who have developed these skills. Finally, meeting with a nurse support group can help the nurse vent feelings and make constructive plans for solving problems.

> *Tension must be released or it will eventually cause a major explosion or (if turned inward) produce anxiety.*

Conclusion

Although transition shock and burnout are realities of the nursing profession, they can be reduced or even avoided altogether. Nurses should be able to recognize the causes and early symptoms of transition shock and burnout to prevent them from developing into a problem. Therefore, nurses should use techniques to prevent these disorders from becoming insurmountable obstacles. In doing so, nurses will be able to practice their profession proficiently and gain the satisfaction that only nursing can provide.

Critical Thinking Exercises

- Make a list of the characteristics that would be found in the "perfect nurse." Make a second list of characteristics found in nurses observed in actual practice. Discuss how and why these lists differ.
- Outline a plan for implementing a preceptor clinical experience for the senior class of a nursing program. Make sure to include how many hours of practice are required, criteria for the selection of preceptors, student objectives from the experience, and methods of evaluation.
- Write at least three long-term and five short-term personal or professional goals. Develop a realistic plan and time frame for achieving these goals. Make sure to include what is required to achieve these goals.
- Complete this statement, using as many examples as possible: "I feel most satisfied when I am done with my shift in knowing that. . . ." Analyze these answers and discuss how they can be implemented in everyday practice.
- Think of at least three situations in which you were asked to do something that you really did not want to do. How did you handle these situations? How could they be handled in a more assertive manner?

References

1. Roberts, K: Nursing's extreme makeover challenge. AJN: 2005 Career Guide:20, 22, 24–28.
2. The citical role of nurses in patient safety. Oklahoma Nurse 49(1):17, 2004.
3. Stanton, M: Hospital nursing staffing and quality of care. Research in Action 14:1–9, 2004.
4. Ruholl, L: Seasoned faculty: To retire or not? One solution to the faculty shortage—begin at the end. Journal of Nursing Education 43(12):529, 2004.
5. Masterson, A: Making sense of nurse numbers. Nursing Older People 16(9):3, 2004.
6. Kimeldorf, M: Using job search portfolios in an uncertain labor market. Retrieved January 21, 2005 from www.amby.com/kimeldorf/portfolio/p_mk-02.html.
7. Trossman, S: The professional portfolio: Documenting who you are, what you do. [Electronic version] The American Nurse (March/April), 1999. Retrieved January 21, 2005 from www.nursingworld.org/tan/99marapr/ portfolo.htm.
8. Peir, JM, et al.: Does role stress predict burnout over time among health care professionals? Psychology and Healthcare 16(5):511–525, 2001.
9. Ekstedt, M: Lived experiences of the time preceding burnout. J Adv Nurs, 49(1):59–67, 2005.
10. Cohen-Katz, J: The effects of mindfulness-based stress reduction on nurse stress and burnout: A quantitative and qualitative study. Holistic Nursing Practice 18(6):302–308, 2004.

Bibliography

Bartram, T: Factors affecting the job stress and job satisfaction of Australian nurses: Implications for recruitment and retention. Contemporary Nurse17(3):293–304, 2004.

Chatterjee, M: Nursing staff shortages are putting patients in danger. Nursing Times 100(45):4, 2004.

Corcoran, J: Learning portfolios: Evidence of learning: An examination of students' perspectives. Nurs Crit Care 9(5):230–237, 2004.

Endacott, R: Using portfolios in the assessment of learning and competence: The impact of four models. Nurse Educational Practices 4(4):250–257, 2004.

Jenkins, R: Stressors, burnout and social support: Nurses in acute mental health settings. J Adv Nurs 48(6): 622–631, 2004.

Leichtling, B: Leadership & management. Preventive medicine for "compassion [sic] fatigue." Caring 23(10): 90–91, 2004.

Lemin-Stone, K: Careers: Learn to manage your stress levels. Nursing Times 100(46):74–75, 2004.

Lipley, N: How many staff is enough? Emergency Nurse 12(7):5, 2004.

Lupoli, J: The impact of technology on the "older" nurse. Home Health Nurse 22(10):668–670, 2004.

O'Dowd, A: Global nurse shortages are "staggering." Nursing Times 100(46):5, 2004.

Raiger, J: Applying a cultural lens to the concept of burnout. Journal of Transcultural Nursing 16(1):71–76, 2005.

Sanner, T: Using telehealth to address the nursing shortage. Home Health Nurse 22(10):695–702, 2004.

Santucci, J: Facilitating the transition into nursing practice: concepts and strategies for mentoring new graduates. Journal of Nurses Staff Development 20(6):274–284, 2004.

Schaffer, M, et al.: Using portfolios to evaluate achievement of population-based public health nursing competencies in baccalaureate nursing students. Nursing Education Perspectives. 26(2):104–112, 2005.

I personally measure success in terms
of the contributions an individual
makes to his or her fellow beings.

3

Leading and Managing

13

Principles of Leadership and Management

Joseph T. Catalano

Learning Objectives

After completing this chapter, the reader will be able to:

- Identify and discuss the three major theories used to explain leadership.
- Define and distinguish between the three styles of leadership.
- Discuss the relationship of transformational and situational theories to leadership style.
- Identify the key behaviors and qualities of effective leaders.
- Distinguish the differences between management and leadership.
- Identify and discuss the two major theories of management.

In today's health-care system, even new graduates who have an "RN" after their name will be placed quickly in positions of leadership and management.

LEADERSHIP

The old saying that "leaders are born, not made" implies that at birth a person either is a leader or is forever relegated to the rank of follower. Not many agree with this statement. Although some people may have an easier time filling the leadership role than others, most experts believe that almost everyone can develop leadership skills.

Many definitions of leadership refer to the ability of an individual to influence the behavior of others. When nurses exert leadership, they inspire other health-care workers to work toward one or more of several goals that include providing high-quality client care, maintaining a safe working environment, developing new policies and procedures, and increasing the power of the profession.

Some leadership theories try to explain why some people are leaders and others are not, but as yet none covers all the possibilities. That may be because leadership requirements differ depending on the situation. In the intensive care unit (ICU), for example, where quick decisions are a matter of life and death, the leader is the nurse with highly developed critical thinking and analytical skills and the confidence to make decisions under pressure. In quality management, where the problems are often long term and complicated, the leader tends to be a nurse who is well organized and can methodically sift through a mountain of information and statistics to develop a policy that covers the widest range of possibilities. Several of the better-known leadership theories are discussed here.

Trait Theory

The trait theory identifies qualities that are common to effective leaders (Box 13.1). Trait theory by itself is limited, because it focuses only

Box 13.1

Leadership Traits

- High level of intelligence and skill
- Self-motivation and initiative
- Ability to communicate well
- Self-confidence and assertiveness
- Creativity
- Persistence
- Stress tolerance
- Risk taking
- Ability to accept criticism

on the traits of the individual and does not take into account how the person acts in specific situations. The question left unanswered is why everyone who has these traits does not become a leader.[1]

> The old saying that "leaders are born, not made" implies that at birth a person either is a leader or is forever relegated to the rank of follower.

Leadership Style Theory

One of the best-known theories of leadership looks at three styles of leadership:

1. Laissez-faire
2. Democratic
3. Authoritarian

Although these theories are discussed separately, they are a continuum of leadership style ranging from a mostly passive approach to a highly controlling one (Table 13.1).

The Laissez-Faire Style

The **laissez-faire** (French for "leave it alone") leadership style is also described as permissive, nondirective, or passive. The laissez-faire style leader allows the group he or she is leading to determine their own goals and the methods to achieve them. There is little planning, minimal decision making, and a lack of involvement by the leader. This style works well in only a few settings, for example, in a research laboratory that is staffed by self-motivated scientists who know what they want to achieve and are familiar with the means of achieving it.

The laissez-faire style works best when the members of the group have the same level of education as the leader and the leader performs the same tasks as the group members. In most situations, however, the laissez-faire leadership style can leave people feeling lost and frustrated because of the lack of direction by the leader. When they do try to achieve some goal, often the only input from the leader is that they are doing it incorrectly. When faced with a difficult decision, laissez-faire leaders usually avoid making a decision in the hopes that the problem will resolve itself.

The Democratic Style

In the **democratic** (also called supportive or participative) leadership style, all aspects of the process of achieving a goal, from planning and goal setting to implementing and taking credit for the success of the

Table 13.1 Comparison of Authoritarian, Democratic, and Laissez-Faire Theories

	Authoritarian	Democratic	Laissez-faire
Degree of freedom	Little freedom	Moderate freedom	Much freedom
Degree of control	High control	Moderate control	Little control
Decision making	By the leader only	Leader and group	Group or no one
Leader activity level	High	High	Minimal
Responsibility	Leader	Leader and group	Abdicated
Quality of output	High quality	High quality/creative	Variable
Efficiency	Very efficient	Moderately efficient	Variable

Source: Tappen, RM, et al.: Essentials of Nursing Leadership and Management, ed. 2. FA Davis, Philadelphia, 2001, p 6.

project, are shared by the group. The democratic leadership style is based on four beliefs:

1. Every member of the group needs to participate in all decision making.
2. Within the limits established by the group, freedom of expression is allowed to maximize creativity.
3. Individuals in the group accept responsibility for themselves and for the welfare of the whole group.
4. Each member must respect all the other members of the group as unique and valuable contributors.[2]

The leader using the democratic style provides guidance to the group, and all members share control. This style works best with groups whose members have a relatively equal status and who know each other well because they have worked together for an extended period. Democratic leadership can be time consuming and inefficient in some situations, particularly when group members disagree strongly, but in the end, when a goal is achieved or a decision made, there is a strong sense of ownership and achievement by the whole group. Many leaders are uncomfortable with this style of leadership because of the minimal control they have over the group.

The Authoritarian Style

The leader with an **authoritarian** (also called controlling, directive, or autocratic) style maintains strong control over all aspects of the group and its activities. Authoritarian leaders provide direction by giving orders that the group is expected to carry out without question. The final decision-making authority rests with the leader alone, although input from the group may be considered.

The Dictator. A leader using a dictatorial authoritarian style has no regard for the feelings and needs of the group members. Achieving the goal is the only thing that matters and the leader will use any means, including harsh criticism, to do so. A military mission to destroy a terrorist group by a SEAL (*sea air land*) assault team is an example of this type of leadership.

What Do You Think?

Have you ever had to be a leader in a group? What type of leadership style did you use? How successful was the outcome of the group work?

The Benevolent Leader. The benevolent authoritarian leader uses a more paternalistic approach to achieving the goal. That leader attempts to include the group's feelings and concerns in the final decision, but ultimately the leader makes the decision. Some group members may feel that the benevolent leader is condescending and patronizing.

The authoritarian leadership style works best in emergency situations, where clear directions are required to save a life or prevent injury, or in situations where it is necessary to organize a large group of individuals. Although highly efficient in achieving goals and completing tasks, authoritarian leadership suppresses the creativity of the group members and may reduce the long-term effectiveness of the group. Authoritarian leadership also reduces the motivation levels of the group and may lead to passive-aggressive behavior by the members that will further reduce the effectiveness of the group. Although some people can accept the need for the total control exerted by an authoritarian leader, most people in a long-term work relationship with this type of leader will become frustrated and even rebellious at some point.

In reality, few leaders use only one style. Most leaders use multiple leadership styles depending on the situation. Many factors may influence what type of leadership style is used at any given time, including external regulations and requirements, the ability of the group members, the work setting, and the problem being solved. For example, a nurse manager on a hospital unit may use a highly democratic style in most of the routine activities of the unit, but when a client goes into cardiac arrest, she may revert to a highly authoritarian style while directing the staff through a code.

Relationship–Task Orientation

High Relationship–Low Task

Another commonly used theory of leadership rates leaders on whether they are oriented more toward establishing relationships or achieving assigned tasks and resolving problems. Leaders with high relationship–low task orientations are usually well liked by their groups because of their acceptance of the group members as individuals, consideration of their feelings, encouragement, and promotion of good feelings among all the group members.

However, this kind of leader often sacrifices the achievement of the task or resolution of a problem when it conflicts with the feelings or goodwill of the group. This leader often allows the group to make its own decisions without regard to the task at hand and ultimately may not achieve the goals the group was organized to do in the first place.

> *The authoritarian leadership style works best in emergency situations, where clear directions are required to save a life or prevent injury, or in situations where it is necessary to organize a large group of individuals.*

What Do You Think?

Think of the best leader you have ever worked with. What traits did that person have? Now think of the worst leader you ever worked with. What traits did that person have?

High Task–Low Relationship

The opposite extreme is the leader with a low relationship–high task orientation. This form of leadership is similar to the authoritarian style, where the leader does all the planning with little regard to the input or feelings of the group, gives orders, and expects them to be carried out without question. Various forms of punishment are used by this leader, ranging from verbal put-downs to poor performance evaluations that are used to determine pay raises.

Both Extremes

The worst leader is the person with a low relationship–low task orientation that simulates the laissez-faire leadership style where the leader is uninvolved, does no planning, has little concern for the group members' feelings, and accomplishes little. On the other hand, the best leader is the one with a high relationship–high task orientation. This leader combines the best of both worlds in that he or she is open to input and actively communicates with the group members, provides constructive direction, quickly resolves conflicts, and ultimately achieves creative and effective solutions to problems.

Certainly, perfect leaders are difficult to find. Most use a combination of styles and adjust them to the circumstances surrounding the problem. Again, think of the nurse manager who uses a high relationship–high task orientation for managing the unit in most day-to-day operations. In the cardiac arrest situation, this nurse manager may quickly change her or his orientation to one of low relationship–high task until the crisis is resolved.

> " *The situational theory recognizes that no one approach works in all situations. A leader needs to acknowledge this and adjust the leadership style and behavior to the situation, considering the many variables that may be involved. Good leaders seem to do this instinctively.* "

RECENT THEORIES OF LEADERSHIP

Although the behavior and trait theories remain popular, researchers have come to the conclusion that leadership is really a more complex process. The situational theory recognizes that no one approach works in all situations. A leader needs to acknowledge this and adjust the leadership style and behavior to the situation, considering the many variables that may be involved. Good leaders seem to do this instinctively. One of the key factors is the type of organization in which the group is located. The environment is always important when exercising leadership.

The transformational theory takes the situational theory one step further. This theory recognizes that multiple intangibles exist whenever people interact. Factors such as sense of meaning, creativity, inspiration, and vision all are involved in creating a sense of mission that exceeds good interpersonal relationships and rewards. Although this is true in most work settings, health care and nursing, where care of human beings is the primary goal, require that nurses do something positive. In many health-care facilities, nursing leaders are expected to inspire excitement and commitment in nurses, who often must provide care to very ill clients in less than ideal circumstances.

KEY LEADERSHIP BEHAVIORS

Traits are characteristics that an individual possesses. Traits may or may not lead to the actions or behaviors that are required for successful leadership. It is also possible to lack leadership traits yet be able to carry out successful leadership behaviors.

Critical Thinking. The ability to think critically is a multistep process similar to the nursing process. Critical thinkers must be able to analyze data, organize and plan, and use creativity in the resolution of problems (see Chapter 6). Leaders must often make important decisions on the basis of incomplete data.

Problem Solving. Being able to use the problem-solving process effectively is essential to effective leadership. Leaders in the health-care setting face problems that arise from many sources, including staffing and personnel, scheduling, and administrative, budget, and client demands.

Acknowledgment and Respect for Individual Differences. Personality is the sum total of people's experiences. Because no two people have identical experiences, each one has different needs, feelings, and orientations. The effective leader recognizes these differences and is able to direct the people to their highest level of achievement given their varying orientations.

Active Listening. To be effective, leaders must be able to not only hear the words that the person is saying but also observe the body language and its underlying emotions and meaning. The experts tell us that only 7 percent of communication is verbal; 93 percent is all the other nonverbal content. Leaders often fail in their leadership roles when they do not listen to the full message of the individuals they are attempting to lead.

Skillful Communication. Communication is a complex process that involves an exchange of information and feedback (see Chapter 14). Mistakes happen on both sides when the information being shared is incomplete or confusing. Providing frequent and positive feedback is one of the best methods for leaders to determine how well they are communicating and how open the communication channels remain. It also can boost morale and improve the working environment. Effective leaders should also be able to give and use negative feedback to improve performance. If negative feedback is given in a nonthreatening and encouraging manner, the person receiving it will often appreciate the chance to improve his or her skills.

Establishment of Clear Goals and Outcomes. The old question, "How do you know when you've arrived if you don't know where you are going?" is a truism that all leaders must address at some point by establishing clear goals and outcomes for the group. Groups who lack clear goals often feel frustrated and lost. Initially, leaders must clearly identify their goals. Then they must identify the goals shared by the group and use them to motivate the group. Successful outcome is often a thoughtful melding of the vision of the leader and the group.

Continued Personal and Professional Development. One of the most valuable lessons that nursing students can learn while in nursing school is that education does not end when they graduate—it just begins. One of the primary goals of the nursing education process should be to teach the student how to learn. Lifelong learning is a goal that effective leaders seek not only for themselves but also for those whom they are leading. Leaders can function as teachers in certain settings, but a more effective means of encouraging others to continue to learn is to set a good example. It is important to recognize that learning takes place not only in a formal school-like setting, but in all those encounters and situations that effect attitudes, beliefs, and behavior.

> *One of the most valuable lessons that nursing students can learn while in nursing school is that education does not end when they graduate—it just begins.*

KEY LEADERSHIP QUALITIES

No matter what style a leader favors, successful leaders have common qualities (Box 13.2).

Integrity. For many years, nursing has been ranked among the top five most respected professions in the annual Gallup Poll (in 2002, nurses ranked second behind firefighters). One of the keys to this respect is the integrity of the profession as it is perceived by

---

Box 13.2

Keys to Leadership

Key Qualities
- Integrity
- Courage
- Initiative
- Energy
- Optimism
- Perseverance
- Well-roundedness
- Coping skills
- Self-knowledge

Key Behaviors
- Critical thinking
- Problem solving
- Acknowledgment of and respect for individual differences
- Active listening
- Skillful communication
- Establishment of clear goals and outcomes
- Continued personal and professional development

Source: Adapted from Tappen, RM, et al.: Essentials of Nursing Leadership and Management, ed. 2. FA Davis, Philadelphia, 2001, p 8.

---

clients and their families. The public expects nurses, as a group, to be honest, trustworthy, ethical, moral, and professional. The American Nurses Association (ANA) Code of Ethics for Nurses (see Chapter 7) is directed toward promoting and maintaining the integrity of the profession. If a group observes less than complete integrity in their leader, that person's ability to lead is markedly diminished.

Courage. Although having the courage to maintain one's convictions in the face of adversity is a quality all leaders must have, certain leadership positions may require a higher degree of courage. Nurses who are in what are called middle management positions, such as unit managers, house supervisors, or quality control coordinators, often find themselves caught in a no man's land between two opposing worlds.[3] For example, higher management may be attempting to implement a plan or procedure that the staff nurses strongly object to, or the

Issues Now

Nurses Carve New Niches in the Health-Care System

The Disappearing Physician

Although nurses have been encouraged to "think outside the box" for many years, only recently has it produced some interesting results, particularly in the area of expanded roles. Nurses can be found in a variety of practice settings that would have been forbidden to them even a few years ago. Nurses are now managing and staffing their own clinics, developing care practices of clients with genetic disorders and working to develop computerized record systems.

The health-care system is beginning to acknowledge that nurses' orientation toward health promotion and prevention works particularly well when nurses, rather than social workers, are assigned as case managers. It works equally as well when providing care for groups such as the elderly or children. When nurses are allowed to be creative in developing and managing their practice, it gives them a sense of empowerment that is often lacking in the more traditional roles that nurses often assume.

Several factors have contributed to these expanded roles for nurses. One has been the gradual decline in primary care physicians that has been ongoing for over a decade. As the reimbursement rates for primary care has declined, more and more physicians have moved toward the more lucrative specialty areas. Managed care also has moved the practice of nurses forward. Managed care's orientation towards the "bottom line" has pushed the need to see more clients in a shorter time to the point where voids have been created in the coverage. Nurses, particularly nurse practitioners, have been able to fill those voids with high-quality and economical care.

The nursing education system has been hard pressed to keep up with the demand for better-educated nurses who can meet the needs of expanding roles. Since the 1980s, the number of nurses obtaining master's degrees and doctorates has tripled. Most of the nonmasters advanced practice programs have been phased out, and the vast majority of nurses who want to be nurse practitioners, nurse midwives, nurse anesthetists or clinical nurse specialists must successfully complete a master's degree program.

A Slow Gain in Respect

Progress has been slow and there is still much to be done. Even after 15 years of working on issues of prescriptive authority for advanced practice nurses (APNs), it is still an uphill fight in some states. The regulations vary greatly from state to state. Some states allow pretty much open prescriptive authority for APNs who meet criteria for pharmacology and allow them to prescribe all medications independently. Other states still require that APNs have a physician's approval before prescribing any medications. One of the underlying problems is one that nurses have experienced, almost since the beginning, lack of respect. Nursing research is funded at a dismal level to medical research. Some physicians still see it as their

(continued)

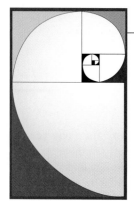

right as "captain of the ship" to verbally abuse nurses and make sure they stay in their places.

Despite these ongoing issues, nurses are making progress. In a health-care system that often overlooks client's needs other than those that are presenting the problem, nurses' orientation toward whole-client care adds an element that many are seeking. As the population ages, many more chronic disease processes require care. Medicine is not well adapted to caring for these. However, nurses have always been there to help and solve problems, and with chronic diseases, this often means spending time with clients, helping them lead healthier lives by changing life styles, and teaching them how to cope with the symptoms and effects of their chronic diseases.

Source: Levine, S, and Marek, A: Nurses step to the front. U.S. News and World Reports 138(4):66–71, 2005.
Hobson, K: Doctors vanish from view. U.S. News and World Reports 138(4):48–54, 2005.

staff nurses may be complaining about some issue, such as staffing, that the middle manager has little control over. The leader in this situation may need to risk offending one or the other of the groups to resolve a difficult problem.

Initiative. Effective leadership demands that the leader be a "self-starter" and have the ability to start projects without pressure from above. Often the group relies on the leader to begin the process of completing a task or resolving a problem.

Energy. Energy refers not only to the ability to do work but also to the display of that energy in the form of enthusiasm for the work. Energetic people are contagious. Charismatic leaders are the ones who are the most energetic and enthusiastic. The group needs to see that the leader is willing to work as hard as they are being asked to work. However, energy has to be rationed carefully to maintain the optimum levels.

Optimism. A positive attitude is also contagious. Conversely, so are negative attitudes, which often lead to discouragement and failure (Table 13.2). A leader who has an overall positive attitude and views new problems as opportunities for success will be much more successful than the leader who constantly complains about each new crisis.

Perseverance. Leaders need to be able to continue to work through difficult problems in difficult circumstances, even when others feel like quitting. Again, if

the leader sets the example for the group with a "there's more than one way to skin a cat" attitude, the group will be encouraged to find new and creative solutions.

Well-Roundedness. Leaders, as well as those they are leading, live multifaceted lives. It is important to develop and foster nonwork relationships with friends and family. The time at work should be balanced with

Table 13.2 Winner or Whiner—Which One Are You?

A Winner Says . . .	A Whiner Says . . .
We have a real challenge here.	This is a big problem.
I'll do my best.	Do I have to do this?
That's great!	That's nice, I guess.
We can do it.	It can't be done, it's impossible.
Yes.	Maybe, when I have some time.

Source: Tappen, RM, et al: Essentials of Nursing Leadership and Management, ed. 2. FA Davis, Philadelphia, 2001, p 8.

recreational, spiritual, social, and cultural activities that complete the person and round out the personality. Time must also be invested in maintaining good health through proper nutrition and regular exercise that will also help prevent burnout (see Chapter 12).

Coping Skills. All jobs have some degree of stress, although people in leadership positions often experience higher levels. Stress can be handled in two ways: unconsciously, through defense mechanisms, or consciously, by bringing learned coping skills into play. A more productive way to deal with stress is to use coping skills developed in dealing with past stressors to promote a positive and healthy resolution to the stress. Some people learn how to use the stress they experience to motivate them and to tap into the energy it generates to achieve at a higher level of functioning.

Self-Knowledge. Leaders who do not know and understand themselves are less able to understand those who are working for them. Self-awareness is the beginning of self-acceptance as a thinking, feeling person who interacts with other thinking, feeling persons. Unless leaders understand and accept their motivations, biases, and perceptions, they will not be able to understand why they feel and react in certain ways to certain individuals and situations.

Charismatic leaders are the ones who are the most energetic and enthusiastic. The group needs to see that the leader is willing to work as hard as they are being asked to work.

MANAGEMENT

Unlike the development of leadership theory, which primarily focused on the leader, the early study of management was aimed toward influencing employees to be as productive as humanly possible. Two schools of thought address and define management.

Time–Motion Theory
Time–motion theory developed out of the early industrial age in which theorists concentrated on ways to complete a task most easily and efficiently. Often their efforts resulted in increased productivity but a decrease in employee satisfaction. From this viewpoint, management can be defined as planning, organizing, commanding, coordinating, and controlling the work of any particular group of employees. The timemotion approach holds that providing the right incentives to the employee, primarily money, can increase employee productivity. Although the weaknesses of this approach make it less desirable in today's society, variations of it served as the harbingers of many of the business techniques currently in use.

Human Interaction Theory
Early on in the study of management, the limits of the time–motion approach became evident. Researchers observed that some lower-paid employee groups had higher levels of productivity than others with higher pay who were doing the same jobs. It appeared that factors such as employees' attitudes, fears, hopes, personal problems, social status in the group, and visions strongly influenced how they worked. From this perspective, management can be defined as the ability to elicit from employees their commitment,

loyalty, creativity, productivity, and continuous improvement.

Managers who favored the human interaction theory were required to develop a different set of management skills, including understanding human behavior, effective counseling, increasing motivation, using effective leadership skills, and maintaining productive communication. Just being a "nice guy" was not enough to guarantee employee cooperation and commitment. To be effective, management needed to be able to recognize and respond to employee concerns and needs, gain acceptance, and protect workers from pressures from higher administration.

It is also important to keep in mind that different management forms are necessary for different work settings. A predominantly time–motion approach may still work best in an area such as manufacturing of automobiles or washing machines. Using the same approach would be inappropriate and probably ineffective when attempting to manage a group of registered nurses (RN) working in an intensive care unit of a busy city hospital.

Motivational Theory

Motivational theory can be defined as the ability to influence the choices people make among a number of possible choices open to them. For example, what factors would motivate a new graduate nurse to work at one hospital when there are four facilities that are offering him or her a job? Are the pay and benefits better? Maybe it is closer to home. Perhaps the shifts are better and the facility does not require mandatory overtime.

Several theorists have attempted to explain this phenomenon. Probably the best known is Abraham Maslow, who developed the Hierarchy of Needs Theory. Although nursing students are taught and use this theory to deal with client needs, the theory also has applications in the realm of leadership and management. Maslow believes that human needs are arranged in a hierarchy from the most basic and essential to those that are more complex. Most basic are the physiological and safety needs, and until these are met in at least a satisfactory fashion, the person is less likely to deal with the higher needs such as social relationships, self-esteem, and self-actualization.

For example, if a nurse was not being paid a salary that would meet the needs for food, housing, and clothing, that would become the nurse's primary concern rather than delivering high-quality client care. Realistically, needs are never fully met, but they have to be accommodated to a degree where the person feels comfortable enough to move up in the hierarchy.

Motivation–Hygiene Theory

Another theory that has become popular is Herzberg's Motivation–Hygiene Theory. Although there are some similarities between Maslow's and Herzberg's theories, particularly in their applications, Herzberg believes that people have two different categories of needs that are fundamentally different from each other.

Hygiene Factors

The first category is referred to as needs dissatisfiers or hygiene factors. According to Herzberg, if these needs are not met, the person feels dissatisfied with his or her job and focuses more on the environment than the work that is supposed to be performed. Hygiene factors are related to the work environment and include, for example, salaries and benefits, job security, status in the organization, work conditions, policies, and relationships with coworkers.

Hygiene factors are related to the conditions under which the work is performed and not to the work itself. They only serve as negative motivators, in that when they are not met, work productivity is reduced. However, if they are satisfied, there is no guarantee that increased productivity and higher quality performance will result.

Needs Motivators

The second category of needs according to Herzberg, is called satisfiers or needs motivators. Unlike the hygiene factors, satisfiers focus primarily on the work. Some of the more important satisfiers that have been identified include elements that tend to expand the work challenges and scope, such as career advancement, increased responsibility, recognition for achievements, and opportunities for professional growth. The satisfiers can have both a positive and negative motivation effect. If they are satisfied, they can motivate workers to increased productivity and higher quality work. If they are not satisfied, they often have the opposite effect.

Motivation in the Hospital Setting

Herzberg concludes that employers must satisfy the hygiene factors as a minimum requirement before there can be any increase in productivity. Programs to promote job enrichment will be effective in upgrading the achievement, roles, and satisfaction of employees. In the hospital setting, career or clinical ladder programs provide nurses with the recognition for achievement and opportunity for advancement, along with financial rewards (hygiene factor), and allow them to remain in direct client care.

It is important for RNs to understand and be able to use motivation techniques, even if they are not in a designated management role. The ability to motivate is one of the keys to success in delegation at any level, and the success of RNs is often assessed by how well people on the health-care team they are supervising perform their jobs. Successful motivation is the door to successful leadership because these are the people who can make things happen in an organization.

> *The ability to motivate is one of the keys to success in delegation at any level, and the success of RNs is often assessed by how well people on the health-care team they are supervising perform their jobs.*

MAKING CHANGES SUCCESSFULLY

Motivating people to change is one of the most challenging and most important functions of leadership. Simply stated, change is the process of transforming, altering, or becoming different from what was before.[4] Although change is a constant in health care and nursing, it is surprising how resistant nurses can be to even minor changes in their work environment.

Internal or External?

Two primary forces bring about change: external forces that originate from outside the person or organization and internal forces that start from within the individual or organization. A primary example of external change is what happens when government agencies pass down new rules and regulations, such as the HIPAA legislation, that affect health care. An example of internal change would be a hospital increasing salaries or eliminating mandatory overtime from the work action of a group of nurses.

Planned or Unplanned?

Change can be planned or unplanned. Planned change is more productive and occurs when there is a directed and designed implementation of some element within the organization. Change can affect all aspects of an organization, including policies, goals, organizational philosophy, work environment, and even structure. Planned change can be used for all sorts of projects, ranging from the minor to the most complex.

Unplanned change, sometimes called reactive change, occurs when a problem forces a person or organization into a situation in which it must respond. These changes are often minor but sometimes can involve projects that are large in scope and complexity. Examples in nursing include changes in staffing because of nurses who call in sick, clients who experience cardiac arrest, or even equipment failures, such as when the electricity fails or a water main breaks.

A Driving Force for Change

Nurses often take on the role of the change agent, that is, the one who brings about the change (Box 13.3). All change requires the ability to overcome resistance to change (called restraining forces) by a driving

Box 13.3

Characteristics of an Effective Change Agent

- Is well organized
- Identifies restraining forces
- Is able to motivate
- Demonstrates and maintains commitment to change
- Develops trusting relationships
- Responds to feedback and negotiation
- Is goal directed
- Communicates well
- Maintains optimistic attitude

force that pushes toward change. When the driving and restraining forces are equal, then no change occurs and the status quo is maintained.

Change can occur only when the driving force is greater than the restraining force. Those who want to change have a tendency to push, but those who are being asked to change tend to push back to maintain things as they were. It is important when attempting to implement change to identify the restraining forces and ways to overcome them. Habit, comfort, and inertia are the three most common restraining forces.

Planned change works best when it is well organized, proceeds at a steady pace, and has a definite date for achievement. There is a level of excitement that raises energy levels when a change is near completion, but postponing the date for the change can drain that energy and lead to disappointment.

> *Those who want to change have a tendency to push, but those who are being asked to change tend to push back to maintain things as they were.*

GROUP DYNAMICS

A Common Goal

All successful leaders and managers understand and are able to use the principles of group dynamics. A group exists when three or more people interact and are held together by a common bond or interests. Groups are open systems that interact with the environment to achieve a goal (see Chapter 4). The individuals who make up the group are its subsystems and interact with each other as well as with the environment. Group dynamics provides the principles that underlie team building, which is essential to the success of nursing units. Establishing and sharing common goals is the starting point for successful team building.

When the common goal is to help one another, effective team building results. Members of the team respond most positively when they feel they are included in the decision making and when they

realize that their input is valued by the other team members. It is important that the leader always ask team members for their ideas about the goal that the team is working toward. A strong team spirit is crucial to the success of the team.

A Common Understanding

Similarly, the team will only function smoothly when the members understand their roles and the roles of the other members. Their roles identify their places on the team and establishes what is expected from each member. To be successful, the leader must establish the belief that all the roles are of equal importance for the achievement of the goals or purposes of the group.

Mutual Support. Team members need to realize they are not merely responsible for their own roles but need to be supportive of the roles of the other members. Although the leader establishes the goals to be achieved, it is important that the team members be allowed to achieve their tasks in ways that are most appropriate for them, particularly when working with self-motivated professionals such as nurses.

Reward for Achievement. Ongoing or complicated projects require a long-term commitment that is sometimes difficult to maintain. Effective team leaders are good at finding accomplishments along the way that the team can celebrate and enjoy. It allows the team to feel good about what they have achieved to this point and motivates them to accomplish more in the future. A good leader also recognizes the accomplishments of others and rewards them appropriately. Often even simple statements of praise can be effective.

Identity and Trust. Finally, establishing a sense of team identity and trust completes the group dynamic and team-building process. Some degree of creativity may be required for establishing team identity, ranging from similar uniforms to buttons or pins. Trust allows the team members to be more open to communications from other members and more willing to take risks. Trust empowers the members, allowing them to make independent decisions and promoting the smooth functioning of the team (Table 13.3).

Table 13.3 Do's and Don'ts of Effective Change Agents

Do's	Don'ts
Do develop a sense of trust.	Don't have a hidden agenda.
Do establish common goals.	Don't be unpredictable.
Do facilitate effective communication.	Don't miss or reschedule meetings frequently.
Do establish a strong team identity.	Don't use threats or bluffs to manipulate members.
Do contribute as much as possible.	Don't volunteer to be the record keeper.
Do find reasons to celebrate and recognize accomplishments.	Don't follow the rest of the crowd.

A good leader also recognizes the accomplishments of others and rewards them appropriately. Often even simple statements of praise can be effective.

CARE DELIVERY MODELS

Nowhere are the elements of group dynamics reflected better than in the nursing units of a hospital or health-care facility. The organizational structure found in the nursing units of a facility reflects how the nursing department interacts with coworkers and participates in the delivery of client care. Various models may be used in the delivery of nursing care. Many health-care facilities have made a transition from one model to another and may even incorporate several different models at the same time. The nurse must recognize which model is being used as well as its strengths and weaknesses. These models include functional nursing, team nursing, primary care nursing, and modular nursing (Table 13.4).

Functional Nursing

Functional nursing has as its foundation a task-oriented philosophy: each person performs a specific job that is narrowly defined according to the needs of the unit. The medication nurse, for example, focuses on administering and documenting medications for the assigned group of clients.

In this organizational unit, the nurse manager is called the charge nurse, whose main responsibility is to oversee the various workers. Charge nurses are also appointed for each shift to manage the care during that time. This model relies on ancillary health workers such as nurses' aides and orderlies. Some believe this model fragments care too much. Because many people have specific tasks, coordination can be difficult and the holistic perspective may be lost.

Team Nursing

Team nursing has a more unified approach to client care, with team members functioning together to achieve client goals. The team leader functions as the person ultimately responsible for the clients' well-being. More cohesiveness is present among the members of the team than is found in the functional model. Rather than having a narrow task to accomplish, team members focus on team goals under the coordination of the team leader. The team conference provides for effective communication and follow-up among team members and is the key to successful team nursing.

Primary Care Nursing

The primary care nursing model provides nurses the opportunity to focus on the whole person. The **primary care nurse** provides and is responsible for all of the client's nursing needs. The nurse manager in this model becomes a facilitator for the primary care nurses. Primary care nurses are self-directed and concerned with consistency of care. The primary care model is similar to the

Table 13.4 Comparison of Common Client Care Models

Model	Nurses Are Called	Description	Where Model is Used
Functional	Charge nurse Medical nurse Treatment nurse	Nurses are assigned to specific tasks rather than specific clients	Hospitals Nursing homes Nurse consultants Operating rooms
Team	Team leader Team member	Nursing staff members are divided into small groups responsible for the total care of a given number of clients.	Hospitals Nursing homes Home care Hospice
Primary Care	Primary nurse Associate nurse	Nurses are designated either as the primary nurse responsible for clients' care or as the associate nurse who assists in carrying out the care.	Hospitals Specialty units Dialysis Home care
Modular	Care pair	Nurses are paired with other less-trained caregivers. Generally involves cross-training of personnel.	Hospitals Home health care Transport teams

case management model, which has one nurse caring for one client. Many home-health-care agencies use this method of assigning an RN to work with an individual or family for the duration of the services rendered.

Modular Nursing

A Response to Downsizing

Modular nursing, also called client-focused care, is one model that was developed in response to professional nursing personnel shortages and to the downsizing of professional nursing staffs. This model is based on a decentralized organizational system that emphasizes close interdisciplinary collaboration. Redesigning the method of nursing care delivery takes much planning and input from the various departments involved, such as nursing, respiratory therapy, physical therapy, radiology, laboratory, and dietary.

Important aspects of modular nursing include relying on unlicensed assistive personnel (UAP), also called unit service assistants, for the provision of direct care; grouping clients with similar needs; developing relative intensity measures (RIM);

and emphasizing team concepts in small groups that remain constant.

Strong, Explicit Leadership

Cross-training of personnel is another important aspect of modular nursing; for example, using this system, respiratory therapists do not just provide respiratory treatments but also help clients to the bathroom and turn bedridden clients. Nurse managers in this system are responsible for providing explicit job descriptions, maintaining the work group's cohesiveness, carefully monitoring each staff person's abilities, delegating tasks as appropriate, and evaluating the effectiveness of care.

The role of UAPs is one area of the client-focused care model that needs more definition, particularly in relation to the RN's accountability and responsibilities in supervising these workers. State boards of nursing across the country are considering possible changes in nurse practice acts necessitated by the use of UAPs.

Benefits of this care delivery model include decreased staffing cost and greater autonomy of cross-trained personnel. The nurse manager must be a strong leader for this model of care delivery to succeed. Consistent collaboration between the nurse manager and physician is of utmost importance in planning client care.

> " *Leadership can be exerted either formally or informally. Often the most effective leaders in a group are not the ones who are officially designated as the leader.* "

LEADERSHIP VERSUS MANAGEMENT

Several questions arise when people speak about leadership and management.

Are They the Same Thing?

Leadership can be exerted either formally or informally. Often the most effective leaders in a group are not the ones who are officially designated as the leader. On the other hand, managers are given the title by some higher authority and have formally designated authority to supervise a group of employees in the achievement of a task. Similarly, managers can be held formally responsible for the quality, quantity, and cost of the work that the supervised employees produce.

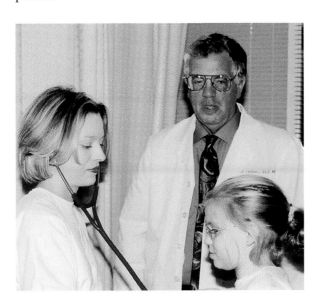

Do Managers Need Good Leadership Skills?

The most effective managers will have highly developed leadership skills; however, by virtue of their title and position, even managers with poor leadership skills are still the official authority, although their effectiveness is reduced. Often, in groups where the manager is not a good leader, unofficial leaders emerge and exert either a strong positive or negative influence on the group. If the unofficial leader is generally supportive of the manager's and administration's goals, then the work group can be highly productive and the organization's goals will be achieved. Conversely, if the unofficial leader's goals are opposed to those of the manager and administration, productivity may decrease to a point where higher-level management asks the manager to leave the position.

Are Leaders Always Good Managers?

A person who has leadership ability may not have good management skills. This phenomenon is often seen in the nursing profession when a highly effective and skilled staff nurse who functions as the unofficial unit leader is taken out of that role and promoted to an official management position. Some do well; others may require additional training in management principles and skills. Some never quite master the skills needed for management.

Management and leadership skills complement each other. As with all skills, they can be learned and require practice and experience to be developed fully. Even new graduate nurses can be effective leaders within their new nursing roles. As they gain experience and develop new skills, their ability and opportunities to provide leadership will also increase. Learning and improving skills in one area will increase the ability in the other.

FUNCTIONS OF THE NURSE MANAGER

Nurse managers often find themselves located on the organizational chart between employees and upper-level management. The functions and duties of nurse managers depend to a great degree on how the institution defines the role. One of the first activities of a new nurse manager is to make sure he or she understands the job description, responsibilities, and level of authority the position has in the institution where he or she is employed. Some of the tasks that have been identified as being a regular part of a nurse manager's position are listed in Box 13.4.

In today's health-care system, nurse managers continue to follow the trend of moving away from the close supervision of the staff nurses' work to a role of helping them complete their work safely and effectively. As this role continues to evolve, the emphasis will shift from traditional management functions to highly supportive functions as are seen in the leadership role

Box 13.4

Common Tasks for Nurse Managers

- Conduct orientation of new staff
- Evaluate staff
- Terminate employees with unsatisfactory work performance
- Develop time schedules that cover the unit safely
- Make team and staff assignments
- Develop a realistic budget for the unit
- Justify the number of nursing hours used by the unit
- Call in nurses on their days off when staffing falls short
- Attend nursing management meetings
- Hold regular meetings with unit staff to resolve problems and implement new policies and procedures
- Set unit goals for staff
- Contribute to facility goals
- Communicate regularly with physicians about unit problems
- Conduct quality assurance studies
- Provide rewards for high-quality care

Conclusion

Over the years, there has been one constant in the changing health-care system, and that is that the RN is still expected to provide leadership and management skills to direct and ensure the high quality of the health care given to clients. Both leadership and management require sets of skills that can be learned. Nurses who learn these skills will become successful managers and the leaders of the health-care system in the future.

Successful leaders and managers understand and often combine the best aspects of the many theories that deal with leadership and management. Knowledge of one's strengths and weakness provides the basis for successful management. Developing effective leadership and management skills is a lifelong, ongoing process. Learning from books and articles, as well as from other successful nurse managers, presents an opportunity for professional and personal growth.

Issues in Practice

Jill, an RN, was recently appointed as the evening charge nurse on a busy postsurgical unit. She has been an active participant in the hospital's quality assurance committee for the past 2 years since her graduation. One of the issues the committee identified as a problem was the higher than average surgical wound infection rate on Jill's unit. After some research, Jill determined that a major component of the high infection rate was the procedures that were used when changing postoperative dressings.

After obtaining permission from the unit manager and hospital education director, Jill developed a new procedure for dressing changes, incorporating the most current research. She presented the changes in a short in-service program to the unit personnel, several times to each of the three shifts to make sure that all the nurses and staff on the unit were familiar with the new changes. The expectation was that there would be a 25 percent reduction in wound infections after using the new procedures for 1 month.

At the end of the first month of using the new dressing change procedures, the postoperative wound infection rate showed no improvement over the previous month's rate. At the monthly staff meeting, Jill discovered that the licensed practical nurses (LPNs) on the unit were refusing to use the new procedures because they "took too much time" and had reverted back to the procedures they had always used before.

Critical Thinking Questions

- What was the style of leadership and management that Jill used when attempting to initiate the dressing procedure change?
- Other than the stated reason, why do you think the LPNs did not want to use the new procedures?
- How can Jill increase the level of compliance by the LPNs on the unit?
- What is the role of the unit manager in initiating the new dressing change procedures?

References

1. Tappen, RM: Nursing Leadership and Management, ed. 4. FA Davis, Philadelphia, 2001.
2. Srsic-Stoehr, K: Success skills for the nurse manager: Cultural debut and sustainment. Nurse Leader 2(6):36–41, 2004.
3. West, B: Evaluation of a clinical leadership initiative. Nursing Standard 19(5):33–41, 2004.
4. Kerfoot, K: On leadership: The shelf life of leaders. Medical/Surgical Nursing 13(5):348–350, 2004.

Bibliography

Bliss, J: Effective team management by district nurses. British Journal of Community Nursing 9(12):524–526, 2004.

Bradley, E: Translating research into clinical practice: Making change happen. Journal of the American Geriatric Society 52(11):1875–1882, 2004.

Isaacson, J: Nursing students in an expanded charge nurse role: A real clinical management experience. Nursing Education Perspectives 25(6):292–296, 2004.

Jeong, S: Innovative leadership and management in a nursing home. Journal of Nursing Management 12(6):445–451, 2004.

Kuzmits, F: 360-feedback in health care management: A field study. Health Care Manager 23(4):321–328, 2004.

Leichtling, B: Leadership & management. Preventive medicine for "compassion [sic] fatigue". Caring 23(10):90–91, 2004.

Owens, J, and Patton, J: Take a chance on nursing mentorships: Enhance leadership with this win-win strategy. Nursing Education Perspectives 24(4):198–204, 2005.

Patterson, P: A few simple rules for managing block time in the operating room. Operating Room Manager 20(11):1, 9–12, 2004.

Robotham, M: How to handle complaints. Nursing Times 97(30):25–28, 2001.

Sanford, K: Become competent in confrontation. Nursing Management 35(7):14, 2004.

Taylor, D, and Pinczuk J: Health Care Financial Management for Nurse Managers: Merging the Heart with the Dollar. Joes & Barlett Publishers, 2005.

Tracy, B: What makes a good leader. The Oklahoman, Jan 9, 2005, p 1H.

Vestal, K: Lessons learned: Making time for leadership. Nurse Leader 2(6):8–9, 2004.

West, B: Evaluation of a clinical leadership initiative. Nursing Standard 19(5):33–41, 2004.

14

Communicating Successfully

Joseph T. Catalano

Learning Objectives

After completing this chapter, the reader will be able to:

- Explain the importance of understanding human behaviors.
- Describe conflict resolution and relationship tools.
- Identify communications styles.
- Analyze and apply problem-solving and conflict-resolution tools.
- Discuss the use of the nursing process in conflict resolution.
- Formulate coping strategies to handle difficult people.

THE NURSE AS COMMUNICATOR

Good communication skills are often advertised as the answer to many of the problems encountered in everyday life. Television personalities, instructors, and psychologists promote improved communication skills as the answer to parental, marital, financial, and work-related problems. The nursing profession recognizes communication as one of the cornerstones of its practice. Nurses must be able to communicate with clients, family members, physicians, peers, and associates in an effective and constructive manner to achieve their goals of high-quality care. Good communication is essential for good leadership and management.

In today's rapidly evolving health-care system, registered nurses (RNs) are called on to supervise a growing number of assistive and unlicensed personnel. One of the keys to good supervision is the ability to communicate to people what they must do to provide the required care and, often, how the care should be given. It is not always easy. Many of the people whom nurses supervise are poorly trained, lack the theoretical and technical knowledge base of the nurse, and may display attitudes that make them resistant to direction. However, nurse supervisors can be and often are held legally responsible for the actions of those individuals who work under their direction.

> " *Change can produce many emotions, ranging from excitement and anticipation to stress, fear, and anxiety. At minimum, change makes most people feel uncomfortable.* "

FACTORS THAT AFFECT COMMUNICATION

Change

Change is one of the few absolute certainties in today's health-care system. Change can produce many emotions, ranging from excitement and anticipation to stress, fear, and anxiety. How people deal with change can affect how they respond to the environment and communicate with others.

At minimum, change makes most people feel uncomfortable. Any change can be simultaneously positive and negative. During the process of learning new skills, treatments, or techniques, most people feel a sense of accomplishment at the same time that they feel afraid of making mistakes, being judged by others, or being labeled as "slow learners."

Fear of the Unknown

Imagine a new graduate nurse starting his or her first day at work, very excited about the new experience and the potential for career development. However, at the same time the nurse is worried about being accepted into the group, being able to practice what was learned in nursing school, and being able to learn the new skills required by the unit. Almost everyone has a sense of dread when moving away from activities with which they have become comfortable. Setting realistic personal goals and time lines for learning new information helps reduce fear and stress when making major changes.

> *People may be afraid to ask questions about new procedures or policies because they fear that they might appear "stupid" in front of their colleagues.*

Change affects communication in various ways. People may be afraid to ask questions about new procedures or policies because they fear that they might appear "stupid" in front of their colleagues. Fear of being criticized closes individuals off to positive suggestions and new ideas. Others may hesitate in sharing ideas because they are afraid of being labeled as confrontational.

For example, a nurse is reassigned from the medical/surgical unit to the intensive care unit (ICU). This nurse will initially be somewhat fearful in the new environment with the highly trained and assertive expert unit nurses who always seem to be in control. A more positive approach would be for the new nurse to take advantage of the unit nurses' expertise and learn from their examples. The new nurse needs to remember that everyone on that unit was a novice at one time. In the current health-care system, almost everyone is fearful much of the time of making mistakes and of falling short of the high standards of the profession.

The Need to Take Risks

Change can have both positive and negative effects. Often when a staff is initially resistant to a change and fights to prevent it, once they have gone through the process, would never go back to the old way of doing things. All change involves some risk taking, and some people are better at risk taking than are others. Consider the following case study:

After analysis of the needs of the clients and the nursing workload of a busy medical unit, the unit manager decided to change the work shift times. In addition to the standard 7 A.M. to 3 P.M., 3 P.M. to 11 P.M., and 11 P.M. to 7 A.M. shifts, she decided to add a 5 A.M. to 1 P.M. shift to increase coverage during the busiest period of the shift. The RN assigned to the new shift recognized the benefits to the unit and clients; thus, she accepted and supported the change with few objections. Also, the change in shift times allowed her to alter her personal schedule so that she could take extra courses toward her master's degree at a local college. For the RN, the change in shifts was a positive experience.

However, the licensed practical nurse (LPN) assigned to this new shift was upset with the change. She was a "late sleeper" and did not want to come in so early. She liked the shifts the way they were and did not see any advantages to changing things needlessly.

After the new shift was initiated, the LPN was usually 15 to 30 minutes late, called in sick frequently, and was "grumpy" and hard to talk to when she did come in to work. For this LPN, the change was negative and unacceptable.

Grief Stages

Nurses need to keep in mind that the communication abilities of clients who are experiencing change will be affected in very much the same way as nurses who are experiencing change. As a result of disease, trauma, or surgery, many clients face sudden and major alterations in their bodies, as well as changes in their ability to function and carry out daily self-care activities. For example, a client with a new colostomy must adapt to major physiological, psychological, and emotional changes.

Most clients who have surgical procedures that result in major body function alterations go through the stages of the grief process: denial, anger, guilt, depression, and resolution. Communication with a client in the anger stage of the grief process, who is hostile, critical of his care, and verbally abusive, will be much different than communication with a client in the depression stage, who is withdrawn, reticent, and sleeps most of the time. Recognition of the communication behaviors of each of the grief stages is essential in understanding why clients are acting in a particular way. A decision must then be made regarding the most effective communication technique to use when providing care.

Stress

Stress is produced by many factors and always affects an individual's ability to communicate. Some common causes of stress for health-care workers include institutional restructuring, group interaction and dynamics, unilateral management decisions, or personal issues and experiences. Regardless of the source, stress usually decreases people's ability to interact and communicate and increases the demands on their coping mechanisms.

A Destructive Circle

When people are unable to cope with a stressful situation successfully, they may experience an increased state of tension or anxiety. They may develop physiological symptoms such as nausea, stomach cramps, diarrhea, or palpitations; in extreme cases, they may even become paranoid or psychotic. Uncontrolled, high levels of stress on a nursing unit may lead to competition among the nurses that affects their teamwork, productivity, and the quality of the care given.

> *At some point, one group's stress always affects another group's stress level, whose stress in turn increases another group's stress. The process becomes a destructive circle of cause-and-effect responses that increases the stress levels for everyone in the facility.*

Physicians who are stressed by worry about a severely ill client or threats to their autonomy, practice, and income from changes in reimbursement policies may become tense and highly critical of or even verbally abusive toward nurses. The hospital management may also experience increased stress owing to the escalating responsibility of maintaining high-quality services with ever-shrinking revenues. Management often deals with its stress by becoming more autocratic, making increased demands on the nursing staff while reducing the control that nurses have over their practice and becoming closed off to input from nurses and physicians.

At some point, one group's stress always affects another group's stress level, whose stress in turn increases another group's stress. The process becomes a destructive circle of cause-and-effect responses that increases the stress levels for everyone in the facility.

Clients Under Stress

Stress in the health-care environment is not just experienced by health-care providers. Stress for clients starts when they first come into contact with the health-care system, peaks when they have to undergo physical examinations, surgery, or invasive treatments, and continues throughout the recovery period. The fear that a nurse may not respond to clients' needs increases clients' stress levels, and they sometimes become more demanding of care, which, in turn, increases the nurse's stress levels. If the nursing staff is experiencing high stress levels, clients often sense this subconsciously, and as a result, clients' stress levels will increase also.

What Do You Think?

List four factors or situations that have produced high levels of stress for you in the hospital or health-care setting. Why did these incidents produce stress? How did you deal with the stress?

_____

_____

_____

_____

_____

_____

_____

_____

_____

_____

_____

Several techniques can be used to reduce clients' stress levels so they can better communicate and become more receptive to teaching. Stress reduction techniques range from very simple measures that everyone can use, such as distraction with music or simple activities, exercise, or reduction in stimuli, to more advanced techniques such as meditation, **biofeedback,** and even antianxiety medications.

Eliminate the Situation

Nurses need to be able to identify situations that produce stress, recognize the symptoms shown by someone in a stressful situation, know how to reduce stress, and be able to use appropriate communication techniques with someone under stress. Of course, if possible, the best way to reduce stress is to eliminate the stressful situation. Consider the following case:

The hospital management has just sent a memo to all the hospital units that a new client assessment form they have developed is to be implemented next week. This new form is in addition to the ones that the nurses already fill out each day. The new form is to be completed by RNs only and must be done each shift on every client and then sent to the house supervisor so that management can track acuity. Because of recent facility restructuring and changes in staffing patterns, often there is only one RN on the 3 P.M. to 11 P.M. and 11 P.M. to 7 A.M. shifts to cover a 42-bed unit. This extra, time-consuming, and seemingly redundant paperwork increases the stress of the staff RNs to an unacceptable level.

They meet as a group with management and propose that the assessment forms they are already using be modified to include the data that management wants on the new forms. Photocopies of the revised form could then be made by the unit clerk for each shift and given to the supervisors, thus eliminating the new form. Management notes the high stress levels of the RNs, recognizes that increased stress lowers the quality of care, and decides to follow the RNs' proposal, thus eliminating the primary source of the RNs' stress.

Although all sources of stress cannot be eliminated completely, in most situations it can be reduced to a manageable level. However, high stress levels should never be used as an excuse for destructive anger and behaviors, failure of communication, or abuse of individuals.

Anger

In addition to being one of the stages of the grief process, anger can be a symptom of personal frustration, lack of control, fear of change, or feelings of hopelessness. Anger is one of the strong primitive natural emotions that help individuals protect themselves against a variety of external threats. Although everyone experiences anger, how it is expressed often depends on a person's family and ethnic background, life experiences, and personal values. In some cultures, loud and physically expressive outbursts are the norm for the expression of anger, whereas in other cultures, anger is internalized and expressed only as a "controlled rage."

Positive or Negative Expression

As with most of the other factors that affect communication, anger can be either positive or negative. When anger is used in a positive, productive manner, it can promote change and release tension. Anger can be used positively to increase others' attention, initiate communication, problem solve, and energize the change process. Sensitivity to internal anger can warn individuals that something is wrong either within themselves or with someone or something in the external environment.

Many individuals have difficulty expressing and using their anger in a positive manner. Anger that is used negatively is very destructive. It hinders communication, makes coworkers fearful, and erodes relationships with others. Anger expressed by abusive behaviors such as pounding on nursing station counters, throwing charts or surgical instruments, verbal outbursts, or even violent physical contact is never acceptable and may lead to civil or criminal actions against the perpetrator.

The negative expression of anger may cause the person who is the object of the anger to retaliate or seek revenge, but probably the most destructive form that negative anger can take is when it is internalized and suppressed. Long-term, suppressed anger has been associated with a number of physiological and psychological problems ranging from gastric ulcers and hypertension to myocardial infarctions, strokes, and even psychotic rage episodes.

What Sets People Off

Nurses who understand what makes both themselves and others angry are better able to either avoid anger-producing situations or cope effectively with their own anger or with that of others. For example, even new graduate nurses soon learn that some situations will almost always evoke an angry response

from hospitalized clients. These include serving meals that are cold or poorly cooked, not answering call lights in a timely manner, waking up soundly sleeping clients at midnight to give them a sleeping pill, or taking 10 attempts to start an intravenous (IV) line.

Similarly, unit managers and hospital administrators quickly learn that some of the things they do will almost always produce angry responses from the staff. These actions include unilateral changes in the work schedule, additional paperwork, reduction in staffing levels, or refusal for requests for vacation or time off.

It is important that nurses understand that anger is a normal human emotion. Once it is recognized, it should be dealt with and then let go. Sometimes situations are not going to change, no matter how angry the person becomes, and sometimes no amount of anger will prevent changes from occurring.

GROUP DYNAMICS

The power of the group over an individual's behavior should never be underestimated. Groups establish and exert their power through a set of unique behaviors or norms that their members are expected to follow. These norms may be formal or informal, written or unwritten, promulgated or merely understood. Unfortunately, in most nursing units the norms are often not clearly expressed, yet they may be used as judgment tools or standards for evaluating work behaviors. When new nurses begin work on a particular unit, they must quickly learn the unwritten unit norms and identify the informal leaders to function effectively.

Unwritten Rules

As with most elements in communication, group dynamics may be positive or negative. Nurses who do not learn and fail to display the expected group behaviors may be ostracized from the group, thus making the work environment psychologically uncomfortable and perhaps even physically difficult. For example, nonconforming nurses may find that there is no one around when they need help ambulating an unsteady client. A particular nursing unit staff may have a strong team approach. If the new nurse is highly independent and prefers to work alone, he or she may not "fit in" and may experience hostility or sarcasm from the other nurses on the unit.

Going Against the Group

Consider the following scenario demonstrating group dynamics:

> The ICU has the responsibility for on-call coverage for the recovery room for unscheduled postoperative clients on the evening shifts, night shifts, and all of the weekend shifts. There is no formal written policy, but coverage has traditionally been handled on a voluntary, rotating basis.
>
> Because it is "voluntary," one of the ICU nurses has decided that he does not want to take call any more. He is the only member of the ICU staff who does not take call. Soon after he announces his decision, he begins to sense anger and experience alienation from his peers. Although he is very knowledgeable, has highly developed nursing skills, and provides consistently high-quality care to assigned clients on his regular shifts, on his semiannual peer evaluation, he receives low ratings from his coworkers on the basis of the informal call coverage standard and expectations. The unit nurses feel that he is no longer a team player.
>
> The nurse becomes angry because he feels that the use of unclear, unwritten standards is an unfair way to evaluate his ability as a nurse. He soon finds that the other ICU nurses accidentally "forget" to invite him to group functions. He also seems to be assigned the most difficult and largest number of clients during any given shift, seemingly to compensate for not taking call.

Group dynamics involves many factors, including methods of communications, professional behaviors, professional growth, flexibility, problem solving, participation, and competition. The ability to understand and use the elements of group dynamics has a direct relationship to the behaviors, cooperation, and effectiveness of the team. Often, when a team labels an individual member as "difficult," it most likely means that the individual is not following one or more of the informal, unwritten group norms.

> *The ability to understand and use the elements of group dynamics has a direct relationship on the behaviors, cooperation, and effectiveness of the team.*

COMPETITION

Competition can be a very powerful element in group dynamics and communication. Depending on how it is channeled, expressed, and used, competition can be a positive or negative force within the group. The various forms of competition can be individual, team, or unit focused.

Peer Evaluation. A common expression of competition in the group setting is peer evaluations. For peer evaluations to be a positive form of competition, the unit must decide ahead of time on the norms and expectations that they value and then design an objective measurement tool to evaluate whether the individual is meeting the norms. Each individual being evaluated must be aware of the criteria before the evaluation is conducted. The evaluation team must be educated on evaluation techniques and must be as objective and professional as possible.

In the health-care setting, it is important for all professionals, unit groups, and management to promote competition in a positive, progressive, and supportive environment. When competition is channeled positively, it leads to new and creative ideas, better programs, increased growth, more productive interactions, and higher-quality client care. When the competition is negative, it often produces failures, depression, sabotage, unit turf conflicts, decreased productivity, and lower-quality care. Consider the following case:

> The competition on a nursing unit turned negative when the nurses on the 7 A.M. to 3 P.M. shift began competing with the nurses on the 3 P.M. to 11 P.M. shift in order to appear more knowledgeable about client care to the nurse manager. To "look better," the nurses on the 7 A.M. to 3 P.M. shift intentionally withheld selected client laboratory test results during shift report.
>
> As a result of this action, several tests scheduled for the 3 P.M. to 11 P.M. shift were not

done, angering the physicians, potentially threatening the safety of the clients, and making the nurses on the 3 P.M. to 11 P.M. shift appear incompetent. In addition, the nurses on that shift had to complete several incident reports on the errors that occurred on their shift.

One informal component of the staff nurses' performance evaluations used by the unit manager is the number of incident reports that a nurse must file. The more incident reports, the poorer will be the nurse's performance evaluation. To the unit manager, the nurses on the 7 A.M. to 3 P.M. shift appear to be more competent because of the seemingly poor care, indicated by a large number of incident reports, that is being given on the 3 P.M. to 11 P.M. shift. However, when the nurses on the 3 P.M. to 11 P.M. shift discovered what really happened, they devised several ways to "get even" with the nurses on the 7 A.M. to 3 P.M. shift.

WORKING ENVIRONMENT

The delivery of health care is currently in a rapid transition from a fee-for-service to a managed care environment. Health care is shifting from acute, inpatient care to long-term outpatient care and from being illness based to a prevention and wellness focus. The changes produced by this transition are creating a high degree of stress at all levels of the health-care system. As discussed earlier, both change and stress are major barriers to effective communication.

Active Involvement in Change

One measure that can be taken to both alleviate some of the stress caused by the current changes in health care and improve unit communication is to encourage all members of the health-care team to participate in the renovation of their work environment. Through active participation, workers have an opportunity to have an impact on and direct the changes that are being made. Some people mistakenly believe that if they do not become involved, the changes will not happen. Unfortunately, when people are not actively involved in the restructuring process, others who are probably less qualified will make the changes anyway.

Increased fear, high stress levels, angry outbursts, and feelings of insecurity all are potential results of a work environment where the workers do not participate in the change process. Difficult behaviors resulting in unclear communication become more evident during times of change and stress. Ugly rumors, feelings of resentment, and increased insecurity often result when intergroup communications are not clear. An open, interactive work environment increases the probability of successful communication and adaptation to change.

Coping With Difficult Behavior

Understanding what motivates a person's behavior permits the individual to design a plan or develop coping mechanisms for communicating on the basis of sound interpersonal techniques. When individuals are able to separate themselves from the difficult situation, they are less likely to take things personally and more likely to begin to focus on the underlying issues causing the problems rather than the other person's difficult behavior. The interaction becomes less judgmental and threatening to the other person. However, understanding the other person's motives never excuses unacceptable behaviors such as sarcasm, angry outbursts, and abusive language. Rather, it allows for direct confrontation of the behavior in a more controlled and less emotional way.

What Do You Think?

Have you ever been in a situation where others have intentionally sabotaged your work? What was the situation? How did you feel? How did you deal with it? Did you try to retaliate?

All professional nurses need to develop coping mechanisms to deal with difficult people. The very nature of the profession exposes nurses to a large number of people who are experiencing change, are under stress, and have a wide range of backgrounds and values as well as varying expectations. By understanding communication, using **behavior modification,** developing **assertiveness,** avoiding submissive and aggressive behaviors, and appreciating diversity, the nurse can develop the coping skills required for problem solving, handling conflict in the work setting, and confronting the unacceptable behaviors of difficult people.

> *Through active participation, workers have an opportunity to have an impact on and direct the changes that are being made. Some people mistakenly believe that if they do not become involved, the changes will not happen.*

UNDERSTANDING COMMUNICATION

Encoding and Decoding

Communication is an interactive sharing of information. It requires a sender, a message, and a receiver. After the sender sends the message, the receiver has a responsibility to listen to, process, and understand (encode) the information and then to respond to the sender by giving feedback (decoding). The encoding process occurs when the receiver thinks about the information, understands it, and forms an idea on the basis of the message.

Several factors can interfere with the encoding process. On the sender's side, these can be factors such as unclear speech, monotone voice, poor sentence structure, inappropriate use of terminology or jargon, or lack of knowledge about the topic. On the receiver's side, factors that may interfere with encoding include lack of attention, prejudice and bias, preoccupation with another problem, or even physical factors such as pain, drowsiness, or impairment of the senses.

For example, a staff nurse is in a mandatory meeting where the unit manager is discussing a new policy that will be starting the next month. However, the nurse is thinking about an important heart medication that her client is to receive in 5 minutes. The

nurse's primary concern is to get out of the meeting in time to give the medication. After the meeting, the nurse has only a minimal recollection of what was said because she did not encode the information well. The following month when the new policy is started, the staff nurse is confused about what she should do and makes several errors in relationship to the new policy.

Verbal or Nonverbal?

There are two primary methods of communication: verbal and nonverbal. **Verbal** communication is either the written or spoken word and constitutes only about 7 percent of the communicated message. **Nonverbal** communication, which makes up the other 93 percent of communication, is everything else, including body language, facial expressions, gestures, physical appearance, touch, vocal cues (tone, pauses), and spatial territory (personal space). When the verbal and nonverbal messages are congruent, then the message is more easily encoded and clearly understood. If the verbal and nonverbal messages are conflicting, the nonverbal message is probably the most reliable. It is relatively easy for people to lie with words, but nonverbal communication tends to be unconscious and more difficult to control.

For example, the nurse suspects that the mother of a newborn infant may be experiencing postpartum depression. The nurse asks the mother how she feels about her new baby. The mother responds in a low volume, very slow-paced monotone voice: "I'm so happy I have this baby," while looking down at her feet in a slouched-over posture. The message from the mother is conflicting. The words are saying she is happy, but all the nonverbal signs indicate that she is depressed. The observant nurse concludes that more assessment for depression is required.

Effective communication requires understanding that the perceptions, emotions, and participation of both parties are interactive and have an effect on the transmission of the message. Nurses often encounter situations that require clarification of the information for accuracy and encoding. The following is an example of client teaching requiring a return demonstration:

A nurse gave a teaching session to a client who was being sent home with a T-tube after surgical removal of gallstones from the common bile duct. After the nurse finished, she asked the client whether he understood how to empty the drainage bottle and measure the drainage.

B o x 14.1

Barriers to Clear Communication	Benefits of Clear Communication
• Unclear/unexpressed • Confusion • Retaliation • Desire for power • Control of others • Negative reputation • Manipulation • Low self-esteem • Biased perceptions • Inattention • Mistrust • Anger • Fear/anxiety • Stress • Insecurity • Prejudice • Interruptions • Preoccupation	• Clear expectations • Understanding • Forgiveness • Recognized leadership • Companionship • Respect • Independence • Realistic self-image • Acceptance • Clear direction • Trusting relations • Self-control • Comfort • Motivation/energy • Security • Increased tolerance • Increased knowledge • Concentration

The client looked very confused, but mumbled "yes," while shaking his head back and forth. The nurse recognized that although the verbal response was positive, the nonverbal responses indicated that he really did not understand. The nurse surmised that further explanation or demonstration was required for proper encoding of the message by this client.

Nurses should recognize the many barriers to clear communication as well as the benefits of clear communication. Once the barriers to communication are identified, they can be overcome and the benefits of clear communication will result. These barriers and benefits that result when they are overcome are outlined in Box 14.1.

Effective communication requires understanding that the perceptions, emotions, and participation of both parties are interactive and have an effect on the transmission of the message.

COMMUNICATION STYLES

There are two predominant styles of communication: assertive and nonassertive. Nonassertive communication can be either submissive or aggressive. Individuals develop their communication styles over the course of their lives in response to many personal factors. Although most people have one predominant style of communication, they can and often do switch or combine styles depending on the situation in which they find themselves. For example, a unit manager who uses an assertive communication style when supervising the staff on her unit may revert to a submissive style when called into the director of nursing's office for her annual evaluation. Recognizing which communication style a person is using at any given time, as well as a person's own style, is important in making communication clear and effective.

Assertive Communication
Assertive communication involves interpersonal behaviors that permit people to defend and maintain their legitimate rights in a respectful manner that

does not violate the rights of others. Assertive communication is honest and direct and accurately expresses the person's feelings, beliefs, ideas, and opinions. Respect for self and others constitute both the basis for and the result of assertive communication. It encourages trust and teamwork by communicating to others that they have the right to and are encouraged to express their opinions in an open and respectful atmosphere. Disagreement and discussion are considered to be a healthy part of the communication process, and negotiation is the positive mechanism for problem solving, learning, and personal growth.

Assertive communication always implies that the individual has the choice to voice an opinion, sometimes forcefully, as well as to not say anything at all. One of the keys to assertive communication is that the individual is in control of the communication and is not merely reacting to another's emotions.

What Do You Think?

Consider the health-care providers whom you have worked with in the recent past. What were their communication styles? How did it affect the way you communicated with them?

_____

_____

_____

_____

_____

_____

_____

_____

_____

_____

_____

_____

Assessing Self-Assertiveness

Answer the following questions to assess your self-assertiveness:

• Who am I and what do I want?
• Do I believe I have the right to want it?

• How do I get it?
• Do I believe I can get it?
• Have I tried to be assertive with a person I am having difficulty communicating with?
• Am I letting my fears and perceptions cloud my interactions?
• What is the worst that can happen if we communicate?
• Can I live with the worst?
• Will communications have a long-term effect?
• How does it feel to be in constant fear of alienation or rejection?

Rules for Assertiveness

Anyone can learn to use an assertive communication style and develop assertiveness. When first developing this skill, people often feel frightened and overwhelmed. However, once individuals become comfortable with assertiveness, it helps reinforce their self-concepts and becomes an effective tool for communication. There are a few rules to keep in mind while developing assertiveness along with an assertive communication style:

• It is a learned skill.
• It takes practice.
• It requires a desire and motivation to change.
• It requires a willingness to take risks.
• It requires a willingness to make mistakes and try again.
• It requires an understanding that not every outcome sought will be obtained.
• It requires strong self-esteem.
• Self-reward for change and a positive outcome is essential.
• Listening to self is necessary for identifying needs.
• Constant re-examination of outcomes helps assess progress.
• Role-playing with a friend prior to the interaction builds skill and confidence.
• Goals for assertiveness growth need to be established beforehand.
• It requires recognition that change is a gradual process.
• Others should be allowed to make mistakes.

" *Assertiveness does not mean that a person will always get his or her way in every situation, and it is likely the individual will handle some situations better than others. Remember that the goal of assertive communication is not to have an "I win, you lose" situation, but rather an "I win, you win" outcome.* "

Personal Risks of Assertive Communication

There are always personal risks involved in learning any new skills or in attempting to change behavior. Learning assertive communication is no exception. People often fear that they may not choose the "perfect" assertive response. However, even seasoned assertive communicators may err from time to time, because every encounter is unique, involving different people and situations. The person who is new to assertive communication needs to recognize that it is a skill that takes practice.

"You really need to work on your verbal skills."

I Win, You Win

Assertiveness does not mean that a person will always get his or her way in every situation, and it is likely the individual will handle some situations better than others. Remember that the goal of assertive communication is not to have an "I win, you lose" situation, but rather an "I win, you win" outcome. A win-win

goal is achieved when both parties have the ability and willingness to negotiate even though they do not get all they want. However, there may be situations when personal goals are not achieved. Some questions to consider when this occurs are:

• How do I feel about losing?
• Did I express my opinion clearly? Why not? How could I make it more clear?
• Did I do the best I could do? How could I have done better?
• Was I in control when responding to the situation? When did I lose control? What should I have done to regain control?
• Did I stay focused on the issues? What side issues distracted me? How could I have avoided distractions?
• Did I allow the situation to get personal? Did the other person initiate the personal attack? How could I have redirected it away from the personal?
• Was what I asked for under my control? If not, why did I ask for it? What would have been more realistic?

Reviewing these questions and analyzing the answers will help when you attempt to be assertive in future communications. For example, if the answer to the second-to-last question was yes, then during the next communication, a special effort can be focused on avoiding personal attacks during the encounter. Learning to communicate assertively is a process of continual improvement.

Familiar Barriers to Change

Another risk factor that quickly becomes evident when changing to an assertive communication style is the impact that it has on those who know the person best. Sometimes family, friends, peers, and coworkers become barriers to change. As mentioned earlier, change always produces some degree of stress. Those individuals who are closest to the person trying to initiate changes may feel uncomfortable because they have become accustomed to the old communication styles and behaviors over a long time. They can no longer anticipate and depend on the person responding and reacting in the usual way. In addition, they will have to develop new communication patterns of their own to match the changes caused by assertive communication.

Sometimes family, friends, peers, and coworkers become so uncomfortable that they may try to sabotage the person's attempts at assertive communication. It is important to recognize why and when these sabotage efforts occur and also to remember that assertiveness is an internal, personal process. Everyone has a right to change, and it must be respectfully communicated to others that their support for these changes is important.

It is also important to know and periodically review the rights and responsibilities of assertiveness to help reinforce the assertive communication process. The rights and responsibilities of assertiveness are listed in Box 14.2.

Practice and reinforcement of assertiveness skills may be required, especially when preparing for an anticipated conflict negotiation or a confrontational meeting with another. Although a confrontational situation always produces anxiety, rather than being feared, it should be recognized as having the potential to be highly productive. Box 14.3 lists several behaviors that, if practiced and used, will help increase confidence and assertiveness skills during anticipated confrontational meetings.

Box 14.2
Rights and Responsibilities of Assertiveness

- To act in a way that promotes your dignity and self-respect
- To be treated with respect
- To experience and express your thoughts and feelings
- To slow down and make conscious decisions before you act
- To ask for what you want
- To say "No"
- To change your mind
- To make mistakes
- To not be perfect
- To feel important and good about yourself
- To be treated as an individual with special values, skills, and needs
- To be unique
- To have your own feelings and opinions
- To say "I don't know"
- To feel angry, hurt, and frustrated
- To make decisions regarding your life
- To recognize that your needs are as important as others'

Box 14.3
Conflict Resolution Tips

In nursing practice, good communication and conflict management skills are essential. The following tips may help resolve communication problems:

Improve Your Conflict Management Skills
- Seminars
- Books
- Mentors

Change Your Paradigm
- Focus on the positive, not the negative.
- Realize that appropriately confronting is a risk-taking activity for:

Better communication
- Improved relationships
- Improved teamwork
- Mentoring

Understand Your Values
- Focus on a win-win.
- Be willing to negotiate and compromise.
- Be direct and honest.
- Focus on the issues.
- Do not attack the person.
- Do not make judgments.
- Do not become the third person; encourage peers to go direct.
- Do not spread rumors.

Set Personal Guidelines
- Confront in private, never in front of anyone else.
- Confront the individual; do not report him or her to the supervisor first.
- Do not confront when you are angry.
- Start with an "I" message.
- Express your feelings and opinions.
- Allow the other person to talk without interruptions.
- Listen attentively.
- Set goals and future plans of action.
- Let it go.
- Keep it private and confidential.

You can use the checklist in Box 14.4 to determine your own degree of assertiveness.

Nonassertive Communication

Two types of interpersonal behaviors are considered to be nonassertive: submissive and aggressive behaviors.

> *Many experts believe that submissive behavior and communication patterns are a protective mechanism that helps insecure persons maintain their self-esteem by avoiding negative criticism and disagreement from others.*

Submissive Communication

When people display submissive behavior or use a submissive communication style, they allow their rights to be violated by others. When people use submissive behavior and submissive communication, they surrender to the requests and demands of others

without regard to their own feelings and needs. Many experts believe that submissive behavior and communication patterns are a protective mechanism that helps insecure persons maintain their self-esteem by avoiding negative criticism and disagreement from others. In other situations, it may be a means of manipulation through a type of passive-aggressive behavior.

Because of their great fear of displeasing others, personal rejection, or future retaliation, submissive communicators dismiss their own feelings as being unimportant. However, at a deeper level, submissive behavior and communication merely reinforce negative feelings of powerlessness, helplessness, and decreased self-worth. Rather than being in control of the communication or relationship, the person is trading his or her ability to choose what is best for the avoidance of conflict. Every communication by a submissive person becomes an "I lose, you win" situation. However, subconsciously it is more of "You may think you win, but I really am winning because I'm getting what I want or need."

Aggressive Communication

Sometimes there is only a very fine line separating assertiveness from aggressive behavior and communication. Whereas assertive communication permits individuals to honestly express their ideas and opinions while respecting the rights, ideas, and opinions of others, aggressive communication strongly asserts the person's legitimate rights and opinions with little regard or respect for the rights and opinions of others.

Aggressive communication can be used to humiliate, dominate, control, or embarrass the other person or lower the other person's self-esteem and creates an "I win, you lose" situation. The other person may perceive aggressive behavior or communication as a personal attack. Aggressive behavior and communication is viewed by some psychologists as a protective mechanism that compensates for a person's own insecurities. By demeaning another person, aggressive behavior allows the person to feel superior and helps inflate his or her self-esteem.

Aggressive communication can take several different forms, including screaming, sarcasm, rudeness, belittling jokes, and even direct personal insults. It is an expression of the negative feelings of power, domination, and low self-esteem. Although outwardly aggressive persons may seem to be in

Box 14.4

Assertiveness Self-Assessment

Evaluation

Statement   **Communication Behavior**

1. I didn't say what I really wanted to say at the last staff meeting.

2. I always express my opinion because it is better than everyone else's.

3. I have the courage to speak up almost all the time.

4. I wish someone else would speak up at the meetings besides me.

5. I am not intimidated by the high-pressure tactics of supervisors, physicians, and/or teachers.

6. I have trouble stating my true feelings to those in authority.

7. I really put that know-it-all aide in her place last shift.

8. After the last meeting with my unit director I felt hopeless, resentful, and angry.

9. I speak up in meetings without feeling defensive.

10. When I need to confront someone, I avoid the problem because it will usually resolve itself.

11. When I need to confront someone, I address them directly.

12. When I confront someone, I let them know in no uncertain terms that they are wrong and need to change their behavior.

13. When I'm reprimanded, I keep silent even though I'm seething inside.

14. The last time I was asked to stay over for another shift, I said "no" and didn't feel guilty.

control, in reality they are merely reacting to the situation to protect their self-esteem.

> *Rather than being divisive, diversity, when recognized and used correctly, can promote teamwork, improve communication, and increase productivity.*

DIVERSITY

Diversity is a multifaceted issue that involves many areas of people's lives, including culture, values, life experiences, instinctual responses, learned behaviors, personal strengths and weaknesses, and native abilities or skills. Each time two people interact, they bring the sum total of all these elements into their communication. To communicate effectively, both parties need to first recognize that the other person is different, then understand how these differences affect the communication, and finally accept and build on these differences.

Building on Differences

Rather than being divisive, diversity, when recognized and used correctly, can promote teamwork, improve communication, and increase productivity. Recognizing diversity helps people better understand each other as well as themselves. The ultimate goal of diversity recognition is to use each individual's strengths, rather than emphasizing the weaknesses, to build a stronger, more self-confident, and productive environment. For example, consider the following scenario:

Anne B, RN, is a nurse in your unit who has a reputation for being a "nitpicker." She is constantly judging her peers and criticizing their actions on the basis of her own personal standards. Her judgments of others are not well accepted by her coworkers, who try to avoid her as much as possible.

Betty A, RN, another nurse on the unit, always seems to be coming up with ideas to change things in the unit, but then avoids joining the committees that are formed to put the ideas into practice. When she does join a committee, she quickly gets bored and does not follow through on her responsibilities. The other committee members become angry and frustrated by Betty's behavior. They feel that because it was her idea in the first place, she should work as hard as everyone else to make the change.

You have been selected as the chairperson for a committee that has been formed to design a new client care documentation tool. Both Anne and Betty are on the committee. The other committee members are upset because Anne and Betty are on the committee. Everyone knows about Anne's and Betty's personality quirks. As chairperson of the team, you need to utilize everyone's strengths while recognizing their diversities to develop a new, comprehensive yet easy-to-use form. If you perform well in your chairmanship role, each team member's self-esteem should be enhanced, and the morale of the group should improve.

At first glance, these may not seem like diversity issues. However, Anne is a detail-oriented person, whereas Betty is a visionary. Although their interests and abilities are very diverse, neither one is right or wrong. Persons who are preoccupied with details are left-brain dominant; creative, visionary individuals are usually right-brain dominant.

Two primary tasks are required to complete the project:

Task 1. Conduct brainstorming sessions with staff members, physicians, and ancillary personnel to develop a general concept of what the documentation should include and how the form should look.

Task 2. Work with the print shop to design the specific layout and content of the final form.

Plan

Task 1. It would be most appropriate to include Betty in the group that directs the brainstorming groups and collects different ideas. She probably has no preconceived form in mind before starting the process and will feel comfortable investigating and researching a variety of different possibilities. Anne would have difficulty with this task. The lack of structure of the brainstorming process would make her feel out of control and would probably frustrate her urge to consider all the details of the project. Anne would most likely already have a good idea of the form she wanted.

Task 2. Anne would be much better at this task because of her orientation to structure and detail. Working with the print shop, she could focus her attention on each item on the form, decide where it should be placed, how much room it should be given, and how it flows in the document. She would make sure the form met all the standards and regulatory requirements of the joint commission as well as ensuring it was error free. Betty, on the other hand, would very quickly become bored with this aspect of the project. To her, all the attention given to the details would seem like a waste of time, and she would probably start recommending changes in other unit forms.

Placing people in the working environments that correspond with their strengths ensure success for the project. The project will be a successful experience for the nurses and will promote positive changes in peer relationships.

A Focus on Strength

For many people, working with diversity can be difficult, especially when individuals feel insecure about their skills or abilities. When people feel insecure, they may revert to submissive or aggressive behavior or communication styles to hide their weaknesses or differences.

Because assertive persons recognize that everyone, including themselves, has both strengths and weaknesses, they feel comfortable with diversity and are more likely to accept and support others by recognizing and using their strengths. Focusing on people's strengths provides them with positive feedback and helps them grow personally and professionally. Focusing on weaknesses and differences tears down an individual's self-esteem, creates an uncomfortable work atmosphere, and makes people defensive and sometimes hostile.

PROBLEM SOLVING

Problem solving is a process that everyone uses all the time. For example, on the way to work, a tire goes flat on a person's car. That is a problem. How the person solves the problem depends partially on critical thinking skills, partially on past experiences, and partially on physical abilities. If the person with the flat tire is a 250-lb, 33-year-old male construction worker in good health, he most likely has changed tires before and will probably be physically able to remove the flat tire and put on the spare without difficulty. However, if the person with the flat tire is a 90-lb, 67-year-old female church organist who is unable to distinguish a lug nut from a tire valve, her solution to the problem will likely be different. She will probably call the automobile association and have someone come and change the flat for her.

One of the primary activities for nurses in the work setting is problem solving using the nursing process. It really does not matter whether the problem is client centered, management oriented, or an interpersonal issue, the nursing process is an excellent framework for problem resolution. It focuses on the goals of mutual interaction and communication to establish trust and respect. Using the process of assessment, analysis, planning, implementation, and evaluation helps the nurse organize and structure interpersonal interactions in a way that will produce an "I win, you win" situation.

The basic problem-solving steps of the nursing process form the framework for successful conflict management. Nurses who are good problem solvers using the nursing process also tend to be good at conflict resolution, and nurses who are good at conflict resolution tend to be excellent problem solvers. Rather than being avoided in the work setting, conflict should be considered an opportunity to practice and grow in the use of problem-solving skills.

> *Everyone experiences conflict at one time or another as a part of daily life. Often people feel more comfortable addressing the conflict that arises in their personal lives than the professional conflicts that arise in the job setting.*

CONFLICT MANAGEMENT

Many people experience less anxiety when practicing personal problem solving than when they are involved in conflict management. Problem solving is often perceived as less emotional and more structured, whereas conflict management is considered to be more emotionally charged with the potential to produce hostility. However, the steps of conflict management are almost identical to those of the nursing process. The one additional element that must be included in conflict resolution is the ability to use assertive behaviors and communication when discussing the issues.

Conflict on the Job

Everyone experiences conflict at one time or another as a part of daily life. Often people feel more comfortable addressing the conflict that arises in their personal lives than the professional conflicts that arise in the job setting.

A common situation that causes conflict is when nurses feel overworked or overwhelmed by their assignments. The overloaded nurse might say something like "I have such a heavy load today, why isn't anyone helping me?" rather than asking a particular individual for help. When the person who is expected to help fails to comply with the implied request for help, the overworked nurse becomes angry and resentful. The other person may not understand where this anger is coming from and often avoids addressing the angry person for fear of making him or her angrier. This type of poor communication and lack of direct, respectful conflict management produces tension among workers, deterioration of working relationships, decreased efficiency, and, ultimately, poor client care.

Individuals are uncomfortable handling or addressing conflict for many reasons, including:

• Fear of retaliation
• Fear of ridicule
• Fear of alienation of others
• Mistaken belief that they are unable to handle the conflict situation
• Feeling like they do not have the right to speak up
• Past negative experiences with conflict situations
• Family background and experiences
• Lack of education and skills in conflict resolution

Conflict Resolution

Several different strategies can be used to resolve workplace conflicts. Depending on a person's communication style and personality traits, different outcomes may occur.

Strategy 1: Ignore the Conflict

• Submissive personality: Person avoids bringing the issue to the other because he or she is afraid of retaliation or ridicule if he or she confronts and expresses honest feelings or opinions.
• Aggressive personality: Person has decided not to pursue the conflict because the other person is "too stupid to understand" or it would just be a "waste of their time."

Strategy 2: Confront the Conflict

• Submissive personality: Person does not handle the situation directly but refers the problem to a supervisor or to another person for resolution.
• Assertive personality: Person sets up a time and place for a one-on-one meeting. At the meeting, the two parties focus on the issues that caused the conflict and negotiate to define goals and problem solve.
• Aggressive personality: Person confronts the other loudly, in front of an audience, and attacks the other's personality rather than the issue. Person either walks away before the other can speak or keeps talking without stopping and does not allow the other person to respond. The communication is strictly one-sided and very negative.

Strategy 3: Postpone the Conflict

• Submissive person: Person keeps track of the issues until they reach a critical point, then dumps all the issues at one time on the offender in a highly aggressive manner. The other person generally has no idea why he or she is being attacked and may respond with anger or submission.
• Aggressive personality: Person waits until he or she can either use the incident as a threat or blackmail or express the conflict in front of an audience.

Professional nurses need to be assertive and feel comfortable when handling conflict situations and confronting others. The conflict situations that nurses may encounter range from uncooperative clients and lazy coworkers to hostile, insecure, but influential physicians and administrators. Practicing assertiveness skills during confrontational situations helps increase the nurse's confidence in handling daily work-related conflicts and allows the honest but respectful expression of opinion and ideas.

Keep in mind that unresolved conflicts never really go away. Ignoring a conflict situation may postpone it, sometimes for a long time, but it will not resolve the issue. Unresolved conflicts often fester until they either reach the boiling point or are manifested in negative behaviors or feelings. Some of the feelings and behaviors that are symptoms of unresolved conflicts include:

- Tension and anxiety manifested as sudden angry outbursts
- Generalized distrust among the staff members
- Gossiping and rumor spreading
- Intentional work sabotage
- Backstabbing and lack of cooperation
- Isolation of certain staff members
- Division and polarization of the staff
- Low-rated peer evaluation reports

Improved Communication Skills

Often, when conflict is handled appropriately, it produces much less anxiety than was initially anticipated. An individual who prepares for a confrontational meeting by expecting the worst-case scenario may be pleasantly surprised when the meeting and discussion take place. Many conflicts turn out to be merely errors in perception, simple misunderstandings, or misquotes of something that was said. If a situation is cleared up at an early stage, this prevents the development of the symptoms of unresolved conflict (listed earlier) and improves staff relationships. Individuals feel more confident and have better self-esteem when they resolve the conflicts in an adult and productive manner.

Another advantage of good conflict management is the improvement in communication skills. As with any skills, the more these skills are practiced, the easier they will become to use. Some tips for conflict resolution are listed in the Issues in Practice box at the end of the chapter.

> *Keep in mind that unresolved conflicts never really go away. Ignoring a conflict situation may postpone it, sometimes for a long time, but it will not resolve the issue.*

DIFFICULT PEOPLE

Identifying the Problem

All nurses recognize that obtaining a thorough history and understanding the underlying disease processes better prepare them for the care of their clients. Similarly, when working with difficult people, a knowledge of their backgrounds and understanding of the underlying personality traits better prepare the individual to deal with the important issues. It would seem that nurses should be better at handling conflict and difficult people, because an understanding of cause and effect and the intricacies of human nature are skills that are used daily in the care of clients.

Shifting the communication paradigm from one of instinctual or reflex "knee-jerk" response to one that uses the nurse's relationship skills should make dealing with difficult people a much less difficult task. Remember that the behavior displayed by a difficult person is really a symptom of a deeper problem, just as an assessment of shortness of breath is a symptom of a respiratory disease. Identification of the cause of the problem permits the nurse to treat the disease rather than just the symptoms. The problem will not be cured by merely ignoring it or dealing only with the symptoms. In the long term, that usually only makes things worse.

Identifying Difficult People

Most of the time, it is easy to identify when a person is being "difficult." However, some behaviors of difficult people may not be evident at first glance. Each type of difficult person requires a different strategy for dealing with his or her behaviors.

There are four basic behavioral pattern types of communication: (1) in control and responsive, (2) in control but unresponsive, (3) uncontrolled and responsive, (4) and uncontrolled and unresponsive.

Anyone who has been employed in or even associated with the health-care setting for any length of time soon becomes aware of a variety of different personality types among the staff members. These personality types can be identified by their predominant behaviors and require different strategies for communication. Keep in mind that these are stereotypes that tend to batch individuals into groups on the basis of predetermined characteristics. In reality, people may have overlapping or combinations of characteristics that may require combining the listed strategies for communication (Box 14.5).

The various types of characterizations, behavioral patterns, and stereotypes all are interrelated and based on individual communication styles. An increased awareness of the various identifying characteristics and strategies for communication will help develop the coping skills and communication techniques necessary for communicating with difficult people.

Box 14.5

Assertive Communications Suggestions

- Maintain eye contact.
- Convey empathy; stating your feelings does not mean sympathy or agreement.
- Keep your body position erect, shoulders and back straight.
- Speak clearly and audibly; be direct and descriptive.
- Be comfortable with silence.
- Use gestures and facial expressions for emphasis.
- Use appropriate location.
- Use appropriate timing.
- Focus on behaviors and issues; do not attack the person.

> *Shifting the communication paradigm from one of instinctual or reflex "knee-jerk" response to one that uses the nurse's relationship skills should make dealing with difficult people a much less difficult task.*

DEVELOPMENT OF COPING SKILLS

Building on Existing Skills

Just as developing communication skills requires a willingness to change and a lot of practice, so does the development of coping skills. Coping skills can be used to resolve crisis situations, deal with anxiety, and resolve difficult issues of communication. Everyone has at least a fundamental set of coping skills that they have developed during their lives, and these can be used as the foundation for adding to or building new coping skills for future problems. Presented here are some strategies that will help in the development of coping skills to use in communicating with difficult people.

Avoid Personal Attacks

First, separate the person from the problem by focusing on the issues without personally attacking the person. Having the facts about the situation makes people much more receptive to resolution of the problem than attacking their personality does. When situations are made into personal attacks, it makes people feel defensive, responsible, or persecuted and either blocks or closes off the communication.

One way to avoid turning a conversation into a personal attack is to use "I" rather than "you" messages. Avoid starting a conversation by saying, "You made a mistake," or "You said this about me," or especially, "You always do this" or "You know what your problem is?" People are less likely to perceive a communication as a personal attack when the conversation begins with an explanation of a personal view of the situation or even how feelings were affected. Statements such as "I thought it was done this way," or "I heard something the other day," or even "I feel hurt when people judge me" are a more productive way to begin an exchange of ideas and information. For example:

During shift report on a particular client, the 11 P.M. to 7 A.M. nurse forgot to tell the 7 A.M. to 3 P.M. charge nurse, Gail L, RN, that the client had fallen out of bed during the night shift. Later in the day, both the client's physician and family confronted Gail to find out what happened and why the client was not placed on "fall protocols." Later, when Gail confronts the night nurse about the omission, she has two options for initiating the discussion of the incident with the responsible night nurse. Which approach would the night nurse probably take as a personal attack?

Option 1. Gail: "I was taken off guard and unprepared when the family and physician asked me about this client's fall, and I felt unprepared to explain the problem or a solution to them. My lack of knowledge about the fall really made me feel incompetent."

Option 2. Gail: "You failed to tell me about his fall last night. Because of you, I was not aware of the incident and was not prepared to answer questions. You always make me look like a fool!"

Another way to avoid making issues into personal attacks is to avoid focusing on what a person should have done based on a personal standard. This type of statement becomes an arbitrary judgment call. Instead, ask the person for his or her ideas on how the situation could have been handled differently or what other options were available. One should especially avoid becoming personally or verbally abusive.

Listen Actively

A second important strategy for developing communication-related coping skills is to be willing to actively listen to and respect the other person's perspectives, ideas, or opinions. Active listening can help minimize the misunderstandings or erroneous perceptions that cause much of the tension seen on nursing units. As mentioned earlier, active listening involves "listening" not only to the words but also to the body language to hear the real meaning of the communication and understand the underlying message.

A person who is focused on the communication is not preoccupied with other issues or mentally preparing a response or a defense. Allowing the other person to say all he or she has to say without interruption before responding creates an atmosphere where honest and open communication can occur. In some situations, merely allowing a person to ventilate emotions by using active listening reduces the levels of anger and animosity and sometimes even solves the conflict situation. Also, when intelligent people are allowed to speak openly and freely, they may be able to develop a new solution to the problem that they had not considered previously.

Before responding to a person, it is important to ask clarifying questions that validate the person's concerns, feelings, and perceptions. Validating will help ensure that the responses address the real issues. Also, avoid reflex type reactions to hostile or aggressive statements. It is a human instinct to become defensive when attacked and to attack back. However, this behavior only escalates the anger and tension and blocks effective communication.

Ignore Trivia

A third strategy that is useful in developing communication coping skills is to always make a conscious decision about the importance of the issue that needs to be discussed. When individuals can identify the issues that really matter and focus their efforts on them, they gain credibility among their peers and develop a reputation for caring and realism. Again, it is a very human tendency to become preoccupied with trivial and unimportant issues. If people spend large portions of their energy dealing with trivia, they will have little energy left to deal with major issues

when they come along. By establishing and analyzing the outcomes to be attained and by being open to negotiations and compromise, both parties will leave the confrontation with a sense of accomplishment and fair resolution even if they did not get everything they wanted.

> *It is a very human tendency to become preoccupied with trivial and unimportant issues. If people spend large portions of their energy dealing with trivia, they will have little energy left to deal with major issues when they come along.*

Setting the Stage

After a decision is made to deal with a difficult issue or person, it is important to set the stage for a positive experience. The location for the exchange should be private. The format of the meeting needs to be established ahead of time, including an explanation to the other person that each party will take turns expressing their opinions and feelings without interruption.

Establishing Trust

An important issue in conflict negotiations is the establishment of trust. In addition to showing respect for the other person's opinions and ideas, trust can be established by talking first and directly to the person about the problem rather than to everyone else on the unit. Being talked about behind one's back tends to make people resentful and defensive.

Trust is reinforced by making it known that all you want is to resolve the issue and then move on. When the threat of retaliation is removed, people are more likely to express themselves honestly, as well as becoming more open to the other side's ideas. Once two people begin to trust each other, even if they disagree about some of the issues, they are much more likely to come to a satisfactory resolution of the problem.

The Exchange

When the exchange takes place, it is important to avoid "I" language and be direct by focusing on the facts and issues. Remember that active listening is a two-way street. A person's body language, tone of

Box 14.6

Seven Principles of Communication

1. Information giving is not communication.
2. The sender is responsible for clarity.
3. Use simple and exact language.
4. Feedback should be encouraged.
5. The sender must have credibility.
6. Acknowledgment of others is essential.
7. Direct channels of communication are best.

Source: Adapted from Tappen, RM: Nursing Leadership and Management Concept and Practice, ed. 3. FA Davis, Philadelphia, 1995, with permission.

voice, and eye contact can say much more than the words spoken (Box 14.6). Showing the other person that his or her opinion is respected, even if not agreed with, helps develop that important sense of trust between the two parties.

After both people have had a chance to express themselves and validate the communication, they begin to address the issues and develop a solution for the problem. Sometimes there is a need to set goals for, or at least agree on, how the issues are to be approached and settled. It is fairly common that some issues will remain unresolved after the first meeting. A decision about when and where the second meeting will take place needs to be made before leaving the first meeting. Also, before leaving the first meeting, both parties should summarize what they agreed to and how they felt about the exchange. This summarization will help clarify any miscommunications and give each party one last chance to introduce any issues that remain unresolved.

Dealing with difficult people and conflict resolution are never pleasant undertakings. However, like most skills, the more they are practiced, the more comfortable you will become using the communication techniques discussed. The importance of handling problematic situations in a timely, honest, and caring manner is self-evident. The anxiety and fear provoked by confrontation are part of the price that nurses must pay to do their jobs well and provide high-quality client care.

Conclusion

A person's professional and personal life is influenced by communication styles and behavioral patterns. The ability to analyze personal strengths, weaknesses, and communication behaviors is particularly important when dealing with difficult people.

Certain specific communication qualities and skills are essential when interacting with difficult people. First, it is important to develop the skill of assertive communication, which allows people to express themselves openly and honestly while respecting other people's opinions and ideas. Being able to identify submissive and aggressive behavior is also essential when trying to resolve problems, as well as recognizing issues of diversity, which underlie many problems in communication. Difficult situations are ultimately resolved through the practice of conflict management. Because it is an outgrowth and extension of the problem-solving method, nurses should be able to quickly grasp its structure and master its use.

Issues in Practice

Julie H, RN, has been working the 7 P.M. to 7 A.M. shift in a busy, 32-bed surgical unit of a large university hospital since her graduation from a small bachelor of science in nursing (BSN) program 6 months ago. Although Julie was told by the unit director when she was hired that she would have at least a full year of training before she had to work as charge nurse, tonight the other two RNs who usually work the shift called in sick, and Julie was left in charge. The 7 P.M. to 7 A.M. shift is always busy because the unit has to discharge clients who are ready to go home after surgery as well as admit clients who are coming in for surgery the next day. Hospital policy requires the RN make and sign both the discharge and admission assessments.

Although Julie is nervous about this new role as charge nurse, she feels that she can handle the responsibility if she has some additional help. Normal staffing for the unit on this shift is three registered nurses (RN), three licensed practical nurses (LPN), and three unlicensed assistive personnel (UAP). Julie calls the house supervisor to see if she can get some help. The only place in the hospital that is not busy that night is the obstetrics (OB) unit, so the supervisor sends two of the OB unit's UAPs to the surgical unit to help Julie.

It was not the help Julie really wanted, but she feels that she can handle the responsibility. However, when Julie begins to make assignments, the older of the OB unit UAPs, Hanna J, informs Julie that she, for the past 15 years, had worked only in the newborn nursery and does not know anything about the care of adult clients who had surgery. In addition, Hanna states that she has a bad back and cannot lift or turn adult clients and is afraid that she might catch some disease from the adults that she would take back to the babies. Julie asks Hanna, "What do you feel you are qualified to do on the surgical unit?" In response, Hanna crosses her legs, folds her arms across her chest, puts her head down and mumbles under her breath, "A lot more than a new know-it-all RN like you."

Critical Thinking Exercises

- What messages, both verbal and nonverbal, are being communicated? How should Julie respond to this comment? What should she do to rectify the situation?
- Using the various tables in the chapter, identify the personality type of each of the persons involved in the situation.
- How can the RN best communicate with this UAP? What were some of the communication mistakes the RN made?
- What background, cultural, and diversity factors played a part in this situation? Develop a strategy for resolution of this conflict.
- Make a list of your values and where they came from. Describe how each value affects your work ethic and life.
- List your communication strengths and weaknesses. Rank them on a scale of 1 to 10 (10 being the highest). Determine which weaknesses you want to change and create an improvement plan.
- Identify your primary communication style and character type.
- Complete this statement, using as many situations or statements as possible:
- "In a conflict situation, I have difficulty saying _____." Analyze reasons that prevent you from saying it. What would have been the worst thing that could have happened to you if you had said it? Create a phrase that you feel comfortable with that you could use the next time you want to say something difficult to the members of your team.
- Identify the communication and behavior characteristics of your work group or team. List areas of diversity for each member, including yourself. Identify their strengths and weaknesses. Identify methods for using the team members' diversity to enhance the team.

Bibliography

Banks, C: Careers: Improving your communication skills. Nursing Times 101(3):48–49, 2005.

Briles, J: Zapping conflict in health care workplace. The Oklahoma Nurse 49(2):43, 2004.

Callister, L: Toward evidence-based practice: How delivery ward staff exercise power over women in communication. MCN 30(1):70, 2005.

Cole, A: Reaping the benefits of teamwork. Nursing Times 101(1):59, 2005.

Dunham, K, and Smith, S: How to survive and maybe even love your life as a nurse. FA Davis, Philadelphia, 2005.

Force, M: Creating a culture of service excellence: Empowering nurses within the shared governance councilor model. Health Care Manager 23(3):262–266, 2004.

Goddard, M: The impacts of knowledge management and information technology advances on public health decision-making in 2010. Health Information Journal 10(2):111–120, 2004.

McHugh, N: Improving staff member satisfaction and productivity through technology. AORN 80(3):523–526, 2004.

McMurray, A: Factors impacting on nurse managers' ability to be innovative in a decentralized management structure. Journal of Nursing Management 12(5):348–353, 2004.

Raiger, J: Applying a cultural lens to the concept of burnout. Journal of Transcultural Nursing 16(1):71–66, 2005.

Rosenstein, A: Disruptive behavior & clinical outcomes: Perceptions of nurses & physicians. AJN 105(1):54–65, 2005.

Sanford, K: Become competent in confrontation. Nursing Management 35(7):14–18, 2004.

Tappen, RM: Nursing Leadership and Management, ed. 4. FA Davis, Philadelphia, 2001.

Tappen RM, et al: Essentials of Nursing Leadership and Management, ed. 2. FA Davis, Philadelphia, 2001.

Weiss, R: Communication strategies: New styles in trustee leadership. Health Progress 85(5):9, 2004.

15

Delegation and Supervision in Nursing

Joseph T. Catalano

Learning Objectives

After completing this chapter, the reader will be able to:

- Apply the principles of delegation to nursing practice.
- Analyze and identify situations where delegation is used improperly.
- Discuss the legal implications of delegation in the current health-care setting.
- Distinguish between delegation and supervision.

AN ESSENTIAL SKILL

In today's health-care system, delegation has become an essential component of client care and management of nursing units. It allows health-care managers to maximize the use of caregivers who are educated at multiple levels in a variety of programs. Delegation, if performed properly, permits nurses to meet the requirements of quality care for all clients and has become a basic skill that registered nurses (RN) must learn. The goal of delegation is to meet the cost restraints of limited health-care budgets by using less-expensive personnel that maximize the use of time by RNs and to promote team building.

DELEGATION OR SUPERVISION?

Although delegation and supervision are closely related concepts, they are different. **Delegation** is recognized as assigning or designating a competent individual the responsibility of carrying out a specific group of nursing tasks in the provision of care for certain clients. Delegation includes the understanding that the authorized person is acting in the place of the RN and may be carrying out tasks that generally fall under the RN's scope of practice. **Supervision,** on the other hand, is the initial direction and periodic evaluation of a person performing an assigned task to ensure that he or she is meeting the standards of care. Although delegation almost always requires supervision, it is possible to have supervision without delegation.

When nurses delegate nursing tasks to non-nurses, the RNs are always legally responsible for supervising those people to ensure that the care given meets the standards of care. However, if the facility, the state board of nursing, or some other official body has a predesignated list of tasks that non-nursing personnel may undertake in the care of clients, then the RN is responsible only for supervising them to make sure the tasks are carried out safely.

Legally, the power to delegate is restricted to professionals who are licensed and governed by a statutory practice act. RNs are considered professionals with state-sanctioned licenses governed by a nurse practice act and therefore are authorized to delegate independent nursing functions to other personnel.

NURSING RESPONSIBILITIES WHEN DELEGATING

Look to All These Things

The concept of delegation has been a part of health care since the time of Florence Nightingale, when she instructed the nurses she educated "... to look to all these things yourself does not mean to do them yourself."[1] In more recent times, the American Nurses Association (ANA) initially addressed and defined delegation in 1991 when it was beginning to become a more widespread practice in health care. They further refined the definition in 1997.

The ANA defines delegation as "the transfer of responsibility for the performance of an activity from one individual to another while retaining accountability for the outcome."[2] The ANA stresses the belief that even though the leader or manager delegates a task to another employee, he or she remains responsible and accountable for the care that is provided.

> *When nurses delegate nursing tasks to non-nurses, the RNs are always legally responsible for supervising those people to ensure that the care given meets the standards of care.*

The Nurse's Responsibilities

Assess the Client. Prior to delegating any task, RNs should give careful consideration to the condition of the client and the client's health-care needs. Assessing clients is a designated **responsibility** of registered

What Do You Think?

Is delegation used in the facility where you have clinicals? Who does the delegation on the unit? Does it work well?

nurses. Without a thorough assessment, it is likely that critical needs will remain unidentified by less-trained personnel, leading to potential errors in care. Clients who are relatively stable and not likely to experience drastic changes in health-care status are the most suitable for delegation. Also, the tasks being delegated must be relatively uncomplicated, routine, performed without varying from policy or procedure, and should not require the use of nursing judgment while being performed.

Know Staff Availability. The delegating nurse needs to know the availability of staff, the education, and competency levels of the personnel to be assigned. These factors must be matched with the level of care required by the client. Key information to obtain in relation to delegation is how often the delegatee has performed the required tasks or cared for this type of client, what units the delegatee has worked on and feels comfortable in, and his or her organizational abilities.

Know the Job Description. The RN needs to know both the institution's official position description for the unlicensed assistive personnel (UAP) as well as the individual UAP's abilities. For example, the position description may state that the UAP can care for postoperative clients who have multiple wound drains. However, when the RN assigns a specific UAP to such a postoperative client, the nurse discovers that the UAP has worked only in the newborn nursery for the past 5 years and has no knowledge of how to care for adult postoperative clients. If the RN assigns this UAP anyway and a major complication develops as a result of the UAP's lack of competence (even though the position description states that this is an appropriate function for the UAP), the RN will be held legally responsible for the poor outcome. When the RN determines that the client's needs match the skills and abilities of the UAP or licensed practical nurse (LPN), only then should that person be assigned.

Educate the Staff Member. RNs who delegate are also responsible for educating the UAP about the task to be done. If the UAP is unfamiliar with the task, the RN is required to demonstrate how the task or procedure is performed and then document the training. Education also includes telling the UAP what is expected in the completion of the task and what complications to watch for and report to the RN. The ANA suggests that the RN watch the UAP perform the designated task at least initially, then make periodic observations throughout the shift to ensure safe and competent care for the client.[3] Furthermore, the RN must always be available to

answer questions and help the UAP whenever assistance is required. Consider the following situation:

> Elsie Humber, RN, is the evening charge nurse on a busy oncology unit of the county hospital. On one particularly busy evening, she discovers during shift report that one of the scheduled LPNs has called in sick and no other LPNs are available to take her place. Ms. Humber assigns the LPN's duties and clients, including a heat lamp treatment for a decubitus ulcer, to a UAP who has worked on the unit for several months. The UAP protests the assignment, but Ms. Humber rebukes her saying, "I have no one else. If you don't care for these clients, they won't get any care this shift." In setting up the heat lamp treatment, the UAP knocks the lamp over and burns the client. Because of his suppressed immune system from chemotherapy and generally debilitated condition, the burn does not heal and develops into an infection. The client later sues the hospital for malpractice. The hospital in turn attempts to shift the legal responsibility for the burn to Ms. Humber. Who is legally responsible for the incident? Does the client have grounds for a successful case?

Predictable and Uncomplicated

When a nurse delegates tasks, the outcomes of tasks should be expected and predictable. For example, when a UAP is assigned the task of feeding a client who has suffered a stroke and has hemiplegia, the predicted outcome will be that the client will eat and not choke on the food. The task should not require excessive supervision, complex decision making, or detailed assessment during its performance. If any of these elements are required, then it needs to be reassigned to an RN.

❝

It is important to remember that when nurses delegate nursing tasks, they are not delegating nursing. ❞

It is important to remember that when nurses delegate nursing tasks, they are *not* delegating nursing. Professional nursing practice is both a science,

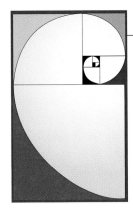

Issues in Practice

Using Evidence-Based Nursing Practice: The Next Step

Although nurses have been using evidence-based nursing practice in some form since the early days of nursing, it is only recently that the process has become formalized and widespread as a methodology. The current use of evidence-based practice (EBP) in nursing requires a transition from the provision of nursing care that is based on opinions, past practices, and precedent to decisions that are based on scientific research and proven evidence. The goal of nurses using EBP is to obtain the best information available and integrate it into nursing practice that includes the client's and the client's family's values and self-determination in providing care. The ultimate outcome sought is improved quality of care.

Evidence Reports

There are a number of sources that nurses can use when incorporating EBP into the care they provide. Research reported in the literature is one of the primary sources of high quality information, but not the only one. Other sources include expert opinion, collaborative consensus, publish standards, historical data, local quality assurance studies, various institutional reports including cost effectiveness and client/family preferences and input. The key to using these various sources of information is the ability to grade or rank them so that nursing practice is on the basis of the *best* information available. An excellent way to sort out the quality of information is to visit the Web site www.guideline.gov. for evidence reports.

The evidence reports contained at this site provide a scientific basis for a disease or nursing practice and then integrate the data into actions used in practice. The reports synthesize previous and current knowledge related to the topic, review the information for quality and documentation, explain how EBP is currently being used, and discuss how useful the EBP is to the clinical practice. The reviews in evidence reports are more detailed than a typical literature review and include broad-based information that is translated into specific approaches to client care. Although currently the data is somewhat limited, new data is constantly being added to the site.

Nurses should look for several key elements in evidence reports when attempting to integrate EBP into their care. The first part of the report should include a structured summary statement of the problem, practice, or disease that describes what is in the evidence report. The second part should include a lengthy and detailed analysis of the published and unpublished data including reviews of various articles and reports, the populations included in the studies, and the nature of the nursing actions investigated. One of the most important elements in the second part of the evidence report is the ranking or grading of the quality of the evidence.

The level of quality of the evidence is sometimes referred to as the "level of recommendation for use" and simply answers the nurse's question, "Should I value this information and use it in my practice?" Integrative reviews in evidence reports should provide both the type of evidence that is included and the strengths and consistencies of the information.

(continued)

Issues in Practice continued

Types of Evidence Used

Five types of evidence can be present in an evidence report, ranked from I (strongest) to V (weakest). They are:

I. Meta-analysis of multiple well-designed controlled studies that examines and synthesizes many studies to find similar results
II. At least one well-designed experimental study with a random sample, control group, and intervention
III. Well-designed, quasi-experimental studies such as nonrandomized controlled, single-group pre-post test group, cohort studies or time series studies
IV. Well-designed nonexperimental studies such as comparative and correlational descriptive studies and controlled case studies
V. Case reports and clinical examples

The strength and consistency of evidence is also ranked on a five-point scale ranging from A (best) to E (poorest). In general, a "B" or higher should be present before integrating the data into a nurse's EBP. The rankings are:

A. There is evidence of type I or consistent findings from multiple studies of types II, II or IV.
B. There is evidence of types II, II, or IV, and the findings are generally consistent.
C. There is evidence of types II, III, or IV, but the findings are inconsistent.
D. There is little or no evidence or there is type V evidence only.
E. Panel Consensus: Practice recommended on the basis of the opinions of experts in the field.

One of the potential problems in using these ranking systems is that they may not be the best method to analyze the strength of the evidence. In nursing, much of the research is qualitative or descriptive or even linguistic in nature because of the difficulty in performing controlled studies with large groups of clients. The nurse needs to look at the consistency of the results, even though there may not be any type I, II, or II studies in the evidence report.

The next section of the evidence report should include recommendations for clinical practice that include practice-focused guidelines or recommendations for specific clinical interventions. Often this section begins with a statement such as "There is very good evidence that …" or "There is no evidence that …" The practices outlined should be specific and relevant to the care being given.

The last section of the evidence report is the report source. These should be specific, current, and from high-quality refereed professional journals.

Evaluating an Evidence Report

The nurse can evaluate the evidence report by asking three questions. Only after answering these questions will the nurse be able to decide what to do with the information.

1. *Is this the best available evidence?* Best sources include peer-reviewed journals and reports no more than 3 to 5 years old.

(continued)

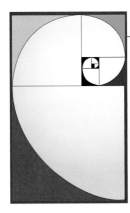

Issues in Practice continued

2. *Will the recommendations work for my practice given the client population and problems?* If the study population is of young adult white males and the nurses primary work population is elderly females, then the data generated may not apply.
3. *Do the recommendations fit well with the preferences and values of the clients I commonly work with?* If the values of the nurse's primary group vary greatly from those of the study group, it is likely the recommendations may not work well.

Nurses can locate evidence reports from a number of sources:
Clinical journals:

Evidence-Based Nursing
Online Journal of Clinical Innovations
Reformatted STTI *Online Journal for Knowledge Synthesis in Nursing*

Other sources:

National Guideline Clearinghouse (U.S. Agency for Healthcare Research and Quality): repository for clinical practice guidelines.
The Cochrane Collaboration (international): develops and maintains systematic reviews
SUNY Web site: lists the best sites for information

When nurses begin to take the next step and integrate EBP into the care they provide, they will make a major leap toward raising the level of professionalism in nursing practice. Through the use of EBP in nursing, the quality of client care will improve when the care provided is based on validated evidence that focuses on what works best.

Source: L. Benefield, Evidence-Based Nursing Practice: How to Dance to the Tune. (Presentation at the NSNA National Convention, Phoenix AZ, 4/23/03)

based on a unique body of knowledge, and an art, guided by the nursing process. It is not merely a collection of tasks. Of all health-care workers, professional nurses are the most qualified to provide holistic care of the client by promoting health and treating disease. Nurses' education and experience provide them with the skills and knowledge to coordinate and supervise nursing care and to delegate specific tasks to others.

Although mastering delegation skills can seem like a daunting task, a nurse can take a number of common sense steps to attain this skill (Box 15.1). Nursing students often have tasks delegated to them from the RNs on the units where they are having clinical rotations. It is easy to identify the RNs who have developed good delegation skills and those who still need to work on those skills.

DEVELOPING DELEGATION SKILLS

Clear Communication
In the process of developing delegation skills, students should try to emulate the good delegators. Develop good communication and interpersonal relationship skills. Make eye contact with the other person, be pleasant, and ask for suggestions. However, avoid allowing the person to whom the tasks are being delegated to control the exchange by intimidation or resistance.

Box 15.1

Five Rights of Delegation

- Right task

    Do the tasks delegated follow written policy guidelines?

- Right person

    Does the person have the proper qualifications for the tasks?

- Right direction or communication

    Are the instructions and outcomes clearly stated? When should the person report changes?

- Right supervision or feedback

    How can the delegation process be improved? Are the client goals for care being achieved?

- Right circumstances

    Are the tasks that are being delegated free from requiring independent nursing judgments?

Sources: Fisher, M: Do you have delegation savvy? Nursing 2000 (9):58–59, 2000.
Tappen, RM: Nursing Leadership and Management, ed. 4. FA Davis, Philadelphia, 2001.
Wheeler, J: How to delegate your way to a better working life. Nursing Times 97(36):34–35, 2001.

After a nurse delegates a task, if one does not already exist, it's a good idea to make a written list of the responsibilities that are expected from the person. The list will help clarify what is expected and head off possible misunderstandings. It is also important to be flexible. Clients' conditions change, new clients may be admitted, and other clients may be discharged. The original assignments may have to be modified in response to changes in the environment.

Careful Monitoring

Effective delegation includes monitoring the delegatees while they are giving care. Are they doing what they should be doing? Do they understand the responsibilities involved in the client's care? Help them if they need help. Effective delegation also presumes that the delegator will teach the delegatees who demonstrate a lack of knowledge. Most important, at the end of the shift, say "Thank you. I appreciate the hard work (good job) you've done today."

Certain delegation situations may place the RN at an increased risk for liability (Boxes 15.2, 15.3). Try to avoid the following when delegating:

- Assigning tasks that are highly invasive or have the potential to cause significant physical harm to clients

- Assigning tasks that are designated under the scope of practice or standards of care as belonging exclusively to the RN (admission assessments, care plan development)
- Assigning tasks that the person is not trained for or lacks the knowledge to safely complete

What Do You Think?

What qualities have you observed in good delegators? What qualities made the poor delegators ineffective?

_____

_____

_____

_____

_____

_____

_____

_____

_____

_____

_____

_____

_____

_____

• Assigning tasks when there is inadequate time to safely monitor or evaluate the practice of the person performing the tasks[4]

The long-term effect of the growing trend to delegation on the quality of client care remains to be seen. However, the knowledge and judgment of the professional nurse will remain essential elements in any health-care system reforms, including clinical integration, case management, outsourcing practices,

Box 15.2

Barriers to Effective Delegation

A. Internal barriers (person delegating):
1. Lack of experience delegating
2. Lack of confidence in others
3. Personal insecurity
4. Demanding perfectionism
5. Poor organizational skills
6. Indecision
7. Poor communication skills
8. Lack of confidence in self
9. Fear of not being liked by everyone
10. Micromanaging management style

B. External barriers (circumstances or person being delegated to):
1. Unclear policies about delegation
2. Policies that do not tolerate mistakes
3. Management-by-crisis model for facility
4. Unclear delineation of authority and responsibilities
5. Poor staffing
6. Lack of competence
7. Overdependence on the person delegating
8. Unwillingness to accept responsibility for one's own practice
9. Immersion in trivia and gossip
10. Work overload

Source: Tappen, RM, et al: Essentials of Nursing Leadership and Management. FA Davis, Philadelphia, 2001.

Box 15.3

Delegation Decision Tree

1. Are there laws and rules in place supporting the rules of delegation?
2. Is the task within the scope of practice of the UAP, LPN/LVN, RN, or new graduate?
3. Has there been an assessment of the client's needs?
4. Is the UAP, LPN/LVN, RN, or new graduate competent to accept the delegation?
5. Does the ability of the caregiver match the care needs of the client?
6. Can the task be completed without requiring nursing judgments?
7. Is the result of the task somewhat predictable?
8. Can the task be safely performed according to directions?
9. Can the task be performed without repeated assessment?
10. Is appropriate supervision available?

Source: Tappen, RM: Nursing Leadership and Management, ed. 4. FA Davis, Philadelphia, 2001.

total quality management (TQM), and **continuous quality improvement (CQI).**

LEGAL ISSUES IN DELEGATION

One area of fallout from the movement to managed care is the increase in nurses' liability for lawsuits in the area of supervision and delegation. In the search for cost-effective client care, current managed-care strategies attempt to make optimal use of relatively expensive RNs by replacing them with less-costly and less-educated personnel. As more and more health-care facilities move toward restructuring, the use of UAPs who have minimal education and experience will continue to increase. Although RNs have always been responsible for the delegation of some tasks and the supervision of less-qualified health-care providers, it is now one of the primary functions of RNs in today's health-care system.

Delegation does have some advantages. It is an RN extender in that it allows more care to be given to more clients than can be given by one RN. Delegation can free the RN from lower-level time-consuming tasks so that more time can be spent planning for care and performing those skills that less prepared individuals would be unable to perform. For those to whom tasks are delegated, it can serve as an incentive to learn additional skills, increase knowledge, develop a sense of initiative, and perhaps to seek further formal education. Delegation, if performed properly, maintains accountability and decision making where they belong—with the RN.

> *From the ethical view, RNs have an obligation to refuse assignments that they are not competent to carry out and to refuse to delegate particular nursing tasks to individuals who they believe are unable or unprepared to perform them.*

WHO CAN DELEGATE—LEGALLY?

An Ethical Obligation
Most state practice acts do *not* give delegatory authority to **dependent practitioners** like licensed

practical nurses/licensed vocational nurses (LPNs/LVNs) or UAPs. In addition, professionals who delegate specific tasks retain accountability for the proper and safe completion of those tasks as well as responsibility for determining whether the assigned personnel are competent to carry out the task. One exception is when the person who is assigned a task also has a license and the tasks fall under that person's scope of practice.[5] Then again, the RN is responsible only for supervision of the other licensed person; this is often seen in situations where LPNs/LVNs are assigned to client care.

The delegation and supervision responsibilities of RNs have been and continue to be a major concern for the nursing profession, both ethically and legally. The ANA Code of Ethics for Nurses states, "The nurse is responsible and accountable for individual nursing practice and determines the appropriate delegation of tasks consistent with the nurse's obligation to provide optimum patient care" (statement 4).[6] From the ethical viewpoint, RNs have an obligation to refuse assignments that they are not competent to carry out and to refuse to delegate particular nursing tasks to individuals who they believe are unable or unprepared to perform them.

"Why don't I get someone else to remove Mrs. Lemke's sutures?"

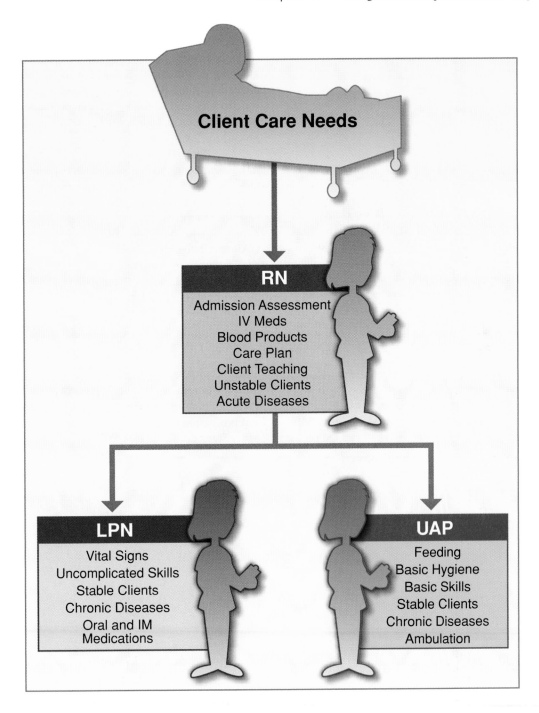

> *Most state practice acts do not give delegatory authority to dependent practitioners like licensed practical nurses/licensed vocational nurses (LPNs/LVNs) or UAPs.*

Direct and Indirect Delegation

The legal side of the delegation issue has also been addressed by the ANA in the *ANA Basic Guide to Safe Delegation*. This document makes a distinction between direct delegation, which is a specific decision made by the RN about who can perform what tasks, and indirect delegation, which is a list of tasks that certain health-care personnel can perform that is produced by the health-care facility.[3]

The **consensus** among many experts is that indirect delegation is really a form of covert institutional licensure. Lists of activities from the facility allowing non-nursing personnel who do not have the education of the RN to carry out professional nursing functions is a de facto permission to practice nursing without a license. Indirect delegation places RNs in a precarious legal position.

Basically, indirect delegation takes away much of the authority of the RN to assign personnel tasks, yet the RN remains accountable for the safe completion of the tasks under the doctrines of **respondent superior** and **vicarious liability.** Although some states are beginning to address the UAP and delegation issues in their nurse practice acts, many states either have no official standards for UAP delegation or include UAP standards under the medical practice act.

Conclusion

With the increased use of less-educated and unlicensed personnel in today's health-care system, it is essential that the nurse develop effective delegation and supervision skills. The nurse needs to be mindful that the tasks that can be delegated can change on the basis of work setting, client needs, position descriptions, institutional training of personnel, and the ever-changing requirements of nurse practice acts and professional standards. Nurses also need to know when delegation is inappropriate.

Critical Thinking Exercises

- Obtain a copy of your state's nurse practice act. Review the section that deals with delegation. Apply those criteria to the case study at the beginning of this chapter.
- As a student, you have had tasks delegated to you. Identify how delegation has changed in regard to your learning and level of skills as you have progressed through your program.
- Obtain a copy of the policy on delegation from at least two of the clinical sites where you have practiced. How do these policies differ? How are they similar? What are the reasons for the similarities and differences?

References

1. Nightingale, F: Notes on Nursing. What It Is and What It Is Not. Harrison and Sons, London, 1859, p 17.
2. American Nurses Association: Position Statement: Registered Nurse Utilization of Unlicensed Assistive Personnel. ANA, Washington, DC, 1997.
3. American Nurses Association: Registered Professional Nurses and Unlicensed Assistive Personnel, ed. 2. ANA, Washington, DC, 1996.
4. Tetuan, T: The effects of budget, delegation, and other variables on the future of school nursing. Journal of Scholarly Nursing 20(6):352–358, 2004.
5. Cohen, S: Managers' fast track. Delegating vs. dumping: Teach the difference. Nurse Manager 35(10):14, 18, 52, 2004.
6. ANA Code of Ethics for Nurses, 2001. Available at: www.ana.org.

Bibliography

American Nurses Association: Policy Series: Regulation of Unlicensed Assistive Personnel. ANA, Washington, DC, 1996.

Creighton, H: Law Every Nurse Should Know, ed. 5. WB Saunders, Philadelphia, 1986.

Curtis, E: Delegation: A key function of nursing. Nurse Manager 11(4):26–31, 2004.

Garvis, M: Advice of counsel: When it's OK for an RN to delegate. RN 66(12):70–71, 2003.

Henderson, L: Nursing delegation. Pulse 41(2):1, 4, 2004.

Khaliullah, K: Professional misconduct: Nurse who compromised patient care through delegating a task. British Journal of Nursing 13(11):668, 2004.

Pearce, C: Careers: Honing the art of effective delegation. Nursing Times 100(29):46–47, 2004.

Tappen, RM: Nursing Leadership and Management, ed. 4. FA Davis, Philadelphia, 2001.

Tappen, RM, et al.: Essentials of Nursing Leadership and Management, ed. 2. FA Davis, Philadelphia, 2001.

Teasdale, K: Tips for the top: Better delegation. Professional Nursing 19(12):56, 2004.

Williams, J: Navigating the difficulties of delegation. Nursing 2004 34(9):32, 2004.

16

Collective Bargaining and Governance

Joseph T. Catalano

Learning Objectives

After completing this chapter, the reader will be able to:

- Define collective bargaining.
- Analyze the key issues that concern nurses in collective bargaining.
- Identify the steps in the contract negotiation process.
- Distinguish between a mediator and an arbitrator.
- Delineate the important elements in a contract.
- Name alternative forms of governance.
- Analyze the effect governance has on collective bargaining.

SHOULD NURSES UNIONIZE?

The image of nursing has always been one of dedication, service to clients, and selflessness. In the past, nurses' pay and working conditions were often secondary considerations, and many nurses felt that too much emphasis on money demeaned the profession. In today's society, nurses are beginning to realize that professionals with a career should have a say in matters that affect their practice, including working conditions, staffing patterns, benefits, and income. They need to be able to express these concerns without loss of status or reputation with the general public and other health-care professionals.

As nursing moves toward achieving its full status as a profession, the issue of collective bargaining becomes more important. Since the early 1960s, the number of nurses who have joined unions has increased steadily, yet the question remains: Is professionalism compatible with membership in a union? Union members still have the image of male workers in blue-collar, heavy industry jobs. However, not only are registered nurses (RNs) joining unions at a faster pace than most other categories of workers, but they are also more militant and aggressive in their demands.[1]

Nursing practices have often been defined and controlled by other groups, such as physicians and hospital administrators. These groups saw the potential power of an organized large group of well-educated and dedicated nurses and feared the time when they would become independent. Even today, in areas of the country where collective bargaining for health-care workers is not a part of the system, many hospital administrators react to any unionization attempts on the part of nurses with hostility and resistance. As the independence, authority, and responsibility of nurses increases, they need to consider whether or not joining a union will help them reach their goal of full professionalism. Without a doubt, this is one of the most highly charged issues that a nurse might face in professional practice.

> *Even today, in areas of the country where collective bargaining for health-care workers is not a part of the system, many hospital administrators react to any unionization attempts on the part of nurses with hostility and resistance.*

PERSPECTIVE ON COLLECTIVE BARGAINING

Collective bargaining is the uniting of employees for the purpose of increasing their ability to influence their employer and to improve working conditions.[2] Collective bargaining is on the basis of the principle that there is greater strength in large numbers. Its primary goal is to equalize the power between labor and management. The primary collective bargaining unit is the union.

Initially unions were formed to protect workers from exploitation by greedy and insensitive employers. Although confronted with much opposi-

tion, they did accomplish their goals and became very powerful entities. Recently, unions have received a more negative image because of the use of destructive and sometimes illegal practices in the quest for additional power. The end result is that the union movement is now in a fight for survival because of decreasing membership.[3] For some, unions and collective bargaining arouse images of picket lines, rowdy strikes, and violence. Many professionals, including nurses, do not regard this as activity that professionals should be involved in and tend to reject the idea of union membership outright.

Legislative Development of Collective Bargaining

The National Labor Relations Act
Although the informal roots of collective bargaining can be traced back to the mid-1800s, formal collective bargaining in this country was first legally recognized in 1935 with passage of the National Labor Relations Act (NLRA). This act granted employees the right to self-organization and to form, and help in the organization of, labor unions that could then bargain collectively through representatives. The representatives would be appointed by the union and bargain with management for the purpose of collective bargaining, mutual aid, and protection.[4] Under the NLRA, the National Labor Relations Board

What Do You Think?

How do you perceive unions? Do unions have any place in health care?

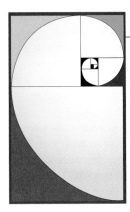

Issues Now

Workplace Violence in the Health-Care Setting

Of all the places on the planet, a person would assume that hospitals and other health-care facilities that are dedicated to promoting wellness and curing disease, would be one of the safest for workers. However, there has been a gradual but steady increase in health-care setting violence. The factors that lead to violence in other settings are also present in the health-care setting. Most violence is a result of unresolved stress that does not have an acceptable outlet. Health-care facilities are full of stress: money worries, demands of the job, short staffing, authority conflicts, and personality incompatibility.

The phenomenon of "going postal" is not isolated to the U.S. Postal Service. Studying the reasons people become violent in the workplace has demonstrated that it is a gradual building process that occurs over many months or even many years. It is often first noted when a person begins to objectify and dehumanize coworkers and administrators. They seem to have "authority issues" and often argue with those who supervise them. They may use profanity and are verbally abusive to those whom they supervise.

If such issues are not resolved early on, the behavior often becomes even more overtly threatening. Individuals caught in this escalating cycle of stress and violence often have very intense and frequent arguments with coworkers and even the clients they are providing care for. They may demonstrate obvious hostility to the organization they are working for including stealing supplies, intentionally violating procedures and policies, and even making sexual or violent threats to others. They fight any attempts to change the organizational structure and react to any attempts to help them identify their problems with blatant resistance.

Left unchecked, the behavior becomes physically violent. They may bring a weapon into the workplace to threaten supervisors or coworkers. They may threaten suicide. Other signs include those that are similar to what is seen in the burnout syndrome: drug or alcohol abuse, decrease in hygiene status, changes in personality, withdrawal from interactions with others and frequent "sick" days off.

All institutions should have a policy addressing the identification of individuals who have a potential for violence and measures to deal with them early on before the problem escalates to overt and deadly actions. These policies should include:

- Zero tolerance for verbal and physical threats of violence
- Identification of early warning signs of individuals who may pose a threat to others
- Training for staff on workplace violence
- Identification of resources that can be used when a person is demonstrating an escalating cycle of violence
- An emergency response plan so workers can know what to do beforehand if a person becomes violent in the work place

As unfortunate as it may be, violence in the workplace is a growing problem, even in the health-care setting. Being able to recognize persons who are manifesting characteristics that indicate an escalating cycle of violence and having a comprehensive plan to deal with them is an essential element in the workplace today.

Sources: Esposito, N, et al.: Preventing violence in an academic setting. Nursing Education Perspectives 26(1):24–28, 2005.
Brinker, D, et al.: Violence in the workplace: Are our units safe? AACN News 20(5):1, 9, 2003.

(NLRB) was established to supervise the implementation of the act.[1]

Originally, the NLRA included nonprofit hospitals and other health-care providers under its authority. In its attempt to protect unions, the NLRA prevented some employers from reducing wages, in hopes that higher-paid workers would spend more and decrease the severity of the Depression. One negative result of the NLRA was that many employers who did not have enough income to pay the higher wages went bankrupt.

The Taft-Hartley Act

The NLRA was amended in 1947 by the Taft-Hartley Act, also called the Labor Management Relations Act (LMRA), with the goal of restoring equality between the unions and management. Taft-Hartley excluded nurses in nonprofit hospitals from coverage under the NLRA, legally preventing nurses from organizing collective bargaining units and going on strike. It was not until 1974 that the Taft-Hartley Act was amended to cover nurses in nonprofit hospitals, thus allowing nurses to form collective bargaining units.[1]

Bargaining Units for Hospitals

In April of 1991, the U.S. Supreme Court ruled that the NLRB had the authority to define bargaining units for health-care providers in all settings, including acute care hospitals. Under this ruling, the NLRB defined eight separate bargaining units that were appropriate for use in hospitals (Box 16.1).[5]

Ultimately, this ruling by the Supreme Court permitted "all registered nurses (RNs) bargaining units" to be formed so that work issues important to

Box 16.1

Eight Bargaining Units for Use in Hospitals

1. Nurses
2. Physicians
3. All professionals except nurses and physicians
4. All technical employees
5. All skilled maintenance employees
6. All business office clerical employees
7. All guards
8. All other nonprofessional employees

professional nurses could be addressed. The current major representative for nurses is the Service Employees International Union, which represents almost 500,000 nurses and health-care providers nationwide. The American Nurses Association (ANA) has been active in the support of collective bargaining throughout its history.

Although the ANA does not serve as a bargaining agent, it does support the state nurses associations (SNAs) to function as bargaining agents. As early as 1944, the ANA ruled that the SNAs could engage in collective bargaining. In response to the attempt to regulate nursing from the outside, the ANA presented a position paper in 1946 that stated the importance for nursing to assume responsibility for advancing the social and economic security of its practitioners rather than leaving it to organizations outside the profession.[6] Today the SNAs represent approximately 140,000 RNs in 840 individual bargaining units across the United States.

Since the ruling by the Supreme Court in 1991, there has been an increased interest in organizing additional bargaining units.[7] The Workplace Advocacy Initiative was also enacted in 1991 to help RNs improve the work environment and gain more control over professional practice.

> " *One of the most important goals of a bargaining unit is to protect the employee against arbitrary treatment and unfair labor practices. These can be anything from working five weekends in a row to being fired because a physician felt the nurse was acting in an insubordinate manner.* "

Goals of Collective Bargaining

Although the basic goal of collective bargaining is to equalize power between management and employees, the inequality of power between the two groups is not so great as it initially appears. In many organizations management relies on employees who are near the bottom of the power structure hierarchy to carry out the work of the organization. Employees are vital to the growth, development, and even the survival of the organization. Employees also far outnumber individuals in management. Collective bargaining takes advantage of these two factors when attempting to produce change in the organization. An individual employee is highly vulnerable when attempting to force the employer to change.

Basic Comforts

The main area of concern of collective bargaining is basic economic issues such as salaries and benefits. In some hospital settings, nurses are paid less than other individuals in the hospital who have less education and fewer responsibilities. Collective bargaining attempts to balance these inequities.

Other concerns of collective bargaining include shift differentials, overtime pay, holidays, personal days off, the number of hours required in a work week, sick leave, maternity and paternity leave, uniform reimbursements, lunch and coffee breaks, health insurance, pension plans, and severance pay.[2] These elements all are found in the employment contract and may vary greatly depending on the hospital and the power of the bargaining unit.

Fair Treatment

One of the most important goals of a bargaining unit is to protect the employee against arbitrary treatment and unfair labor practices. These can be anything from working five weekends in a row to being fired because a physician felt the nurse was acting in an insubordinate manner. Other issues that might be considered unfair labor practices include being passed over for promotion without an explanation, unreasonable staffing and scheduling policies, excessive demands for overtime, rotating shifts, unfair on-call time, transfers, layoffs, seniority rights, and failure to post job openings.

The collective bargaining unit establishes a grievance procedure by means of which the employee can bring a complaint against management without fear of reprisals. These grievance procedures also allow a mechanism for the employee to follow up on the complaint to a satisfactory conclusion.

Professional Practice

An important goal of collective bargaining is to maintain and promote professional practice. Often overlooked by management, this goal is one way nurses can keep and increase control over their own professional practice. For example, some nurses'

bargaining units have been able to include the entire ANA Code of Ethics into the contract with the hospital. Other units have been able to address issues such as staffing, standards of care, and quality of care in the contract negotiations.

Interest-Based Bargaining

Traditionally, collective bargaining has been viewed as a struggle between two groups, one (usually employees) attempting to gain more power and another (usually management) attempting to retain power. This type of struggle often resulted in hurt feelings or impasses in negotiations.

An Open Environment

Interest-based bargaining, also called mutual gains, win-win, and best-practice bargaining, is based on the idea that the way to achieve a mutually beneficial contract is to create an environment in which all parties can openly discuss all issues to the fullest extent. In interest-based bargaining, a highly structured six-step process is followed:

1. Selection of issues
2. Discussion of interests
3. Generation of options

What Do You Think?

Who are the people who hold governing power in your clinical institution? What process can employees in health-care facilities use to affect the quality of care that they provide?

_____

_____

_____

_____

_____

_____

_____

_____

_____

_____

_____

_____

4. Establishment of standards to measure the options
5. Measurement of the options
6. Development of solutions

This step-by-step process prevents the parties involved in bargaining from reverting to the traditional power struggle. All steps are done jointly, and even the 2-day training session that precedes negotiations requires participation by both management and labor.

The Role of the RN. An issue that is central to the contract negotiations is ensuring that the role of the RN as the primary assessor and planner of care be maintained. The contract spells out what the RN's role will be, including activities such as assessing, planning, and evaluating the client's nursing care needs. To ensure that nursing issues are addressed adequately in contracts, RNs need to participate in facility committees that establish priorities for labor-management relations, nurse staffing, client-care standards, and health and safety policies. This partnership between nurses and hospital administrators allows for joint decision making when issues of nursing practice and delivery of care are involved.

A Trend for the Future. Interest-based bargaining seems to be gaining momentum and may be the trend for the future, particularly in the health-care industry. Traditional collective bargaining methods are primarily adversarial and often leave the parties involved with deep-seated feelings of hostility toward each other. The old methods sometimes result in strikes or other types of work actions that harm the reputations of both nurses and the hospitals. Interest-based bargaining allows participants to negotiate without hostility and, after negotiation of the contract, promotes the development of a more positive relationship.

> *An issue that is central to the contract negotiations is ensuring that the role of the RN as the primary assessor and planner of care be maintained. The contract spells out what the RN's role will be, including activities such as assessing, planning, and evaluating the client's nursing care needs.*

NURSES' QUESTIONS ABOUT COLLECTIVE BARGAINING

Although large numbers of RNs have successfully unionized, there remain some fundamental questions about collective bargaining. These questions are at the heart of what makes collective bargaining an ethical issue for many nurses.

> *The NLRB defines nurses as professionals because their work requires advanced and specialized education and skills. They also make critical judgments that affect the health and well-being of others.*

Is It Unprofessional?

Nurses have a great deal of difficulty in adjusting their image to that of a union member or a striker. It just does not seem to be professional. For many nurses it seems that there must be other ways to achieve the same goals without collective bargaining.

> *The collective bargaining unit establishes a grievance procedure by means of which the employee can bring a complaint against management without fear of reprisals. These grievance procedures also provide a mechanism for the employee to follow up on the complaint to a satisfactory conclusion.*

Organizers of collective bargaining units stress that many other professionals, such as pilots, teachers, and even physicians, are members of unions. The NLRB defines nurses as professionals because their work requires advanced and specialized education and skills. They also make critical judgments that affect the health and well-being of others. Union organizers contend that it is even less professional to accept low pay and poor working conditions than it is to join a union to improve these elements. They also feel that collective bargaining will give nurses control over their practice, which is one of the keys to professionalism.

Is It Unethical?

One of the major beliefs of nurses is the priority of the clients' health and well-being over the personal needs and gains of the health-care provider. This concern conflicts with the methods commonly used by collective bargaining units, such as strikes or work slowdowns. There is a feeling among many health-care providers that these types of actions constitute abandonment of their clients and therefore violate the code of ethics.

Those who support collective bargaining stress that poor working conditions, such as lack of qualified staff, are as much a threat to clients' health and well-being as the work actions taken to correct these conditions. The ability of nurses simply to threaten to strike, even though it may never materialize, is often powerful enough to bring about change.[8]

Law requires that a 10-day notice must be given before a strike takes place. This gives the hospital a chance to prepare for the strike and to make changes to ensure client safety, such as transferring critical care clients to another hospital, eliminating elective surgeries, and refusing to admit new clients. If the hospital fails to take appropriate measures when they have received adequate notice, then the issue of client abandonment becomes their responsibility, not that of the nurses who have gone on strike.

In the few times when nurses have gone on strike, client safety and well-being have not been affected. The institutions involved were always given enough lead time to discharge or transfer the majority of the clients. The few remaining clients were cared for by management personnel, who are not covered by unions.

Is It Divisive?

Nurse Against Nurse

Does the process of collective bargaining set nurse against nurse? Collective bargaining is adversarial by nature. It sets two groups, management and employees, against each other. Although this relationship can result in conflict, it allows the staff nurses to be heard and to initiate changes that affect the practice of nursing. Nurses have been attempting for years to improve working conditions in the health-care setting and to achieve **comparable worth.** Administrators pay little attention to an individual nurse or to a small group of concerned nurses. When a collective bargaining unit speaks for all of the nurses, however, administration will listen.[1]

The chief executive officer (CEO) of a large home-health-care agency in a southwestern resort area called a general staff meeting. She reported that the agency had grown rapidly and was now the largest in the area.

"Much of our success is due to the professionalism and commitment of our staff members," she said. "With growth comes some problems, however. The most serious problem is the fluctuation in patient census. Our census peaks in the winter months when seasonal visitors are here and troughs in the summer. In the past, when we were a small agency, we all took our vacations during the slow season. This made it possible to continue to pay everyone his or her full salary all year. However, with the pressures to reduce costs and the large number of staff members we now have, we cannot continue to do this. We are very concerned about maintaining the high quality of patient care currently provided, but we have calculated that we need to reduce staff by 30 percent over the summer to survive financially."

The CEO then invited comments from the staff members. The majority of the nurses said they wanted and needed to work full-time all year. Most supported families and had to have a steady income all year around. "My rent does not go down in the summer," said one. "Neither does my mortgage or the grocery bill," said another. A small number said that they would be happy to work part-time in the summer if they could be guaranteed full-time employment from October through May. "We have friends who would love this work schedule," they added.

"That's not fair," protested the nurses who needed to work full-time all year. "You can't replace us with part-time staff." The discussion grew louder and the participants more agitated. The meeting ended without a solution to the problem. Although the CEO promised to consider all points of view before making a decision, the nurses left the meeting feeling very confused and concerned about the security of their future income. Some grumbled that they probably would begin looking for new positions "before the ax falls."

The next day, the CEO received a telephone call from the nurses' union representative. "If what I heard about the meeting yesterday is correct," said the representative, "your plan is in violation of our collective bargaining contract." The CEO reviewed the contract and found that the representative was correct. A new solution to the financial problems caused by the seasonal fluctuation in patient census would have to be found.

(Tappen, RM, et al.: Essentials of Nursing Leadership and Management, ed. 2. FA Davis, Philadelphia, 2001, pp 106–107, with permission.)

Closed or Open Shop?

Different collective bargaining units have different requirements for membership, which are often included in the negotiations. Many unions negotiate a *closed shop or agency shop* clause in the contract. A closed shop institution requires that all the employees pay membership dues whether they belong to the union or not. The rationale behind the closed shop approach is that because all the employees benefit from the union's negotiations, they should all pay for it. It also encourages employees to join the union because they are already paying the dues.

However, many states have *right to work* laws that make closed shop contracts illegal. In these states, the *open shop* collective bargaining model is used, and only those employees who desire to be members join the union and pay dues. There is more chance for nurse-to-nurse conflicts in open shop institutions because of the divisions between those who belong to the union and those who do not.

Collective bargaining does not have to be adversarial, and in facilities where the administration is open to change and the collective bargaining unit is realistic in its requests, the process can be very smooth and amicable.

> ❝ *Collective bargaining does not have to be adversarial, and in facilities where the administration is open to change and the collective bargaining unit is realistic in its requests, the process can be very smooth and amicable.* ❞

Is There a Threat to Job Security?

Although the main goals of collective bargaining are improvement of working conditions and protection from unfair labor practices, it can itself pose a threat to job security. In some cases, employees who are active in the collective bargaining process become well known to management and may become the targets of reprisals, particularly if the collective bargaining fails. Facilities sometimes suggest that granting RNs higher wages and benefits will cause bankruptcy and closure of the facility or that the higher RN wages will at least drain the organization's resources so much that it has to cut back the number of other employees.

In reality, recent changes in contract law have resulted in some job losses. Nurses can be replaced during strikes, and even if a settlement is reached, they are hired back only after new employees leave or openings occur. If no settlement is reached, striking nurses may never be hired back.

Taking action always carries risk. Nurses involved in collective bargaining have to consider the risk-to-benefit ratio before they take action. Are the working conditions so poor and the pay so inadequate that they overshadow the risk of possible job loss? The first attempts at organizing a collective bargaining unit are usually the most dangerous in terms of job security.

Initial attempts at organizing nurses are usually made outside the hospital between representatives of the SNA and the union. This type of activity may prevent individuals from becoming targets of management's anger and makes management's reprisals more difficult for a short time. However, it is virtually impossible to keep knowledge of collective bargaining activities secret. Hospital information and rumor "grapevines" are very well developed, and at times it seems the administration hears of the activities almost before they start.

Some legal protections exist for nurses who organize collective bargaining. Grievance procedures against vengeful administrators can be initiated under the unfair labor practices rules that vary somewhat from state to state. However, even if successful, nurses may pay a heavy toll in both financial and emotional terms in the process of proving they were in the right.

> *Taking action always carries risk. Nurses involved in collective bargaining have to consider the risk-to-benefit ratio before they take action.*

THE CONTRACT

Negotiation

After a collective bargaining unit has been selected, the next important step is to develop or negotiate a contract between the nurses and the hospital. The contract is a legal document that is binding for both management and the union.[2] Contracts can be very specific and include just a few items or very broad and include many. Contracts often contain requirements for union membership by the employees and set the cost of dues for that membership.

Representation. Negotiating teams are selected by both management and employee groups. One member of each of these teams is designated as the spokesperson who will be the main representative for the group. Before negotiations start, each team meets separately to decide on its position on various issues and on what they are willing to compromise. A list of demands is exchanged by the two sides; it should include everything each might possibly want.

Power and Benefits. Generally, management is reluctant to give up power or relinquish money. The employees' group tries to gain some of management's power and gain benefits for its members. Often many meetings between the two groups are required before they discover the key issues and determine where compromise is possible. Posturing and showmanship play a big part in the initial negotiations. Later, when serious issues are discussed and dealt with, final agreements may be reached behind closed doors.

Good-Faith Bargaining. The law requires that each side bargain in good faith. Good-faith bargaining requires that both parties must agree to meet at reasonable times, to send individuals to the negotiations who can make binding decisions, and to be willing to

bargain with the other side.[2] A lack of willingness to negotiate is not bargaining in good faith.

Mediation or Arbitration?

Working With a Mediator

When the sides are unable to reach a settlement, a stalemate occurs. Stalemates are sometimes resolved through mediation, in which a neutral third party provided by the Federal Mediation and Conciliation Service meets with each side. After determining the nature of the conflict, the mediator brings the two sides together to attempt to work out a settlement. Both sides must work with the mediator, but they are not required to accept the mediator's recommendations.

If mediation fails, the Federal Mediation and Conciliation Service may appoint a fact-finding panel to investigate the conflict and to make recommendations. The panel's report is made public and can exert pressure on both sides to accept the recommendations of the mediator.

Binding Arbitration

In some situations, an arbitrator with binding power may be appointed. This person is a neutral third party who, like the mediator, investigates the conflict, meets with both sides, and makes a recommendation for settlement. However, the arbitrator's recommendation, unlike that of the mediator, must be accepted by both sides. Both labor and management try to avoid binding arbitration because it limits their negotiating powers and they may lose something gained during previous negotiations.

The Prospect of a Strike

When all else fails, the final step in the contract negotiation process is work slowdowns or stoppages (strikes). Although strikes are usually the tool used by employees to gain power, management can use a form of enforced strike called a lockout, whereby employees are not permitted to enter the work facility.

The prospect of a strike is usually accompanied by more intense negotiations that may lead to a last-minute settlement. Strikes are detrimental to both sides. Employees lose pay and benefits during a strike, and management loses income. In addition, the overall public image of strikes is negative, and they have little support. Some collective bargaining units have developed alternative ways of achieving their goals without a strike. Methods such as disruption of services on a random basis or boycott of an organization can achieve the same effects as a full-blown strike without damaging the image of the union.

What Do You Think?

Did you ever sign a contract for employment? Did you read the contract? Were all the elements of a good contract present?

Box 16.2
Elements of a Good Contract

- A statement outlining the objectives of both management and the employees
- A description of the official collective bargaining group
- A description of the benefits included in the contract, such as wages and salary, overtime pay, holiday pay, shift differentials, differentials for advanced education or certifications
- A description of other benefits, such as health insurance, life insurance, retirement, and legal benefits, among others
- A description of acceptable in-house labor practices, such as transfers, promotions, seniority, layoffs, **grievance** procedures, and work schedules
- A description of the procedure to be used when employees have disciplinary problems or when there is a **breach of contract**
- A description of the grievance procedures and the due process to be followed
- A description of what is expected of the professional, including standards of care and codes of ethics

Ratifying the Contract

After a settlement has been reached, the contract must be ratified. The collective bargaining unit takes the contract back to the employees, who must approve it (Box 16.2). Once it is approved by a majority of the employees, the contract becomes legally binding for both management and the employees.

CONCERNS

Representation

One of the most difficult decisions that nurses have to make is who will represent them as a collective bargaining unit. It is reasonable to conclude that only a professional organization, such as the state nurses' association (SNA), that understands the complex and varied needs of the profession will be able to represent that profession in a collective bargaining situation.

Over the years, SNAs have developed into skilled representatives able to negotiate contracts with considerable success. However, nonprofessional unions have years of experience with negotiations and large sums of money to spend on developing skilled individuals whose only job is negotiating contracts. The union must be able to convince the group of nurses that it is able to represent their interests more effectively than the SNA.

Union groups that attempt to represent nurses soon find that nurses have difficulties forming a consensus concerning problems and issues. Individuals outside the nursing profession have difficulty understanding issues such as quality and standards of care, ethical dilemmas, or even the different levels of nursing education.

Nurses should also be concerned about the public image of the collective bargaining unit they select to represent them. Some nurses' groups have been represented by a machinists' union, a teamsters' union, or even a meat cutters' union. Although these unions are highly proficient at negotiating contracts to gain benefits for their members, some feel the image of nursing is tarnished in the process.

> *Nurses should also be concerned about the public image of the collective bargaining unit they select to represent them. Some nurses' groups have been represented by a machinists' union, a teamsters' union, or even a meat cutters' union.*

Nursing Supervisors: Employees or Management?

Everyone is familiar with the idea of the traditional nursing supervisor. This is the older, more experienced nurse who guides the less experienced nurses. Nursing supervisors make sure staffing is adequate for their assigned shifts, resolve problems that are beyond the skills of the staff nurse, act as mediators between physicians and nurses, and use their higher skill levels to assist the staff nurses with code blues or complicated procedures. The term *nursing supervisor* also includes nurse educators, directors of nursing, head nurses, unit supervisors, assistant head nurses, and sometimes even charge nurses on the 3 P.M.to 11 P.M. or 11 P.M. to 7 A.M. work shift.

Redefining the Supervisor

Under the amendments to the Taft-Hartley Act of 1974, a supervisor was defined as any individual with authority to hire, transfer, suspend, lay off, promote, assign, reward, or discipline another employee.[2] From this legal viewpoint, nursing supervisors were no longer employees but really members of the management. Management cannot be involved in collective bargaining activities and is therefore prevented from joining unions. A careful reading of the definition of a supervisor as presented in the Taft-Hartley Act makes the category of supervisor open to interpretation. Anybody who assigns a task to another nurse could be considered a supervisor.

Management has sometimes used this provision in the Taft-Hartley Act in an attempt to control the organization and function of collective bargaining units. Management, if so inclined, can use this distinction to induce tension between nursing staff and supervisors, thus reducing the cohesion of the group. Supervisors often serve on important hospital committees to develop standards of care, foster professional recognition, and support nurse advancement. When contracts are negotiated, the supervisors are on the opposite side of the table from the staff nurses. Often in the heat of negotiation, things are said that foster negative feelings. After the negotiations have ended, it is difficult to re-establish that sense of unity that contributes to high-quality client care.

Some health-care institutions have attempted to categorize all of their RNs and licensed practical nurses (LPNs) as supervisors, thus preventing any of them from organizing into a collective bargaining unit.

A Supreme Court Decision

In a 5 to 4 vote, the Supreme Court of the United States supported the decision that LPNs at the Heartland Nursing Home in Urbana, Ohio, should be considered supervisors because they directed the work of nurses' aides "in the interest of the employer." Under this ruling, these LPNs were not protected under the NLRA. This ruling has been of great concern to all nurses, but particularly to the ANA's Department of Labor Relations and Workplace Advocacy committee.

The implications of this decision are far-reaching and pose a direct threat to the ability of RNs to pursue collective bargaining. Employers have already begun to use this ruling to fight nurses in collective bargaining units from Alaska to Washington, DC.

The ANA has been working toward developing language that would follow the description of a supervisor as found in the NLRA and the Taft-Hartley Act (see earlier discussion). Since the passage of the NLRA, nurses who provide client care have been considered to be acting within the professional nature of nursing and not in the interests of the employer (as a supervisor would primarily be).

Under the ANA's proposed revisions, the scope of the definition of supervisor would be narrowed to include only employees of health-care institutions. This change would allow the NLRB to continue to determine, on a case-by-case basis, whether nurses were supervisors or professional or technical employees. This legislation, introduced to Congress in 1996, was initially tabled. Although never officially acted upon, recent court rulings have supported the position that not all RNs are supervisors, with resulting successful work actions and strikes nationwide.[4]

GOVERNANCE

The term *governance* has a variety of meanings in different contexts. In general, the term describes the arrangement of the hierarchy of power within an organization and how that power flows through the organization.

A System of Control

In relationship to nursing, governance has been defined as "the establishment and maintenance of social, political, and economic arrangements by which nurses maintain control over their practice, their self-discipline, their working conditions, and their professional affairs."[9] The traditional structure of authority in the health-care industry has been on the basis of the triad of the board of directors, the administrator, and the medical staff.

Authority is a type of power that has its origins in the position that an individual holds within an organization.[2] This individual has this power only because others are willing to accept the decisions made by the person in that position. This allows relatively few people in the organization's hierarchy to control large numbers of employees as well as the directions and functions of the rest of the organization.

The Board of Directors. At the top of the governance hierarchy is the board of directors, also called the trustees or governors. The board of directors is usually composed of influential business people who are considered community leaders. Although they retain the ultimate legal and ethical responsibility for the operation of the organization, generally the day-to-day operation is delegated to the administrator. The board's main function is to set general policies and to plan for the long-range development of the organization. Most boards become directly involved in the facility's operations only when there is a crisis, such as a financial shortfall or a major lawsuit.

The Administrator. The administrator is usually the highest ranking member of the hierarchy to be involved in the daily operation of the facility. The administrator has the education and knowledge required to direct the highly complex and technologically advanced elements that are an essential part of today's health-care system.

The Medical Staff. In most health-care facilities, the medical staff exerts a great deal of control over the governance structure. The medical staff also has its own internal governance structure with higher- and lower-level members. Traditionally, the physicians in a facility had a great deal of influence in the facility because they were neither employed nor controlled by the facility. However, the advent and spread of managed care has markedly altered the traditional physician–institution relationship in many facilities. In a managed care setting, physicians are hired and salaried employees just like nurses, housekeepers, administrators, and security personnel. Their practice and productivity are monitored and evaluated, and they can be terminated from the facility for poor performance.

> *Some health-care institutions have attempted to categorize all of their RNs and licensed practical nurses (LPN) as supervisors, thus preventing any of them from organizing into a collective bargaining unit.*

Nurses' Role in Governance

In the recent past, nurses had little say in the governance of their facility or agency. Because of their traditional ideology of professionalism, nurses were more oriented toward loyalty and respect than autonomy of practice and independent decision making about the quality of care.[1] Nurses often accepted the work hours assigned to them without question, withstood disrespect and abuse from physicians and administrators as part of the work environment, and were satisfied with the meager salaries paid to them because theirs was a profession of caring and dedication. This situation has, however, changed drastically since the 1970s.

The AMA Example

Self-governance is a concept that is important to all professions. The most powerful professional groups are those that maintain a strong sense of self-governance for their members. The American Medical Association (AMA) is a classic example of the power that an organized group can exert. Much of the physicians' power to affect institutional governance, and even broader issues such as managed care, comes from the AMA.

Membership in a powerful organization can be an alternative to unions. Up to this time, the ANA has split its activities and focus between self-governance and collective bargaining. It has been successful in most of its efforts at collective bargaining but somewhat limited in its success at self-governance.

Autonomy for the Nurse

As nursing responsibilities increased with advancing technology and changes in the health-care system, nurses began to recognize that their responsibilities far exceeded their authority to influence their practice. They started to view professional autonomy, authority, and accountability as essential elements in high-quality client care. One approach to gaining these elements was to change the organizational structure of the health-care facilities where they were employed.

Nurses have challenged the traditional governance structure at a number of levels with varying amounts of success. Nursing service administrators are the leaders of the largest single group of health-care professionals in most health-care organizations—generally about 50 percent of all the employees.[2] Because of their education and experience, many nursing administrators have moved into positions of power in the health-care system and are no longer willing to accept the traditional role to which nurses were once relegated.

As middle managers, nursing administrators are often caught in the middle of conflicting expectations. For example, the chief administrator may want to cut the budget by reducing staffing, whereas the nurses on the units recognize that they can no longer provide high-quality nursing care because the staffing levels are already too low.

Positional Authority

Staff RNs often view themselves as located at the bottom of the hierarchy with very little power. This is rarely the case. Depending on the organization of the facility, RNs have positional authority over LPNs, nursing assistants, and individuals from the laboratory and radiology department.

Nurses have gained greater control over their practice by fostering change in the organizational structures of health-care facilities and agencies. The changes include decentralization of authority, identification of professional nurses as peers, agreement on the philosophy and goals of nursing care, and increased responsibility for directing and planning the care given to clients while they are in the facility.[10]

Self-governance is a concept that is important to all professions. The most powerful professional groups are those that maintain a strong sense of self-governance for their members.

Alternative Models for Governance

In an attempt to redistribute power and authority within health-care organizations, several alternative forms of governance have been developed. Some of these work better than others, depending on the facility and the willingness of the individuals involved to cooperate.

Board of Nursing

In this model of governance, the nursing staff structure is similar to the medical staff structure. There is a general board of trustees at the top and, immediately below, at the same level, a medical board of

directors, a nursing board of directors, a board of directors representing other professionals, and the hospital administration itself.[2] The nursing board of directors deals with such matters as credentials and standards of care and promotes cooperation between nurses and the other professionals of the facility.

Although this type of structure places nurses on an equal administrative footing with the physicians, administration, and other professionals in the facility, it does have the tendency to create a large number of administrative personnel. A tendency for conflicts to arise between the different board members does exist.

Nurses have gained greater control over their practice by fostering change in the organizational structures of health-care facilities and agencies. The changes include decentralization of authority, identification of professional nurses as peers, agreement on the philosophy and goals of nursing care, and increased responsibility for directing and planning the care given to clients while they are in the facility.

Contracting for Nursing Services

The **fee-for-service** model proposes that clients be billed for nursing care as a separate item, much the same way that they are billed for medical care by the physicians. Currently, when a client receives a hospital bill, the care provided by nurses is included in the overall room charge. To make this model work, nurses select individual clients for whom they wish to care and then accept responsibility for providing that care. Some type of scale would need to be developed so that the nurse could charge a higher rate for taking care of more seriously ill clients with more complex health-care needs. Nurses would take responsibility for scheduling and for self-management. As with physicians, there would have to be a **peer review** mechanism to monitor the quality of health care provided.

Although this model supports primary care and the expansion of the nurse's role and responsibility, it would be very difficult to implement. Some of the problems include establishing acceptable pay scales, ensuring adequate staffing, and paying ancillary help such as orderlies and nursing assistants. Probably the most significant single factor that affects the implementation of this model is the hospital administration's loss of control over the nursing staff. If the nurses' pay were to come directly from the client, rather than the hospital, nurses would tend to place the client's needs before the needs of the facility. This model is still unacceptable to most facilities.

Shared Governance

In the shared governance model, power and authority are transferred to the nursing staff rather than being seated primarily in nursing administration. The key to shared governance is decentralization of the nursing administration structure. Its goal is to involve professional nurses in the decision-making process at all levels to ensure that their knowledge and expertise are used to deliver the highest quality care possible.[1]

Shared governance is a model that the staff is willing to undertake, rather than being forced into it by the administration. Unfortunately, many facilities that profess a shared governance structure really are using a traditional hierarchy structure with somewhat more open lines of communication.

Shared governance gives the nurse autonomy in decisions about nursing practice, working conditions, staffing levels, standards of care, and other areas. It gives professional nurses the chance to be held accountable and responsible for their clinical judgment and the care they give to clients. It allows their peers a chance to recognize their knowledge and competence as true health-care professionals.

In general, shared governance locates the source of power in clinical areas rather than in **administrative** areas. Several different types of shared governance exist.

Congressional Model. In the congressional shared governance model, a group of professional nurses is organized into a congress. This congress develops bylaws, elects representatives, and forms committees to govern the activities of the nursing staff.[9] Composed entirely of professional nurses, the committees oversee professional practice, evaluate quality of care, provide continuing education, plan for staffing, conduct research, and discipline errant nurses. Although this is a highly effective method to provide nursing care and to increase the autonomy of nurses, it does require a tremendous initial expenditure of time, effort, and money. Many institutions are not willing to make that commitment.

Unit-Based Model. In the unit-based model, the shared governance is on a smaller scale. Groups of nurses on each unit form councils for professional practice that perform many of the functions that the professional congresses perform. To make this model succeed, there must be a real transfer of decision-making power from the head nurse or unit supervisor to the staff nurses.

Shared governance is a model that the staff is willing to undertake, rather than being forced into it by the administration. Unfortunately, many facilities that profess a shared governance structure really are using a traditional hierarchy structure with somewhat more open lines of communication. The test of a true shared governance model quickly becomes evident when difficult decisions have to be made. For example, if the staff nurses decide that more staffing is needed for their unit, but the administration refuses to make money available for new nurses, then it is not a true shared governance model.

In the shared governance model, power and authority are transferred to the nursing staff rather than being seated primarily in nursing administration. The key to shared governance is decentralization of the nursing administration structure.

Governance and Collective Bargaining

Forms of governance directly affect which issues are likely to be involved in nurses' collective bargaining. Although salary and benefits are important considerations in professional nursing, issues of autonomy, accountability, and control of practice are gaining importance for many nurses.

In a health-care facility with a form of governance that allows nurses to have a relatively large degree of control over their practice, the issues discussed at the bargaining table are more likely to revolve around a professional agenda. In facilities with rigidly structured hierarchies of authority that gives nurses little autonomy, accountability, or control over their practice, collective bargaining is more likely to center on control and power issues.

Nurses are highly educated professionals. They recognize that they can practice autonomously and can make sound decisions about client care. They also recognize that an increased understanding of the governance process requires many of the same skills used in collective bargaining. Key elements in both processes are an understanding of negotiation, compromise, and consensus building to attain one's goals. Changes in methods of governance also will require major changes in the health-care system. Professional nurses have the power to produce those changes and the ability to deal with the future of health care successfully.

Conclusion

Although few issues elicit such strong emotions among nurses as collective bargaining, it is a reality in today's health-care system. Nurses are beginning to realize that they are not in a strictly altruistic profession, but rather one in which they use their knowledge and skills to provide high-quality services to clients. The knowledge and skills used in client care are gained at the cost of years of expensive education in schools of nursing and dedication to an often underappreciated profession. Nurses no longer need to apologize or feel guilty about seeking payment for their work on a level commensurate with their knowledge and skills.

Negotiation is the process of give and take between groups with the goal of reaching an agreement acceptable to both sides. Negotiations may be formal or informal, hostile or friendly. A cooperative atmosphere fostered by both sides that recognizes the similarity of each side's demands will be the most productive in reaching a satisfactory contract.

Although not a new concept for nursing, collective bargaining is an issue that is still hotly debated among professional nurses. Collective bargaining is viewed by some as unprofessional, unethical, divisive, and a fundamental threat to job security. However, the goals of collective bargaining, including improvement of economic benefits, better staffing and scheduling, fair treatment for all nurses, and improved quality of care for clients, are common to all health-care providers.

Nurses must decide at some point in their careers whether joining a collective bargaining unit will best help them to achieve these goals. This is not an easy decision to make, and each nurse should gather as much information as possible about the situation before making a decision.

Nurses need to recognize that the time has arrived to elevate the profession to a new level. Change in forms of governance is one method that nurses can use to change the health-care system. Nursing as a profession now has the opportunity to gain tremendous power and take its rightful place as an indispensable force in the health-care system. All that is required is for nurses to become educated in the issues involved and to take an aggressive stance in shaping the future.

Issues in Practice

Deciding to Go on Strike

Sharon S, RN, was completing her charting on another busy 3 P.M. to 11 P.M shift. While she was walking down the hall toward the time clock, she wondered who would be taking her place for the rest of the week. Like most of the other nurses at the medical center, she had decided to go on strike starting with the 7 A.M. to 3 P.M. shift the next day. The decision to strike had not been an easy one and had been reached only after many hours of meetings and conferences with the hospital negotiators and animated discussion among the nurses' negotiating team.

Sharon could see both positive and negative sides to a strike. On the positive side, increased salaries, better fringe benefits, and improvements in working conditions and staffing would be a plus for all the nurses and clients at the medical center. Sharon herself had felt increasingly stressed during the past year because of the hospital's measures to reorganize. From what Sharon was able to see, reorganization meant saving money by cutting professional staff and partially replacing them with less-trained, unlicensed individuals. This pattern of restaffing had led to longer hours, increased responsibilities for the RNs, and fewer support services. She also felt that the overall quality of care had decreased noticeably.

On the negative side, Sharon was experiencing a real ethical and emotional dilemma about going on strike. The quality of care was sure to deteriorate even further because of the reduced services caused by the strike. Was it really fair to decrease the services and care for clients who had nothing to do with the issues that brought on the strike? Of course, during the past 3 days, the clients who had been well enough were sent home early in anticipation of the strike. Some whose conditions were too complicated for them to be cared for at home were sent to other facilities. The hospital had severely restricted admissions, reducing the census to an all-time low.

Yet there were several clients who were too ill to transfer or send home. Mrs. Anderson, a 78-year-old client with renal failure, congestive heart failure, and a recent colostomy for a bowel obstruction, came to mind. Mrs. Anderson and a number of other clients like her, who had no family nearby and few resources, were highly dependent on the nursing staff to meet their needs of care. Mrs. Anderson was just beginning to be taught how to care for her colostomy. Even if she was discharged to a nursing home, there was no way to ensure that she could receive the teaching needed for her eventual self-care. Although there was to be a skeleton crew of nurses left in the facility, they would be stretched very thin in trying to care for the remaining clients.

Sharon also thought about the ANA Code of Ethics for Nurses she had been taught in nursing school, particularly the passage that stated "the nurse participates in the profession's effort to establish and maintain conditions of employment conducive to high-quality nursing care." The reason for the strike was to bring about improved working conditions that would benefit future clients in the hospital, but should these measures be carried out when nursing services were already operating at a reduced level of care and at a minimal level of safety? Didn't that somehow contradict the first statement in the code, that "the nurse provides services with

(continued)

Issues in Practice continued

respect for human dignity"? When Mrs. Anderson was admitted to the hospital 4 days before, she came with the expectation of the best possible care under any circumstances. The code seemed to have a split personality on strikes. While calling for service to the profession to maintain high standards and quality of care, the code also insisted that the health, welfare, and safety of the clients should be the nurse's first consideration.

What should Sharon do? Does the overall welfare of the profession ever supersede the obligation to provide client care?

Critical Thinking Exercises

- Develop a position paper either supporting or opposing collective bargaining.
- A nurse on your unit states one day, "Membership in the state nurses' association is a waste of time and money. They can't help you make a better living!" How would you respond to this nurse?
- Develop an ideal contract for nurses. Which elements would receive the highest priority?
- Develop a plan for shared governance in a facility you are familiar with. How would the organizational process take place? What are some of the major difficulties in developing this plan?

References

1. Gordon, S: Collective thinking. Nurse Manager 11(2):8, 2004.
2. Tappen, RM: Nursing Leadership and Management, ed. 4. FA Davis, Philadelphia, 2001.
3. Szczepanski, A: Cutting deals on the side: Is your employer trying to go through the illegal back door? Michagan Nurse 77(2):15, 2004.
4. DeMass-Martin, S: Striking nurses win from coast to coast. American Nurse 34(2):8–10, 2002.
5. Budd, K: Traditional and non-traditional collective bargaining: Strategies to improve the patient care environment. Online Journal Issues in Nursing 9(1):1–6, 2004.
6. Tappen, RM, et al.: Essentials of Nursing Leadership and Management, ed. 2. FA Davis, Philadelphia, 2001.
7. Bissett, L: Perspectives in leadership: The manager's list. Nursing Spectrum 5(2):9, 2001.
8. Costa, L: As union activity surges, it pays to be alert to workplace disruptions. Patient Care Management 16(4):10–11, 2001.
9. McKeown, C, and Thompson, J: Clinical governance: Implementing clinical supervision. Nursing Management 8(6):10–13, 2001.
10. Forman, H: Effective labor relations. The "New Age" of union organizing. J Nurs Adm 34(3):120–124, 2004.

Bibliography

Briles, J: Zapping conflict in the health care workplace. The Oklahoma Nurse 49(2):23, 2004.
Cross, LL: Protected whistle-blowing or a legal firing? The Oklahoma Nurse 47(1):14–16, 2002.
Curtin, L: Ethics in management: case study. A showdown over overtime. Journal of Clinical Systems Management 6(5/6):14, 2004.
DeMass-Martin, S: Striking nurses win from coast to coast. American Nurse 34(2):8–10, 2002.
Green, A: Common denominators: Shared governance and work place advocacy—strategies for nurses to gain control over their practice. Online Journal Issues in Nursing 9(1):1–7, 2004.
Kennedy, MS, et al.: To supervise or unionize? That is the question: A Supreme Court ruling may limit nurses' ability to form unions. Am J Nurs 101(8):21, 2001.
Oregon nurses strike for pay, health care. American Nurse 34(1):7, 2002.
Rigiero, D: Empowering nurses to raise their voices in unity. Mass Nurse 75(3):1, 3, 2004.
Sanford, K: Become competent in confrontation. Nursing Management 35(7):14, 2004.
Trossman, S: Illinois nurse loses job for helping Sept. 11 victims. American Nurse 34(1):1–2, 2002.

17

Health-Care Delivery Systems

Nicole Harder

Learning Objectives

After completing this chapter, the reader will be able to:

- Analyze the evolution of the health-care delivery system in the United States.
- Analyze the evolution of the health-care delivery system in Canada.
- Evaluate the factors that influence the evolution of the health-care delivery system.
- Synthesize the concerns surrounding the uninsured in this country.
- Analyze industry efforts to manage health-care costs.
- Evaluate the efforts being made to ensure high-quality cost-effective health care.
- Describe and list the levels and types of health-care delivery.

THE NEW FACE OF HEALTH CARE

Traditionally, the primary purpose of health care was to provide services to those who were ill or injured. These services were typically delivered in a hospital or clinic-like setting. Currently, an awareness and interest in maintaining optimal health are resulting in a movement toward preventative care and primary care as a means to promote health. This focus has produced substantial changes to the way health-care services are delivered and how health-care professionals interact with these systems. As health-care professionals, nurses need to understand these systems. Nursing practice is influenced by societal and cultural realities and needs to adapt to the changing world that affects everyday practice. Today's health-care institutions are heavily impacted by cost delivery, access to services, and health-care professionals.

DEMOGRAPHICS AFFECTING HEALTH-CARE DELIVERY

Age

Between now and the year 2050, the number of persons 65 years of age or older is expected to double, so that by 2050, one in five people living in Canada or the United States will be elderly, and their numbers will reach an estimated 80 million.[1] Of this number, many will eventually become more dependent on the health-care delivery system as a result of chronic health problems.

Although an aging population constitutes a sizable number of persons who will potentially require expensive long-term health care, their community activism and powerful influence at the ballot box may provide them with better access to health care than other less vocal and politically savvy groups. Additional at-risk groups consist of persons residing in urban areas with limited incomes as well as individuals living in remote rural areas where access to care is limited.

Chronicity

Another factor influencing the climate of health-care delivery is the long-term and expensive nature of many health problems. Although significant strides have been made in the treatment of some acute infectious diseases, many challenges still exist in the management of health concerns such as cancer, heart disease, Alzheimer's disease, diabetes, chronic obstructive lung disease, and human immunodeficiency virus (HIV). Additional concerns include environmental and occupational safety, drug abuse, and mother and child health care.

HEALTH CARE AS AN INDUSTRY

In most developed countries, health care is one of the largest industries. According to the World Health Organization, total expenditures on health accounted for 9.6 percent of the gross domestic product in Canada and 14.6 percent in the United States.[1] These numbers alone indicate the significance of health care and health-care spending to the people of these two countries.

In the United States, with the introduction of managed care, the organizations that pay for health care have the capacity to dramatically influence who provides care, how the care is furnished, and who receives compensation.[2] The significance to the economy, along with other factors, is evident.

> *In most developed countries, health care is one of the largest industries.*

> *According to the World Health Organization, total expenditures on health accounted for 9.6 percent of the gross domestic product in Canada and 14.6 percent in the United States.*

Health Care in the Global Context

Understanding the approach to health care in comparison to other countries is important in assessing the challenges to and potential of health care delivery. How and why health-care systems differ is a function of multiple influences. These may include societal values and beliefs, sociocultural climate, the state of the economy, political realities, geographic density, international influences, historical realities, established practices and programs, and other factors. For health-care systems to develop, several factors must come into play at different points. This development is similar for health-care systems throughout the world, as can be seen by examining the contexts in which various health-care systems were developed.

One way to think about system differences is to consider that Western countries provide for health-care in a variety of ways, all of which involve variable combinations of private or public funding of services and private or public delivery of services.[3] Table 17.1 shows the degree of public involvement in financing health services and the essential role envisioned for the health care system.[4]

Type I Systems

In the type I health care system, private approaches to health services predominate and physicians and other caregivers (such as midwives) and clients have

Table 17.1 Types of Health Care Systems in the Western World

Type I	Type II	Type III	Type IV
Private health insurance	National health insurance	National health service	Socialized health system
Primary goal: preserve autonomy	Primary goal: egalitarian	Primary goal: egalitarian	Primary goal: essential service
Secondary effect: acceptance of social differences	Secondary effect: preserve autonomy	Secondary effect; public management	Secondary effect: physicians as state employees

Najman, J, and Western, J: A comparative analysis of Australian health policy in the 1970's. Social Science and Medicine 18(1):949–958, 1984.

maximum autonomy. In this plan, individuals who can afford private health insurance, or who simply can pay for their health care, chose their care providers and receive health services. Those who cannot pay do not have choice or benefit.

In the pure form of the type 1 system, there would be no option other than to pay for service. In reality, most countries have adopted a mixture of system types. For example, although the United States has a mainly private payment system of health care, some publicly funded programs assist elderly and poor people. Even with these programs, it is estimated that 45 percent of Americans have no health insurance and therefore are limited in their ability to access health care.

Type IV Systems

On the opposite end of the spectrum from type 1 is type IV. This type of health-care system focuses on keeping the general public healthy so they can continue to contribute to society and the economy. Health care is considered an essential service or even a right, not necessarily involving compassionate motives, and the goal is to keep the population healthy so that national productivity will remain high. Physicians are considered agents of the state who work to keep others working efficiently.

In Canada, the type IV structure is seen in such organizations as the military, hockey teams, and other sports teams. Physicians are hired by these organizations to ensure the players stay healthy and can do their part to achieve the goals of the group.

Type III Systems

Between the extremes of type I and type IV health-care systems are two less extreme types. The type III system is funded and operated by the government as was seen in the health-care system of Great Britain some years ago. With this system, the state-operated and state-funded health services were on the basis of an egalitarian value. Public management of each service was considered key to efficient and effective operation.

Type II Systems

The type II system is a hybrid of type I and type III systems, wherein egalitarian values are given high priority but so is practitioner and client autonomy. The type II health-care system uses tax dollars to pay for health services through health insurance available from a nonprofit agency (e.g., government).

Each health service is operated more or less autonomously by others including municipalities,

citizen groups, physicians, nurse practitioners, or physiotherapists in private offices, group practices, or other groups. All services rendered to clients are then paid from the central pool of health insurance funds created through taxation. This type of system is used in Canada and embodies the collective sharing of burdens and benefits while allowing a degree of autonomy in delivery.[5]

Third World Alternatives

It is important to note that the four systems described above exclude a group of third world countries that cannot afford the type of health care that is enjoyed in most developed countries. Yet, many third world countries have managed to develop primary care systems that are not as institution dependent as the systems found in Canada and the United States. In their systems, primary care includes preventive health care, first point of contact, and continuing care. However, in some countries, their primary and preventive systems have been undermined by the influence of Western countries promoting high technology and institutionalization.

What Do Taxes Cover?

Even in countries that finance health insurance through tax dollars, there are variations in services provided. For example, some fund home care but others do not; some provide coverage for prescription

---

What Do You Think?

What type of health-care system was used the last time you accessed health care? Did you use the health-care system for preventive care or illness care?

Issues in Practice

Numbers of Americans without Health Insurance Continues to Rise

The United States does not offer universal health insurance coverage to its citizens as Canada and many European nations do. Most Americans receive coverage through their employers or purchase it from private insurance companies.

The Institute of Medicine estimates that over 18,000 Americans die each year because they lack health insurance. Even with coverage, approximately 14 percent of families in the United States have accumulated enough debt from medical expenses to place a significant strain on their financial resources.

The Centers for Disease Control (CDC) has been collecting health insurance data since 1997, when the rate of uninsured adults in the United States was 12.8 percent. By 2002, that number had risen to 19.1 percent, and in 2003, the last year for which data is available, 20.1 percent lacked health insurance. Notably, the increase in uninsured people occurred during a downturn in the economy when the country was experiencing a rise in unemployment. Of the 43.6 million Americans without health insurance, Hispanics have rates three times higher than whites and almost twice that of blacks.

On the positive side, the United States improved its health-care coverage for children. The rate of children without health insurance coverage decreased from 13.9 percent in 1997 to 10.1 percent in 2003. Officials at the CDC's National Center for Health Statistics cite efforts by states to increase coverage for children living at or near the poverty line as the most significant factor in this increase.

1. Do you think the United States should have universal health care insurance? Why or why not?
2. Do you know anybody who does not have health insurance and had to use the ER or go to the hospital? How are they paying the bills?
3. If a person without health insurance goes to the hospital and cannot pay the bill, how are those expenses covered?

Source: Reuters, CNN.Com Wednesday, July 1, 2004.

drugs and others do not. Regardless of the type of system, it is important to reflect on the influences that have created it and continue to maintain it.

ADMINISTRATION AND FUNDING OF HEALTH-CARE SYSTEMS

Financing and administering health-care systems can be an overwhelming responsibility. The Canadian government spends $2048 on health per year for each of its citizens. The United States government spends $2368 per citizen per year. The total expenditure on health, including both private and pubic spending is $2222 per person in Canada and $5274 in the United States. With these staggering numbers, it is easy to see how this billion-dollar industry can be difficult to manage.

Health Care in Canada

In Canada, health-care services are provided under the Canada Health Act. The Canadian federal government collects funds through taxes and gives the responsibility of administering health care services to the provinces. As in the United States, the cost of financing health-care services has risen tremendously since the first Medical Care Act was introduced in 1967–1968. In Canada, medical insurance premiums became an increasing burden for the federal government as a result of the improved services promised to all Canadians.

Federal Transfer Payments

In an attempt to control the costs to be paid to all provinces, the Canadian government proposed a system of block funding. In 1977 the Federal-Provincial Arrangements and Established Programs Financing Act was established after lengthy negotiations with all provinces. The formula for federal transfer payments consisted of four components:

1. Per capita payments were made, on the basis of previous expenditures and adjusted regularly in relation to the gross national product (GNP).
2. Tax points were transferred by the federal government, allowing provinces to reduce their tax contribution to the federal government and at the same time increase the portion of tax collected at the provincial level.

3. Equalization of tax points was distributed among poorer provinces.
4. Additional per capita payments were indexed to help pay for nursing home care, residential care, home care, and ambulatory care.

This new act changed the funding formulae from a 50-50 cost sharing arrangement to one that gave taxation points to the provinces in exchange for lower cash transfer payments. The provinces were initially very receptive, as this meant they had more taxation power in an economy that was very healthy. However, with rising costs of health care, owing in part to an aging population and increased technology, some physicians and provinces struggled with health-care coverage. With extra billing or balance billing becoming prevalent, there was a heated public debate, and the new Canada Health Act was passed in 1984.

The Canada Health Act

Although the Canadian federal government has a limited constitutional basis for making health-care decisions, it has considerable economic clout to develop and shape a national health-care plan. To support their positions on health care, the federal government enacted the Canada Health Act (CHA). The purpose of the CHA is to "establish criteria and conditions in respect of insured health services and extended health care services provided under provincial law that must be met before a full cash contribution may be made."[6]

The insured health services defined by the CHA include all medically necessary hospital services and medically required physician services, as well as medically or dentally required surgical-dental services that needed to be performed in a hospital for safety. New criteria, conditions and provisions were formulated to eliminate extra-billing and user charges.

For the provinces to qualify for full cash refunds from the federal government under the Canada Health and Social Transfer agreement (CHST), they must meet five basic criteria and conditions. These criteria and conditions must be met for each fiscal year and include:

1. Public Administration: The health-care insurance plan must be administered and operated on a non-profit basis by a public authority, responsible to the provincial government and subject to audit of its accounts and financial transactions.

2. Comprehensiveness: The plan must ensure all insured health services provided by hospitals, medical practitioners, and dentists and, where permitted, services rendered by other health-care practitioners.

3. Universality: One hundred percent of the insured population of a province must be entitled to the insured health services provided for by the plan on uniform terms and conditions.

4. Portability: Residents moving to another province must continue to be covered for insured health services by the home province during any minimum waiting period imposed by the new provinces of residence not to exceed three months. For insured persons, insured health services must be made available while they are temporarily absent from their own provinces on the following basis:

   • Insured services received out of province, but still in Canada, are to be paid for by the home province at host province rates unless another arrangement for the payment of costs exists between the provinces. Prior approval may be required for elective services.

   • Out-of-country services received are to be paid, as a minimum, on the basis of the amount that would have been paid by the home province for similar services rendered in the province. Prior approval may be required for elective services.

5. Accessibility: The health-care insurance plan of a province must provide for:

   • Insured health services on uniform terms and conditions and reasonable access by insured persons to insured health services not precluded and unimpeded, either directly or indirectly, by charges or other means

   • Reasonable compensation to physicians and dentists for all insured health services rendered

   • Payments to hospitals in respect to the cost of insured health services

Although discussion and debate continue surrounding the federal and provincial responsibilities for health-care funding and the escalating costs associated with health care, the Canada Health Act of 1984 continues to be the model that the Canadian health-care system operates under.

> *According to the World Health Organization, the United States spends more per person on health care than any other country, yet in overall quality its care ranks 37th in the world.*

U.S. Health-Care Systems

The United States has a far different method of funding and administering health-care services. According to the World Health Organization, the United States spends more per person on health care than any other country, yet in overall quality its care ranks 37th in the world. This disparity is attributed in large part to the cost of health-care services, not the quality of the services available.

In the attempt to contain some of these costs, professional standards review organizations (PSROs) were introduced to review the quality, quantity, and cost of hospital care through Medicare. The primary goal of PSROs was to review the care provided by physicians to determine if the best diagnostic and treatment approaches were being used. Another measure was the introduction of utilization

What Do You Think?

Review the bill from your last hospitalization or the bill of a family member. What do you think about the charges listed? Does the bill seem excessive?

_____

_____

_____

_____

_____

_____

_____

_____

_____

_____

_____

_____

_____

_____

review committees requiring Medicare-qualified facilities to review admission, diagnostic testing, and treatments provided to clients with the goal of eliminating overuse or misuse of services.

Prospective Payment Systems

Although these measures have assisted with cost containment to some degree, one of the most significant factors that has influenced cost control was the prospective payment system (PPS) that was established by the U.S. Congress in 1983. This system required facilities providing services to Medicare clients to be reimbursed using a fixed-rate system and included monetary incentives to reduce the length of hospital stays. Medicare clients are classified using a diagnosis-related group (DRG), and the facilities are reimbursed a predetermined amount. Clients may be classified into one of 468 DRGs, and reimbursement occurs regardless of the length of stay.

If the client is discharged sooner than anticipated, the facility keeps the difference. If the client requires a lengthier hospital stay, the hospital pays the extra cost. Under the PPS, the emphasis is on the efficient delivery of services in the most cost-effective manner.

Capitated Payment Systems

Capitation, or a capitated payment system, is a health-care payment structure that was introduced to encourage cost effectiveness in a growing health-care system. In a capitated payment system, participants pay a flat rate, usually through their employer, to belong to a managed care organization (MCO) for a specified period of time. The health-care providers who serve the participants receive a fixed amount for each participant in the health-care plan.[7]

Controlled Access

The goal of capitation is to have a payment plan for selected diseases or surgical procedures that provides the highest quality of care, including essential diagnostic and treatment procedures, at the lowest cost possible. Any expenses that are in excess of the capitated rate are the responsibility of the MCO. If the MCO spends less on the care of a client than it is given for delivery costs, it can keep the excess as profit, providing it with a strong incentive to reduce the cost of services.

> *The effectiveness of the MCO plan rests on the theory that health-care costs can be reduced by decreasing the number of hospitalizations, shortening the length of inpatient stays, providing less-expensive home care services, and keeping people healthy through health promotion and illness prevention services.*

Another goal of managed care is to enhance the efficiency and effective use of health-care services. A key underlying concept of managed care is to maintain administrative control over access and provision of primary health-care services for the members of the plan. The MCO controls all aspects of care including delivery, financing, and the purchase of health-care services for clients who are enrolled in the program. Clients are allowed to use only the services of primary care physicians who are approved by the organization. Any referrals to other medical specialists must be approved by the MCO. The MCO contract determines what treatments or procedures will be reimbursed.

A Spending Increase

The effectiveness of the MCO plan rests on the theory that health-care costs can be reduced by decreasing the number of hospitalizations, shortening the length of inpatient stays, providing less-expensive home care services, and keeping people healthy through health promotion and illness prevention services. It is logical to conclude that if people stay healthy, the cost of health-care services should decline.

Although much debate surrounds managed care and its advantages and disadvantages, the reality is that managed care has *not* reduced health-care costs nationally. The Centers for Medicare and Medicaid Services (CMS),[1] reports that although health-care spending evened out during the late 1990s, total health-care expenditures grew from $888 billion in 1993 to $1299 trillion in 2002. This increase in spending is attributed to rising health-care wages, legislation that increased Medicare

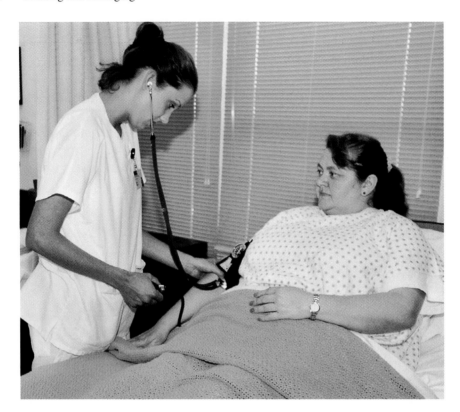

spending, increasing insurance premiums, technology, and consumer demands for less restrictive plans.

QUALITY ASSURANCE

Continuous Quality Improvement

Quality assurance initiatives are essential when efforts are being made to cut costs and, at the same time, maintain high standards of care. To ensure high-quality care, the health-care industry borrowed the philosophy of **continuous quality improvement (CQI)** from the business world. The **Joint Commission on Accreditation of Healthcare Organizations (JCAHO)** was so impressed with its potential to improve health-care delivery that in 1994 it began requiring hospitals to implement CQI strategies.

Exceeding Expectations

CQI, also known as **total quality management (TQM),** is on the basis of the belief that the organi-

zation with the higher-quality service will capture a greater share of the market than competitors with lower-quality services. Emphasis is placed on not only meeting the expectations of the customer (in this case, the health-care consumer) but exceeding those expectations.

According to the CQI philosophy, there are internal customers and external customers. The external customers are clients and their families; internal customers are individuals working within the health-care setting. Delivering high-quality services is valued above all else, and the ideal goal is that every constituent be completely satisfied with the services provided.

A Proactive Approach

Continuous quality improvement requires that the process used to deliver services receive close and constant scrutiny, and everyone is encouraged to generate ideas for improving quality. Although change on the basis of systematically documented evidence is encouraged, standardization of the process is also valued so that efficiency is maximized. CQI is proactively oriented so that emphasis is placed on anticipating and preventing problems rather than reacting to them after the fact.

Nurses are in an excellent position to implement CQI strategies. On a daily basis, they assess the functioning of the health-care delivery system and the effectiveness of specific treatment approaches. For example, on the basis of evidence that inexpensive saline is as effective as heparin in keeping intermittent intravenous catheters patent, nurses at one hospital implemented a new protocol and saved $70,000 within 1 year.[8]

Case Management Protocols

Another mechanism that has been instituted for monitoring cost-effective quality care is outcomes-based case management protocols, also known as **clinical pathways.** The development of clinical pathways grew out of a need to assess, implement, and monitor cost-effective high-quality client care in a systematic manner.

Clinical pathways were an outgrowth of nursing care plans but have the advantages of streamlining the charting process, encouraging documentation across multidisciplinary team members, and systematically monitoring variances from prescribed plans of care. The ability to identify how client care and progress varies from a predetermined plan

enables more accurate assessment of client care costs and maintenance of quality control measures. Integration of clinical pathways into practical usage has been enhanced by computerization of client records and on-line bedside documentation.

Overview of Health-Care Plans

See Boxes 17.1 through 17.5 to compare the principal features of different health-care models.

HEALTH-CARE LEVELS AND SETTINGS

Even though there are many methods for providing and funding health care, providing high-quality health care services remains the highest priority. Consumers who have access to multiple types of health care may not always understand the differences among them.

> " *It is believed that a focus on wellness and a population living a healthier lifestyle will reduce the number of people who require expensive illness-care services.* "

Box 17.1

Managed Care Organizations (MCOs)

Definition: Provide comprehensive, preventive, and treatment services to a specific group of voluntarily enrolled persons.

Managed Care Structures

Staff model: physicians are salaried employees of the MCO
Group model: MCO contracts with single group practice
Network model: MCO contracts with multiple group practices and/or integrated organizations
Independent practice association (IPA): MCO contracts with physicians who usually are not members of groups and whose practices include fee-for-service and capitated clients.
Characteristics: Focus on health maintenance and primary care. All care provided by a primary care physician. Referral needed for access to specialists and hospitalization.

Medicare MCO

Definition: Program same as MCO but designated to cover health-care costs of senior citizens
Characteristics: Premium generally less than supplemental plans

Box 17.2

Provider Organizations

Preferred Provider Organization (PPO)

Definition: One that limits an enrollee's choice to a list of "preferred" hospitals, physicians, and providers. An enrollee pays more out-of-pocket expenses for using a provider not on the list.

Characteristics: Contractual agreement exists between a set of providers and one or more purchasers (self-insured employers or insurance plans). Comprehensive health services at a discount for companies under contract.

Exclusive Provider Organization (EPO)

Definition: One that limits an enrollee's choice to providers belonging to one organization. May or may not be able to use outside providers at additional expense.
Characteristics: Limited contractual agreement; less access to specialists.

In the past, health-care services were primarily illness or institution based and focused primarily on treating the ill or injured. The emphasis is now shifting slowly toward prevention and health promotion of the population. It is believed that a focus on

Box 17.3

Medicare

Definition: Federally funded national health insurance program in the United States for people over age 65. Part A provides for basic protection for medical, surgical, and psychiatric care costs based on DRGs. Part B is a voluntary medical insurance plan that covers physician and certain outpatient services.

Characteristics: Payment for plan deducted from monthly individual Social Security check; covers services of nurse practitioners (varies by state); does not pay full costs of certain services; supplemental insurance is encouraged.

Box 17.4

Medicaid

Definition: Federally funded, state-operated program of medical assistance to people with low incomes. Individual states determine eligibility and benefits.

Characteristics: Finances a large portion of maternal and child care for the poor; reimburses for nurse midwifery and other advanced practice nurses (varies by state); reimburses long-term care facility funding.

wellness and a population living a healthier lifestyle will reduce the number of people who require expensive illness care services.

Levels of Service

Health-care services are frequently categorized according to the complexity or level of the services provided, and this complexity relates to the kinds, or levels, of services: primary, secondary, and tertiary.

Primary Care

In nursing, primary care refers to health promotion and preventative care including programs such as

Box 17.5

Private Insurance

Traditional Private Insurance

Definition: Traditional fee-for-service plan. Payment computed after services are provided on basis of the number of services used.

Characteristics: Policies typically expensive; most policies have deductibles that clients must meet before insurance pays.

Long-term Care Insurance

Definition: Supplemental insurance for coverage of long-term care services. Policies provide a set amount of dollars for an unlimited time or for as little as 2 years.

Characteristics: Very expensive; good policy has a minimum waiting period for eligibility, payment for skilled nursing, intermediate or custodial care, and home care.

immunization campaigns. Primary care focuses on health education and on early detection and treatment. Maintaining and improving optimal health is the overriding goal.

Secondary Care

In the secondary level, the focus shifts toward emergency and acute care. Secondary services are frequently provided in hospitals and other acute care settings, with an emphasis on diagnosis and the treatment of complex disorders.

Tertiary Care

The tertiary level emphasizes rehabilitative services, long-term care, and care of the dying. Nursing services are essential in all three levels of health care, including both hospital and community settings.

What Do You Think?

Have you ever received care in a "nontraditional" health-care setting? What was it? What role did nurses play in the delivery of care?

_____

_____

_____

_____

_____

_____

_____

_____

_____

_____

Health-Care Settings

While nursing care is provided in traditional settings such as the hospital and the community, nursing services are also delivered in a growing number of nontraditional locations. One growing trend in care is seen in the outpatient departments attached to some hospitals. Outpatient services are used by clients who require a relatively high level of skilled health care

but who do not need to stay in a hospital for an extended period of time. An inpatient is a person who enters a setting such as a hospital and remains for at least 24 hours. Whether the client is an inpatient or outpatient, they often need assistance from the nurse to identify which services best suit their needs.

Today, the scope of public health, while retaining its contagious disease and prevention mission, has expanded to areas such as child health, obstetrical and pregnancy care, and more recently into the early detection and treatment of terrorist acts, particularly bioterrorism.

Public Health

Public health departments are government agencies that are established at the local, provincial or state, and federal levels to provide health services. The goal of early public health departments was to prevent and control communicable diseases that were rampant in the eighteenth and nineteenth centuries, producing epidemics that killed millions of people. Today, the scope of public health, while retaining its contagious disease and prevention mission, has expanded to areas such as child health, obstetrical and pregnancy care, and more recently into the early detection and treatment of terrorist acts, particularly bioterrorism (see Chapter 22).

School-Based Services

Nurses provide a variety of services within local school systems. These services include screenings, health promotion and illness prevention programs, and treatment of minor health-care problems. Emphasis is placed on physical, social, and psychological well-being. Concerns relating to self-esteem, stress, drug abuse, and adolescent pregnancy are frequently addressed by the school nurse. In addition, children and adolescents with long-term health problems often attend school, and it is not uncommon for the nurse to be consulted about such issues as seizure management, colostomy care, or gastric tube feedings.

    Students who have health concerns are frequently referred to providers within the community, and an important role of the school nurse is that of community liaison. For this reason, the nurse must be knowledgeable about community resources and adept at getting clients into the system in a timely and efficient manner.

Community Health Centers

Community health centers are being more frequently used in many communities. Most centers use a team approach involving physicians, nurse practitioners, and community nurses working together to provide health services. Most centers have diagnostic and treatment facilities that provide medical, nursing, laboratory, and radiological services. Some centers may also provide outpatient minor surgical procedures that allow clients to remain at home while accessing health services as needed.

Physician's Offices and General Clinics

The physician's office continues to be the location where most North Americans access primary health care. The majority of physicians in North America continue to work either in their own office, or with a group of physicians in a group practice. Services range from routine health screening to illness diagnosis and treatment and even some minor surgical procedures.

The responsibilities of nurses who work in physicians' offices or in general clinics include obtaining personal health information and histories of current illness and preparing the client for examination. Nurses also assist with procedures and obtain specimens for laboratory analysis. Teaching clients basic health information and home management of treatments and medications is also a responsibility of the clinic nurse.

Occupational Health Clinics

Maintaining the health of workers in their workplaces to increase productivity has long been recognized as an important role for nurses. In response to rising health insurance costs, today's employers are increasingly supportive of workplace health promotion, illness prevention, and safety programs. Many companies provide wellness programs and encourage or even require their employees to participate. These services range from providing exercise facilities and fitness programs, to health screenings and referrals. Illness prevention focuses on topics such as smoking cessation, stress management, and nutrition.

Although some companies may hire health educators to manage their clinics, community health nurses often provide these services.

In Canada, occupational health nurses are registered nurses (RNs) holding a minimum of a diploma or BS degree in nursing. Many may also have occupational health certification, or a degree in occupational health and safety from a community college or university. Nurses who are certified in occupational health nursing must meet eligibility requirements, pass a written examination, and be recognized as having achieved a level of competency in occupational health. The certification is granted by the Canadian Nurses Association.

Hospitals

Hospitals, the traditional provider of health-care services, are still an essential part of the health-care system and still provide the majority of nurses with employment. Hospitals range in size from small, rural facilities with as few as 15 to 20 beds to large urban centers that may exceed a bed capacity of several thousand.

Depending on the services they provide, hospitals will have varying classifications. General hospitals offer a variety of services such as medical, surgical, obstetric, pediatrics, and psychiatric services. Other hospitals may offer specialized services such as pediatric care. Hospitals can be further classified as acute-care or chronic care, depending on the length of stay of the client and the services available. Large hospitals may be designated as specific centers for treatment, such as a trauma or cardiac center because they can offer specialized services.

Long-Term Care Facilities

The majority of senior citizens in North America continue to live in their own homes. However, a growing group of seniors have health needs that require long-term care or extended care services. Some individuals may require rehabilitation or intermediate care, while others require extended, long-term care. These services are provided for both the elderly and younger clients who have similar needs, such as clients with spinal cord injuries.

The current trend in extended care facilities is to provide care in a home-like atmosphere and have programs that are based on the needs and abilities of the clients, or residents as they are commonly called, of the facility. Many of these residents require personal services such as bathing and assistance with activities of daily living. Others may require higher-level skilled nursing care such as tube feedings and catheter management or even occasional medical attention. Because of the range of needs of clients, some facilities will admit clients with specific needs to specific areas of the facility where the appropriate services are provided.

In Canada, admission to long-term care facilities must meet specific guidelines. Assessments of client needs and the nursing services available must be completed prior to admitting the client to the facility. Frequently, there are waiting lists for admission to extended care facilities.

In the United States, many long-term care facilities are for-profit institutions that rely heavily on Medicaid and Medicare reimbursements.[8] When Medicare coverage is limited, the resident must use private insurance or personal resources to pay the difference in cost.

> *Hospitals, the traditional provider of health-care services, are still an essential part of the health-care system and still provide the majority of nurses with employment.*

Retirement and Assisted Living Centers

As the population continues to age, assisted living centers are increasing in popularity because they allow clients, or residents, to maintain the greatest amount of independence possible in a partially controlled and supervised living environment. These centers consist of separate apartments or condominiums for the residents and provide services such as meal preparation and laundry services.

Many centers work closely with home care and other social services to provide the resources required for maintaining a degree of independence. Case coordinators, often nurses, assist residents with navigating their way through the complex paperwork usually involved in obtaining required services. Some assisted-living centers are attached to long-term care facilities. Depending on the level of care required, residents may be transferred to various facilities as their care needs change.

Rehabilitation Centers

In many acute care facilities, discharge planning and rehabilitative needs are discussed at the time of admission. Rehabilitation centers or units are similar to some extended care facilities where the client goal is to restore health and function to an optimum level. Often clients are admitted to rehabilitation units after recuperating from the acute stage of an injury or illness. The rehabilitation unit then provides services to complete the recovery and restore a high degree of independence.

Some common types of rehabilitation units include geriatric, chemical dependency, stroke, and spinal cord injury units. Nurses who work on these units have the responsibility of coordinating health-care services, providing skilled care when required, supervising less-educated personnel, and ensuring client compliance with treatment regimes.

Day-Care Centers

Day-care centers can be used by any age group. Traditionally, day-care centers have referred to the care of children; however, over the past 10 years, adult day-care centers have become relatively common. Adult day-care centers provide services for elderly adults who cannot be left at home alone but are not at point where they require institutionalization.

Services provided by adult day-care centers include health maintenance classes, socialization and exercise programs, physical or occupational therapy, rehabilitative services, and organized recreational activities. Nurses who are employed in adult day-care centers may administer medications, give treatments, provide counseling and teaching, and coordinate services between day care and home care.

Rural Primary Care

A Problem of Distance

Delivering health-care services to the rural areas of North America is a challenge because of the great distances between homes. In many rural towns, it is common to have small hospitals or other health-care facilities available to provide basic health-care services. Most of these facilities have basic laboratory and radiological services available.

In the far north of Canada, aboriginal communities have nursing stations or health centers in the community to provide basic health services. The centers are staffed by nurses. Visiting physicians come in occasionally to provide additional services. The nursing stations also provide emergency services to people who require stabilization before being transferred to a larger facility.

A Problem of Cost

In the United States, paying for health-care services in rural areas is a concern. Many of the residents in rural areas are farmers or employees of small businesses that do not offer health insurance. A type of group insurance called health insurance purchasing cooperatives (HIPS) is now available to Americans who are self-employed or who do not have health insurance for other reasons. This program allows larger groups of people or employers to band together to purchase health insurance at a reduced cost.

However, even with this health insurance option, approximately 45 million Americans (15.6% of population) do not have health insurance.[9] In April 2005, the U.S. Senate proposed a bill to promote the development of health-care cooperatives that would allow small businesses owners to join together with the goal of increasing their power for the purchase of health insurance. If this bill passes, it should increase the number of Americans with health insurance.

Hospice Services

Hospice care originated in Great Britain and has changed the way end-of-life care is delivered. Disillusioned with health-care services that focused on technology and the preservation of life at all costs, the hospice movement gained momentum in the 1970s. Hospice care emphasizes physiological and psychological support for clients who have terminal diseases. Hospice care provides a variety of services in a caring and a supportive environment to terminally ill clients, their families, and other support persons. The central concept of hospice care is not on saving life, but on improving or maintaining the quality of life until death occurs.

Telehealth and E-health

Telehealth, or telephone health, advice services have experienced major growth in Canada in recent years. These services are generally available 24 hours a day, seven days a week. Nurses man the phones, supply answers to health-related questions and advise callers on how to handle nonurgent health situations.[3]

"For animal bites, please press 3."

Although telehealth activities have grown significantly in the past 3 to 4 years, its full potential has not yet been reached. The success of telehealth rests on a full and seamless integration of the service as part of the health-care delivery system. Understanding and eliminating barriers to telehealth's use while capitalizing on the opportunities it presents will eventually improve the acceptance and mainstreaming of telehealth technologies. Telehealth is discussed in detail in Chapter 18.

E-health, electronic health advice, takes the telephone into the computer age. Rather than calling a resource center for information, the client can use a computer to access any number of sites that provide health-care information. Unfortunately, some of the information available on-line may not be completely accurate. Persons who use these resources need to evaluate their quality and the accuracy of the information they provide.

Parish Nurses

It is estimated that approximately 2000 parish nurses throughout the United States are attempting to meet the needs of individuals who are without adequate primary care or who are experiencing escalating health-care costs. Many of these nurses work part-time or are volunteers, and some work in conjunction with community-based programs. Churches engage parish nurses to:

• Serve as health educators and counselors
• Do health assessments and referrals
• Organize support groups
• Visit parishioners who are sick or elderly
• Serve as client advocates or case managers

Parish nurses are in a unique position to exercise their skills as case managers. As nurses, they possess clinical knowledge and skills, understand the health-care delivery system in their communities, and know many of the key health-care providers. As members of their parish, they are intimately familiar with their communities, understand the cultural climate of their clientele, and are familiar with the services that are available. Moreover, as members of the church community they serve, they are likely to be familiar with the spiritual, psychosocial, and financial needs of their clients. However, direct reimbursement is not yet available for parish nurses.

Voluntary Health Agencies

Since their inception in 1892, voluntary health agencies have experienced steady growth to the point where they currently number more than 100,000. The first voluntary health agency was the Anti-tuberculosis Society of Philadelphia. Some of the more well-known agencies that exist today include the American Cancer Society, The American Heart Association, The National Foundation for the March of Dimes, The National Easter Seal Society for Crippled Adults and Children, and the Alliance for the Mentally Ill.

These agencies provide many valuable services, including fundraising in support of cutting-edge research and public education. Some, such as the American Cancer Society, which has a strong emphasis on education and research, also help individuals secure special equipment such as hospital beds for the home and wigs for chemotherapy patients. The Alliance for the Mentally Ill is very politically active and organizes support groups for the mentally ill and their families. These groups are not-for-profit organizations, so that all revenue in excess of cost goes toward improving services.

Independent Nurse-Run Health Centers

Similar to community health centers, nurse-run health centers tend to focus on health promotion and disease prevention. Historically, they have been service rather than profit oriented and remain so today. Nurses who are interested in autonomous practice often work in these settings.

Several types of nurse-run health centers have been identified. Among these are community health and institutional outreach centers. These facilities may be freestanding or sponsored by a larger institution, such as a university or public health agency. Primary care services are generally offered to the medically underserved, and these centers are typically funded by public and private sources.

Wellness and health-promotion clinics are another type of nurse-run clinic that offer services at work sites, schools, churches, or homeless shelters. Many of these centers are affiliated with schools of nursing, providing health-care services while offering educational experiences for nursing students.

A final type of nursing center includes faculty practice, independent practice, and nurse entrepreneurship models. These facilities are owned and operated by nurses and may be solo or multidisciplinary practices. Services are typically reimbursed through fee-for-service, grant monies, and insurance. The ability of nurses in these centers to secure payments through the newly emergent and complex health-care reimbursement network will in large part determine the future financial viability of these types of clinics.

HEALTH-CARE COSTS AND THE NURSING SHORTAGE

A Cost-Cutting Measure

The origins of the current nursing shortage can be traced directly back to the implementation of managed care in the 1990s as a method of controlling health-care costs. Managed care companies required many procedures to be performed outside the hospital, leading to clients being sicker when they do enter the hospitals.

An Expensive Mistake

Health-care facilities trying to cut costs hired fewer expensive RNs in favor of less-expensive personnel. Nursing service at most facilities is the largest single budget item, averaging between 50 and 60 percent of the overall operating budget. At first glance, this seemed like a promising way to control health-care costs, but in the long run it turned out to be a very expensive mistake. RNs who were employed in acute care settings moved in droves to the home-health-care and primary care settings. At the same time, the population was aging, resulting in a need for more nurses who can deliver high-quality specialized care in the acute care facilities.

As a result, the health-care industry has seen a trend of closing hospital units because of a lack of RNs. It is estimated that a closed 20-bed general medical/surgical unit will cost a hospital approximately $3 million in lost revenue per year.

Stress on the Nurse

The nurses who remain are finding working conditions to be less than ideal. Mandatory overtime, short staffing, and increased acuity of client conditions all are adding to the stress these nurses experience. As a result, they call in sick more often or leave for other facilities that have fewer demands. Sick time, recruitment, and orientation costs for many facilities have skyrocketed as a result.

Stress on the Facility

The other area where health-care institutions feel the cost of the RN shortage is in lawsuits and rising insurance costs. During periods when there is a shortage of RNs, the quality of health care decreases, clients become dissatisfied with the care they are receiving, and serious mistakes are made in care, resulting in injury or death of clients. It only takes a relatively few of these cases with awards in the range of tens of millions of dollars to re-emphasize the correlation between RN care and quality care.

Staffing Ratio Laws

One proposed solution to the nursing shortage problem is the passage of mandatory staffing ratio laws. Of course, hospital associations see these as increasing operating costs. However, the presumption is that more RNs will equate higher quality of care and ultimately reduced long-range health-care costs.

Although laws have been passed in California, Florida, and other states, their implementation seems to be inconsistent. Hospital association groups in several states have challenges to the laws that have effectively blocked their implementation for the time being. However, nursing groups generally support these laws and see them as a way to solve staffing shortages by enticing inactive nurses or nurses who

have sought employment in other health-care areas to return to the bedside in acute care facilities.

A Lack of Information

Not everyone, including some in the nursing profession, is convinced that enforced staff-to-client ratios will cure an ailing health-care system. One of the key issues is a lack of documented research that demonstrates that more RNs per clients equals higher-quality care. Intuitively, it would seem that putting more RNs back into the hospital would improve client care, yet more than 6 years ago the Institute of Medicine identified a dearth of information about the quality of care being delivered in the nation's acute care facilities.

The documentation and research have been slow to develop, although an increasing body of knowledge is now available. Leaders in the nursing profession hope the new staffing ratio laws will help demonstrate the important and critical part nurses play in providing high-quality care.

Beyond the Numbers

Some in nursing are concerned that managed care facilities will use the mandated staffing ratio as a ceiling number rather than the minimum number of nurses required to provide safe care. There is also a fear that the facilities will look only at the numbers and not at the educational, skill, and experience levels of the nurses they use to meet their quotas. Without consideration of the acuity of client conditions on a unit and the care needs related to their illnesses, staffing ratios may actually lower the quality of care and threaten the safety of the clients. In addition, some fear that facilities that find the staffing ratio laws unworkable will merely close units where sicker clients are being treated, thus reducing access to care.

A More Acute Problem

Some farsighted nursing leaders see the passage of staffing ratio laws as an important, but short-term, solution to a much broader problem. Decreasing nurse-to-patient ratios are just a symptom of a much more acute systemic problem in the health-care industry. The underlying problem revolves around an overly aggressive policy of cost cutting by managed care, often at the expense of the very clients who support the system with their insurance premiums.

Issues Now

More RNs Equals Better Care

To most people, it would seem logical to conclude that a hospital with more RNs would be able to provide higher-quality care than a hospital with fewer RNs. However, some managers in the health-care industry have refuted the logic behind this deduction.

A new study, funded primarily by the U.S. government, set out to determine whether there was a correlation between RN-to-client staffing and the quality of the care provided. The massive study reviewed the outcomes of more than 6 million clients at 799 hospitals in 11 states, 5 million of whom had medical problems and 1 million who had surgery.

The results show that in regard to certain elements of care, the presence of more RNs increased the quality of care. A comparison between those hospitals with the highest RN-to-client ratios to those with the lowest RN-to-client ratios revealed the following results:

Client Care Area	Results of Increased RN Staffing
Length of stay (surgical)	Reduced by 3–5%
Postoperative complications	Reduced by 2–9%
Length of stay (medical)	Reduced by 3.5%
Urinary tract infections	Reduced by 9%
Gastrointestinal bleeding	Reduced by 5.1%
Pneumonia	Reduced by 6.4%
Cardiac arrest	Reduced by 9.4%
Survival after serious complications	Increased by 2.5%

This study is one of a series of studies that looked at RN staffing ratios and client outcomes. It validates what the American Nurses Association has been saying since the early 1990s—that there is a direct correlation between the care provided by RNs and positive client outcomes. The American Hospital Association (AHA) has formally acknowledged that RNs are critical to ensuring good client care. However, the AHA still resists the move toward mandatory staffing ratios, characterizing them as an "oversimplistic" solution to a complex problem. It is evident, however, from this study that in hospitals with low numbers of RNs, clients are more likely to stay longer, suffer more complications, and die from complications that, if they were identified and treated sooner, would be survivable.

Passing staffing ratio laws may be a quick fix to an emotional and dramatic concern, but it does not address a much wider range of problems hospitalized clients face every day. What is needed to ultimately cure the industry is a long-range plan for systemic reform on the basis of client needs, not the needs of a profit-motivated insurance industry.

Clients educated to understand what quality care is, and how it can best be achieved, will ultimately be the most powerful force for attaining the care they require. When managed care facilities begin to really listen to the clients they are supposed to be serving, nurse staffing ratio laws will no longer be necessary. The facilities will meet the quality expectations by making sure that the needed number of nurses are there to provide the care the client expects.

Although laws may not be the ultimate solution to a much deeper problem, clients in the states with staffing ratio laws will be reassured to know they will have a well-educated, skilled professional nurse nearby who can act as an advocate for their needs and monitor the care they are receiving when they are most vulnerable.

Conclusion

Health-care delivery systems are complex and multifaceted. Nurses continue to provide the majority of health-care services to North Americans and they need to understand the important role they play in the system. Changes in the health-care system are never ending. By understanding the various health-care systems and how they are related to each other, nurses put themselves at the forefront of change and advocate changes that benefit the health of all people.

Nursing is as complex as the health-care systems. It occurs in a wide variety of locations, and the role of the nurse will vary just as much as the health-care systems do. How a nurse functions in a hospital is different from how a nurse functions in parish nursing, but the caring and compassion that nurses bring to their roles will not vary. Nurses need to understand and develop their roles, and they will undoubtedly continue to have a significant impact on the further development of the health-care system.

Critical Thinking Exercises

- Select three clients you are familiar with who have different health-care needs. Describe these clients' medical histories, current problems, and future health-care needs, then determine which health-care setting and which health-care practitioners would be most appropriate for them. Identify any difficulties that might be encountered during their entry into the health-care system. How can the nurse facilitate the process?
- Skilled nursing facilities, subacute care facilities, and assisted living facilities all are forms of long-term, or extended, health care. Identify five specific problems that nurses working in such facilities encounter. What is the best way to resolve these problems?
- Identify cost-cutting measures used at a health-care facility with which you are familiar. Have these measures affected the quality of client care? What other measures to cut costs can be implemented? How have changes within the health-care delivery system altered nursing practice?
- Identify four health-care priorities that may be initiated by the year 2010. How are these likely to affect the profession of nursing?
- Describe the advantages and disadvantages of various health-care reimbursement plans. Which ones will produce the highest-quality care? Which ones are best for the profession of nursing? Are there any payment plans that do both?
- Identify the most necessary elements in health-care reform. Should nurses support these changes? Why?

342 Unit 3 Leading and Managing

References

1. Centres for Medicare and Medicaid Services National health expenditures and human services. 2002. www.cms.hhs.gov/stats.
2. Choudry, S: The enforcement of the Canada Health Act. McGill Law Journal, 41, 461–508, 1996.
3. Health Canada: Canada's health care system. 2002. www.hc-sc.gc.ca/datapcb/iad/hcsystem-e.htm.
4. Najman, J and Western, J: A comparative analysis of Australian health policy in the 1970's. Soc Sci Med 18(1), 949-958, 1984.
5. Storch, J: Foundational values in Canadian health care. In Stingl, M, & Wilson, D (eds): Efficiency vs. Equality: Health Reform in Canada. Fernwood Publishing Co., Halifax, Canada, 1996.
6. Bagshaw, P: Managerialism in public hospitals and universities in New Zealand. New Zealand Medical Journal, 2000.
7. Bhimji, A: Managed care by any other name is still managed care. Hospital Quarterly 2(2):6, 1996.
8. Higgs, Z: Health care access: A consumer perspective. Public Health Nursing, 18(1):3–12, 2001.
9. National Health Information Center, U. S. Department of Health and Human Services. Income Poverty, and Health Insurance Coverage in the United States: 2003. Washington, DC, 2003.

Bibliography

Bradford, N: Commissioning Ideas: Canadian National Policy Innovation in Comparative Perspective. Oxford University Press, Toronto, 1998.
Brittain, B: Who is being accountable for the well-being of the patient? Hospital Quarterly 1(2):56–58, 1998.
Dwivedi, O, and Gow, J: From Bureaucracy To Public Management: The Administrative Culture of the Government of Canada. Broadview Press, Toronto, 1999.
Evans, R: Going for the gold: The redistributive agenda behind market-based health reform. J Health Polit 22(2):426–465, 1999.
Kernaghan, K, and Langford, W: The Responsible Public Servant. Institute for Research on Public Policy, Montreal, 1999.
Singer, P, and Mapa, J: Ethics resource allocation: Dimensions for healthcare executives. Hospital Quarterly 1(4):29–31, 1998.

18

Nursing Informatics

Kathleen Mary Young

Learning Objectives

After completing this chapter, the reader will be able to:

- Discuss the impact of the information revolution on society in general and on health care specifically.
- Define nursing informatics.
- Explain the importance of nursing informatics to nursing practice.
- Analyze the availability of resources and references in the practice site.
- Evaluate the importance of human factors engineering on equipment design.
- Compare the electronic health record to the paper record system.

INFORMATION CHANGES EVERYTHING

The information revolution continues to expand exponentially, pushing the systems of modern culture to the breaking point. The information revolution is changing both the way teachers teach and the way learners learn. It is changing the way people work, communicate, and play. Teaching in public schools, and even in colleges, now demands fast-moving, entertaining lessons that capture the students' attention, because classroom teachers must compete with television and the computer games with which this generation has been raised.

School children and college students no longer read as extensively as they once did. Technology has accustomed them to 30-second "sound bites" of information. Libraries are evolving from repositories of hardbound volumes and journals to providers of Internet access to on-line journals and books. Many people spend 8 to 10 hours a day in front of a computer. People who have lost traditional jobs in manufacturing and service industries are finding that to become marketable in today's workplace, they must have computer skills.

> *Not only does technology change the way in which people communicate and work, but it also creates a new decision-making process that affects all aspects of industry and commerce, including health care.*

TECHNOLOGY AND COMMUNICATION

The information revolution has changed both the form and the format of communication. Before the advent of the telephone, people communicated through the written word. Letter writing was an art. Before television and the computer were invented, people gathered together in neighborhoods and developed a sense of community.

Today the whole world is the community and every corner can be reached from a home computer. Senior citizens use their computers not only to chat but also to organize get-togethers and other social activities. Teenagers use their cell phones and text-messaging to meet friends and stay connected, even when they are in the bathroom with their pajamas on.[1]

Asymmetrical Information

Not only does technology change the way in which people communicate and work, but it also creates new decision-making processes that affect all aspects of industry and commerce, including health care. Informed decisions produce better outcomes. When people are able to sift through and use the vast amount of information available to them, it gives them a decided advantage in conducting business.

The use of multiple sources of data in economics and business is called asymmetrical information. Many businesses currently are characterized by asymmetric information: individuals on one side of the transaction may have much better information than those on the other. Borrowers know more than lenders about their repayment prospects, managers and boards know more than shareholders about the firm's profitability, and prospective clients know more than insurance companies about their accident risk.[2] The fact that the person with more information has an advantage seems like common sense, but a grasp of the impact of asymmetric information will lead to a better understanding of day-to-day economic activity.

Competitive Health Care

Competition has become a driving force in the pricing and marketing of health care. Payment methods that promote competition are encouraged by Medicare and Medicaid prospective payment systems (PPSs), health maintenance organizations (HMOs), preferred provider organizations (PPOs), and managed care. For an organization to offer competitive and high-quality services, information must be available to make decisions. More information is available to decision-makers with information technology.

Technologically driven organizations have a competitive edge through the collection of large amounts of information and its application to decision making in health care. To stay competitive in national and international health care, the health-care delivery system, and specifically nursing, must open itself to new information and ideas.

The health-care information revolution is progressing at the speed of light. Computers are involved in almost every area of client care today including the assessment of the quality of care, decision making, management, planning, and medical research.[3]

DEFINING INFORMATICS

Two definitions of informatics are commonly used in health care. The term *medical informatics* was coined in the mid-1970s. Borrowed from the French expression *informatique medicale,* it included all the informational technologies that deal with the medical care of the client, medical resources, and the decision-making process.[4]

Health informatics is a more comprehensive term that is defined as the use of information technology with information management concepts and methods to support the delivery of health care.[5] Health informatics includes the medical, but also encompasses nursing, dental, and pharmacy informatics as well as all other health-care disciplines. The definition of health informatics focuses attention on the recipient of care rather than on the discipline of the caregiver.

Models for Nursing Informatics

The nursing community has been working toward developing a discipline of informatics that is specific to the delivery of nursing care based on the science of nursing. Nursing has distinct and discrete information needs. The content and application of nursing information is substantively different from that of other disciplines. Data gathered by the nursing profession presents unique problems for the use of information in the delivery of nursing care on the basis of critical thinking.[6]

Three Basic Elements

An early model for nursing informatics can be traced back to 1989. Although somewhat simplistic, it viewed nursing informatics primarily as combining computer science, information science, and nursing science in a manner that would help the nurse in the planning and delivery of care to clients. These technologies aid in the collection and analysis of data so that the nurse can make informed and accurate decisions about the type of care required by clients.[6]

In this early definition of nursing informatics, computer science was seen primarily as the computer and the institution-wide system to which it was connected. Information science refers to the computer software, including how data or tasks are processed, how problems are solved, and where products are produced. Nursing science is all the research data from nursing and other associated disciplines that relate to and support nursing practice.[7]

More Complex Elements

In newer models of nursing informatics, a fourth element, cognitive science, has been added. Cognitive science combines psychology, linguistics, computer science, philosophy, and neuroscience in a way that is useful for the delivery of client care. Cognitive science is also concerned with perception, thinking, understanding, and remembering. This model unites information science, computer science, and cognitive science into a framework of nursing science.[8]

It is also believed that wisdom should be added as a component of nursing informatics in addition to data, information, and knowledge. With wisdom, the nurse is able to know how and when to use the available information in managing clients' problems and meeting their needs.[9]

The nursing community, however, has been working toward developing a discipline of informatics that is specific to the delivery of nursing care based on the science of nursing. Nursing has distinct and discrete information needs.

Data, Information, and Knowledge

In most theories of nursing informatics, *data* is defined as raw and unstructured facts. For example, the numbers 102 and 104 are raw data: by themselves, these numbers have little meaning because they lack interpretation. *Information* consists of data that have been given form and have been interpreted. If the number 102 is given additional data so that it becomes a 102°F oral temperature of a 25-year-old man taken at 9 A.M., it becomes information that has meaning to the nurse.

What Do You Think?

Have you used computerized health-care records? Describe your experience

Knowledge takes the process one step further because it is a synthesis of data and information. Combining the information that an oral temperature of 102°F is higher than normal for a 25-year-old man with an understanding of human physiology and pharmacology, the nurse is able to decide what treatment should be given. This process relies on critical thinking and decision making and can be used in research to create new knowledge.

The data to information to knowledge model of informatics is linear in design, but the process of synthesizing data into information to create knowledge is circular. New knowledge creates new questions and areas of research, which in turn lead to more new knowledge. To answer any research question, new data are required that must be processed into information to create more knowledge. The goal of this process is to provide the most accurate and current information so that nurses can make informed decisions in their daily practice.

Areas of Focus in Informatics

Over the years, the specialty of nursing informatics has evolved through three levels of special interest: technology, concepts of nursing theory, and function.[8]

Technology. The earliest attempts to define nursing informatics focused solely on the use of technology. A commonly used early definition of nursing informatics stated that it existed whenever the nurse used any type of information technology in delivering nursing care or in the process of educating nursing students.[10] Some of the key points in the use of technology and/or computer systems to store, process, display, retrieve, and communicate health-care information quickly in the health-care setting include:

• Administering nursing services and resources
• Managing the delivery of client and nursing care
• Linking research resources and findings to nursing practice
• Applying educational resources to nursing education

Nursing Theory. As nursing informatics has evolved, it began to combine nursing theory and informatics. Without a well-articulated theoretical basis to guide the gathering of data, nurses soon become overwhelmed with meaningless data and information. Obviously, there is a need for common definitions, a standardized nursing language, and criteria for organization of the data.

Function. An additional step in the evolution of nursing informatics is the inclusion of the concept of

function. The function of nursing informatics is to manage and process data to help nurses enter, organize, and retrieve needed information. Technology is then developed to achieve specific purposes related to client care needs. Although technology forms the foundation of informatics, the nurse's ability to use that technology and make it function to meet clients' needs is the real test of the system's effectiveness.

In reality, nursing informatics includes all three of these areas—technology, nursing theory, and function. However, the field of informatics has become so large that it is difficult for any one person to be an expert in all three areas.

> " *Although technology forms the foundation of informatics, the nurse's ability to use the that technology and make it function to meet clients' needs is the real test of the system's effectiveness.* "

INFORMATICS AS A SPECIALTY

A Broader Definition

A broader definition of nursing informatics is provided by the American Nurses Association (ANA). It defines nursing informatics as

> A specialty that integrates nursing science, computer science, and information science in identifying, collecting, processing, and managing data and information to support nursing practice, administration, education and research; and to expand nursing knowledge. The purpose of nursing informatics is to analyze information requirements; design, implement and evaluate information systems and data structures that support nursing; and identify and apply computer technologies for nursing.[11]

Nursing informatics is now recognized as a nursing specialty for which a registered nurse (RN) can receive certification. The catalog of the American Nurses Credentialing Center (ANCC) states that the nursing informatics practice

> . . . encompasses the full range of activities that focus on the methods and technologies of

information handling in nursing. It includes the development, support, and evaluation of applications, tools, processes, and structures that assist the practice of nurses with the management of data in direct care of patients/clients. The work of an informatics nurse can involve any and all aspects of information systems, including theory formulation, design, development, marketing, selection, testing, implementation, training, maintenance, evaluation, and enhancement.[12]

Nursing informatics supports all areas of nursing, including practice, education, administration, and research. It facilitates and guides the management of data.

Informatics is no longer just an elective subject. In today's competitive and rapidly changing health-care delivery system, mastery of informatics is a basic requirement.

Articulation

Informatics is no longer just an elective subject. In today's competitive and rapidly changing health-care delivery system, mastery of informatics is a basic requirement. The importance of the role of informatics is apparent in the need for the articulation of nursing practice. Articulation is an important way for nursing to demonstrate its accountability and credibility so that it can remain an essential element of the health-care system.

The Need for a Standard

Historically, the nursing profession has had difficulty in locating relevant nursing information quickly because there was no universally agreed upon nomenclature and taxonomy for either nursing clinical information or management data. In the past, this lack of access to information has presented several seemingly insurmountable challenges for nurse executives, including being able to identify what the nursing staff actually does, determining the impact nurses have on outcomes, and establishing appropriate reimbursement for nursing activities.[13]

For example, how does a nurse interpret the term *weak grasp* when it is seen in the chart of a client? The meaning of weak grasp differs widely depending on the client. If the client is a premature infant with a weak grasp, the term has an entirely different meaning than if it is applied to a 25-year-old professional football player with a head injury or even a 60-year-old client with a stroke. Imagine the difficulty that a researcher will have when investigating the phenomenon of weak grasp because of the lack of a standardized definition among the nursing community. Because of the need to standardize nursing language to name and communicate what nurses do, nursing classification schemes, taxonomies, and vocabularies have come to the forefront with the evolution of nursing informatics.

What Do You Think?

Think of four terms, not defined actions, carried out by nurses that have multiple meanings. How could these terms be clarified?

Unified Nursing Language System

The American Nurses Association Database Steering Committee was formed in 1991 to develop a common nursing language called the Unified Nursing Language System (UNLS). UNLS maps concepts and identifies common terms from different vocabularies and acknowledges them as synonyms of the same concept.

Twelve classification systems are recognized by the ANA as uniquely developed to document

Box 18.1

Standards and Scoring Guidelines for Nursing Languages

1. Terms in data dictionaries and tables are appropriate to the domain of nursing.
2. Terms from ANA-recognized languages for nursing are used as a core for the nursing vocabulary.
3. The system allows for the development and addition of new terms as needed, without duplicating existing terms or disrupting the integrity of existing languages.
4. When using a "local" language, those terms are mapped to appropriate ANA-recognized nursing languages, which may include using reference terminologies.
5. The system accommodates the use of reference terminologies to map nursing languages with other existing standardized data sets, classification systems, or nomenclatures.

nursing care. They are designed to record and track the clinical care process for an entire episode of care for clients in the acute, home, and/or ambulatory care settings. Standards and scoring guidelines for nursing languages can be found in Box 18.1.

Nursing Minimum Data Set

Standardization of the data in a client's record is the first step toward unifying information to make it usable to the bedside nurse. The second step is the development of criteria to determine the necessary elements that must be included in every client record or encounter. The Nursing Minimum Data Set (NMDS) developed in 1985 and accepted by the ANA in 1998 is a list of the data elements necessary in any computerized client record system or national database. The NMDS is considered to be the umbrella for other nursing process schemes. The purpose of the NMDS is to:

1. Describe the nursing care of clients and their families in various settings, both institutional and noninstitutional
2. Establish comparability of nursing data across clinical populations, settings, geographical areas, and time
3. Demonstrate or project trends regarding nursing care provided and allocation of nursing resources to clients according to their health problems or nursing diagnoses
4. Stimulate **nursing research** through linkages of detailed data existing in nursing information systems and in other health-care information systems
5. Provide data about nursing care to influence health policy and decision making[14]

The NMDS has 16 elements divided into 3 main categories: nursing care (e.g., nursing diagnosis, intervention, outcome, and degree of nursing care), client demographics (e.g., the client's personal identification, date of birth, sex), and service elements (e.g., the unique service agency number, the admission and discharge dates, client's condition, and expected payer).

Accountability

Intuitively, the nursing profession has long known that the presence of RNs improves the quality of care and client outcomes, while decreasing the cost of health care. According to the Congressional Office of Technology Assessment,[15] better use of nurse practitioners could result in savings for clients, employers, and society owing to the cost-effectiveness of both their training and their services. Nurses affect client outcomes positively and contribute measurably to the goals of a competitive health-care delivery system. However, nurses traditionally have not been very good at documenting their worth and effectiveness.

In order to measure effectiveness with accurate information about client care and outcomes, nurses must use standardized language in both practice and documentation. The ability to measure the resources used and the client outcome achieved will help distinguish one health-care provider from another. This process forms the basis for evidence-based practice (EBP).

As nursing practice becomes more efficient and can demonstrate improved client outcomes, the quality of care will increase and health-care organizations will become more financially stable.

> *If the nursing profession cannot artic-
> ulate and measure the unique contri-
> butions that nurses make to the client's
> health and well-being, then the profes-
> sion will continue to have difficulty
> justifying its higher costs over less-
> educated and less-qualified health-
> care providers.*

Credibility

The credibility of the nursing profession rests on its
ability to document how nursing care improves
clients' health and saves money for health-care institutions. Nurses must be able to measure their effectiveness with accurate information about both the
care given and the client outcomes achieved. Having
control over the process of care as well as the information and assessments of the quality of care is an
important element in achieving this goal.

Improvements in quality do not occur in
isolation. Improvements in quality result from a continual process of assessing care and measuring outcomes that produces improvements in treatments,
changes in care procedures, and an increased number
of support services.[16]

A standardized language will facilitate the
nursing profession's ability to delineate the costs and
benefits of nursing care from the costs and benefits
of other health-care providers. If the nursing profession cannot articulate and measure the unique contributions that nurses make to the client's health and
well-being, then the profession will continue to have
difficulty justifying its higher costs over less-
educated and less-qualified health-care providers.

Accessing Information

An Information Explosion

Health-care journals and textbooks form a key element in the information explosion. The amount of
health-care information contained in scientific journals has grown to a point where no individual is able
to read all of the material. With just a nightly perusal
of the latest journals, even the most conscientious
practitioners will have difficulty keeping up with all
the current research and new developments in their
specialty field.

Coping with the volume of biomedical and
nursing literature is an enormous task. In 1994,
34,000 references from 4,000 journals were added
each month to the National Library of Medicine
Medline database from among the more than
100,000 scientific journals published.[17] In the past 20
years, the number of articles indexed annually in the
Medline database has nearly doubled, the number of
clinical trials in cardiology has increased five times,
and the number of clinical trials in health services
has increased 10 times. One new article is added to
the medical literature every 26 seconds.

Conflicting Paradigms

Although a large amount of new information is available, only a small portion is read by and incorporated
into the practice of many health-care professionals.
The traditional paradigm that still seems to guide the
decision-making process for many nurses is to:

- Refer back to the knowledge learned in school
- Confer with a colleague
- Look up the problem in any textbook or reference
  book available in the work setting
- Use previous experiences and "gut" instincts

Although this process is useful and has
some merit, it is questionable whether it is adequate
for the delivery of high-quality care in today's complex health-care system. EBP is more appropriate for
the information age.[18] This process includes:

- Accessing current literature concerning the latest
  diagnostic techniques and treatment modalities
- Conferring with a knowledgeable colleague
- Evaluating the effectiveness of previous experiences

Research on the Job

Ironically, even though EBP produces higher-quality
care, the nursing profession has only recently
embraced its use. However, with increasing client
care responsibilities, nurses rarely have time to go to
the library to research solutions to client care problems. Furthermore, nurses still are not being
rewarded for taking the initiative to use EBP.

One development that is encouraging the
use of EBP is that nurses no longer have to leave the
practice setting to access relevant information. Literature can be searched from the nurses' station or
even the client's bedside using available information
systems. Nurses find that having access to literature

Box 18.2

Principles for Access to Library and Information Services

1. All nurses should have access to a free library service funded by their employer that contains appropriate literature and multimedia resources.
2. Library services should have flexible opening hours and be staffed by qualified librarians.
3. Nurses should have equal rights, similar to those of other health-care professionals, to paid study time to update their practice.
4. Every nurse should have access to training on the Internet and appropriate databases.
5. Every nurse should be educated in electronic systems and services to support evidence-based practice.

Source: Urquhart, C, and Davis, R: The impact of information. Nursing Standard 12(8):23–31, 1997.

about clinical issues increases their confidence levels in dealing with clients and other health professionals. It also allows them to contribute more fully to the multidisciplinary health-care team.[19]

Nurses must continue to make time for information searches that promote improved client care (Box 18.2). The creation of workplaces in which nurses can easily access client information, including research information, is essential to high-quality nursing practice.

> *The creation of workplaces in which nurses can easily access client information, including research information, is essential to high-quality nursing practice.*

THE HUMAN FACTOR

Is the System Friendly?

When information tools, machines, and systems are developed, they must include recognition of human factors, including knowledge about human capabilities, human limitations, and characteristics that may affect the use of the system. The terms *human factors, human engineering, usability engineering,* and *ergonomics* are often used interchangeably.

The study of human factors examines how to make the interaction of people and equipment safe, comfortable, and effective. Cognitive science,

one of the components of informatics discussed earlier, forms part of the foundation for the study of human factors. Cognitive science includes the human acts of perception, thinking, understanding, and remembering.

In order to manage and process information, especially with an automated system, the individual must be able to understand and remember a great deal of data. The more logically this information is arranged, the easier it is to use the system. "User friendly" systems are intuitive, self-evident, and logical, even if they are complicated.

Does the System Make Sense?

Every day in their client care, nurses use complex machinery, including many types of monitors, ventilators, intravenous (IV) pumps, feeding pumps, suction devices, electronic beds and scales, lift equipment, and assistive devices. The directions for use of many of these machines are not self-evident and may be highly complicated. Although hospital equipment producers are becoming better at incorporating the human factor in the design and use of this complicated equipment, it would seem that consulting with practicing nurses or "field testing" equipment in the workplace prior to its mass production would make it more user friendly.

Confusing Technology

New computer systems present many learning challenges for health-care providers. Many computer systems are not user friendly. Computer systems designers are notorious for supplying computers with numerous advanced but obscure functions. These systems often seem to make relatively simple daily tasks much more complicated.[20] Millions of dollars have been wasted on computer systems that are not used or are underused because the user's needs were not considered before the systems were designed.

Individuals encountering complicated computer systems for the first time commonly feel that they are stupid, incompetent, or too old to learn because they cannot quickly master the new technology. However, the fault often lies not with the individual but with the design of the technology.

Nurses, through their education and philosophical orientation, are generally more in tune with the human factor than computer designers, particularly as it relates to client care. Nurses can use their human factor orientation in the process of evaluating new technology before it is purchased. Also, nurses may be able to make suggestions to medical equipment producers to help improve the equipment after it has been used for some time.

Is the System Well Designed?

There has been an ongoing concern in the United States about the problem of health-care error and the large number of client deaths attributed to it. Estimates of how many people die annually in the United States as a result of medical error range from 44,000 to almost 100,000. Based on these numbers, medical error ranks as the eighth leading cause of death in the United States.[21]

Medical Error

The most common type of health-care error was related to medications, followed by wound infections; technical complications were ranked in third place. The proliferation of new medications and the increasing complexity of medication therapy have dramatically increased the risk of medication errors and adverse drug events both inside and outside hospitals.

Also, the increased use of "fast tracking" medications through the testing process has led to withdrawal of several medications from the market because of long-term complications not seen in the initial shortened testing phase. Well-designed computerized physician-order entry systems can reduce serious prescribing errors by more than 50%.[22]

Poor Design

Poor user design is responsible for thousands of health-care "accidents" each year. Complex medical devices are often used under extremely stressful conditions in which the user's cognitive abilities are not as focused as they might be in a less stressful situation. Often the users are not considered during the design phase, because the designers believe they know what is needed.

Errors Increase

The inevitable result of poor design in all types of equipment, ranging from laboratory forms to life-support devices, is an increased error rate.[23] Cognitive science studies have shown that the average person's memory can retain only six to eight pieces of information at a time. A well-designed system takes these elements into account (Box 18.3) and should reduce the number of errors. However, a poorly designed system can just as easily increase the number of errors rather than reduce them.

Training Doesn't Compensate

Employees are commonly trained to use an information system to reduce errors. Although training is important, by itself it may not be adequate. In one study, there was no reduction in the number of errors even with an increase in training time. However, well-designed computer-based reminder systems did help clinicians reduce errors significantly. Even after the clinicians received additional training, errors returned to the previous level when the computerized reminder system was removed.[24]

Box 18.3

Elements of a Good Technology Design

- Can be operated intuitively with minimal reliance on complicated manuals
- Easy-to-read displays that are logically arranged
- Easy to use and reach controls
- Positive and safe electrical and mechanical connections
- Alarms that sound only when there is a real problem so that they are not turned off because of annoyance
- Long-life reliability with few malfunctions
- Easy and quick to repair and maintain

When automated and computer systems are made user friendly by incorporating engineering techniques based on human needs, they can make a valuable contribution to monitoring and preventing error in clinical practice. As nursing professionals, it is important to understand that human performance is not perfect and cannot be perfected through education and training. Professionals must look for well-designed systems that can reduce and even eliminate errors.

> *Estimates of how many people die annually in the United States as a result of medical error range from 44,000 to almost 100,000. Based on these numbers, medical error ranks as the eighth leading cause of death in the United States.*

THE ELECTRONIC HEALTH RECORD

A health record serves multiple purposes. It is used primarily to document client care. It also provides communication among health-care team members. It acts as a financial and legal record and is used for research and continuous quality improvement (CQI). Although the health record can take many forms, the most common forms are either paper or electronic. Both forms have advantages and disadvantages (Box 18.4).

Advantages
Electronic health records (EHRs) have many advantages. Multiple care providers can access them simultaneously from remote sites. They can provide reminders about completing information or carrying out protocols as well as providing warnings about incompatibilities of medications or variances from normal standards.

Redundancy is reduced with the EHR. Rather than every health-care worker asking a client for his or her health history, allergies, and current medications, the information is captured once and then transmitted to every record requiring the information. EHRs require less storage space, are more difficult to lose, and are much easier to research.

Box 18.4

Advantages and Disadvantages of the Paper Record

Advantages
- People know how to use it.
- It is fast for current practice.
- It is portable.
- It is nonbreakable.
- It accepts multiple data types, such as graphs, photographs, drawings, and text.
- Legal issues and costs are understood.

Disadvantages
- It can be lost.
- It is often illegible and incomplete.
- It has no remote access.
- It can be accessed by only one person at a time.
- It is often disorganized.
- Information is duplicated.
- It is hard to store.
- It is difficult to research, and CQI is laborious.
- Same client has separate records at each facility (physician office, hospital, home care).
- Records are shared only through hard copy.

Improved communication, increased completeness of documentation, and reduction in error are the most important advantages of the EHR.

Disadvantages
EHRs have some obvious disadvantages. There is a high front-end cost in buying an electronic system and converting from a paper system. Employees may have problems adapting to the new system because of the steep learning curve involved. EHR systems are becoming more portable with the advent of the wireless network; however, they are also subject to all the glitches of electronic systems.

Decisions must be made about who can enter data into the system and when the entries should be made. The Health Insurance Portability and Accountability Act (HIPAA) regulations currently creating so many headaches for health-care providers were written specifically to address the many legal and ethical issues involving privacy and access to client information (see Chapter 9). Some issues still remain to be resolved.

The Ideal Record

The ideal EHR would be a lifelong continuous record of all the care that the client has received, rather than the episodic, piecemeal data that it now provides. This one record would reflect an individual's current health status and lifetime medical history. It would be unique to the person and not to the institution. This record would reside in multiple data sites and would accept multiple data types (e.g., graphs, pictures, x-rays, text) and be accessible worldwide.

Several Places at Once

The information on the EHR does not physically have to reside in one place, like a paper record. When viewed from a computer workstation, the EHR only appears to be in one place. In reality, the individual records are retrieved from many information systems, such as laboratory, radiology, document imaging, anatomic pathology, anesthesiology, bedside, and accounting.

With proper authorization, this record could be accessed from anywhere in the world, at any time. Many people around the world could look at the same record at the same time. If an individual became critically ill on a cruise ship or in a foreign country, the local health-care provider would be able to access the medical record to facilitate the client's diagnosis and treatment.

New Forms of Access

Health-care providers and technology designers are still working to resolve the many barriers to implementation of the ideal EHR. The issues of maintaining confidentiality and security are now closer to resolution. The high cost of starting up the system is still a barrier.

Access to the system would probably require a universal ID code or a unique client identifier.[25] Many organizations may resist a universal ID because they now use either their own client numbering system or social security numbers to identify individual records. Neither of these systems is adequate for the global access of the future. Fingerprinting, iris and retinal imaging, face prints, and voice-

prints all are identification methods under investigation for use as the universal ID.

Bedside or Point of Care?

Bedside System. Some currently used systems allow nurses to enter information through bedside systems. A bedside system, as the name implies, is a computer terminal installed in each client's room or next to each bed.

Point-of-Care System. A point-of-care system has a broader meaning and includes not only the bedside but also many other points of care in the health-care environment and community, including the laboratory, radiology department, outpatient clinics, and even the home for home-health-care providers. Many facilities currently have a unit system that can be accessed at only one terminal in the client care area (e.g., the nurses' station).

A Process Redesigned

Taking a paper record and typing it into a computer does not, in itself, constitute a modern electronic record. Automating the paper record in its present form only automates inefficient practices based on outdated requirements. Modern systems go beyond merely computerizing paper records. These new systems gain control over the generation of information and develop new techniques for using it creatively.

One of the most important characteristics of a bedside or point-of-care system is that client information can be input directly from the terminal rather than the nurse having to keep notes or chart from memory at the end of the shift. Documenting at the time of care is an important change in workflow for most health-care workers, who are accustomed to documenting at the end of a shift in a workroom with other professionals.

The re-engineering and streamlining of departmental workflow is accomplished by the automatic and continual routing of electronic documents and medical images from one person or department to another throughout the shift. With this system, traditional manual tasks are now automated, increasing the efficiency of management decisions and improving the distribution and evaluation of complex client records and electronic documents by authorized staff. This redesign of the old manual processes that provides the real return on investment for implementing the electronic health record.

One of the most important characteristics of a bedside or point-of-care system is that client information can be input directly from the terminal rather than the nurse having to keep notes or chart from memory at the end of the shift.

ETHICS, SECURITY, AND CONFIDENTIALITY

Information for Sale

Most people assume that all doctor–client communications are strictly confidential. However, in the new electronic world, confidential information has become a commodity that is bought and sold in the electronic market place.[26] Although the HIPAA laws have tried to deal with this issue (see Chapter 9), people who use the Internet or e-mail quickly realize that their personal information is no longer so personal.

Examples of violations of client confidentiality abound. In 1996, a convicted child rapist working as a technician in a Boston hospital rifled through 1000 computerized records looking for potential victims. He was caught when the father of a 9-year-old girl used caller ID to trace a call back to the hospital.

A banker on Maryland's State Health Commission pulled up a list of cancer clients from the state's records, cross-checked it against the names of his bank's customers, and revoked the loans of those clients diagnosed with cancer. At least a third of all Fortune 500 companies regularly review health information before making hiring decisions. More than 200 subjects in a case study published in *Science and Engineering Ethics* reported that they had been discriminated against as a result of genetic testing.[27]

A Question of Ownership

One of the key ethical questions is "Who owns the client's health-care data?" Does the individual's health-care information belong exclusively to the individual? Does it belong to the organization (e.g., insurance company, PPO) that paid for the care or should it belong to the physician who directed and ordered the care? What about the facility in which the care occurred—can they claim some ownership to the information, particularly if it is stored there? Do all these groups and individuals own a part of the information?

Should Society Benefit?

Those who argue the "individual rights" end of the ethical spectrum believe that each individual should have total and exclusive control over the information concerning his or her health and the care rendered. Those on the utilitarian, or "social good," end of the ethical spectrum believe that society as a whole benefits from shared information about disease occurrence and treatment. Therefore, the information should be available to all interested parties. As with most ethical dilemmas, a single definitive answer has not been proposed regarding who owns the data.

However, public policy debates have increased concerning the collection of health-care information for use as aggregate databases to underpin health-care planning. Many consumers are concerned about the status of future physician–client relationships. Driving the development of data collection policy is the public's fear about the damage that may result from excessive and uncontrolled health-care information disclosures through automated information systems.[28]

The Implications of Consent

When clients enter the health-care system, they are generally asked to sign consent forms so that other organizations can obtain information about their health status and the care that they received (particularly insurance companies so that bills can be paid). They are usually unaware that this information can be supplied to many other organizations or institutions.

For example, reports to the trauma registry are made about injuries resulting from accidents. The tumor registry collects information about benign and malignant tumors, and infectious disease reports are made to the Public Health Department. Currently, health-care information is shared to develop payment systems, examine access to care, identify cost differences of treatment modalities, research disease trends and epidemiologic implications, and expand consumer information.

The Evolution of HIPAA

HIPAA policies attempt to base the collection, development, and use of client data on issues of confidentiality and security. In 1996, the federal government started to develop the guidelines that have become HIPAA. The primary objectives of HIPAA include:

• Ensuring health insurance portability
• Reducing health-care fraud and abuse
• Guaranteeing security and privacy of health information
• Enforcing standards for health information

In 2000, rules governing the exchange of electronic administrative health-care information were developed and added to HIPAA. The object of these rules was to simplify and standardize the electronic forms required for claims for services rendered. Every organization must now use the same form.

Rules for Disclosure

In 2001, HIPAA was modified by the addition of rules that address the use and disclosure of individually identifiable health information in any form, electronic or paper. Health-care providers and facilities must obtain client consent before using or disclosing client information for treatment, payment, or health-care operations. The full HIPAA was enacted in 2004.

What Do You Think?

Who do you think owns health-care information? How does your decision affect health-care policy in the future?

> " . . . *most health-care institutions have policies prohibiting unauthorized access to confidential information. Individuals can lose their jobs because of unauthorized access or sharing of client information and, under recently enacted HIPAA laws, may be convicted of a crime.* "

Even with HIPAA regulations, confidential client information can be legally used for such purposes as quality assurance, institutional licensing and accreditation, biomedical research, third-party reimbursement, credentialing, litigation, regional and national databases, court-ordered release of information, and managed care comparisons. Although automated information systems did not cause these information uses, automation does make acquiring this information much easier.

Threats to Security

Unauthorized Access

Unauthorized sharing of health-care information is generally unethical and, now, always illegal. The code of ethics for most health-care professionals prohibits unauthorized or unnecessary access to client information. In addition, most health-care institutions have policies prohibiting unauthorized access to confidential information. Individuals can lose their jobs because of unauthorized access or sharing of client information and, under recently enacted HIPAA laws, may be convicted of a crime.

Unauthorized access or sharing of information is not a new problem associated only with the electronic age. It is just as easy to gain unauthorized access to a paper record as it is to the automated electronic record. The professional codes of ethics that stress client confidentiality have always been the primary protector of client information. Still, access to the paper record is available to anyone who picks up the chart.

In some ways, the automated electronic record provides greater privacy. Access to the automated record is generally restricted to employees who have been issued a password. Also, most organizations have periodic **audits** that can track each person who has accessed a record, and some systems can even detect unauthorized access at the time of entry into the system.

Accidents

Threats to the security of information can be either accidental or intentional and affect both paper and electronic systems. Accidental threats involve naturally occurring events such as floods, fires, earthquakes, electrical surges, and power outages.

The paper record has little security against natural events. Typically, paper records are secured in a locked file cabinet or medical records room. Although current safety regulations require fire detection and suppression systems in these areas, even a small fire can destroy a large number of paper records very quickly. There is little that can be done to protect paper records against major flooding. Once the charts are destroyed, they cannot be reproduced.

Facilities with automated systems usually have well-developed natural disaster plans built into the system design. These plans include the automatic production and storage of a backup tape of the data at a protected location some distance from the health-care facility. The frequency of data backup varies with the organization's requirements. Most systems automatically save all the data in the system every 24 hours, although this time interval can be shortened or increased to meet the facility's needs.

Although these measures provide a high degree of protection from major natural events such as floods and fires, power surges and outages create problems for electronic systems that leave paper systems unaffected. Anyone who works with computerized equipment recognizes the major disruptions in service and work that occur when the system goes down. Again, some safeguards can be built into the system so that not all the most recent information is lost when the power goes out. Power surges can be controlled with surge protection devices.

Intentional Acts

Intentional threats to the security of information involve the actions of an individual or individuals who wish to damage, destroy, or alter the records. In most cases, it is difficult to protect paper records from intentional tampering. It is a rather simple task for a determined individual to gain access to paper records and either erase, add to, or rewrite sections of the chart. These changes are often very difficult to detect. In addition, a person could simply remove the chart and destroy it so that there would be no record left at all. Although automated electronic records are vulnerable to several kinds of intentional threats, they are, overall, more secure than the paper record. All current automated systems have computer virus–checking programs that protect the automated record from both intentional and accidental introduction of destructive computer viruses into the system.

Once data have been entered into the automated system, the data are difficult to alter. Modern automated systems are designed with "write once, read many" (WORM) programs. If a legitimate change in the electronic record needs to be made, it must be added as an addendum. Any changes made in the electronic record are logged by the time and the person who made them and can always be tracked to the point of origin.

Although it is true that a determined and gifted hacker can still obtain access to almost any electronic database, electronic security systems are becoming more and more difficult to breach. However, terrorist acts ranging from detonation of bombs in key locations to developing "superviruses" to destroy electronic records are difficult to defend against and present an ever-increasing threat.

> *Although automated electronic records are vulnerable to several kinds of intentional threats, they are, over all, more secure than the paper record.*

USES OF THE INTERNET

For nursing professionals, the Internet has become a valuable resource for communicating with colleagues and professional organizations, researching clinical information, and educating consumers about health resources and information.[29] Because of the lack of standardization and regulation, it is important that the nurse evaluate each site for accuracy of information, authority, objectivity, currency or timeliness, and coverage.[30]

A Resource for Professionals

Most professional organizations maintain a Web site containing information about the organization. Many include policy statements and lists of publications. **Continuing education units (CEU)** can be obtained via the World Wide Web to help nurses remain current and retain licensure. The Nursing Network (www.nursingnetwork.com), for example, is a site that lists education courses, position vacancies, conferences, and other pertinent information. News groups such as those listed at www.nursingworld.org provide professional information and access to experts in specific areas of interest.

Disease-specific Web sites publish clinical information for both the consumer and the professional. OncoLink is an example of a resource for information about cancer. Often the most recent information about a disease is found on the Internet. Publishing is quicker and easier on the World Wide Web than in a peer-reviewed journal. Web-based support groups disseminate information on both technical and consumer levels. Protocols and policies are shared through Web sites and news groups.

A Guide for Consumers

Today, consumers are more knowledgeable about health care through use of the Internet. Clients are better informed than they were in the past, because they now have easy access to a wide range of health-care information. Preventive and wellness services are available electronically through articles, chat groups, and health risk assessment surveys posted on consumer Web sites.[31] Clients can now purchase medications over the Web, often at a much lower cost than they can get from their local pharmacist.

Healthfinder is a consumer health and human services information Web site created and maintained by the federal government. The site links the user with on-line government publications, clearinghouses, databases, Web sites, support and self-help groups, as well as the government agencies and not-for-profit organizations that produce reliable information for the public. The goal of this information source is to help consumers make better choices about their health and human services needs for both themselves and their families.

TELEHEALTH

Health Care at a Distance

From its fledgling beginnings almost 40 years ago, clinicians, health services researchers, and others have been investigating the use of telecommunications and information technology to improve health care. Physicians examine and treat clients from distant sites with video cameras, thus saving money by exchanging office visits for on-line appointments.

The terms *telehealth* and *telemedicine* are often used interchangeably.[33] As defined here, telehealth is the use of electronic information and communications technologies to provide and support health care when distance separates the physician and the client. Telehealth includes a wide range of services and technologies, from "plain old telephone service" (POTS) to highly sophisticated digitized cameras, telemetry, and voice systems. Telemedicine is just one of the services provided by the overall telehealth system that primarily involves consultation with a physician.

Telehealth is being used in emergency rooms across the United States. The University of Pittsburgh offers neurological consults to physicians at seven linked hospitals. In Baltimore, providers are using cellular telephone technology to transmit live video and client data back to home base.[32]

Some uses of telehealth, such as emergency calls to 911, are so common that they are often overlooked when considering telehealth systems. Other applications such as telesurgery involve exotic technologies and procedures that are still in the experimental stage.

Serving Remote Populations

Historically, consumer concerns about access to health care have been the driving force behind the development of many clinical telehealth systems. Early applications focused on remote populations scattered across mountainous areas, islands, open plains, and arctic regions where medical specialists, and sometimes even primary care practitioners, were not available.

Many telehealth projects from the 1960s through the early 1980s failed because they were expensive, awkward to use, and often not guided by the strategic plans of the facilities using them. However, as the technology has become more common, the costs of many systems have decreased dramatically. With the development of cellular technology, many of the newer systems are tapping into the systems already in place for telephone service.

Renewed interest in telehealth has been spurred by managed care initiatives seeking to reduce health-care costs while maintaining or increasing the quality of and access to care. Overall costs have decreased for many of the information and communications technologies used by telehealth systems. In addition, the ever-developing National Information Infrastructure is making these technologies more accessible and user friendly. Medicare reimburses some types of telehealth care, although other third-party payers have been slow to include reimbursement for telehealth services.

Telehealth in an Emergency

Telehealth offers many advantages that will affect the cost of and access to the health-care system of the future. The telehealth system allows access to centralized specialists who can support primary care providers in outlying areas. Outlying areas can be either rural or urban areas that lack access to the full range of health-care services. Outlying clinics staffed only with nurse practitioners or physician assistants have immediate access to physician referrals through the telehealth system.

> *Nurses who practice in rural and underserved urban areas will have more autonomy and provide higher-quality care when linked electronically with the support services of a large medical center.*

University medical centers can offer specialist consulting services to primary care physicians at distant locations, thus reducing unnecessary travel and increased cost to clients. Here is an example of how the telehealth system functions in an emergency situation:

In 1996, a 72-year-old man with a collapsed lung walked into the emergency room (ER) in

Issues Now

Tomorrow's Technology Today

Almost any health-care provider with even a passing familiarity with the *Star Trek* movies or television shows has been envious of the tricorder used by fictional medical personnel to diagnose and treat a variety of ills by just waving the device over the client in distress. Although present technology is not quite to that point, it certainly is a lot closer than even a few years ago.

Wearable computers, initially developed for use in the military as a type of flak jacket/telemetry vest, are currently being tested. The Massachusetts Institute of Technology has improved upon the technology by developing a heart brooch that sends heart sounds back to the health-care provider. It looks like an elegant piece of jewelry that anyone can wear. The Japanese are beginning production of "smart" toilets that can collect, process, and transmit data based on their contents.

A technology company called BodyMedia has developed an integrated program that combines principles of wellness with technology. People who wish to join the program are fitted with a BodyMedia SenseWear Armband, a personal body-monitoring apparatus. It is a little smaller than an arm radio, weighs about 3 ounces, and is worn on the back of the right triceps. The brain of the unit is a computer, memory chip, and sensors that continuously monitor body motion, skin temperature, heart rate, evaporation heat loss, and the amount of heat being dissipated by the body. The device, when programmed with the wearer's sex, age, height, and weight, provides data on the expenditure of energy during various activities. The armband can be used to treat clients with congestive heart failure, improve client compliance, and alter lifestyle habits.

Nurses will soon be exposed to these smart devices. They will provide more data for integration into the health-care record, allow comparison of client's progress not only from day to day, but hour to hour or even minute to minute, and provide highly accurate and detailed information.

Another technology that nurses will be experiencing sooner rather than later is voice-activated information systems. We are used to seeing sportscasters, singers, and others in the media with the headset/microphone devices. Nurses will soon be wearing something very similar, a voice-activated headset that will allow them to dictate their documentation as they go about their daily tasks. Nurses have long realized that most of their work is highly activity directed and performed on the run. Sitting behind a computer, or even standing in a room at a computer console, is not the reality of nursing. This technology will allow for more timely documentation and free up some time now devoted to paperwork.

These are just two areas of many that are around the corner in health care. One important element in any developing health-care technology is input from the people who are going to use it. Too often new technology is developed by people who are experts in computers but have very little experience with health care. Unless a technology is user friendly, it is not going to be effective. Nurses need to play an active role in designing and testing new systems.

a small town in North Dakota. The general practitioner who usually saw routine emergency cases immediately called the trauma II medical center in Bismarck and arranged a teleconsult with an ER physician and a thoracic surgeon. The man would die without a thoracotomy. Following the surgeon's instructions, the physician was able to insert the chest tubes needed to safely transport the client by helicopter to Bismarck.[32]

> *Telehealth services often save lives and prevent permanent disability, especially when time is a factor in treatment.*

Telehealth services often save lives and prevent permanent disability, especially when time is a factor in treatment. For example, health-care providers know that if thrombolytic medications are given within 3 hours after the onset of symptoms of a stroke, the likelihood of death or permanent disability is reduced by 50 percent. Using telehealth technology, neurology specialists can evaluate a client's condition while he or she is still in the ambulance en route to the hospital, thus saving valuable time in making the decision about using lifesaving medications. The ER is prepared to administer the medications as soon as the client enters the department rather than having to wait several hours for all the routine evaluations and consults to be completed.

Issues for the Future

A Boost for Home Care

In the future, home care may benefit the most from telehealth. By investing in telehealth technologies, home care providers should be able to balance cost reductions with increased quality of care.

Clients can be monitored at home using a combination of telephone calls, home visits, video visits, and in-home monitoring via the telehealth system. In-home monitoring devices for conditions ranging from congestive heart failure and diabetes to cancer and cardiac conditions can send information from the client's home to a central base for assessment by professionals.

Future Challenges

System Design. Many of the older systems are poorly designed and may be totally incompatible with the systems used in modern health-care facilities. The human factor design and user assessments must be carefully considered when developing any new technologies.

Expense. Although the overall costs of electronic systems continue to gradually decrease, initial expenditures are still a barrier to implementation, especially in smaller facilities. Lack of **third-party payment** for telehealth systems also limits their development and use.

Legal Issues. Several legal issues still need to be resolved, including health-care provider licensure when consults are given across state lines and the liability incurred by providers who examine a client by television rather than in a face-to-face, hands-on encounter. Federal and state policies protecting privacy and confidentiality need to be developed with specific provisions for telehealth systems.

Effects on Nursing Practice. The telehealth system also affects nursing practice. Nurses are the primary users of telephone triage systems that rely on computerized decision-making trees to suggest appropriate actions when given a set of client symptoms. Nurses who practice in rural and underserved urban areas will have more autonomy and provide higher-quality care when linked electronically with the support services of a large medical center. The use of remote monitoring devices provides nurses with immediate information about changes in their clients' conditions, improves outcomes, reduces complications, and lowers the number of re-admissions to the hospital.

Education and Conferencing. The same types of technology used for telehealth can be used for distance and **nontraditional education** applications. Widespread use of **continuing education** is achieved through distance technology. Courses are video-conferenced with two-way interaction. Continuing education credits can be earned through courses on the Internet. Even college credits can be earned via Internet access. Grand rounds are conducted at multiple sites with video conferencing equipment, and in-services are beamed to multiple locations.

Conclusion

The information revolution affects every aspect of health care, not only in the United States but also throughout the world. Advanced communications technology and its increased availability worldwide promotes ties between people and nations, bridging the gap between isolated rural communities and major metropolitan areas.

The nursing profession needs to be actively involved in developing clinical information systems and the electronic health record, establishing care standards, safeguarding client privacy, using the Internet, and researching better ways of improving access and the quality of care through technology. The nursing profession is transformed, enhanced, and enriched as nurses become active participants in the information revolution.

Critical Thinking Exercises

- Debate the ethical issues of personal privacy and the greater social good in relation to availability of health-care information.
- Discuss how the design of equipment increases or decreases error rates.
- Discuss uses of telehealth for patient teaching and monitoring of home health clients.
- Write a vision paper describing your view of technology in health care in the year 2030.
- List all the pieces of data you had to give at your last visit to the doctor or hospital.
- Was all of the information necessary for your care?
- Who needed the information?
- How was the information recorded or transmitted?

References

1. Emerging technologies center: Informatics competencies. Nursing Education Perspectives 25(6):312, 2004.
2. The 2001 Sveriges Riksbank prize in economic sciences in memory of Alfred Nobel @ The Bank of Sweden Prize in Economic Sciences press release. Retrieved March 20, 2002, from www.nobel.se/economics/laureates/2001/press.html.
3. Simpson, R: Nursing informatics. The softer side of technology: How IT helps nursing care. Nursing Administration Quarterly 28(4):302–305, 2004.
4. Wright, C: Orienting the clinician to point of service systems. Home Healthcare Nurse 22(10):687–694, 2004.
5. Jiang, W: Important computer competencies for the nursing profession. Journal of Nursing Research 12(3):213–225, 2004.
6. Delaney, C: Forum supports unified voice for nursing informatics in the United States. Computer Information Nursing 22(5):298–999, 2004.
7. Featherly, K: News & trends. Nursing informatics: Nurses champion clinical technologies. Healthcare Information 21(8):10–12, 2004.
8. Turley, RJ: Toward a model for nursing informatics. Image J Nurs Sch 28(4):309–313, 1996.
9. Nelson, R, and Joos, I: On language in nursing: From data to wisdom. PLN Visions, Fall 1989, pp. 6–7.
10. Fischetti, L: A framework for strategic action: The report from HHS's Secretarial Summit on Health Information Technology, cornerstones for electronic health care. Caring Newsline 3rd Quarter; 19(3):1, 3–4, 2004.
11. American Nurses Association: Scope and Standards of Nursing Informatics Practice. American Nurses Publishing, Washington, DC, 2001.
12. American Nurses Credentialing Center Catalog. American Nurses Publishing, Washington, DC, 2001.
13. Currell, R: Nursing record systems: Effects on nursing practice and health care outcomes. The Cochrane Library, 2005, n. 1.
14. Prophet, CM: Nursing interventions classifications. In Grobe, SJ, and Pluyter-Wenting, ESP (eds): Nursing Informatics: An International Overview for Nursing in a Technological Era. Elsevier, Amsterdam, 1994, pp 692–696.
15. Simpson, R: Nursing informatics. Recruit, retain, assess: Technology's role in diversity. Nursing Administration Quarterly 28(3):217–220, 2004.
16. Ferguson, L, and Day, R: Evidence-based nursing education. Myth or reality? Nursing Education 44(3):107–116, 2005.
17. Erickson, P: Privacy measures cause headaches: 1 year later [HIPAA] laws draw mixed response. The Oklahoman April 4, 8, 2004.
18. Grace, P: Patient safety and the limits of confidentiality. AJN 104(11):33–37, 2004.
19. Miller, D, et al: A study of personal digital assistants to enhance undergraduate clinical nursing education. Nursing Education 44(1):19–27, 2005.
20. Rogerson, W, and Tremethick, M: Turning the tide on medical errors in intensive care units. Dimensions of Critical Care Nursing 23(4):169–175, 2004.
21. Beyea, S: Patient safety first: The 2005 National Patient Safety Goals. AORN Journal 81(1):207, 209–211, 2005.
22. Brommeyer, M: E-nursing and e-patients. Nurse Manager 11(9):12–13, 2005.
23. Edwards, M: Reducing medical errors through better documentation. Health Care Manager 23(4):329–333, 2004.
24. Gardner, R: Using computer technology to detect, measure, and prevent adverse drug events. Journal of the American Medical Information Association 11(6):535–536, 2004.
25. Jeffries, P: Technology trends in nursing education: Next steps. Nursing Education 44(1):3–5, 2005.
26. Hassol, A: Patient experiences and attitudes about access to a patient electronic health care record and linked Web messaging. Journal of the American Medical Information Association 11(6):505–513, 2004.
27. Coleman, R: Multidimensional analysis: A management tool for monitoring HIPAA compliance and departmental performance. Journal of Digital Imaging 17(3):196–204, 2004.
28. Carney, L: Was HIPAA a hurricane or just hot air? We sort it out for you. HIV Clinician 16(2):12–14, 2004.
29. Cassidy, B: Using web technology. Journal of AHIMA, June 2000. Available at: www.ahima.org/journal/features/feature.0006.4.html.
30. Alexander, J, and Tate, M: The Web as a research tool: Evaluation techniques. Available at: www.science.widener.edu/~withers/alaslides/pptfirst.htm.
31. Schneider, P: Patient informatics is growing. Healthcare Informatics, August 1997, p 14.
32. Swan, B, and Dickey, E: Perspectives in ambulatory care. Access to quality health care: Links between evidence, nursing language, and informatics. Nurse Econ 22(6):325–332, 2004.
33. Feldman, P: Charting the course for home health care quality: Action steps for achieving sustainable improvement: Conference proceedings. Home Health Care Nurse 22(12):841–850, 2004.

Bibliography

American Nurses Association: Scope and Standards of Nursing Informatics Practice. American Nurses Publishing, Washington, DC, 2001.
Bartholomew, K: High-tech, high-touch: Why wait? Nurse Manager 35(9):48, 50–54, 2004.
Curran, C: The informatics nurse: Helping to build the knowledge infrastructure for nursing. Nurse Leader 2(3):26–29, 2004.

Englebardt, S, and Nelson, R (eds): Health Care Informatics: An Interdisciplinary Approach. Mosby, St. Louis, 2002.

Nicoll, LH: Nurses' Guide to the Internet, ed. 3. Lippincott, Philadelphia, 2001.

Puskar, K: Implementing information technology in a behavioral health setting. Issues in Mental Health Nursing 25(5):439–450, 2004.

Roscoe, T: An assessment tool for medical informatics skills. Health Information Journal 10(2):155–159, 2004.

Shifman, M: Exploring the portability of informatics capabilities from a clinical application to a bioscience application. Journal of American Medical Information Association 11(4):294–299, 2004.

Young, KM: Informatics for Healthcare Professionals. FA Davis, Philadelphia, 2000.

Every person is born into the world to do something unique and something distinctive, and if he or she does not do it, it will never be done.

Benjamin Mays (1895–1984)
American educator

4

Issues in Delivering Care

19

The Politically Active Nurse

Donna Gentile O'Donnell

Learning Objectives

After completing this chapter, the reader will be able to:

- Explain why it is important for nurses to understand and become involved in the political process.
- Discuss how a bill becomes a law.
- Identify the major committees at the federal level that influence health policy.
- Identify four points at which nurses can influence a bill.
- Give examples of how nurses may become politically involved.
- List and describe four methods of lobbying.

A NUTS-AND-BOLTS APPROACH

The word *politics* conjures up various images—some positive and some negative. There are images of great statesmanship, like the inaugural speech of John F. Kennedy, who exhorted the nation, "Ask not what your country can do for you, but what you can do for your country." There are also images of ignoble moments, like the national tragedy of Watergate, the resignation of Richard Nixon, the impeachment proceedings against Bill Clinton, the dubious election practices that put George W. Bush in office, or the numerous negative campaign commercials vilifying political opponents. Politics touches people's lives at all levels, crossing national boundaries, affecting individual states, and permeating local governments.

This chapter will provide a foundation for understanding the political basics by using a nuts-and-bolts approach and will motivate nurses to become active in the political world. Politics is examined both within the profession of nursing and within society at large. In addition, this chapter discusses the forces that drive politics and the three concepts that comprise it: partisanship, self-interest, and ideology.

Almost everyone, ranging from political candidates, academicians, and members of the press to regular citizens, has something to say about politics. People define politics in many ways. One of the most cynical definitions of politics is offered by Ambrose Bierce in *The Devil's Dictionary,* where it is described as "a strife of interests masquerading as a contest of principles. The conduct of public affairs for private advantage." Other, more widely accepted definitions include "the art or science of government," "the art or science concerned with guiding or influencing government policy," or "the total complex of relations between [people] in society."[1]

THE NURSING SHORTAGE

The nursing shortage is a good example of where nurses' concerns intersect with the political process. In many areas of the United States, the nursing shortage has reached crisis levels, and there do not appear to be any permanent cures on the near horizon. Different areas of the country are attempting to deal with the shortage in the short term with quick, stop-gap political measures that may have an adverse effect on the nursing profession in the long term.

> *Politics touches people's lives at all levels, crossing national boundaries, affecting individual states, and permeating local governments.*

Foreign Recruitment

One quick and easy solution some hospitals are initiating is recruitment of nurses from outside the country. Hospitals in various parts of the country have started programs to bring nurses from countries such as the Philippines. These foreign nurses generally receive the same pay and benefits as the American registered nurses (RNs). They also often receive permanent resident visas and housing if desired. These foreign nurse recruitment plans do not address obtaining U.S. licensure, an issue that affects the state boards of nursing and nurse practice acts.

The importation of foreign nurses to meet nursing shortages is not a new idea. It has been a potential solution for nursing shortages stretching back as far as World War I. Health-care facilities, especially hospitals, strongly favor this approach to solve the nursing shortage.

It is also a very good deal for the nurses who come into this country. They can easily make up to five times the salary they receive in their own countries in addition to upgrading their living conditions and lifestyles. However, as a profession, nurses need to examine this practice very closely because it seems to be an end-run around existing regulations in the nurse practice act.

The primary concern is not one of quality of care. Nursing programs in foreign countries such as the Philippines are often 5 years long and require considerable clinical practice. Although often based on a medical model rather than nursing models, foreign schools usually produce nurses whose technical nursing skills are at levels comparable to those of new graduates from the United States.

Institutional Licensure

The issue American nurses should be concerned with about the importation of foreign nurses is legislative in nature, namely institutional licensure (see Chapter 3). The practice of institutional licensure has been universally rejected by every major nursing organization; however, health-care facilities continue to attempt "back-door" institutional licensure. When foreign nurses are allowed to practice in specific institutions without taking the American licensure examinations, de facto institutional licensure exists even if it is not called by name.

What's so bad about institutional licensure? The primary problem is the lack of external standards to determine the level of competency. Obviously, when the representatives of hospitals planning to hire foreign nurses interview candidates, they are looking for certain characteristics or qualities. What were these qualities? Ability to speak English? Not having a family? Knowledge in critical care, obstetrics, or pediatrics? The hospital establishes the criteria and no one outside the administration really knows how the finalists are selected.

Without external standards, the designations of RN or LPN/LVN (licensed practical nurse/licensed vocational nurse) become relatively meaningless. In addition, without an American nursing license, these foreign nurses would not be under the control of the state board of nursing. What if the foreign nurse was practicing unethically or made grievous negligent errors that caused harm to the client? Who would be responsible? Who would discipline the nurse?

Nurses practicing in states where the importation of foreign nurses is being planned or actually practiced need to contact their state board of nursing. It is highly probable that the practice violates a standard in the nurse practice act, and the facilities conducting the practice should be investigated.

Luxury Health Care

Guest Suites for Gourmets

Some nurses are attempting to deal with the consequences of the nursing shortage, such as understaffing, mandatory overtime, supervision of undertrained personnel, and erosion of the quality of care, by seeking employment in what have become known as "luxury health-care centers."

Luxury health-care centers are for-profit facilities that specialize in specific, high-revenue health care. In addition to offering high-end perks for the clients, such as gourmet meals, well-decorated, "resort-like," comfortable rooms that are sometimes called "guest suites," and one-room stays rather than moving from the intensive care unit (ICU) to a medical/surgical unit, these facilities attract nurses who are tired of the working conditions in traditional hospitals.

Profitable Procedures

The luxury health-care centers focus on providing specific services for particular procedures that generate high profits. Heart and orthopedic hospitals, cancer centers, and freestanding surgery facilities currently are the most common focus for this type of health care. The heart hospitals offer the services usually found in a general hospital, such as angioplasty, pacemaker insertion, and bypass surgery, but with a much higher level of care. These hospitals use the client-focused care model in which a client stays in one room throughout the stay and is provided care by the same nurses until discharge.

These facilities generate revenue by offering only certain high-end medical procedures that have a large profit margin and are covered by insurance. The luxury facilities save money by having a minimal number of administrators and allowing the nurses more input into the policy decisions and day-to-day provision of care.

In many of these facilities, up to 60 percent of the nursing staff is involved in direct client care, whereas the average in general hospitals is about 40 percent. Nurses are also cross-trained so they can function in multiple roles. In addition, the facilities reduce costs by shortening the length of client stays. Several limited research studies have shown that in luxury facilities where the client-centered model is used, client stays are routinely reduced by 25 to 50 percent.

> *Nurses employed at magnet hospitals have a high degree of job satisfaction and a much lower than average turnover rate compared to nurses in other hospitals of similar size.*

What Do You Think?

What experiences have you encountered, either as a client or a health-care worker, related to the nursing shortage? How might the political system help solve the shortage?

_____

_____

_____

_____

_____

_____

_____

_____

_____

_____

_____

_____

_____

What Attracts the Nurse?

Nurses find a luxury health-care environment attractive for several reasons. They feel that they can provide a higher level of continuity of care because the same nurse admits the client, cares for the client during the stay, and then handles the discharge when the client goes home.

Nurses feel that the quality of care is much higher in luxury facilities. They work primarily with adequate numbers of well-trained professionals. Cross-training allows nurses to practice in several different settings, reducing the monotony of practice sometimes experienced in general hospitals. Also, by having a bigger say in the work environment, policies, and care they provide, one of the primary elements of burnout—lack of control—is significantly reduced.

Finally, nurses in luxury care facilities earn on average $5.00 to $7.00 more per hour than nurses in traditional hospitals. Retirement and health insurance plans are often better, and some even offer stock options as part of the benefit package.

The Downside

Revenue Siphoning

What is the downside to luxury hospitals? One significant problem is the siphoning off of the highest revenue procedures from the general hospitals. Most general, not-for-profit hospitals do a continual financial juggling act in an attempt to balance services that lose money or make little money (trauma centers, burn units, obstetric units) with areas that have a high income (cardiac centers, orthopedic centers, one-day surgery). Some analysts believe that the competition from luxury hospitals will force general hospitals to improve the quality of their care so they can draw in more clients, but the reality is that if the general hospitals run at a deficit for too long, they will be forced to close.

Increased Shortages

Another concern is that the most experienced and most qualified nurses are being lured away from general hospitals. The nursing shortage has made it an employees' market. Luxury hospitals, because of their higher pay, can pick and choose from the best of the best. Heart hospitals are particularly interested in hiring ICU and critical care unit (CCU) nurses, as well as nurses with surgical and recovery room experience. This group represents some of the best-educated and most skilled nurses in any facility. As a result, the staffing shortages in the general hospitals will increase, and the quality of care will suffer more from the loss of experienced nurses.

Magnet Hospitals

Another more positive approach to the nursing shortage is the establishment of "magnet hospital" status for hospitals that retain a high percentage of the nurses they hire. In 1980, the American Academy of Nurses conducted a study to identify those elements that were present in hospitals that attracted and retained nurses. Several key factors were identified in hospitals that seemed to fulfill the magnet status, including a participative management style, allowing the nurses a relatively high degree of autonomy in practice and decision making, high-quality leadership at the unit level, a horizontal organizational structure, allowing nurses to practice as full professionals, offering opportunities for career development, and high-quality client care. Nurses employed at magnet hospitals have a high degree of job satisfaction and a much lower than average turnover rate compared to nurses in other hospitals of similar size.

The magnet hospital program has grown markedly since the original study. The ANA has established rather rigorous standards for hospitals to meet to obtain the magnet designation. Most hospitals have found achieving magnet status to be very challenging and only a small percentage are able to achieve it on the first try. However, hospitals that do obtain magnet status have achieved a well-deserved level of prestige among their peers. Nurses working at these hospitals have more control over their practice, and the end result is that higher-quality care is provided to the clients.

A Long-Term Solution

None of the above-mentioned measures really address the underlying problem of the nursing shortage. The long-term solution is to increase the supply of nurses by encouraging more young men and women to enter schools of nursing.

National trends in nursing school enrollments have shown a gradual increase in enrollment over the past few years, offering some hope for a long-range cure. However because of an acute shortage of nursing faculty, many nursing schools are turning away qualified students. For those who do choose to enter the nursing profession and manage to get into nursing school, the future looks bright. There are many opportunities, and health-care facilities are beginning to appreciate and reward nurses at the level they deserve.

Legislating Nurse-to-Client Ratios

A recent example of the power of an alliance occurred in California in relation to the nursing shortage. The California state legislature made the precedent-setting move to establish minimum nurse-to-client ratios by enacting legislation in late 1999. The regulations are to be phased in over several years and took effect in July 2003.

Although the initial results have been mixed, nurses' unions and consumer advocacy groups, such as the American Association of Retired Persons (AARP), support the proposal as a step toward increasing client safety and reducing the nursing shortage. Other states are following the development of this legislation closely. As always, there is political opposition to bills of this type, generally by the state hospital associations and often the physicians' association too.

The nursing shortage and the various attempts to resolve it are health-care issues that have become political. They have the potential to

Issues Now

The Need for Organization at the State Level

Why do nurses need to organize at the state level? A debate that just starting in nursing about the political activity of the ANA at the federal level. The ANA over the past several years has successfully raised money through telemarketing in every state in the country. Many nurses do not realize that the ANA Political Action Committee (PAC) is now the second largest federal PAC in Washington. In the last election cycle, they raised $1.2 million, which was spent on political activities exclusively at the federal level. However, it is important to realize that many of the political battles nurses have to fight are at the state level.

There is an ongoing discussion between the federal and state governments about what constitutes a legitimate course of action for the federal government and what constitutes a legitimate course of action for the state government. The 10th Amendment to the Constitution essentially says that any powers that are not expressly articulated to be part of the federal government mandate go to the states. This amendment underlies the current debate about Medicaid and Medicare and whether or not the states should be responsible for its administration.

The Role of State Nursing Organizations

The concept of unfunded mandates has come to the forefront in the past few years as a result of the states' rights push. There is an ongoing discussion among members of the National Governors' Association demanding that the federal government give governors more latitude in governing their states. They are saying, "Don't give us mandates. Give us the opportunity to set our own standards, our own regulatory actions, and our own legislative and governmental agenda." The nation is moving toward greater state control governmentally. It would be great if nurses could organize and just concentrate on issues at the federal level in Washington, but because most of nursing's issues are at the state level, this strategy is probably not going to work.

For nursing organizations to be effective, there has to be organized political action among nurses and by nurses in every state in this country. In states where nurses are not active and organized politically, there is going to be in trouble, and the nurses in them will fare badly. Nurses need to realize that the trend is toward state nursing organizations becoming more active politically and determining their own fate. Consequently, nurses need to organize politically at the state level to increase their political power.

Another thing to keep in mind is that nurses' licensure, as well as the certification and regulation of hospitals, is a function of the state. Again, it does not make sense to concentrate all of nursing's resources at the national level. Of course, there are some issues and programs, particularly with respect to funding, in which federal action is necessary, but most of the issues nurses are going to be dealing with occur at the state level, and that is where attention needs to be focused. The reality is that the states have the capacity to define and regulate objective standards for both nurses and hospitals. The mandate for nursing is to define how those standards are established and then develop an achievable agenda for political action by nurses at the state level.

significantly affect the profession of nursing, and nurses need to get out in front of the issues if they want to have a say in what is decided about their future.[2]

GOVERNMENT AND POLITICS

Keep in mind that *government* is a very broad term that refers to almost any type of hierarchical structure that functions to organize and direct an organization. From this context, the governance structure of any health-care facility can be considered a type of government that has its own politics. At this level, nurses have the potential to have a considerable amount of political influence.

Relevance to Nursing

Historically, most nurses avoided becoming engaged in government, perhaps because they agree with definitions similar to the one presented by Bierce. However, nurses, both as individual citizens and as a professional group, need to recognize that their personal lives and professional practice are affected by the political world. Some recent trends in health care, particularly the nursing shortage, managed care, and cost containment, have made nurses increasingly susceptible to the "bottom line."

In addition, because of politics, nurses are confronting major changes in health care on a daily basis. They have experienced the erosion of the profession through their replacement with less-educated personnel and have seen the quality of client care deteriorate. Nurses, if they decide to act, are not powerless against such trends.

The Sleeping Giant

As a large group of voters, nurses have the power, influence, and skill to take an active role in the political process. Senator Daniel Inouye of Hawaii referred to nurses as the "sleeping giant in health care." Nurses can gain much by using the tools of political action, and now more than ever their professional survival depends on it.

Individual nurses can take attainable, deliberate actions that can create a powerful, political force. However, before nurses can realize their full potential, a basic knowledge and understanding of the political system is necessary. Henry Adams stated long ago that "knowledge of human nature is the beginning and end of a political education." If he is correct, it is logical to conclude that nurses, who are among the most astute observers of human nature, are in many ways ideally suited to the art and science of politics.

WHY SHOULD NURSES BE INVOLVED?

Every Aspect of Life

A widely accepted definition of politics is the process of influencing *public policy,* including all forms and levels of governmental regulations. The effects of politics are pervasive and related to almost every aspect of life.

On a personal level, politics influence where children go to school, the quality of food, the water that flows from your kitchen tap, what medications are prescribed, and the speed limit on roadways. On a professional level, politics influences where nurses work, what they do and how they do it, the ability to organize professionally, and even the nurse's professional status through licensure and certification. The effects of politics on a person's life would seem to have no limits.

Is Acceptance Necessary?

Nurses experience the effects of governmental regulations both directly and indirectly. Examples of directly experienced government regulations include some recent reforms that many states have initiated. Some state legislatures have considered nurse-to-patient ratios. All states now have granted advanced practice nurses prescriptive privileges, although the regulations governing their implementation vary widely from state to state.

Earlier attempts at national health-care reform resulted in massive restructuring of the health-care system that led to dramatic decreases in the number of nurses employed in acute care hospitals. These reforms, initiated to forestall proposed legislation, continue to influence health care today. Many nurses respond to these changes with sad acceptance and believe that they are beyond their control.

Saul Alinsky provides useful pointers regarding tactics that nurses can use. Box 19.1 summarizes and gives examples of Alinsky's Rules for Radicals.[3]

POLITICS AND POLITICAL ACTION

Politics

As a dynamic process, politics plays a key role in all forms and levels of government, including federal, state, and local. It can be seen as the complex interaction between public policy and various public and constituent interests.

Politics is directly and indirectly influenced by the self-interest of political officials, both elected and appointed. The mass media also have both a direct and indirect impact on the political process through numerous political commentators, political commercials, and investigations into the backgrounds of selected political figures.

Political Action

Political action is a set of activities, methods, tactics, and behaviors that affect or have the potential to affect governmental and legislative processes and outcomes.[4] Examples of political action include grassroots efforts to change policies, the activities of lobbyists to change elected officials' opinions or votes, the give and take of political compromise within legislative bodies, and even the power of veto by the chief executive of a governmental structure.

A Series of Processes

Government is often thought of as a series of processes used to maintain society. As both an element of and result of politics, government is also influenced by the forces that drive politics and the three concepts that constitute it:

- Partisanship
- Self-interest
- Ideology

Partisanship

Partisanship refers to membership in a political party. Because of the limited nature of this chapter, it focuses on Democrats, Republicans, and to a lesser extent, independents.

Self-Interest

Self-interest is almost always the most important factor in politics. It dictates the kind of issues that legislators become involved in and present to their constituencies as the key issues. For instance, a congressman who resides in a blue-collar industrialized district that has a majority who support unionization will most likely be pro-union. The legislative structure in the United States was designed so that elected officials represent the people in their districts

Box 19.1

Alinsky's Rules for Radicals (with O'Donnell's Comments)

- Power is not only what you have but what the enemy thinks you have.

This concept is widely used in political organizing. Fundraising reports are a classic example. Candidates work very hard to get their financial commitments before filing their candidacy, to inform people of their ammunition.

- Never go outside the experience of your own people.

This is the fundamental mistake that has been made in some efforts to organize nurses. The American Nurses Association (ANA) and the state associations too often reflect an elite group not connected to the real world. Their leadership tends not to be nurses from the bedside or those intimately connected with front-line nursing. Their concerns, although legitimate, do not reflect the experience of the nurses entrenched in patient care issues.

- Wherever possible, go outside the experience of your enemy. Pick your battlefields.

During a press conference around the March on Washington in 1996, nurses talked about their experiences that were foreign territory to the press. They presented a compelling picture. Most of the press were not accustomed to listening to nurses talk about high-tech procedures and gained a new level of respect for what nurses do. To the extent to which you can impress people with your knowledge and go outside their experience, it forces them to compete.

- Make them live up to their own book of rules.

An example of this rule happened many years ago. Bob O'Donnell, former speaker of the Pennsylvania House, tells a story about when he was first breaking into the political world. There was a party machine that was not interested in supporting the common interests of the neighborhoods. Undaunted, O'Donnell learned the rules by which the next ward leader and committee person election would be held.

Ward leaders and committee people are the smallest unit of the partisan political system. Usually committee people are responsible for districts. The districts add up to the ward. The ward leader oversees the committee people who manage those districts and register people to vote.

Standing within the system is necessary to be successful in a political system. The way to do that in the ward structure is to either be ward leader or to have significant influence over the ward leader. Over a period of several years, O'Donnell assisted his allies in obtaining committee positions. When there was an election for the ward leader, the committee people elected O'Donnell to the position. The party machinery refused to seat the ward leader. O'Donnell used their own rule book to bring the issue to federal court and forced them to seat him as the new ward leader. He beat them at their own game.

- Ridicule is man's and woman's most potent weapon.

This is also known as the Dan Quayle phenomenon. Dan Quayle has been repeatedly characterized as a political buffoon. Dan Quayle is not as unintelligent as people assume him to be. Unfortunately for him, Vice President Quayle did some uninformed things while he happened to be standing in front of a magnifying glass with the national press behind it. More recently, Bill Clinton became the focus of many a political joke because of his involvement with Monica Lewinsky. His Republican enemies seized on the incident to the point where they made it an issue of impeachment.

(continued)

B o x   1 9 . 1

Alinsky's Rules for Radicals (with O'Donnell's Comments) (conitnued)

- A good tactic is one that your people enjoy.

The 1996 March on Washington is a wonderful example. Laura Gasparis Vonfrolio did a wonderful job of tapping into the anger disseminated all over the country. Nurses enjoyed the national forum that permitted a massive demonstration for their voices to finally be heard.

- A tactic that drags on too long, becomes a drag; use the concepts of reward and momentum.

This is the most dangerous pitfall for nurses attempting political organizing. The process is difficult and takes time to reach a successful conclusion. Nurses can become discouraged by the slow pace of the change process in the political arena. Rather than focusing only on long-range goals, it is important to concentrate on smaller objectives such as achieving a significant role in a city council race.

- Keep the pressure on. Become the constant by which all other variables are defined.

Currently, the ANA defines issues and concepts at the national level. The ANA has raised money in every state and has translated that money into a political power base in Washington. When a senator or congressman who has been a beneficiary of the ANA's largess takes a position, it is with the ANA in mind. Nurses need to become the standard by which all related variables are measured in their states. State legislators need to consider nurses' opinions the same way they do now with the teachers' association.

- The threat is usually more terrifying than the thing itself. Threat is multiplied by the unknown and the imagination of someone under attack.

This principle can be used very effectively over time. Imagine if someone opposed pro-nursing legislation and nurses threatened to demonstrate. The public image of thousands of nurses donning their uniforms would be a very powerful image for legislators to contend with.

- The major premise for tactics is the development of operations that will maintain a constant pressure on the opposition. The pressure must be sustainable over time.

This is the concept of "if what, then what." In a tactical plan, you have to be able to look beyond and determine what happens after you reach the end of this tactic.

- Pick the target. Freeze it. Personalize it. Polarize it. And use a focused and strategic attack.

Essentially, nurses need to be focused in their political activities. For example, imagine that nurses have considerable support from various legislative groups for objective standards and want to pass a law. A solid bill has been drafted, but a Democrat or Republican will not introduce your bill.

The strategy is to target the one person who is slowing it down, whether it is the speaker, the senate pro tem president, or the majority leader. Pick the target. Freeze it. Go after it with a vengeance. Personalize the attack and look at the person's constituencies. If he or she has a large senior citizen constituency, proclaim to the media that the prevention of the passage of your legislation is putting senior citizens in your legislative district in danger. The legislator will have to respond. Remember the one cardinal tenet of legislative action: never hurt "Mom," "Pop," or the "little guy." That is a focused and strategic attack.

Source: Alinsy, S: Rules for Radicals: A Practical Primer for Realistic Radicals. Random House, New York, 1971.

rather than having the whole population of the United States trying to make policy decisions. If a candidate does not represent the beliefs of the district, it is unlikely that he or she will succeed in that district.

In the larger world of electoral politics, the principle of self-interest often means that an elected official will not make legislative or political decisions that could lead to professional damage, namely loss of an election. Occasionally, there are exceptions to this rule. There have been a few cases in which elected officials were so ideologically committed to an issue that they defied conventional wisdom and made decisions that went against their self-interest. Generally, to be effective in politics, a person needs to understand and accept the self-interests of his or her constituents and use these self-interests as the driving force in political decision making.

Ideology

Ideology is a broad concept that embodies the beliefs and principles of an individual or group. Conservatives, liberals, populists, libertarians, and radicals represent five examples of ideologies.

Conservatives

Traditionally, conservatives support less governmental regulation, less involvement in everyday life, fewer taxes, and smaller social programs. The general characterization of the conservative belief system is "less government equals better government." Applied to the current range of issues, conservatives tend to be antiabortion, anti–gun control, anti–stem cell research, anti–socialized health care, and pro-choice on education.

However, after the election in 2004, the conservative movement has become closely identified with fundamentalist Christian and Mormon values. Its past focus on financial conservatism also appears to be changing with the accumulation of huge federal deficits that will affect the national economy for many years to come.

Liberals

Traditional liberals believe that government has a moral responsibility to do good for society and that government intervention is necessary for the greater good of the citizens. This ideology traditionally translates into larger government structures, increased taxes, and more spending for a wide range of social programs. Liberals are traditionally pro-choice, pro–gun control, pro–government-regulated health care, and anti-choice on education.

Populists

Populists are probably the most dominant political force in the United States at a grassroots level. Although populists in general do not like paying high taxes, ideologically they may represent a variety of positions on any particular issue. For instance, one group of populists may be antiabortion, whereas another may be pro-choice.

The common bond among all populists is that they have a sense of being burdened by a large, oppressive government structure. "The middle class is under siege" is a major theme that has resonated throughout several recent presidential campaigns.

Libertarians

Libertarianism is both a political party and an ideology. As a political partisan group, they represent an electoral fringe element. Ideologically, Libertarians differ from populists because they do not have the underlying middle-class anger that often drives the populists to take political action. Although they do believe in fiscal conservatism and dislike paying high taxes, Libertarians tend to be "laid back" in their approach to politics. Typically, they avoid ideological battles because they do not want to be burdened with decisions about choice on gun control, health care, schools, or abortion.

Radicals

Radicals exist at both ends of the ideological spectrum in both of the major parties. It is important to recognize that although most voters tend toward the middle of the political spectrum between conservatism and liberalism, radicals attempt to force their parties to the extreme ends of the spectrum.

For instance, Republicans are challenged by the radical right, which consists of the anti–big government and pro-life forces that make conspicuous demands on the party. To counteract the rhetoric of the radicals, the Republican party tries to find candidates who are ideologically near the middle of the spectrum because they know that most Republican voters have similar opinions.

UNDERSTANDING THE PLAYING FIELD

Structure

The three branches of the government are the executive, judicial, and legislative branches. These branches exist simultaneously at the federal, state, and local government levels.

The Executive Branch

At the federal level, the executive branch consists of the president, vice president, cabinet, and various executive administrative bodies. The executive of a state is the governor. Boards and commissions can also be construed as part of the executive branch because they are appointees of the chief executive. In county government, one or more county commissioners function as executives. Larger cities usually have a mayor. Smaller cities and townships sometimes also elect mayors (Fig. 19.1; Box 19.2).

The Judicial Branch

The judicial branch is the court system. It is important to note the distinction between state court and federal court; appeals and supreme courts are found at both levels. At the state level, there are supreme courts, appeals courts, and the lower courts. At the federal level, there is the Supreme Court, federal courts of appeal, and district or circuit courts. Additionally, many cities and counties have a local court system.

The judicial branch of government should not be discounted as unimportant to nurses. Over the years, courts have decided several important issues that have an effect on the practice of nursing. These include the Supreme Court's decision regarding the right of nurses to organize into collective bargaining units (see Chapter 16), the requirement of health-care providers to report potentially violent patients to the police, the obligation of nurses to refuse to carry out physician orders they deem dangerous, and criteria for when nurses can withdraw life support measures. New test cases that are continually being brought before the Supreme Court have the potential to dramatically change the way nurses are perceived and what they are permitted to do in the workplace.

The Legislative Branch

At the federal level, the legislative branch of government consists of the House of Representatives and the Senate. Each state also has a legislative branch of government, and, except for Nebraska, all states have a bicameral legislature with both a house of representatives and a senate. The primary function of the legislative branch of government is the formation of policy by the making of laws.

Key Players in the Legislative Process

Members of the legislative branch of government have a wide range of ability and influence. It is important to remember that legislators are human

Box 19.2

Know the Structure to Play the Game

One of the keys to creating power is understanding the organizational structure of the government. The Constitution of the United States establishes three separate branches of the federal government: legislative, judicial, and executive. The Constitution also ascribes certain auxiliary powers to the individual states. It is the role of the state governments to serve their citizens within these parameters and to delegate discrete areas of activity to local governments.

Beneath the federal and state level of government in the United States, there exist five layers of local government identified by the U.S. Census Bureau: county, municipal, township, school district, and special district governments (which include various utility, construction, and facility authorities). The qualifications for the classification of these local government structures are generally determined by the parent state governments. State governments are defined by their individual state constitutions and in turn delineate responsibility for the local governments.

It is important for nurses to understand that there are three levels in each governmental sector: federal, state, and local. These distinctions are important and are the most common source of confusion for nurses.

Figure 19.1 The organizational structure of the government.

and they respond to the same forces that all people respond to, including interpersonal dynamics, peer pressure, and both internal and external factors.

The Majority Leader
The majority leader in the House is the person who generally supervises and directs the activities on the House floor. Some consider it to be the most powerful job in politics. The majority leader has control over the legislative calendar, which ultimately determines when many of the House session activities take place and even when bills are introduced for consideration. The majority leader is also the central figure in crafting the budget, which is the most important activity the legislature performs on an annual basis.

The Majority Whip
The majority whip is responsible for collecting votes when legislators may be leaning toward voting against their party. At the same time the majority leader is supporting a bill, the whip is negotiating on the House floor for the votes necessary to successfully pass the bill. The whip is responsible for collecting support and votes for various issues both during the legislative session and when they are in recess.

The Minority Leader
The minority leader represents the party that does not have a numerical majority in the House and helps organize support against bills introduced by the majority leader. The minority leader presents an alternative point of view. There is an expression in the legislature: "The majority will have their way, and the minority will have their say."

In most cases, the majority party has the capacity to pass almost any bill they support over the objections of the minority. The minority leader usually only has the capacity to speak against it. However, there are some issues that legislators will almost never vote against: "mom," "pop," and the "little guy." When these issues are included in a bill, most legislators will support it even if they must vote against their party.

The Conference Committee
The conference committee attempts to reconcile differences in bills from the House and the Senate. The

What Do You Think?

Who do you know in the legislature of your state government? Who is your representative or congressperson? Make a list of the things you would want that person to do for health care.

rules governing the structure, composition, and function of the conference committee vary from state to state. Generally, they consist of an equal number of appointed members from both the House and the Senate. Often a specified combination of votes, such as two votes from the House and two votes from the Senate, is necessary to approve a compromise bill and move it out of committee.

Caucuses
Caucuses are formed when the legislature divides into groups consisting of people with mutual interests. These groups operate as a unit, trading on their capacity to bring a block of votes for or against an issue or bill, rather than an individual vote. Examples are the Black Caucus, the Women's Caucus, the Hispanic Caucus, and the Business Community Caucus.

Although caucuses may be bipartisan, many are partisan in nature. For example, the largest caucus groups are the Democratic Caucus and the Republican Caucus. Each caucus develops its own internal governance structure and leadership, including a speaker who leads the caucus and speaks for the group. After a group member achieves a leadership role, he or she must try to balance the wishes of the group against his or her own political survival in the caucus and the political pressures exerted by the larger world.

> *The media have become a tangible power in government, often driving and shaping public opinion that eventually evolves into a legislative agenda.*

THE POWER OF THE MEDIA

When Is It News?

The media and the voters are external forces that influence policy makers. The media have become a tangible power in government, often driving and shaping public opinion that eventually evolves into a legislative agenda. The public often perceives media personalities as the people who know, write, and speak about important public issues and matters of substance. Although they claim to be objective, the major news organizations decide what is and what is not news. The Fox news network has made it publicly known that they support the Republican conservative positions and slant all their news to favor those positions.[5]

One study performed at a large research university investigated how the media reported political campaigns from the years 1975 to 1995. The study compared the number of words recorded in writing or spoken on television by the candidates with the number of words spoken or written by the media about the candidate, which acted as a filter, translator, or commentator for the public. The results showed that the media consistently out-communicated the candidates at all levels. Recent experience would tend to reinforce these findings.

Election by Media

Before media campaigns became the norm, with millions of dollars being spent on television and radio advertising, the printed news media used to publish what the candidate said and often printed whole speeches. This approach allowed the public to read the speeches and make up their minds about which issues the candidate supported. Today, the trend is to give a 30-second sound bite of a speech, then have 10 minutes of political analysis by a well-known commentator who tells the public what the candidate is saying.

Some of the printed media have adopted a similar approach to political issues. In newspapers, it is not unusual to see a lengthy editorial comment positioned next to a statement made by a candidate. Elected officials have a great respect for the power of the media to influence public opinion. Those who learn to use the media to their advantage get elected.

Legislator Beware

Legislators, while recognizing and using the power of the media, have also become wary of it. They know that although they can use the media to proclaim their message, the media also pose a risk to their political survival, depending on the vulnerability of their position. Some legislators have a false sense of invulnerability because of the nature of their constituency base.

A Story with Legs

For example, a legislator may have a large population of senior citizens in his district who have supported him for many years. The legislator publicly supports senior citizen issues and believes that the senior citizen support will always be there. However, during an election campaign, a political opponent's investigation uncovers information that the legislator voted against several bills that would have increased senior citizens' benefits. In addition, the opponent discovers that the legislator is having an affair with his married secretary.

The opponent leaks this information to the media, which immediately put it on television and report it in the newspapers. If the story develops "legs," meaning it takes on a life of its own and continues to grow even without further information from the opponent, it will be on television news programs and in the newspapers every day. The major networks will do investigative reporting on the issues, and eventually the talk show and television tabloid programs will become interested and begin interviewing people who know or have heard about more "dirty little secrets" about the legislator.

At this point, the legislator who is the subject of that story is in political jeopardy. There is little that a politician fears more than being the subject this type of negative story.

THE POLITICAL PROCESS

Who Introduces Legislation?

Where Laws Begin

Laws serve to maintain order in a complicated society and regulate the interactions of its citizens. As society becomes more complex, more laws are needed to ensure the survival and smooth functioning of the population.

For example, although computers and electronic communications have increased the quantity of information individuals can process and the speed at which it is transmitted, they have also added to the complexity of the world. Just a few years ago, there were no laws that dealt with hacking, computer fraud, computer theft of bank funds, or on-line pornography. Today, there is an ever-growing body of law that deals with computers, and whole sections of police agencies, such as the Federal Bureau of Investigation's Computer Crime Unit, are dedicated to enforcing these laws. Where do ideas for laws and policies come from, and how do these ideas become laws?

Elected Officials

Any elected official, including governors, mayors, county commissioners, and city council members, can propose a program or initiative that requires passage by the legislature (i.e., a *bill*). The elected official will go to the legislative leadership in the parties and ask them either to submit the bill or to help move the bill through the legislative process.

Lobbyists, constituency groups, and advocates are a major source of proposed legislation. They represent various interests ranging from public interest groups to corporate lobbyists. Lobbyists frequently craft legislation and then pass it on to a friendly legislator. Consumer groups are often visible at the legislature through demonstrations and lobbying.

Constituency groups can best be described by example, such as the AARP. These groups are made up of individuals interested in advancing an agenda that promotes a range of issues based on self-interest. Advocates, in contrast, are groups that have a single issue or point of view that they are trying to advance, such as housing or abortion rights.

Government Agencies

Legislation is also generated from government agencies. When agencies are seeking fee increases or another type of policy reform, they can introduce legislation. For example, policy reforms in the Internal Revenue Service (IRS) are a type of agency-initiated legislation. Frequently the employees of the agency will draft the legislation and then direct it toward a supportive legislator.

What Drives Legislation?

Funding. Because almost all government agencies depend on legislative funding to sustain their operations, they become actively engaged, overtly or covertly, in seeking the passage of a budget that will sustain their survival.

Public Demand. Legislators are very careful to listen to the demand of their voters and avoid voting against an issue to which the public is emotionally attached. A classic example of this process was seen in New Jersey, where a child was sexually molested and murdered by a known convicted sex offender who moved into the child's neighborhood. The tragedy prompted a public outcry: How could this happen? Something needs to be done! Ultimately, the outcry produced the now famous Megan's Law, which requires public disclosure of a known sex offender's residence.

Program Issues. These issues recur periodically and require legislative attention. Requests for increases in television cable rates constitute an example of a programmatic issue. The cable industry will be very interested in the outcome of legislation that may affect what they can charge for their services. Both cable and consumer group lobbyists actively seek the ear of key legislators at these times.

Constituent-Specific Issues. Groups of voters may have specific interests that can lead to introduction of a bill. For example, in legislative districts where a large population of senior citizens reside, the escalating cost of prescriptions may be an important issue. Legislation specific to that constituency will be introduced at a greater rate than in areas with fewer senior citizens.

How Bills Become Law

The Tracking Number

Any legislator can introduce a bill from any source. Additional legislators can sign on as the bill's cosponsors. A bill is considered to be strong if it has

Contact your state legislature's Web site and identify two bills that deal with health care. How do you feel about these bills? How should your representative vote on this issue?

_____

_____

_____

_____

_____

_____

_____

_____

_____

_____

_____

strong sponsorship, including a number of powerful cosponsors, a high degree of bipartisanship, and the interest of powerful individuals, both political and nonpolitical. After the bill is introduced, it is taken to the chief clerk, who assigns it a number that permits it to be tracked throughout the process.

The Committee

After the bill is assigned a number, it is referred to a **committee.** The house and senate leaders decide which committee considers the bill. This decision, greatly influenced by politics, is critical to the survival and ultimate passage of a bill.

It is no coincidence that most bills die in committee. Invariably, the leadership discusses their expectation for the bill with the committee chairs, and if the leadership wants a bill to fail, it is referred to a committee where it will never be voted on or passed on to the House.

Full Committee Hearing

At the federal level, bills are referred to a full committee and, generally, because of the enormous number of bills being introduced, to a subcommittee. Most of the work of Congress takes place within the committee structures. Committee action is perhaps the most important phase of the congressional process, for this is where the most intensive consideration is given to proposed measures and where people are provided with an opportunity to be heard.

Subcommittee Hearing

The subcommittee studies the issue carefully, holds hearings, and reports the bill back to the full committee with recommendations. There are numerous standing committees in the House and Senate. In addition, there are several select committees and several standing joint committees. Each committee has jurisdiction over certain subjects and often has two or more subcommittees.

In the U.S. Congress, the committees with greatest jurisdiction over health matters and their subcommittees are:

- **House Ways and Means Committee:** Social Security and Medicare (health-care subcommittees)
- **House Commerce Committee:** Health legislation including Medicaid (Subcommittee on Health and the Environment)
- **Senate Finance Committee:** Medicare and Medicaid (health subcommittees)
- **Senate Labor and Human Resources Committee:** Health legislation in general; also works cooperatively with the Senate Finance Committee in considering issues involving Medicare and Medicaid
- **House and Senate Appropriations Committee:** Authorizes all money necessary to implement action proposed in a bill (subcommittees for labor, education, and health and human services)

The Next Step

As a result of full committee hearings, several things may happen to a bill. It may be:

- Reported out of committee favorably and be scheduled for debate by the full House or Senate
- Reported out favorably, but with amendments
- Reported out unfavorably
- Killed outright

For example, a bill reforming the way judges are elected ideally would go to the judiciary committee; however, there is no legal requirement that the speaker or the Senate pro tem president send the bill to any particular committee. For political reasons, the speaker may refer the bill to the committee on intergovernmental affairs, where it will languish and die.

Can the Bill Survive?

For a bill to survive, the bill's sponsor must have the knowledge and the political standing to move the bill out of committee. If sponsors are truly committed, they will trade on their political capital. *Political capital* generally refers to some type of favor or action that a politician can exchange for something he or she wants. It is an extremely important element in the legislative process and consists of, but is not limited to, votes, amendments to bills, appointments, and support from constituency groups. Political capital often consists of an "If you vote for my bill, I'll vote for your bill" type of exchange.

A Scheduled Debate

After a bill has been reported out of a House committee (with the exception of ways and means or appropriations committees), it goes to the Rules Committee, which schedules bills and determines how much time will be spent on debate and whether or not amendments will be allowed. In the Senate, bills go on the Senate calendar, after which the majority leadership determines when a bill will be debated.

After a bill is debated, possibly amended, and passed by one chamber, it is sent to the other chamber, where it goes through the same procedure. If the bill passes both the House and the Senate without any changes, it is sent to the president for signature.

Opposing Versions

If the House and Senate pass different versions of a bill, however, the two bills are sent to a conference committee, which consists of members appointed by both the House and the Senate. This committee seeks to resolve the differences between the two bills; if the differences cannot be resolved, the bill dies in committee. When the conference committee reaches agreement on a bill, it goes back to the House and Senate for passage. At this juncture, the bill must be voted up or down, because no further amendments are accepted.

Passage or Veto?

If the bill is approved in both houses, it then goes to the chief executive—at the federal level, the president

or at the state level, the governor—who makes determinations about bill. Governors can do one of two things: sign the bill into law or actively **veto** the bill. At the federal level, the president has the same options, with the addition of the pocket veto. Pocket vetoes, found only at the federal level, occur when the president, rather than actively vetoing a bill, simply does not sign it so that it does not become law. If vetoed, it is sent back to the House and Senate. To override the veto, a two-thirds vote by both chambers is required.

The Fiscal Note

Clearly, the passage of a law can be a long and difficult process. This is often quite frustrating for action-oriented nurses who are used to seeing immediate outcomes—forming plans and making things happen quickly.

All bills that are passed need a fiscal note attached to them. Therefore, the appropriations committee is operationally very powerful. A piece of legislation that is passed without a fiscal note attached will never become a law. Over the years, many pieces of legislation have been passed by the legislature but have been starved to death financially. These are called unfunded mandates.

Housekeeping Bills

Major regulatory change occurs in laws in the form of housekeeping bills. Legislators can use this tactic to move a piece of legislation through the process, especially when the bill is more significant than the leadership acknowledges it to be. Although regulatory reform and change may seem tedious, they are important to the legislative process and have the capacity to do enormous public good or harm.

Executive Orders

Executive orders provide the chief executive, the governor or the president, with a means for moving an agenda item forward. Executive orders are in many cases a convenient way to formulate policy with minimal involvement of the legislature. They also allow the executive to make a statement about an issue that can be entered on the public record.

The legislature can leave executive orders uncontested or challenge them, by characterizing them as beyond the scope of the executive branch. This may involve turning to the third branch of government, the judiciary.

Regulatory Agencies

Regulatory agencies are also arenas where policies are made and amended. For instance, the role of the Intergovernmental Regulatory Reform Commission (IRRC) is to examine regulatory issues across the state.

HOW TO BE POLITICALLY ACTIVE

Why Be Active?

The first step in becoming politically active is to identify the specific goals that nurses, as a group, want to accomplish. Nurses recognize many important issues in today's health-care system, including:

• Increasingly acute conditions of hospitalized clients, who require higher levels of care and more complex levels of support than ever before
• Increasing responsibilities for nurses in supervision of rising numbers of unlicensed health-care personnel
• Loss of control of the work environment caused by managed care organizations
• Ever-shortening hospitalizations resulting in clients being sent home "quicker and sicker"

Any one of these issues can become a focal point at which nurses aim their considerable political power.

For example, most nurses are concerned that RNs, who have traditionally been at clients' bedsides, are being replaced by individuals who are less prepared and less able to deal with high-acuity clients. Nurses believe that when they are replaced in large numbers by unlicensed assistive personnel, including nursing assistants, as well as with personnel who provide specific services, such as monitor technicians who sit in front of cardiac monitors, the quality of client care decreases. Nurses know that these technicians often take on responsibilities for which they have had little training. Rarely are there established national standards that require these assistive personnel to demonstrate their ability to provide a specific level of care or even standards that protect the public safety.

Feeling Powerless

Nurses are usually employees at will and can be fired for any reason. Although some efforts have been made in this direction, whistle-blower protection is generally not available to protect nurses who wish to speak out against unsafe staffing levels or employment practices.[6] Nurses are, at times, torn between their obligations to maintain high standards of safe, ethical care and their obligations to their families.

Although nurses often feel powerless against a monolithic health-care bureaucracy, in reality they have the potential to be a potent political force. Nationally, with almost 3 million nurses licensed to practice, the nursing profession constitutes the largest single body of health-care providers in the country.

Finding a Voice

Nurses in all health-care settings are saying, "Somebody's got to do something about this situation." The reality of the situation is that the "somebody" is nurses themselves. Once nurses identify exactly what it is that needs to be accomplished and understand what is possible within the political framework, then they can use their considerable political power to make changes that will benefit both the clients and the profession.

Rules for Radicals

Saul Alinsky, in *Rules for Radicals,* hypothesizes that human beings are divided into three groups: "the haves, the have nots, and the have a little and want mores." Nurses typically fall in the last group.[3]

Have a Little

One problem nurses in this group encounter is the ongoing conflict between the status quo and progress. They want to obtain more power and control, gain more benefits, earn more money, and have more respect as professionals. However, the strong desire to advance is counterbalanced by fear of jeopardizing their current jobs and their professional standing. Their motivation to be something more, to do something new, or to believe in something bigger is held back and pulled in another direction by their fear of change. The result of this internal tug-of-war is an attitude of inertia and ambivalence that has prevented nurses from organizing politically and effectively using their numerical power.

Want More

Despite the inertia and ambivalence problems of individuals in the "have a little and want more" category, some of the most notable revolutionaries in history have come from this group, including Thomas Jefferson, Napoleon Bonaparte, Martin Luther King, Jr., and Vladimir Lenin. Each of these individuals came from the working middle class with a belief that it could be made better. Nurses can use their actions as examples of what individuals can accomplish to raise their own motivation levels to a point where they overwhelms the inertia of the status quo.

Sit Back and Watch

A fourth group of people, who seem to come from the inertia found among the "have a little, want more" group are the "do-nothings." These individuals can be heard saying things like, "I agree with what you are saying, I just don't agree with your means," "I'm not going to get involved in this," or "I'm too busy to belong to the organization." The do-nothings tend to watch the activities of others, and if their efforts are successful, then they will join in as a beneficiary because they feel they have supported the effort from an ideological standpoint. However, they avoid any active involvement in politics. The eighteenth century British politician Edmund Burke recognized the danger of the do-nothings. He said, "The only thing necessary for the triumph of evil, is for good men [and women] to do nothing."

What Can One Nurse Do?

It is important to remember that politics is a free market enterprise open to anyone who is willing to become involved and play the game. Success in the political arena is contingent on three elements:

1. Knowledge and understanding of the process
2. The ability to offer something of value to the political figure
3. The capacity to identify what will be necessary to accomplish the objective

Anyone who is interested in becoming politically active must recognize that all candidates and elected officials need three things: resources to run their political operation (money and volunteers), votes, and a means to shape public opinion.

Resources

Money

Sufficient resources are essential to running a political campaign. The first and most necessary resource is always money. Would-be candidates soon discover that a lack of money to fund a campaign will inevitably lead to political failure. An unfunded candidate cannot travel, send mailings, produce radio and television commercials, post signs, or organize a telephone bank.

Voters often fail to realize that political candidates are only as available as finances permit. Frequently, good candidates lose because they fail to garner the financial resources necessary to run an effective campaign. Nurses can gain a candidate's support for issues by donating to his or her campaign chest.

Volunteers

A second important resource in an election campaign is volunteers. Volunteers work in campaigns by manning telephone banks, making literature drops, placing signs, and conducting voter registration drives. Usually political candidates are very glad to have free help for their campaigns.

Although nurses may not be able to make large monetary contributions to a candidate's campaign, they can always volunteer some time. Working closely with a candidate on a volunteer basis allows individuals to discuss important issues and helps candidates who support issues important to nurses. Most candidates need a considerable amount of education about health-related issues because of their lack of knowledge about medical and nursing concerns.

Votes

Obviously, votes are essential to any candidate. If a candidate does not have votes, he or she will not be elected. One of the most significant activities nurses can become involved in is to join and support a political party. The chosen party should reflect the nurse's value system and fundamental beliefs.

Keep in mind that there is never a perfect fit with any political party. Almost everyone who belongs to a political party will disagree at some point with some element of the party, usually with the extremist views. However, differing opinions and beliefs should not be a barrier to membership in a political party. The only way to change a view or opinion is by active participation from within the party.

The ultimate political power is the vote. Nurses need to be registered to vote and go to the polls on election day to cast their ballots for the candidates who support legislation that empowers nurses and who recognize what is needed for beneficial health-care reform.

Shaping Public Opinion

Public Trust in Nurses

Candidates need endorsements from their constituents so they can build their support base. They generally consider endorsements from nurses as one of the most valuable assets to their campaign. By careful selection of candidates who support legislation favorable to nursing and health care, endorsements can give nurses the capacity to shape public opinion. The periodic polls conducted by national news magazines asking readers to rank various professions by how much they are trusted have consistently shown that the public views nurses very highly, in the same category as police officers, firefighters, and teachers.

Why the Governor Matters

Nurses should use endorsements by choosing candidates in campaigns that have an impact on important issues. Often the campaign for governor falls into this category, because governors, as chief executives, have a great deal of political power and can appoint people to a number of boards, committees, and other positions. Nurses need to recognize that the members of the board of nursing in their state, as well as other important appointed positions in health departments and other regulatory agencies, may be appointed by the governor and that this board has the final decision on the way that nurses practice.

When nurses establish a working political relationship with the governor, the governor is more likely to look favorably on them as those who have sustained him or her, provided financial supported, and given endorsements during the political campaign. They will be the people the governor is going to appoint to a board position.

Targeting endorsements will prevent nurses from making blind political decisions. Candidates should be assessed first on their willingness to be supportive to issues that nurses are interested in and then on their capacity to win the election.

Grassroots Effort

A model for individual political development that encourages grassroots involvement in local issues is based on the belief that grassroots efforts may be more fulfilling than involvement in partisan politics.[7] This model is an activity-oriented ladder, including activities at four distinct levels:

- Rung 1: Civic involvement. Children's sports, parent-teacher association (PTA), neighborhood improvement group
- Rung 2: Advocacy. Writing letters to public officials and newspapers and making organized visits to officials to discuss local issues
- Rung 3: Organizing. Independent organizing on local issues, incorporation of single-issue citizens' groups, and networking with similarly situated citizens' groups
- Rung 4: Long-term power wielding. Campaigning for oneself or another, local government planning, and agenda setting

Nurses in Office

Nurses usually shudder at the thought of running for political office. They tend to perceive political campaigns as something underhanded and tawdry, and they just do not want to be involved. However, it is not impossible for nurses to achieve high status in public office.

One way that nurses can direct their political activities is to develop a political relationship with a legislator or a political operative who can mentor and guide the nurse in finding a route through the political maze. As discussed earlier, the principle of self-interest is one of the most critical elements in politics, and to establish a relationship with a political figure, nurses must demonstrate that the issues they support have value to both themselves and to the politician.

Making Alliances

There are several ways that a nurse can decide whom to support when becoming involved in the political process. A first step is to begin identifying the issues particular legislators are interested in and will vote for. Editorial opinion pieces in newspapers can provide a sense of the issues of concern to legislators.

It is a good idea to begin with local legislators and candidates, like the state representative, state senator, or the councilperson serving the neighborhood. Call their offices and find out when and where they are scheduled to speak, then go and listen to the speech to get a sense of who they are and what issues they support. Their speeches and the way they answer questions will reveal their ideology and partisanship. Also, during question and answer periods, ask elected officials what they think about issues important to you.

Another way to become familiar with prominent political figures is by attending some of the many partisan events that occur during an election season. A good way to visualize the local political landscape is by observing who is talking to whom at the event. Nurses can make their own assessments of political candidates by observing the candidates in action, calling their offices for information, reading published literature, and talking to people who know the candidate.

Beginning the process may seem difficult, but once you decide to become politically active, you'll become more confident.

Know the Issues

For nurses to be successful in the political process, they must know and understand the issues. At times an issue may be readily apparent in the nurses' community, for example, an increased number of homeless people. Other issues are easily identified by reading newspapers. Issues are generally presented in the editorial section; most newspapers also have a political watch section, which reports the results of any significant votes at the state and federal levels.

The American Nurses Association (ANA) newspaper, *American Nurse,* is an excellent source of information on issues of concern to the profession. In addition, the *American Journal of Nursing* Newsline feature and *Nursing and Health Care's* Washington Focus are excellent, easily readable sources of information in journals. *Capitol Update,* the ANA legislative newsletter for nurses, reports on the activities of its nurse lobbyists and on significant issues in Congress and regulatory agencies. This publication requires a subscription but is available in most nursing school and hospital libraries.

State nurses' associations and many specialty-nursing groups also publish newsletters or legislative bulletins. Many of these are free to members but may be sent only when requested. Action alerts may also be sent to inform members of vital issues and the action needed by nurses. Most state legisla-

tures now have on-line access to their proceedings so that bills of interest to nurses can be tracked as they progress through the legislative process.

Tactics

Tactics, essential tools for those who desire to be politically active, are the conscious and deliberate acts that people use to live and deal with each other and the world around them. In a political sense, tactics usually means using whatever resources are available to achieve a desired goal.

Hannibal, one of the great tacticians in political history, said, "We will either find a way or we will make a way." Nurses, with their long history of accomplishing much with few resources, are natural tacticians. As nurses learn how to organize themselves for political purposes, they can use their well-developed tactical skills to achieve important political goals. Listed below are some easy-to-use tactics for political action.

Use Powerful Resources

As an example, there are approximately 270,000 licensed nurses in Pennsylvania. By enlisting 25 percent of those nurses and collecting minimal dues, a powerful political force can be organized. If 25 percent of 270,000 nurses contribute $75 to a political action committee each year, approximately $5 million in annual revenue will be produced. In most states, $5 million would almost guarantee a win in any election.

Engage in Bipartisan Tactics

Both republican and democratic nurses need to be politically active to achieve unified goals. Political action across the spectrum of issues and across partisan lines is necessary to achieve the goal of bipartisanship. Nurses should understand that only by supporting candidates who favor nursing and its agenda, whether Democrat or Republican, can the profession make changes that will advance its agenda. The most important thing, always, is the issue being addressed, not the personality or party of the candidate.

Lobbying

Sometimes communication with legislators takes the form of lobbying. Lobbying may be defined as attempting to persuade someone (usually a legislator or legislative aide) of the significance of one's cause or as an attempt to influence legislation. Lobbying methods include letter writing; face-to-face communication or telephone calls; mailgrams, telegrams, or e-mail; letters to the editor; and providing testimony (verbal or written).

To lobby effectively, one should be both persuasive and able to negotiate. Lobbying is truly an art of communication, an area in which nurses can become skilled. Before beginning any lobbying effort, it is vital to gather all pertinent facts.

In politics, getting the facts and laying the groundwork are analogous to developing a nursing care plan. Before visiting or writing a legislator, gather facts, delineate a problem or concern you wish to discuss, and develop a plan to articulate your concerns. Determine a method for evaluating your effectiveness.

If the plan is to visit the legislator's office, an appointment should be set up in advance. Usually, the meeting will actually be with the legislative aide, particularly at the federal level. This should not be discouraging, because this individual is often responsible for assisting in the development of position statements and offering committee amendments for the legislator.

To ensure that legislators listen to your concerns, it is important not only to be well prepared but also to show that others support your position. When

one person speaks, legislators may listen, but when many people voice the same concern, legislators are much more likely to pay attention.

Collaborate with Constituency Groups

Nurses can increase their political power by making alliances with other powerful constituency groups that support similar issues, such as the AARP. The AARP is very interested in health-care issues, particularly managed care, national health insurance, and the decreased quality of care from the increased use of nonlicensed personnel. Nurses who are organized into collective bargaining units can use an alliance with powerful unions. Unions are traditionally concerned with issues such as working conditions, including staffing patterns in hospitals, wages, job security, and benefits. Nurses are concerned about the same issues.

How to Organize

"Know thine enemy" is one of the most fundamental rules that tacticians must follow, whether it is in war or politics. Napoleon was successful as a tactician and general because before he fought any battle, he walked the battlefield. He knew what the terrain was like and he knew where the rocks and crevices were. He knew what to anticipate when he arrived on the battlefield. Nurses who want to be successful in a political battle must first learn the hills, valleys, rocks, and crevices of the primary political battlefield, their own state demographics.

Comparing numbers helps define the political landscape of a state. Important demographics for organizing nurses at the state level include:

- Total population of the state. This provides a demographic overview of the political arena.
- Total number of registered voters.
- Total number of registered voters by political party.
- Total number of likely voters in any given election cycle. To determine this number, the difference between an on-year election cycle and off-year election cycle should be understood. An on-year election cycle occurs when there is a major race in the state, usually during a presidential or gubernatorial race. An off-year cycle is when a major race is not being run. Lower levels of political activity are seen in an off-year election cycle.

• Total number of registered nurses. This information can be obtained from the state board of nursing. Comparing the number of actual voters with the number of registered nurses in a state provides an indication of the potential power of an RN voting block. For example, if there are 800,000 people who regularly vote in a state and there are 100,000 nurses in the state who are organized into a voting block about a particular issue, then that group of nurses represents a significant percentage of voters, and candidates running for statewide office will be interested in having nurses' support. Nurses must be encouraged to register and vote to increase the power of the block.

Important Characteristics of an Organizer

Many of the characteristics of an organizer listed in Box 19.3 are the same characteristics that are required of nurses on a daily basis in the practice of their profession. Although these characteristics may have varying degrees of value for the organizer, the one critical element a political organizer has to have is the capacity to communicate. Although nurses usually have a well-developed ability to communicate at the bedside, they may lack the confidence to communicate in the larger public and political arenas. Nurses need to recog-nize that the communication skills they use on a daily basis, such as when explaining complicated medical jargon to clients, are the same skills they can use in translating health-care issues into language that the public and elected officials can understand (Box 19.3).

One way to gain the public's interest and elected officials' support is to personalize health-care issues by stressing the fact that nurses are the professionals who provide the bulk of direct care for their mothers, fathers, brothers, and children. Communication of issues that touch people personally is usually the most effective method.

WHAT FOLLOWS ORGANIZATION?

Drafting Legislation and Creating Change

Certain critical questions must be asked. The first question always must be, "Who is the decision-maker?" For example, if an issue needs to be resolved in the state board of nursing, the first step is to identify who makes the decisions at the board. Although the board members make decisions, it is important to remember that the people who sit on the board are appointed. Who appoints them and what is the basis of those appointments? If they are political appointees, they usually have some sort of political benefactor or a political relationship with someone in power.

Understanding these types of relationships makes it easier to determine the appointees' ideological and partisan positions on many issues. For example, if a nursing board is newly appointed by a recently elected Republican governor, it is probably safe to assume that most of the board members are Republicans who agree with the governor on many key issues.

The second question to address is, "How accessible is the appointee's benefactor?" Sometimes board members are appointed by the legislative leadership and not the governor. It is important to discover who appointed the board and whether or not individual voters have access to them. Generally, access by individual voters to the power figures who make these types of appointments is very limited. Organized groups, like the ANA, provide the best avenue of access at the federal level.

B o x   1 9 . 3

Characteristics of an Organizer

Curiosity
Motivation
Reverence
Realism
Flair for the dramatic
Sense of humor
Charisma
Self-confidence
Communication skills
Clear vision of the future
Capacity to change
Persistence
Ability to organize
Imagination

Nurses need to recognize that the communication skills they use on a daily basis, such as when explaining complicated medical jargon to clients, are the same skills they can use in translating health-care issues into language that the public and elected officials can understand.

Questions About Health Care

Other questions that need to be answered include:

- How successful have nurses been in the past in achieving specific goals?
- What positions do nurses hold in government?
- What does the state board look like politically?
- Which legislators have supported nursing issues in the past?
- Which legislators traditionally oppose nursing and health-care issues?

Because of the failure to ask and answer these questions, numerous pieces of pro-nursing legislation have died in committee or lacked sponsors to move the bill through the process. In states where nurses are in tune with the political issues and powers, they have more success moving bills through the legislative process so that they become law than in states where nurses are apathetic about the political process.

If a Bill Doesn't Pass

Even if a bill favorable for nurses or health care does not pass the first time, the fact that it was brought to a vote is important for several reasons. First, it has brought an issue to the attention of the whole legislature that they might otherwise have dismissed as unimportant.

Second, the legislative process brings to light the proponents and opponents of the issue and allows nurses to specifically target legislators who voted against the bill. One of two approaches can be used at this point. Nurses can either communicate with the legislators to explain why the bill is important in hopes of changing their minds, or they can organize as a voting block and attempt to vote the opposing legislators out of office.

Third, after a bill has gone through the process the first time, it becomes much easier to identify the obstacles and sticking points in the language of the bill. Before the bill is re-introduced in a later session of the legislature, it can be modified and amended to eliminate those parts that may have caused ideological problems for specific legislators.

The Nurse as Political Ally

Very few nurses have sought or been elected to governmental positions. However, it is important to realize that not all nurses who hold elected positions are allies for nursing. Unless elected nurses identify themselves as nurses and support the profession, they may not be willing to support nursing issues politically.

For example, a nurse currently elected to Congress from a Southern state refused to speak to the nurses who participated in the March on Washington Nurses. Although she is a nurse and has had a number of articles published in nursing journals in the past, she refused to support the nurses who marched. Elected officials must always be judged by what they do and what they deliver, and not by what they say, or look like, or think, or what people think they think.

Conclusion

There is nothing magical about nurses becoming involved in politics. It is simply a matter of hard work and use of the critical thinking skills nurses already possess. It is clear, however, that nurses can and do make a difference in the political arena. Nurses must ask how and where they can make a difference and how they can become involved in the process. Not every nurse will choose to run for political office, but each nurse can and should make a contribution. The willingness of nurses to become involved in politics is the key to developing legislative respect for the profession and improving health care.[8]

Issues in Practice

How Do Politics Affect You and Your Family?

Why should nurses be involved in politics? Does it really make a difference who is elected and who makes the laws? Take a minute to go through the questions below and check the items you think may be affected by politics.

Between the time you wake up and the time you leave the house, several things usually happen to you. Do you think any of the following subjects are affected by politics?

• The water with which you wash your face and brush your teeth
• The electricity that lights the room
• The price and quality of food you have for breakfast
• The safety of the products you buy

As the average person's life span grows longer and the retirement age is lowered, these later years become more meaningful. Are any of the following decisions affected by our political systems?

• The age at which you can retire
• The income that you get during retirement
• The quality and cost of health care
• Our life expectancy

We value our leisure time and the chance to get away from it all. Are any of the following areas affected by politics?

• The parks and lakes where vacationers fish and swim
• The air you breathe
• The radio and television programs that entertain you

Take some time to think about these questions. The answers will make you think some more.

References

1. Webster's New Collegiate Dictionary, Simon & Schuster, New York, 2005.
2. Keating, SB, and Sechrist, KR: The nursing shortage in California: The public policy role of the California Strategic Planning Committee for Nursing. Online Journal of Issues in Nursing 6(1):14, 2001.
3. Alinsky, S: Rules for Radicals: A Practical Primer for Realistic Radicals. Random House, New York, 1971.
4. O'Donnell, DG: Unpublished material, 1996.
5. Stoff, Rick: Filtering Fox. St. Louis Journalism Review, 35(275):7, 2005.
6. Cross, LL: Protected whistle-blowing or a legal firing? Oklahoma Nurse 47(1):14–16, 2002.
7. Chalich, T, and Smith, L: Nursing at the grassroots. Nurs Health Care 13:242–244, 1992.
8. Greene, J: Wanted: Nurse political action leaders. American Nurse 37(3):10, 2005.

Bibliography

Brewer, C, and Kovner, CT: Is there another nursing shortage? What the data tell us. Nurs Outlook 49(1):20–26, 2001.

Burke, RJ: The ripple effect: Staffing post restructuring. Nursing Management 33(2):41–43, 2002.
Carlson, ED: Welfare reform: Policy implications for health. Texas Journal of Rural Health 19(2):42–48, 2001.
Clemons, T: Highlights from the Hill: NIWI 2000: Issues and opportunities. ORL-Head and Neck Nursing 19(2):22–23, 2001.
Des Jardin, K: Political involvement in nursing: Politics, ethics, and strategic action. AORN J 74(5):614–618, 2001.
Frank, IC: Policy perspectives: The nursing shortage. Journal of Emergency Nursing 27(4):391–393, 2001.
Higgs, ZR, et al.: Health care access: A consumer perspective. Public Health Nurs 18(1):3–12, 2001.
Malone, B: Making nursing's presence felt at the political party conferences. Nursing Standard 16(5):22, 2001.
O'Grady, ET: Health policy and politics. Access to health care: An issue central to nursing. Nursing Economics 18(2):88–90, 2001.
Rains, JW, and Barton-Kriese, P: Developing political competence. Public Health Nurs 18(4):219–224, 2001.
Roit, SM: When money talks, politicians listen. American Nurse 34(1):22, 2002.

20

Spirituality and Health Care

Roberta Mowdy

Learning Objectives

After completing this chapter, the reader will be able to:

- Develop a working definition of spirituality.
- Distinguish spirituality from religion.
- Describe what is meant by the nursing diagnosis spiritual distress.
- Describe research that supports the health benefit of spiritual practices.
- Describe the relationship between spirituality and one alternative healing modality used within nursing.

ROUGH SPOTS ON THE TRAIL

The road of life often is filled with twists and turns, ups and downs, and precipitous waysides. People who are facing potentially long-term or debilitating illnesses, confronting acute health crises, or suffering from loss and grief may find themselves reexamining the foundational beliefs they have held since childhood. Usually, at no other time in a person's life is he or she so focused on evaluating the spiritual self than during such crises. Yet the times when clients are most vulnerable also can be opportunities for personal and spiritual growth.

Nurses have the unique task of working with clients at various points throughout their life journeys. Often, nurses encounter clients during the "rough parts of the trail." The holistic nursing perspective requires nurses to view each person as a biopsychosocial being with a spiritual core. Each component of the self (physical, mental, social, and spiritual) is integral to and influences the others (Fig. 20.1). Thus, nurses must be sure to address the spirit along with the other dimensions to provide holistic care.

> *Nurses have the unique task of working with clients at various points throughout their life journeys. Often, nurses encounter clients during the "rough parts of the trail."*

NURSING AT LIFE'S JUNCTURES

It is universally true that the human life cycle is marked by a rhythm of transitions: birth, the entry of a child into society, puberty, sexual

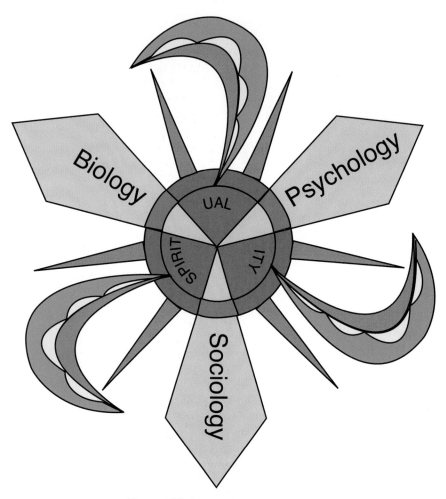

Figure 20.1 Components of the self.

awakening, entry into adulthood, marriage, parent-hood, illness, loss, old age, and death. In all cultures there are other rhythms that people honor, such as the solar and lunar cycles, the agricultural cycle, and the reproductive cycles. These cycles constitute the rhythm of human life.

Developmental Crisis

All people recognize the importance of each of these transitions and in some way have ritualized them through their religions. People learn from their own cultural groups how to behave during each transition, and each cultural group has conceptualized an understanding of these human experiences; however, their importance is universally recognized.

Nurses primarily have contact with clients in the health-care setting within the context of these transitions. Developmental crisis theory holds that these transitions are times of anxiety and vulnerability for families. Therefore, nurses are required to treat people who are going through these transitions with great tenderness and care. It is a sacred trust for nurses to be allowed into a family system in transition. During these transitions, clients and families may seek spiritual support or they may feel spiritual abandonment. Ideally, nurses can help people identify and find the spiritual support they require.

Science as Magic

Over a long period of time, from the enlightenment of the seventeenth century to the dawn of the twenty-first century, political leaders and educated people in Western cultures came to believe that all the answers to human suffering could be found in science and technology. For example, early in the twentieth century, antibiotics were thought of as "magic bullets" that cured diseases and reduced suffering. People were eager to take part in research studies to solve their health-care problems.

It was in this context that the nursing profession embraced the Western scientific method as the measure for defining itself. Nurses believed, and some still do believe, that rigorous research involving testing of hypotheses would provide the theoretical base for the practice of professional nursing.

SOCIAL AND SCIENTIFIC EFFECTS ON SPIRITUALITY

To Be Fully Human

More recently, the horrors of terrorism, the harnessing of nuclear power, space exploration, and the mapping of the human genome are among the new capabilities that have given urgency to reconsideration of the question, "What does it mean to be fully

What Do You Think?

Make two lists: a list of the problems that science and technology have caused during the last 20 years and a list of the problems that have been solved by technology and science. Which list is longer? Why?

human in the universe as it is now understood?" It is evident that science and technology cannot offer the solutions to all human problems; in fact, they have contributed to many of them.

Science, electronic communications, and the great social experiments of the past two centuries are among the influences directing humans to a consciousness of the individual's connectedness to the whole of creation and all peoples. One of the ways in which both consumers of health-care professionals are responding to this realization is by reintegrating spirituality and spiritual modes of healing into health and illness practices. Another response is the growing inclination to examine and adopt the spiritual wisdom of traditions other than one's own.

Phenomenology

A feature of postmodernism is the realization that the concept of truth is a relative one, allowing for an appreciation of diverse perspectives on what is true. Science, including nursing science since the mid-1980s, has expanded its ways of discerning truth, leaving behind traditional hypotheticodeductive, quantitative research. The emergence of **phenomenology** within the discipline of philosophy is one major influence that has led to an appreciation of qualitative methods of discovery within nursing. As a philosophical approach to understanding truth, phenomenology parallels and is closely related to existentialism, advocating the view that consciousness determines reality and truth in space and time.

In the health-care setting, a phenomenological approach appreciates the belief that the client's observations may be more objective than those of the nurse, because they are attached to the client's past experiences and knowledge, which includes rich descriptions of the person's experiences of life transitions. In nursing, intuition has emerged as a phenomenon worthy of further investigation. This change in viewpoint coincides with increased interest in complementary and alternative therapies and with the importance of spirituality in healing and wellness.

> *Spirituality may be regarded as the driving force that pervades all aspects of and gives meaning to an individual's life.*

THE NATURE OF SPIRITUALITY

What Is Spirituality?

Spirituality is a broad and somewhat nebulous concept that has to do with people's search for answers to questions and issues such as those listed in Box 20.1. Similar concerns have been identified among children of various cultural backgrounds in research on the development of spirituality.

A Diverse Heritage

A rich heritage of spiritual practices, including systematic reflection for growth toward wholeness, is found in all the major religions of the world. The roots of the great traditions, including each religion's prayer practices, can be traced to the shift in human consciousness that occurred around 500 B.C. During this period, many great teachers and spiritual leaders emerged, including Confucius; Lao-tzu; Siddhartha Gautama, who became the Buddha; Zoroaster; the Greek philosophers Socrates, Plato, and Aristotle; and the Hebrew prophets Amos, Hosea, and Isaiah.

St. Augustine, a Roman Catholic bishop who lived in North Africa during the fifth century, is credited with first identifying the relationships among contemplation, action, and wisdom within the Christian tradition. For Augustine, the contemplative life was properly focused on the discernment of truth and was open to all people. Augustine equated truth, ultimately, with God.

Hope Through Compassion

Spirituality is often defined as integrative energy, capable of producing internal human harmony or holism. Other definitions refer to spirituality as a sense of coherence. Spirituality also entails a sense of transcendent reality, which draws strength from inner resources, living fully for the present, and having a sense of inner knowing. Solitude, compassion, and empathy are important components of spirituality for many individuals.

The concept of hope is central to spirituality. Spirituality may be regarded as the driving force that pervades all aspects of and gives meaning to an individual's life. It creates a set of beliefs and values that influence the way that people conduct their lives. Spiritual activity involves introspection, reflection, and a sense of connectedness to others or to the universe. For many people, this connectedness focuses ultimately on a supreme being who is sometimes called God.

When providing spiritual care to their clients, nurses must base their actions on compassion, or sensitivity to the suffering of others. Compassion is a way of living born out of an awareness of one's relationship to all living creatures, a sensitivity to the pain and brokenness of others. The Greek word for compassion literally means "to feel in one's innards." Given this definition, one can easily see how compassion is part of spirituality and the life journey.

A Sense of Meaning

Traditionally, the term *spirituality* has been defined as a sense of meaning in life associated with a sense of an inner spirit. However, it is difficult to identify what such a spirit is like and how it can be observed. Spirituality can be defined from both religious and secular perspectives. A person with spiritual needs does not necessarily need to participate in religious rituals and practices.

Despite the lack of consensus regarding the definition of spirituality, several themes emerge from an interdisciplinary review of the literature:

- All human beings have the potential for spirituality and spiritual growth.
- Spirituality is relational.
- There is a necessary link among religion, moral norms, and spirituality.
- Spirituality involves lived experience; it is a way of life.

Box 20.1

Spiritual Questions

Why are we here?
How do we fit into the cosmos?
What power or intelligence created and orders the universe?
What is the nature and meaning of divine or mystical experiences?
How are we to make meaning of suffering?
How are we to behave toward other people?
How are we to deal with our own shortcomings and failures?
What happens to us when we die, and where were we before we were born?

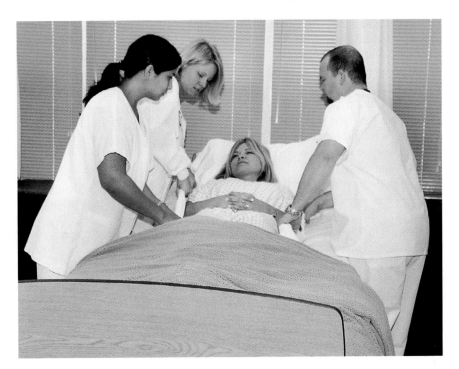

In some ways spirituality is a mystery. Although human beings can experience spirituality, appreciate it, and grow in it, there is much about spirituality that cannot be explained or reduced to human language.

Based on these themes, spirituality is defined as a way of life, informed by the moral norms of one or more religious traditions, through which a person relates to other persons, the universe, and the transcendent in ways that promote human fulfillment (of self and others) and universal harmony.

The Religious Perspective

From the religious perspective, spirituality can be defined as encompassing the ideology of the *imago dei* (image of God), or soul, that exists in everyone. The soul makes the person a thinking, feeling, moral, creative being able to relate meaningfully to a supreme being and to others. This being or force may be called God, Allah, the divine creator and sustainer of the universe, the divine mystery, or other names that convey a profound sense of transcendence and awe. A religious perspective often entails a set of beliefs that help explain the meaning of life, suffering, health, and illness. These beliefs can be crucial to a believer's well-being.

Beyond Religious Practice

Spirituality is often mistakenly understood to mean just religious practice; however, it should be considered in the broader sense of the term. Religion can be an approach to or expression of spirituality, and spirituality is a component of religion, but the two concepts are different.

It is quite possible for the members of a specific religion to be quite limited in their spirituality. Most people have known individuals who dutifully follow the rules of their religious tradition. They strongly believe that if they have adhered to the rules correctly, God will reward them with blessings such as health, success, affluence, social status, and power. For these individuals, adverse events like disease, death of a loved one, or loss of investments can be devastating, because they are perceived as a failure in religious practice or punishments from God. On the other hand, there are many deeply spiritual persons who do not belong to any organized religion but who may be profoundly reflective about the meaning of their life and experiences.

Specific Values and Beliefs

Current religious leaders attempt to help a diverse population appreciate religious traditions other than their own. They point out that all the world's major religions seek to answer the same questions: "Why are we here?" "What does it all mean?" and "What, if anything, are we supposed to be doing with our lives?" All religions taken together can be perceived like a stained-glass window that refracts the light in different colors and offers reflections of different shapes. Each of the world's religions is different because it has evolved to respond to unique histories and different cultural developments.[1]

Definitions of religion usually identify a specific system of values and beliefs and a framework for ethical behavior that the members must follow. Religion can be thought of as a social construct that reflects its cultural context and specific philosophical influences. A religion evolves within a specific cultural group, situated in history, and attempts to discern what the group beliefs are and how the group has come to understand God's commandments.

Religion, as an institutionally based, organized system of beliefs, represents only one specific means of spiritual expression. Participation in a religion generally entails formal education for membership, an initiation ceremony, participation in worship gatherings, adherence to a set of rules of behavior, participation in prescribed rituals, a particular mode of prayer, and the study of that group's sacred texts. Religious groups vary widely in their tolerance of intragroup diversity of beliefs and behaviors as well as their respect for the belief systems of others. In addition, within a specific religious group there may be a wide range of understanding of what their practices represent.

Occasionally, health-care professionals may encounter individuals whose spiritual practices are highly questionable or discomforting to witness (e.g., worshipers of Satan or those who seek to invoke harm to others through their prayers and rituals).

> *Occasionally, health-care professionals may encounter individuals whose spiritual practices are highly questionable or discomforting to witness (e.g., worshipers of Satan or those who seek to invoke harm to others through their prayers and rituals).*

The Secular Perspective

From a secular perspective, spirituality is seen as a set of positive values, such as love, honesty, or truth, chosen by the individual to ultimately become that person's supreme focus of life and organizing framework. These values have the capacity to motivate the individual toward fulfillment of personal needs, goals, and aspirations, leading ultimately to self-actualization.

Manifestation of Spirituality

The religious and secular perspectives can exist together in the totality of a person's life. A person's spirituality may be nourished by the ability to give and receive touch, caring, love, and trust. Spirituality may also entail an appreciation of physical experiences such as listening to music, enjoying art or literature, eating delicious food, laughing, venting emotional tension, or participating in sexual expression. A series of four developmental stages have been proposed for human spirituality:

- Stage 1: The chaotic (antisocial) stage, with its superficial belief system
- Stage 2: The formal (institutional) stage, with its adherence to the law
- Stage 3: The skeptic (individual) stage, with its emphasis on rationality, materialism, and humaneness
- Stage 4: The mystical (communal) stage, with its "unseen order of things"[2]

A SPIRITUAL TRADITION IN NURSING

Modern nursing has a rich legacy of the appreciation of spirituality in health and illness. Florence Nightingale's views of nursing practice were based on a spiritual philosophy that she set forth in *Suggestions for Thought.* She was the daughter of Unitarian and Anglican parents, and among her ancestors were famous dissenters against the Church of England. The skepticism fostered by her Unitarian upbringing may have influenced her to question and critique established religious doctrine. Her search for religious truth caused her to become familiar with the writings of Christian mystics (e.g., St. Francis of Assisi, St. John of the Cross) and also with various Eastern mystical writings, including the *Bhagavad-Gita.*

What Do You Think?

How would you define your spirituality—religious or secular?

_____

_____

_____

_____

_____

_____

_____

_____

_____

_____

_____

_____

The Lady of the Lamp

Most modern nurses consider Florence Nightingale (1820–1910) to be the mother of the nursing profession (see Chapter 2). Most know her as "the lady of the lamp," who almost single-handedly brought about sweeping changes in British medicine, care delivered on battlefields, and public health. Nightingale realized a call to care early in her life. She was a sickly child, and as the recipient of care from family members, she began to reciprocate in kind by nursing other sick relatives.

A Modern Prophet?

Nightingale sought places where she could learn to care for the sick and dying in a way that distinguished what she did from the work of common chambermaids. She attended the Institution of Deaconesses at Kaiserwerth in Dusseldorf, Germany. This was a Protestant training hospital that taught something akin to nursing as a call from God and a diaconal function. Through her time at Kaiserwerth and her contacts there, she learned that all persons on a mission or quest to become Christ-like are given certain gifts and talents. Some say Nightingale was a modern prophet of God and saw herself as a liberated human being.

For Nightingale, spirituality involved a sense of a divine intelligence who creates and sustains the cosmos, as well as an awareness of her own inner connection with this higher reality. The universe, for Nightingale, was the embodiment of a transcendent God. She came to believe that all aspects of creation are interconnected and share the same inner divinity. She believed that all humans have the capacity to realize and perceive this divinity. Nightingale's God can be described as perfection or as the "essence of benevolence."[3]

The Thoughts of God

Nightingale saw no conflict between science and mysticism. To her, the laws of nature and science were merely "the thoughts of God." Spirituality, for Nightingale, entailed the development of courage, compassion, inner peace, creative insight, and other "God-like" qualities. Based on this belief, Nightingale's convictions commanded her to lifelong service in the care of the sick and helpless.

Nightingale endorsed the tradition of contemplative prayer, or attunement to the inner presence of God. All phenomena, Nightingale believed, are manifestations of God. A spiritual life entails wise stewardship of all the earth's resources, including human beings. She saw physical healing as a natural process regulated by natural laws, and as she stated in her *Notes on Nursing,* "What nursing has to do...is to put the client in the best condition for nature to act upon him."[3]

Spirituality and Religion in Nursing Theory

As nursing sought to establish itself as a profession with a legitimate knowledge base, the concern with human spirituality was downplayed and even consciously ignored until the early 1980s. Typically, the spiritual domain is assigned to the art rather than to the science of nursing, because of its seemingly subjective nature mistakenly equated with aesthetics and intuition. Paying attention to the spiritual domain in providing holistic care depends on the beliefs and values of both the nurse and the client.

> *Nightingale saw no conflict between science and mysticism. To her, the laws of nature and science were merely "the thoughts of God."*

There are 26 major nursing theories and conceptual frameworks that have been developed since the 1960s. Although 14 of them recognized the spiritual domain of health somewhere in their assumptions, only 2 theories mention it by name.

Energy Fields

Martha Rogers' Science of Unitary Human Beings is an example of a profoundly spiritual view of humanity that does not directly name the concept of spirituality. Rogers' framework suggests that there are unbounded human energy fields in interaction with the environmental energy field. Rogers' spiritual definitions can apply as well to the concept of the soul (discussed later). Rogers, who grew up in Tennessee amidst fundamentalist Christians, was loath to be interpreted in that light; moreover, she had to establish her credibility at New York University during the 1950s, before nursing was accepted as a scientific discipline.

An Aspect of Holistic Health

Betty Neuman, in the later development of her theory, and Jean Watson are the only theorists who clearly acknowledged the impact of spirituality in the development of their theories (see Chapter 4). Watson alone defined and explained the spiritual terminology she used to discuss the spiritual aspect of holistic health.

Watson specifically identifies the awareness of the clients' and families' spiritual and religious beliefs as a responsibility of a nurse.[4] She advocates that nurses should appreciate and respect the spiritual meaning in a person's life, no matter how unusual that person's belief system may be. Watson states that nurses have an obligation to identify religious and spiritual influences in their clients' lives at home and to help clients meet their religious requirements in inpatient settings. For example, nurses can facilitate clients' use of measures such as the lighting of candles (real or electric), put flowers and personal objects in the room, ensure privacy, and play music to promote increased comfort and to relieve anguish.

> *At times clients make health-care decisions that conflict with the beliefs of their religious communities. These often produce high levels of spiritual distress that may affect the client's mental and physical well-being.*

Spiritual Distress

Since 1978, the North American Nursing Diagnosis Association (NANDA) has recognized the nursing diagnosis of spiritual distress.[5] It has most recently been defined as "disruption in the life principle that pervades a person's entire being and integrates and transcends one's biological and psychosocial nature."

Defining characteristics of spiritual distress include concerns with the meaning of life and death, anger toward God, concerns about the meaning of suffering, concerns about the person's relationship to God, questions about the meaning of life, the inability to participate in preferred religious practices, seeking spiritual help, concerns about the ethics of prescribed medical regimens, black humor, expressing displaced anger toward clergy, sleep disturbances, and altered mood or behavior. Spiritual distress may occur in relation to separation from religious or cultural supports, challenges to beliefs and values, or intense suffering.

Illness as Punishment

Nurses should be aware that some individuals have been seriously harmed by their religious communities. Examples of harm might include being shunned or excommunicated, being told that they are evil, being forced into a rigidly controlled lifestyle by a cult, or being physically or sexually assaulted by members of the religious community. For these people, illness may be seen as punishment for some sinful action, and they may perceive any offer of spiritual support from the religious community as profoundly threatening. They may believe that God has abandoned them or that the idea of God is foolish or even destructive.

Given the rapid turnover of clients in most health systems, there may be little that the nurse can do other than to acknowledge their spiritual pain and accept them, with the assurance that "I am here for you now." If there is more time for contact, the nurse may be able to refer a client or family to appropriate support groups or clergy.

Going Against Tradition

At times clients make health-care decisions that conflict with the beliefs of their religious communities. These often produce high levels of spiritual distress that may affect both the mental and physical well-being of the client. Consider the following case study:

> When I was a nursing student in the early 1970s, I cared for a woman who was

undergoing a therapeutic abortion because of several medical complications of her pregnancy. She had her first child before RhoGAM was available, and she, an Rh-negative mother, had borne an Rh-positive baby. She had only one kidney, and her physicians were concerned that the immunological complication of carrying a second Rh-positive baby would jeopardize that kidney's function. The decision was difficult for the woman and her husband to make, but they believed the first priority was to care for and raise their 7-year-old son. She needed to protect her kidney so that she could live and participate fully in the child's upbringing.

The night before I cared for this woman, her clergyman came to the hospital and told her that she would go to hell for her decision. Being a devout church member, the woman was extremely distressed the next day. The primary nurse assigned to this woman recognized the spiritual distress caused by the clergyman and requested that a hospital chaplain spend time with her. The chaplain talked and prayed with the woman for several hours. These actions brought great comfort to the woman, who proceeded with the abortion.

Clients often make choices that are difficult for nurses to accept. For instance, based on religious beliefs, clients may refuse commonplace treatments, such as blood transfusions, medications, and even minor surgeries. End-of-life decisions are often based on family members' spiritual beliefs and can be controversial among the health-care personnel who are involved in the decision. In some acute care settings, chaplains and psychiatrists conduct regular group sessions with staff nurses to assist them in understanding and accepting controversial client decisions. The recent Schiavo case in Florida demonstrates how well-meaning people with strong religious beliefs can be diametrically opposed when it comes to end-of-life decisions.

The Human Energy System and the Soul

Most religious traditions include a concept called "the soul." Religious traditions usually offer explanations of what the soul is, how and when human beings acquire a soul, and what happens to the soul after death, but soul need not be a religious concept.

Images of the Soul

Thomas Moore, a psychotherapist who has written extensively about spiritual development, describes the soul "not as a thing, but a quality or a dimension of experiencing life and ourselves. It has to do with depth, value, relatedness, heart, and personal substance…[not necessarily] an object of religious belief or…something to do with immortality."[6] Yet Moore observes that the soul must be nurtured, and religious practices can provide that nurturance. For Moore, spirituality is the effort a person makes to identify the soul's world view, values, and sense of relatedness to the whole of the person and of creation. The work of the soul is the quest for understanding or insight about major life questions.

Some people may depict the soul as an image of the person that extends several feet beyond the physical self, or the soul is characterized by color and energetic movement. The soul enters the body at some point during gestation and leaves the body at approximately the moment of death. Reincarnation, or the return of a soul for many earthly lifetimes, is a concept encountered in many religious frameworks, including certain mystical traditions within Judaism and Christianity, although not all denominations ascribe to it. The reason for the soul's return to earthly life is to learn, to develop, and to be purified. Some traditions express this process in terms of earning an improved position in the spiritual world to become closer to God after the final judgment.

The soul would seem to be an exquisitely precise and vast center for communication. Souls have the capacity to communicate with one another, with all living things, and with the divine source of all energy. Their capacity is not limited by the laws of physical matter. Some alternative modalities of healing rely on energy movement through the soul.

Examples of therapies that capitalize on knowledge of the soul and the movement of a divinely generated energy, life force, or grace (*chi* in Chinese, *ki* in Japanese, or *prana* in Indian traditions) include therapeutic touch, Reiki, and shiatsu. Energy can move in many directions. When a person needs it, energy can be drawn from the divine source of energy into the person; excess energy can be moved from one person to another, and the flow of energy throughout the person's energy field can be balanced to achieve a state of health.

Human Energy Centers

Some alternative healing practices that use colors, herbs, aromas, and crystals can be regarded as consistent with a paradigm of repatterning the human energy field or altering the flow of energy throughout the person's body. The circulation of divine energy may be thought of as coming from God and circulating through all living things, the earth, and all the celestial bodies, thus interconnecting all creation.

Religious traditions of India and other Eastern cultures teach that the human energy system contains seven energy centers, or chakras. These might be considered as the primary openings in the human energy system through which energy flows. Each center has or controls a unique type of energy and spirituality that it allows to enter or leave the body. The root chakra is located at the base of the torso, or the perineum, and its energy has to do with the material world. The crown chakra, the highest level of energy at the top of the head, relates to spirituality.

Examining the religious art of many cultures, over many centuries, artists depict these areas of their subjects' bodies in similar ways. For instance, holy people are depicted with vivid, large, or colorful hearts, and their heads are surrounded by halos. At the very least, the chakras represent a paradigm for ordering the archetypal issues of human life.

What Do You Think?

What sources of religious energy do you have? When and how do you use them?

Communication Between Worlds

Some individuals seem to be more aware of the non-physical or spiritual realms than others. Many people have had a precognition or déjà vu experience during their lives. However, nurses may have more opportunities to glimpse a different reality than laypeople. Nurses have been involved in research on the near-death experience for more than 20 years.

The Near-Death Experience

Across religious and cultural traditions, and throughout history, a common near-death experience has been documented, but it has been only since the early 1980s that it has gained credence among Western health professionals.

Many clients describe the experience of near death as a sensation of floating in the air while visualizing their body lying below on a hospital bed, at the scene of an accident, or where the near death occurred. They often watch health-care personnel who are working to resuscitate the body. The person then experiences being drawn into a tunnel, perhaps accompanied by other forms or spiritual beings, and moving toward a bright light that emanates great energy or love. They also describe a communication with the light being, generally identified as God, about whether they are to remain there or return to the earthly body.

"Sir, the bright light you see is my penlight, not the afterlife."

Obviously, in cases of near death, the decision is made to return. Individuals who have experienced near death often report that they have developed a great inner peace, that they no longer fear death, and that their lives have been transformed by what they have experienced.

Nurses who spend much of their time working with clients who are near death, like hospice nurses, are most likely to have witnessed the experience of deathbed visions and gained a glimpse of a different realm of reality. Dying clients who are having a deathbed vision are often aware of multiple realities: the tangible here and now that family members and caretakers can observe, and "the other side," where they see loved ones who have died and are waiting for their arrival.

Some medical researchers attribute near-death and deathbed experiences to progressive hypoxia in specific brain centers. However, others give the experiences a spiritual interpretation. Could a husband, for example, really come to meet his wife of many years past? There is a vast amount of literature on angels and spiritual guides emphasizing that people need not feel alone or frightened by future situations or crises. Angels and other spiritual guides are available to comfort them just for the asking.

A Gown of Glowing White

Some authorities believe that children are more open to communication from the spiritual world than adults because they have not yet been contaminated by the laws of natural science that are generally accepted by Western society. For example, a young child related the following experience: When she was about 7 years old, she awoke in the middle of the night to find a beautiful lady in a gown of glowing white watching her. She had the experience at least one other time, but her mother, whom she called into the room at the time, was unable to see the lady.

Mysticism

Mystics are believed to be people who have a different relationship to time, space, matter, and energy than most of the population. It seems that they are able to understand the real nature and full capability of their souls and can apply that knowledge and ability to the physical world, producing changes that science has difficulty explaining and that some call

miracles. For example, a current-day Hindu holy man in India, Sai Baba, generates ash that has brought miraculous healing to some people who have touched it. Also, many healing miracles were documented by physicians and scientists during the lifetime of the Italian Franciscan priest Padre Pio before his death in 1968.

The common message of mystics from around the world is that people are to live lives of love and compassion for all. The extraordinary love and compassion that most marks the early life of the Dalai Lama, a Buddhist holy man, is depicted in the historical films "Seven Years in Tibet" and "Kundun."

> *Some authorities believe that children are more open to communication from the spiritual world than adults because they have not yet been contaminated by the laws of natural science that are generally accepted by Western society.*

SPIRITUAL PRACTICES IN HEALTH AND ILLNESS

Nurturing the Spirit

The way that nurses care for and nurture themselves influences their ability to function effectively in a healing role with another person. The spiritual path is a life path. Attentiveness to one's own spirit is a key component of living in a healing way and is foundational to integrating spirituality into clinical practice. Care of their spirit or soul requires nurses to pause, reflect, and take in what is happening within and around them; to take time for themselves, for relationships, and for other things that animate them; and to be mindful about nourishing their spirits. The many ways to nurture their spirits and respond to their spiritual concerns are the same as those that they suggest to their patients.

A Professional Responsibility

Care of the spirit is a professional nursing responsibility and an intrinsic part of holistic nursing. Nurses must become confident and competent with spiritual care giving, expanding their skills in assessing the spiritual domain and in developing and implementing appropriate interventions.

A persistent barrier to the incorporation of spirituality into clinical practice is the fear of imposing particular religious beliefs and values on others. Nurses who integrate spirituality into their care of others need to recognize that, although each person acts out of and is informed by her or his own spiritual perspective, acting from this foundation is not the same as imposing these beliefs and values on another. In fact, many practitioners believe that the more grounded they are in their own spiritual understandings, the less likely they are to impose their values and beliefs on others.

A number of organizations and agencies encourage the incorporation of spiritual practices into health care (Boxes 20.2 through 20.5).

Prayer and Meditation

Prayer and meditation are spiritual disciplines practiced in many traditions, both cultural and religious. Appreciating the personal nature of these disciplines, the nurse, with respect and sensitivity, can help clients remember or explore ways in which they reach out to and listen for God or the absolute. Recalling the place and meaning of prayer and the ways in which they experience the presence of and communion with God or the absolute provides clients with a rich resource.

In the clinical setting, both the nurse's and the client's understanding of prayer will determine the role of prayer. Clarifying the client's understanding of and need for prayer is part of holistic nursing. Some clients want others to pray with or

---

Box 20.2

American Holistic Nurses' Association

The American Holistic Nurses' Association (AHNA) was founded in 1980 by a group of nurses dedicated to bringing the concepts of holism to every arena of nursing practice. They define holism as wellness, that state of harmony between body, mind, emotions, and spirit in an ever-changing environment.

The AHNA offers certification in holistic nursing and has endorsed programs in aroma therapy, interactive imagery, and healing touch.

Visit the AHNA Web site at www.ahna.org.

Box 20.3

Parish (Congregational) Nursing

Parish (congregational) nursing is a movement of the past decade in which churches, synagogues, mosques, and other faith communities designate nurses to serve their membership. Parish nursing is viewed as a healing ministry, and parish nurses are attuned to spiritual issues raised by health transitions, as well as the healing nature of spiritual practice. They may assist people to remain in their own homes; they may connect them with other health services for which they are eligible; they may provide needed health teaching and support; and at times their role is to simply be present with them.

The International Parish Nurse Resource Center is located in St. Louis, Missouri. They can be contacted at 314-918-2559, 314-918-2527, 877-627-5653, or on the World Wide Web at www.parishnurses.org.

---

for them, while others do not believe in prayer. Nurses should support each client's request and needs for prayer, which may mean inviting others to take part in various forms of prayer with and for the client, or simply praying with the client themselves. Facilitating the appreciation and practice of prayer in a client's life is an important aspect of caring for the spirit.

Box 20.4

Office of Alternative Medicine

The Office of Alternative Medicine (OAM) was initiated at the National Institutes of Health in 1992 to evaluate the effectiveness of alternative medical treatment modalities. In addition to funding studies, they have developed a research database and a clearinghouse for disseminating information to the public.

The OAM's Web site is located at www.altmed.od.nih.gov/oam.

Box 20.5

International Center for the Integration of Health and Spirituality

The International Center for the Integration of Health and Spirituality (ICIHS) in Rockville, Maryland, disseminates research on the benefits of spiritual practices to health professionals through their publication, conferences, and speakers.

For further information about this resource, contact ICIHS at 310-984-7162, or visit their Web site at www.icihs.org.

Relief Through Imagery. When a person is physically confined to a hospital room, the practice of imagery may enable him or her to experience another space. Imagery can take a person to a temple, an ocean, a place of religious worship, a breakfast nook, or any "sacred space," that is, a life-giving and healing place for the client. In this other space, the client may feel more comfortable in spirit and more able to engage in prayer. Family and friends, as well as other clients and other staff, may be resources in this practice of imagery.

Exploring as many aspects of the prayer experience as possible enriches both the nurse's and the client's understanding of the nature and place of prayer. Sacred or inspirational readings, music, drumming, movement, light or darkness, aromas, and time of day are among the many factors that may be important considerations in one's prayer life.

The client's prayer life, in all of its fullness and meaning, nurtures the spirit, and the nurse may be able to support the client's prayer needs by facilitating changes in the environment or schedule. It is wise to remember that merely the process of listening to and appreciating the prayer life of another nurtures the spirit and acknowledges the spiritual dimension of that person.

> *Care of the spirit is a professional nursing responsibility and an intrinsic part of holistic nursing.*

Relaxation Response

Remembered Wellness

The relaxation response and prayer have been demonstrated to affect illnesses. The ability of people to participate in their own healing through prayer or meditation may use a source of healing power called "remembered wellness,"[8] sometimes also called "the placebo effect." It is based on the belief that all people have the capacity to "remember" the calm and confidence associated with emotional and physical health and happiness. As a source of energy that can be tapped into, remembered wellness should not be regarded suspiciously but instead used for healing. However, its effectiveness depends on the individual's belief system.

Remembered wellness depends on three components: belief and expectation of the client, belief and expectation of the caregiver, and belief and expectation generated by a caring relationship between the client and the caregiver. A warm and trusting relationship seems to enhance the effectiveness of the care that is provided.

Everyone involved in providing health care is in a position to use remembered wellness as an energy source to enhance the healing process. One thing health-care providers can do to promote healing is to speak positively of treatments and medications being used. For example, positive reinforcement occurs when the nurse refers to the clients' medication as the "drug your doctor prescribed to help your heart" or the food tray as "nutrition to help your body fight your infection."

The Nocebo Effect

In contrast, the "nocebo effect" is the fulfillment of an expectation of harm. It is also an effect that health professionals can cause. Examples of the nocebo effect include advising clients that a medicine will probably make them sick, telling them that chemotherapy will drain their energy and cause their hair to fall out, or informing them that a certain percentage of people die from a given procedure. Such warnings can actually bring about the complications.

A Quiet Focus

The relaxation response entails 20 minutes, twice each day, of quiet meditation on a word or image that is spiritually meaningful to the person. When an intrusive thought enters the person's consciousness, the person should lightly dismiss it, as if gently blowing a feather away, and return to the meditation word or image. Over time, individuals who use this method have lowered blood pressure, decreased incidents of dysmenorrhea, reduced in chronic pain, and brought about improvement in a number of illnesses.

Peace Through Awareness

Relaxation, meditation, visualization, and hypnosis can help seriously ill clients, including many with cancer. Meditation is a technique of listening. However, listening is not a passive process. Rather, it is a way of focusing the mind in a state of relaxed awareness to pay attention to deeper thoughts and feelings, to the products of the unconscious mind, to the peace of pure consciousness, and to deeper spiritual awareness.

Some teachers of meditation suggest that the person select a spiritually symbolic word (e.g., God, love, beauty, peace, Mary, Jesus) on which to focus, whereas others suggest watching a candle flame. Still others teach practitioners to focus on their breathing. All these methods are intended to bring the person to a deeply restful state that frees the mind from its usual chatter. This is the experience of being centered. People may experience spiritual insights, but more often they experience a gradual enhancement of well-being.

> *Therapeutic touch (TT) is an active alternative healing modality that involves redirecting the human energy system.*

Visualizing an Outcome

Visualization is the practice of meditating with an image of a desired outcome or the process of attaining it. It is preferable that the image be selected by the person rather than someone else. For example, a person with a tumor might visualize miniature miners mining the unhealthy tissue and carting it away. Hypnosis is a process of suggesting an image of a desired reality to someone. Both these techniques have been demonstrated to stimulate the immune system.

Researchers have also observed that some seriously ill people believe that they deserve their illness as a punishment for something they did in the past. Helping them forgive themselves often brings about dramatic improvements in their conditions. Releasing fear and hate has a similar effect. This process reflects back to Nightingale's belief that nurses need to help clients get out of the way of their own healing.

It might seem logical to conclude that clients who do not recover from illness, or who die, have failed to help themselves or did not adequately use their spiritual powers. That is not the case. Spiritual modes of healing do not always lead to cure. Spiritual healing takes a much broader view and includes enhanced comfort and an inner peace with disability or death.

Therapeutic Touch

Therapeutic touch (TT) is an active alternative healing modality that involves redirecting the human energy system. In recent years, TT has been retrieved from ancient traditions, studied, and refined.

Altered Wave Patterns

As a healing practice, TT is consistent with the Science of Unitary Human Beings developed by Martha Rogers. The Science of Unitary Human Beings defines people as energy fields interacting with the larger environmental energy field. The energy fields are characterized by patterns of waves. One way of altering the wave patterns of the human energy field is to use TT to move energy into and through it in deliberate ways.

The practitioner of TT acts with the intent of relaxing the recipient, reducing pain and discomfort, and accelerating healing when appropriate. Early controlled studies of the effects of TT showed that the hemoglobin levels of a group of clients who received TT increased significantly more than the levels in a control group who did not receive TT.

The TT practitioner should approach the client with compassion and the intent to heal, and the recipient of care ideally approaches the healing encounter with receptivity and openness to change. The practitioner of TT first centers and then assesses the state of the recipient's energy field, noting energy levels and movement around the chakras. Cues may be determined through physical sensations in the practitioner's hands, direct visualization, inner awareness, or other intuitive modes of insight.

Issues in Practice

Religious Issues versus Care Issues

Angie and Edward are a young couple with two teenage children. They are a close and loving family who have a large network of family and friends. The entire family is active in their church, school, and other community groups.

Alan, fifteen years old, has just been severely injured in a high school soccer game. Angie and Edward are summoned to the hospital where they are told that Alan has multiple fractured bones and possible internal injuries. While they are waiting for the surgical team to arrive, the couple keeps vigil at their son's bedside in the pediatric intensive care unit (PICU). The surgeon informs the distressed parents that there is evidence that Alan's injuries are more serious than previously diagnosed. Alan has active internal bleeding and will need a blood transfusion to survive. Although genuinely devastated, the parents adamantly refuse to sign for the lifesaving blood transfusion, stating that they are Jehovah's Witnesses and receipt of blood is against their religion. The surgeon asks you, Alan's nurse, to get the parents to change their minds. You talk with the couple, but they continue to refuse to sign the surgical consent form.

- What are the primary underlying spiritual principles involved in this dilemma?
- Do Alan's parents have the right to refuse their consent for a blood transfusion based on religious beliefs?
- Do you think that the fact that Alan is a minor (under 18 years old) may make a difference in this situation?
- What actions do you think the charge nurse should take?
- How would you resolve this dilemma?

Source: Reprinted with permission: FA Davis, manuscript for *Foundations in Nursing.*

After assessing the recipient, the TT practitioner, working from the center of the client's energy field to the periphery, directs energy from the environment into the client's field as needed, stimulates energy flow through the client's field, clears congested areas in the energy field, dampens excess energetic activity, and synchronizes the rhythmic waves of the energy flow depending on the client's needs. The practitioner is not diverting his or her own energy into the client because it would be detrimental to the practitioner. Rather, the TT practitioner redirects the client's energy field or directs energy from the environment outside the client.

An Expression of Care

Families and friends may need encouragement to share physical expressions of care and concern in the sometimes intimidating hospital environment. Nurses may encourage them with statements such as "It's OK to hold her hand; you won't interfere with the tubes." "He mentioned that you give a wonderful backrub; would you like to give him one today?" "She seems to know when you are in here holding her hand." "I can show how to massage her feet." "Would you like to brush her hair?"

Persons vary in their degree of comfort with touch and the conditions in which they may want to share touch. The nurse's own personal feelings about and comfort with touch help in assessing the place and potential use of touch in the client's situation. At times when words cannot be found, or in circumstances where people are more comfortable with physical expression than with words, touch is a powerful expression of spirit and instrument of healing.

NURSING PRACTICE AND SPIRITUAL WELLNESS

Profession or Vocation?

Although the nursing profession is deeply rooted in religious traditions, modern nursing has spent considerable energy attempting to distance itself from this aspect of its history. Nursing as vocation has given way to nursing as profession (see Chapter 1). The current health-care system has required nurses to shift their identity from vocation to profession in order to achieve appropriate value in a system that is increasingly economically oriented.[7]

> *People working in the helping professions, whose work is rooted in compassion and concern for others, are prone to depression and burnout.*

Nursing as Spiritual Calling

Nursing is much more than the mere secular enterprise the modern world perceives it to be. Perhaps it is time that nurses re-evaluate the work they do and consider it a vocation, that is, a life calling in the spiritual sense of that word. The world's religions consistently allude to the symbolic and deep meaning of the work that nurses do. Nursing practice has the capacity to be richly imaginative and to speak to the soul on many levels. Nursing practice can be carried out mindfully and artistically, or it can be done routinely and unconsciously, like any other job. When nursing is practiced with deep consciousness and purpose, it nurtures the nurse as well as the client.[8]

Some experts perceive that nursing is directly connected to the nurse's fantasy life, family myths, ideals, and traditions. The profession of nursing may be one way nurses sort out their major life issues. Although the choice of nursing as a career may often seem to have been serendipitous, in the spiritual context, it is reasonable to question whether anything really happens by accident. As nurses practice nursing, they craft themselves, undertaking the soul's lifetime work of self-definition and self-identification.

When the Well Runs Dry

As with most professions, at times it may become difficult, even impossible perhaps, to feel good about the work that one is doing. Negative attitudes about work are detrimental to a person's self-development and tend to cause people to become overly invested in the surface trappings of work, such as money, power, and success. The phenomenon of burnout among nurses has been identified and studied for many years (see Chapter 12). Burnout can be viewed from a spiritual perspective, in which the well runs dry, energy fields become imbalanced, or the person experiences a prolonged "dark night of the soul," or even a finding that the nurse's life work is devoid of meaning.[9]

People working in the helping professions, whose work is rooted in compassion and concern for others, are prone to depression and burnout. A concerted effort at spiritual development, or the nourishment of the soul, is essential to nurses' overall mental and physical well-being.

Maintaining Balance

Self-restoration

In the attempt to maintain an internal state of balance, the first thing nurses need to do is take time to feed their spirit. Daily prayer or meditation is an important source of insight and energy. Belonging to a group or community that actively pursues spiritual growth is also a powerful source of spiritual nourishment. Many individuals find that their spirits are nourished within the setting of a formal religion, although not necessarily the one in which they were reared. It is not uncommon for people to seek a faith community in midlife or later life, perhaps after being away from one for many years. The experience of trying various religions and modes of worship is, by itself, a broadening, nurturing experience.

A Sense of Sacredness
Periodic retreat from the hustle and bustle of modern living can be highly restorative to the spirit. A retreat may be for a few hours, a half-day, a weekend, a

week, or longer. For some people, keeping a journal is a retreat-like experience. For others, it may be a stroll through a beautiful park, a few hours watching waves on a beach, or a trip to the woods. Retreat is most effective when time is consistently set aside for introspection and reflection rather than for tasks.

> *Only when nurses begin to slow down and start centering their energy fields will they have the capacity to be fully present and be able to attend with complete consciousness to their loved ones, colleagues, and clients and focus completely on the present moment.*

A sense of sacredness can infuse everyday life with meaning and zest if nurses open themselves to it. It is a part of normal human activity to celebrate seasonal and family holidays with specific rituals, music, decorations, group gatherings, and foods. These types of activities honor life cycles that are greater than the individual and nurture important relationships that serve as a **support system.**

> *Burnout can be viewed from a spiritual perspective, in which the well runs dry, energy fields become imbalanced, or the person experiences a prolonged "dark night of the soul," or even a finding that the nurse's life work is devoid of meaning.*

Enjoy Special Moments
Many people have routines for their weekends or days off that allow time for self-restoration. These special activities may include a large country breakfast while listening to favorite music; baking cookies, bread, or a pie; sitting for an extended period of time in a favorite easy chair; or even playing a physically demanding sport like basketball. Many people have favorite coffee mugs or dishes or special objects in their homes that are not only beautiful but may remind them of loved ones, wonderful trips, religious

experiences, or other events that nourish them each time they view the object.

One of the most spiritual aspects of a person's life is the enjoyment of beauty. It costs little or nothing to plant or cut flowers or to listen to music. It is in these moments that a person's creativity and insight are most evident.

Regaining the Center

The hectic modern world continually urges people to enhance their capacity for dealing with multiple concerns at the same time. Some people even define success by looking at how many tasks they can juggle simultaneously. *Multitasking* is the new buzzword for the health-care environment of the twenty-first century. Nurses must be able to talk on the telephone, send faxes and e-mail, surf the net, and use a word processor for entering client data at the same time that they are developing care plans, evaluating clients, answering call lights, supervising unlicensed assistive personnel, and providing physicians with information.

Although this is highly productive, the more nurses multitask, the more disconnected they become from themselves. Multitasking can be thought of as the antithesis of spiritual nurturance. Spirituality is about personal wholeness, whereas multitasking is about fragmentation.[10] Only when nurses begin to slow down and start centering their energy fields will they have the capacity to be fully present and be able to attend with complete consciousness to their loved ones, colleagues, and clients and focus completely on the present moment.

Conclusion

Spirituality within the nursing context needs to be seen as a broad concept encompassing religion but not equating it. Fundamental to this concept is a search for meaning within life and its particular events such as ill health. Nursing students need to be made aware of the many forms that spiritual distress may take.

For nurses to be able to focus clearly on patient spiritual needs they must first consider their own spirituality; this would appear to be the most appropriate starting point for educational input. The means of supporting clients with spiritual problems would then need to be explored. Teaching methods need to be participatory and student-centered; the means of assessing and meeting spiritual needs hinge on effective communication skills and determine the difference between the nurse "being with" the patient as opposed to merely "being there."

Critical Thinking Exercises

Mrs. Jan Steiner, 73 years old, has outlived two husbands. Ted, her second husband, died 20 years ago. Reared in the Roman Catholic faith, Mrs. Steiner converted to Judaism when she married Ted. Her two daughters by her first husband were also reared in the Roman Catholic tradition. One of them, Kathy, continues to practice her religion. The other daughter, Judith, is Unitarian.

Mrs. Steiner experienced a stroke 2 years ago that left her moderately disabled. At that time she moved into a long-term care facility. She was still able to read and to enjoy visits with friends and family, but a second stroke 3 months ago left her incontinent and aphasic.

Mrs. Steiner has just had a major heart attack. Although bypass surgery could extend her life, she has never articulated any end-of-life desires. Her daughters are in conflict over how Mrs. Steiner's medical management should proceed. Kathy strongly believes that as long as Mrs. Steiner is alive, life should be actively supported. It would be morally wrong to do less than that. Judith, on the other hand, believes that what had been the "life" of Mrs. Steiner is essentially over and it is a waste of resources to merely delay the inevitable. The nursing staff, as they attempt to facilitate communication between the family and the medical staff, feel caught in the middle.

• What are your own spiritual beliefs about the proper approach to Mrs. Steiner's medical management?
• Analyze the positions of Kathy and Judith from both their ethical and spiritual contexts.
• What resources are likely to be available in the hospital or the community to help the daughters come to a decision?

Bypass surgery is not performed, and Mrs. Steiner returns to her long-term care facility. Her overall condition continues to deteriorate, and within 3 months she is very near death. She seems to have little awareness of her surroundings and she does not consistently recognize or respond to her daughters.

• Knowing the religious divergence within Mrs. Steiner's family, how might the nursing staff facilitate their preparation for the death of their mother and her funeral?
• What would happen within Mrs. Steiner's circle of family and friends if any "side"—Catholic, Jewish, or Unitarian—"won" in planning her end-of-life care?
• Have you seen blending of religious traditions in rituals of marriage or burial? What are the advantages and disadvantages of such an approach?
• What might be the outcomes of handling their mother's death in a strictly secular or nonsectarian way and allowing all relatives and friends to mourn privately in accordance with their own spiritual traditions?

References

1. Smith, H: The Illustrated World's Religions: A Guide to Our Wisdom Traditions. HarperCollins, New York, 1994.
2. Dossey, BM, et al.: Holistic Nursing: A Handbook for Practice. Aspen Publications, Gaithersburg, MD, 2000.
3. Nightingale, F: Notes on Nursing. Dover, New York, 1969. (Originally published in 1860)
4. Watson, J: Nursing: Human Science and Human Theory of Care. Theory of Nursing. National League for Nursing, New York, 1988.
5. North American Nursing Diagnosis Association: Nursing Diagnosis: Definitions and Classification, 1997–1998. NANDA, Philadelphia, 1998.
6. Moore, T: Care of the Soul. HarperCollins, New York, 1992.
7. Bendit, LJ: The spirit in health and disease. In Kunz, D (ed): Spiritual Healing. Quest Books, Wheaton, IL, 1995, pp 92–100.
8. Jackson, J: The challenge of providing spiritual care. Professional Nurse 20(3):24–26, 2004.
9. Van Dover, L: Trusting God: Foundation for spiritual care. Journal of Christian Nursing 22(1):18–21, 2005.
10. Narayanasamy, A: Responses to the spiritual needs of older people. J Adv Nurs 48(1):6–16, 2004.

Bibliography

Brillhart, B: A study of spirituality and life satisfaction among persons with spinal cord injury. Rehabilitation Nurse 30(1):31–34, 2005.
Chesnay, M: Caring for the Vulnerable: Perspectives in Nursing Theory, Practice and Research. Jones & Bartlett, Boston, 2005.
Dameron, C: Spiritual assessment made easy…with acronyms! Journal of Christian Nursing 22(1):14–16, 2005.
Leininger, M: Culture Care Diversity & Universality: A Worldwide Nursing Theory. Jones & Bartlett, Boston, 2005.
McSherry, W: Meaning of spirituality: Implications for nursing practice. Journal of Clinical Nursing 13(8):934–941, 2004.
Ollier, C: Spirituality in nursing: An idea whose time has returned? Patient Care Staff Representative 4(12):4–5, 2004.
O'Mathna, DP, and Quiring-Emblen, JD: Making sense of complementary and alternative therapies. Journal of Christian Nursing 18(4):8–15, 2001.
Pesut, B: Developing spirituality in the curriculum. Nursing Education Perspective 24(6):290–294, 2003.
Sethness, R: Cardiac health: Relationships among hostility, spirituality, and health risk. Journal of Nursing Care Quarterly 20(1):81–90, 2005.
Wisnefske, K: The joy of parish nursing. Nursing Matters 15(12):3, 9, 2004.

21

Cultural Diversity

Joseph T. Catalano

Learning Objectives

After completing this chapter, the reader will be able to:

- Define culture and identify its expression.
- Compare and contrast the "melting pot" and "salad bowl" theories of acculturation.
- Identify the components of an accurate cultural assessment.
- Distinguish between primary and secondary cultural characteristics.
- List and define the key aspects of effective intercultural communication.
- Name two sources of information about transcultural nursing.

TRANSCULTURAL NURSING

Culture is a powerful influence on how nurses and clients interpret and respond to health care. Both nurses and clients expect to be treated with respect and understanding for their individuality no matter what their cultural origins. Nurses who understand essential characteristics of transcultural nursing will be able to provide competent and culturally sensitive care for clients from all cultural backgrounds.

WHAT IS CULTURE?

Culture is defined and understood in ways. Culture may be seen as a group's acceptance of a set of attitudes, ideologies, values, beliefs, and behaviors that influence the way the members of the group express themselves. Cultural expression assumes many forms, including language; spirituality; works of art; group customs and traditions; food preferences; response to illness, stress, pain, **bereavement,** anger, and sorrow; decision making; and even world philosophy.

A Powerful Influence
An individual's cultural orientation is the result of a learning process that literally starts at birth and continues throughout the life span wherein behaviors, beliefs, and attitudes are transmitted from one generation to the next. Although expressions of culture are primarily unconscious, they have a profound effect on an individual's interactions and response to the health-care system.

> Mrs. Su Sung, who is 74 years old, is brought into the emergency room (ER) by her family because of "very bad indigestion that won't go away." Three family members (a middle-aged man and woman and a younger woman) accompany the elderly lady. They

are discussing her condition in a mixture of English and another language the nurse does not recognize. Because the client does not seem to understand any English, the nurse attempts to address the family. The younger woman speaks only broken English but manages to explain that the client is her grandmother and she is accompanied by her mother and father, who speak even less English than she does.

By default, the granddaughter serves as the translator. After much prompting, she explains that her grandmother arrived in the United States for a visit only 2 days ago from a small mountain village in Korea where she has lived all her life. She had been having periodic episodes of "indigestion" for several weeks before the visit and used traditional herbal teas prescribed by the local healer to treat her condition. On the basis of further assessment and a diagnostic test, it is determined that Mrs. Sung had an extensive myocardial infarction at least 1 week before her trip and is currently in a mild state of congestive heart failure (CHF).

She is given medications for the chest pain and CHF and is started on anticoagulant medications in the ER. She is then transferred to the coronary care unit (CCU), where she is scheduled to have coronary angiography the next day. The angiogram shows multiple blockages in her coronary arteries and extensive myocardial damage. Because of her age and the extensive damage to her heart, the physician thinks it would be too risky to attempt bypass surgery and decides to monitor her closely and treat her medically until she is stable enough to have a balloon angioplasty.

When the CCU nurse assigned to Mrs. Sung enters the room at the beginning of her shift the day after the angiogram, she finds the client covered with four heavy blankets and a bedspread and sweating profusely. When the nurse attempts to remove the excessive bed covers, the client's daughter protests vehemently in Korean and puts the blankets back on as soon as the nurse leaves the room. The daughter seems to think that her mother is sick because she is too cold and gives the elderly woman hot herbal drinks from a thermos bottle that she had brought from home.

When the granddaughter arrives, the nurse explains to her why excessive heat is harmful to the client's cardiac status and the need to follow the diet restrictions prescribed by the physician. The ingredients of the herbal drinks are unknown, and there may be some serious interactions with the numerous medications the client was receiving. The granddaughter translates this information to her mother, who seems to become even angrier with the nurse. Although she outwardly seems to comply with the restrictions, she continues the traditional folk treatments in secret, believing the Western hospital food is bad for her mother's health.

Mrs. Sung is very quiet and hardly ever asks for help. When she does talk to her family, the conversation is usually about the airplane flight to the United States and the belief that high altitude probably caused all Mrs. Sung's problems.

Her condition gradually deteriorates during her hospitalization, despite all the medical treatment. The nurse and physician tell the family about the client's worsening condition and the likelihood that she will not survive the hospitalization, but they refuse to relay the information to the client.

Although this situation is fictitious, it demonstrates some of the potential problems that may be encountered when interacting with clients who come from a strong traditional cultural background. Culture, among other things, is a belief system that has been developed over a person's lifetime and, like all strongly held belief systems, is difficult to change. In the case of Mrs. Sung, it is easy to see the futility of attempting to change her belief system in a short period of time with a limited number of interactions. Another important aspect of the situation is the effect of the family. Rather than being helpful to the care of this client or attempting to alter her belief systems to follow care recommendations, the family reinforced the client's beliefs.

"

Culture is not a monolithic concept. Any individual probably belongs to several subcultures within his or her major culture. "

Concepts of Culture

Culture is not a monolithic concept. Any individual probably belongs to several subcultures within his or her major culture. Subcultures develop when members of the group accept outside values in addition to those of their dominant culture. Even within a given culture, many variations may exist. For example, it is logical to conclude that people who live in the United States all belong to the American culture and would be very similar in most ways. However, teenagers living in the rural areas of Oklahoma may find it difficult to relate to teenagers raised in the inner city of Philadelphia. Even though they speak the same language and share some similar interests, they have so many different past experiences that change their perspectives on life that it may be difficult for them to relate to each other.

Culture can be considered a type of flawed photocopy machine that makes duplicates of the original document with minor differences. As a society attempts to preserve itself by passing down its values, beliefs, and customs to the next generation, slight variations in the practices inevitably occur. The key parts of the culture remain similar, but other parts change greatly owing to effects from both within and outside of the group.

Diversity

Diversity is a term that is used to explain the differences between cultures. The characteristics that define diversity can be divided into two groups: primary and secondary.

1. Primary characteristics are those that tend to be more obvious, including nationality, race, color, gender, age, and religious beliefs
2. Secondary characteristics, such as socioeconomic status, education, occupation, length of time away from the country of origin, gender issues, residential status, and sexual orientation, may be more difficult to identify, even though they may have an even more profound effect on the person's cultural identity than the primary characteristics.

When individuals make generalizations about others based on the obvious primary characteristics and do not take the time to consider the secondary characteristics, they are stereotyping the other person. Stereotyping is an oversimplified belief, conception, or opinion about another person (or group) based on a limited amount of information.

MELTING POT VERSUS SALAD BOWL

The United States has traditionally been considered a melting pot of world cultures. Early in the history of the United States, most people who came from distant lands were eager to be assimilated into American culture. Many people Americanized their names, shed their traditional dress, learned American manners and customs as quickly as possible and made heroic attempts to learn English without the benefit of formal schooling—all so they could "fit in" to their new homeland. Until recently, most people who immigrated to this country were very willing to acculturate (i.e., to alter their own cultural practices in an attempt to become more like the new culture). The end result was a blending, or melting pot, of cultures.

Multiculturalism

Since the early 1970s, the practice of intentional acculturation by immigrating cultures seems to have fallen by the wayside. Many individuals who migrate to the United States from other countries now cling tenaciously to their traditional cultural practices and languages, resulting in a phenomenon called multiculturalism. Rather than blending smoothly into the bigger pot as former immigrants had done, the modern immigrants maintain their own unique flavors and textures, much like the ingredients in a large tossed salad. As an ever-growing phenomenon, multiculturalism is something that health-care providers need to be aware of; they must learn ways of adapting their health practices to allow for these differences.

> " *Many individuals who migrate to the United States from other countries now cling tenaciously to their traditional cultural practices and languages, resulting in a phenomenon called multiculturalism.* "

Drawbacks and benefits. There are drawbacks and benefits to both approaches. In the era of the melting pot, individuals who attempted to retain their native beliefs, customs, and languages were often ridiculed, scorned, and generally made to feel they were outsiders to the mainstream culture. When they did become homogenized into the American culture, learned the language of the dominant society, and made an effort to be seen as belonging, they were more likely to be accepted as equals and quickly advanced up the socioeconomic ladder.

Cultural Relativism

The current salad bowl trend has the advantage of allowing individuals in the dominant culture to gain an appreciation of other cultures for their unique

contributions to society. The drawback of the salad bowl is that it tends to create pockets of culturally different individuals who live in, but only have minimal interaction with, mainstream American society. Because they do not speak the language or refuse to accept the customs of the dominant culture, it may be more difficult for them to advance their socioeconomic status.

What Do You Think?

Identify and rank by priority at least five of your own health-care values (e.g., exercise, immunizations). Identify five health-care values of a culture with which you are familiar. How do these values compare with your own?

_____

_____

_____

_____

_____

_____

_____

_____

_____

_____

_____

_____

The salad bowl process has also given rise to cultural relativism among some groups. Cultural relativism occurs when members of a strong cultural group understand their culture and group members only from their own viewpoint rather than from that of the larger culture. They do not try to understand its unique characteristics, values, and beliefs.

Heritage Consistency

Some cultural groups manage to blend the melting pot and the salad bowl together through a rather complex process that is sometimes called heritage consistency. Outwardly, they may become acculturated to the point where they wear business suits, speak passable English, eat fast food, and go to movies. However, when they are at home, or with groups from their traditional culture, they speak their native language, wear their traditional clothes, eat ethnically correct meals, and generally follow their native customs.

This approach to acculturation has the advantages of allowing them to fit in and advance in the larger culture while retaining many of the elements of their traditional culture that provide a sense of stability to their lives. It does, however, create in some individuals a type of cultural confusion that may lead to increased tension and anxiety.

U.S. ETHNIC POPULATION TRENDS

A Population Shift

Rapid population growth in ethnic groups has been the trend in the United States for many years. The last comprehensive national census was conducted in 2000. According to U.S. Bureau of Census statistics, in the year 2000 approximately 30 percent of the U.S. population was composed of minority groups. If current trends continue, it is projected that by the year 2080, the white population will be a minority group constituting 48.9 percent of the total population of the United States.

Contributing to the rapid growth in minority populations is the increasing number of immigrants coming to the United States. Between 1920 and 2000, the number of legal immigrants each year increased from 500,000 to more than 6 million. Currently the largest numbers of immigrants are from Asia, Mexico, and Central and South America. Fewer immigrants have come from Africa and Europe than in previous years.

Despite the relatively low number of minority nurses, it is expected that nurses from one culture should be able to give culturally competent care to individuals from any other culture.

The Need for Transcultural Nursing

Culturally Competent Care

The percentage of minority nurses does not reflect the national population trends. Despite efforts on the part of the National League for Nursing (NLN), American Association of Colleges of Nursing (AACN), and other organizations concerned with nursing education, minority nurses have remained constant at approximately 10 percent of the RNs practicing in the United States. The latest reported statistics from the NLN demonstrate a leveling off of the number of minority students enrolled in basic nursing programs at about 15 percent. In a perfect world, the percentage of RNs from various minority groups would mirror society as a whole to better meet the needs of a culturally diverse country.

Despite the relatively low number of minority nurses, it is expected that nurses from one culture should be able to give culturally competent care to individuals from any other culture. Being on the front lines of health care, nursing is the one profession that is continually confronted with cultural changes that result from ethnic shifts in the population. Nurses now recognize they can no longer use traditional ethnocentric models to guide their practice and protocols. Nurses are beginning to promote an understanding of individuals from other cultures and improve the overall quality of health care.

Coverage for Minorities

The Medicare and Medicaid laws that evolved out of the social programs of the 1960s have increased the number of culturally diverse clients with whom nurses come in contact. Historically, many minority groups tend to be among the poorest segments of the population. Before the Medicare and Medicaid legislation that expanded government-funded health care to cover all welfare recipients, some ethnic minorities were unable to afford health care and were seen in the health-care setting only when severely ill. Ethnic minorities are now covered by these laws and, by their increasing numbers in all levels and areas of health care, have prompted nurses to become more sensitive to the transcultural aspects of health care.

Since the 1970s, transcultural nursing has become an important subject in most nursing programs. However, nursing education has taken only the first unsteady steps on the path to seeking a true integration of cultural competence into daily practice. As technological and transportation advances bring more and more people from different cultures closer together, there will be an increased demand for nurses who can practice effectively in a culturally diverse society. Many challenges still lie ahead.

Issues Now

Minority Nurses Needed for the Future of Nursing

Recruiting, retaining, and reshaping the role of minority nurses has been a primary concern of the health-care industry for almost a decade. Initiatives have been implemented by both the private sector and governmental agencies to increase the numbers of minority nurses and meet the needs of the ever-shifting client demographics.

Recent studies have shown that there has been a 10% increase in the number of minority nurses. The number of minority nurses increased at a faster rate than the overall number of RNs. Based on the estimated number of 2.5 million licensed RNs in the United States, the following percentages are found in each minority group:

- African American, 4.2 percent (107,500)
- Asian, 3.4 percent (86,000)
- Hispanic, 1.6 percent (40,600)
- Native American, 0.5 percent (12,000)

Hospitals have been the primary employer of minority nurses and recognize that their employment is a matter of survival. In the competition to attract clients, hospitals cannot afford to have clients feel uncomfortable because of cultural diversity issues. A recent survey showed that 88 percent of minority nurses are employed in nursing, whereas only 82 percent of nonminority nurses are. Also, 85 percent of minority nurses are working full-time, but that number drops to 70 percent for nonminority nurses.

Although hospitals and health care in general acknowledge the need for more minority nurses, some nurses are experiencing barriers to their career mobility. Although the core issues are not unlike those that all nurses experience—understaffing, frustration with paperwork and regulations, and unappreciative administration and physicians—they also feel that their ethnic background may be hindering their chance for promotion. Sometimes their capabilities are questioned because of their differences, and that is a big deterrent.

The role of minority nurses continues to develop as an issue for the twenty-first century. Not only are they necessary because of the changing demographics of the population, but many in the health-care system believe that it is a sound economic policy to have more minority nurses. To help recruit nurses and retain those who are already practicing, several organizations have been established that nurses can contact. The national Coalition of Ethnic Minority Nurses Association and the Tennessee Hospital Association's Council on Diversity are available for assistance.

Source: Cooper, S: Diversity requires more from role of minority nurses. Oklahoma City Nursing Times, May 6, 2002, p 17.

DEVELOPING CULTURAL AWARENESS

Developing cultural awareness is the first step in becoming a culturally competent nurse. One of the main challenges for nurses who practice in a culturally diverse environment is to understand the client's perspective of what is happening in the health-care setting. From a cultural viewpoint, it may be very different from what the nurse believes is occurring.

Awareness Begins at Home

A nurse develops cultural awareness only when he or she is able to recognize and value all aspects of a client's culture, including beliefs, customs, responses, methods of expression, language, and social structure. However, merely learning about another person's culture does not guarantee that the nurse will have cultural awareness. Nurses must first understand their own cultural background and explore the origins of their own prejudiced and biased views of others. Several tools have been developed to measure a person's cultural awareness.

Cultural awareness begins with an understanding of one's own cultural health-care beliefs and cultural values. To those unfamiliar with a particular culture's health-care beliefs, many of the health-care practices may appear meaningless, strange, or even dangerous.

Beliefs about health care are based in part on knowledge and are often related to religious beliefs. For example, if a particular society has no knowledge of bacteria as a cause of infection, then the use of antibiotics may seem useless in achieving a cure for the disease. On the other hand, if a society believes that illness is caused by evil spirits entering the body as the result of curses by witches or medicine men, then practices such as incantations, use of ritualistic objects like bones, feathers, or incense, and even blood-letting and purgatives to release the spirit from the body are very logical approaches to achieving a cure.

Cultural Belief Systems

The Purpose of Tradition

Cultural belief systems are highly complex. For example, some Native-American groups attributed twin births to witchcraft and believed that one of the twin infants had to die so the other might live. These beliefs and practices are usually kept as closely guarded secrets among the group's members, and there may even be some type of sanction or punishment for members who reveal the belief.

Many cultural beliefs develop over time from a trial-and-error process that has both benefits and drawbacks. For instance, several Native-American tribes that live in the Western desert have developed the practice of keeping infants in cradle boards until they begin walking. This practice, from a safety viewpoint, protects the crawling infant from injury and bites from creatures that are commonly found in the desert, such as scorpions, rattlesnakes, and poisonous insects or lizards. However, the practice tends to delay the leg muscle development of the child and increases the incidence of hip dysplasia because of the child's position in the cradle board.

Some cultural beliefs have a primary purpose of explaining unusual or unpredictable events. For example, many traditional Vietnamese-Americans believe that mental illness results from some action that offended one or more of the gods. They also believe that a family member who is mentally ill brings disgrace upon the family, and thus knowledge of the illness must be kept secret, especially from strangers. As a result, traditional shamans or priest-doctors are sought to attempt to appease the offended deity through rituals and prayers. Only with great reluctance will a traditional Vietnamese-American family seek therapy or medication for a mental illness.

Cultural Values

The several sources of the development of cultural values include religious beliefs, worldview and philosophy, and group customs. The values that underlie any particular culture are powerful forces that affect all aspects of a person's life, ranging from individual actions and decision making to health-care behaviors and life-goal setting. Values, which are discussed in Chapter 7, are the ideals or concepts that give meaning to an individual's life. They are deeply ingrained, and most individuals will strongly resist any attempt to change their value structure.

Cultural values are neither right nor wrong; they exist in a culture as the result of a long-term process of development that can often be traced back to a need for group survival. However, when judged from the perspective of other cultures, they may seem strange or perhaps harmful. Because it makes nurses feel secure and even superior, there is a tendency to transfer to clients health-care expectations based on the nurse's own cultural framework. This approach often leads the nurse to failure when trying to change health-care behaviors.

> " *The values that underlie any particular culture are powerful forces that affect all aspects of a person's life, ranging from individual actions and decision making to health-care behaviors and life-goal setting.* "

Recognizing Health-Care Practices

Changing the Client's Values

It is important to recognize that one of the primary functions of nurses is to change clients' values, particularly values about health care. It is not an easy task. The first step, always, is to recognize that the nurse comes from a particular culture that has its own set of health-care values. Like all values, these have developed over time and are dependent on the nurse's education, upbringing, religious beliefs, and cultural background.

The next step is to identify the culture of the client and recognize specific health-care practices that are both similar to and different from those of the nurse. The nurse must then make a decision about whether it is desirable or possible to change the client's values and if the end result would be worth the effort.

When Is Persuasion Appropriate?

For example, many cultures have strong values concerning pregnancy and the birth of children. In traditional Middle-Eastern families, the birth process is valued as an event strictly involving women, and the father is usually not present to either witness or assist in the delivery. However, midwives and obstetric nurses from the current American culture place a high value on the father's participation in the birth event as a way of promoting stronger family ties and starting the bonding process as soon as possible. The nurse who takes care of a Middle-Eastern family must decide whether or not to try to convince the father to stay in the delivery room during the delivery. In any event, the ultimate outcome remains relatively unchanged. Even without the father in the delivery room, the child is delivered safely, and only the bonding process with the father is delayed.

Some African cultures have discovered over time that a woman who delivers a small infant will have a much easier time during labor and delivery. Small infants usually have fewer traumatic birth defects, and there are fewer stillbirths and a higher maternal survival rate. In some traditional central African homeland settings where there is little skilled health care available, the value of having small infants helps in the survival of the group. The custom of feeding pregnant women only a corn-mush cereal throughout their pregnancies ensures small babies at birth.

In the United States, where good prenatal nutrition is highly valued, this traditional practice is seen as dangerous to both the mother and the infant. Poor prenatal nutrition has been related to developmental delays, mental retardation, and skeletal deformities in infants as well as maternal malnutrition that can lead to infectious diseases and inability to breastfeed. In this situation, changing such practices of traditional African-American women would be rewarded by healthier babies and mothers.

Assessing Culture

Obtaining accurate cultural assessments can be time consuming and difficult. However, the only way nurses can avoid imposing their cultural values and practices on others and develop plans of care based on their knowledge about others' beliefs and customs is to make a concerted effort to obtain this information. Several cultural assessment tools for clients have been developed—some short and directed, others lengthy and complicated. One of the most thorough cultural assessments developed to date is on the basis of Purnell's Model of Cultural Competence (Box 21.1). Although this tool is lengthy, it can provide a good overview of the client's culture. Nurses should not neglect completing an assessment of their own culture, as well.

Beginning the Assessment

Most busy nurses do not have the time to complete this assessment on every client from a different culture. However, the following key questions can serve as a starting point for a cultural assessment:

Box 21.1

The 12 Domains of Cultural Assessment: Purnell's Model for Cultural Competence

I. Overview, Inhabited Localities, and Topography
   Overview
   Heritage and residence
   Reasons for migration and associated economic factors
   Educational status and occupation

II. Communications
   Dominant language and dialects
   Cultural communication patterns
   Temporal relationships
   Format for names

III. Family Roles and Organization
   Head of household and gender roles
   Prescriptive, restrictive, and taboo behaviors
   Family roles and priorities
   Alternative lifestyles

IV. Workforce Issues
   Culture in the workplace
   Issues related to autonomy

V. Biocultural Ecology
   Skin color and biological variations
   Diseases and health conditions
   Variations in drug metabolism

VI. High-Risk Behaviors
   High-risk behaviors
   Health-care practices

VII. Nutrition
   Meaning of food
   Dietary practices for health promotion

VIII. Pregnancy and Childbearing Practices
   Fertility practices and views toward pregnancy

IX. Death Rituals
   Death rituals and expectations
   Responses to death and grief

X. Spirituality
   Religious practices and use of prayer
   Meaning of life and individual sources of strength
   Spiritual beliefs and health-care practices

XI. Health-Care Practices
   Health-seeking beliefs and behaviors
   Responsibility for health care
   Folklore practices
   Barriers to health care
   Cultural responses to health and illness
   Blood transfusions and organ donation

XII. Health-Care Practitioners
   Traditional versus biomedical care
   Status of health-care providers

Source: Purnell, LD, and Paulanka, BJ: Transcultural Health Care. FA Davis, Philadelphia, 1998, with permission.

- Why do you think you are ill? What was the cause of the illness?
- What was going on at the time the illness started?
- How does the illness affect your body and health?
- Do you consider this to be a serious illness?
- If you were at home, what type of treatments or medications would you use? How would these treatments help?
- What type of treatment do you expect from the health-care system?
- How has your illness affected your ability to live normally?
- If you do not get better, what do you think will happen?

Because clients from different cultures may feel uncomfortable revealing information about cultural beliefs, values, and practices to strangers, it is a good idea to begin your assessment by asking some general questions. A client is more likely to trust a nurse who demonstrates interest in that person as an individual. Only after a warm and trusting environment has been established will a client be willing to reveal the more hidden aspects of his or her culture to the nurse.

Understanding Physical Variations
Physical assessments made on individuals from other cultures require a certain level of cultural awareness

and competence. Although the assessment techniques used for different individuals may be identical, the nurse needs to know the basic biological and physical variations among ethnic groups. The interpretation of assessment findings may be affected by ethnic variations in anatomic structure or characteristics (e.g., children from some Asian cultures may fall below the normal growth level on a standardized American growth chart because of their genetically smaller stature).

Changes in skin color may also affect the interpretation of assessment findings (e.g., with regard to an assessment of cyanosis in people with a light versus a dark complexion). To determine whether the client's skin color is normal or abnormal, the nurse must know what constitutes the normal color for a particular ethnic group. In assessing for cyanosis, the nurse may need to examine the client's oral mucosa and may also need to measure capillary refill times to determine whether the client has cyanosis.

What Do You Think?

Using Purnell's cultural assessment tool, assess your own cultural background. In what areas of your own culture are you lacking knowledge?

The ultimate goal of cultural assessment, as with all assessments, is to provide the best care possible for the client. A fundamental belief that nurses hold to strongly is that all clients have a right to self-determination, including the customs, practices, and values that emanate from their culture. By considering both the cultural and ethnic variables of each client, nurses will avoid practice that is ethnocentric and conducted strictly from the nurse's cultural viewpoint.

" *A client is more likely to trust a nurse who demonstrates interest in that person as an individual. Only after a warm and trusting environment has been established will a client be willing to reveal the more hidden aspects of his or her culture to the nurse.* "

PROVIDING CULTURALLY COMPETENT CARE

Transcultural Understanding

Cultural competence has become a buzzword in the health-care system. The term has several divergent definitions, with little consensus among cultural experts. However, cultural competence as it relates to nursing can be regarded as the provision of effective care for clients who belong to diverse cultures, based on the nurse's knowledge and understanding of the values, customs, beliefs, and practices of the culture.

Provision of culturally competent care requires the development of certain interpersonal skills that allow nurses to work with individuals and groups in the community. The primary skills required for cultural competence include communication, understanding, and sensitivity. Although the basic types of cultural skills are similar, their application within and between cultural groups may differ greatly. The development of cultural competence is not a one-time skill to check off on a skills checklist; rather, it is an ongoing process that continues throughout the nurse's career.

Transcultural Communication

The ability to communicate is the foundation on which culturally competent care is built. The most obvious barrier to culturally competent care for the non-English-speaking client is the lack of a common language (Box 21.2). Communication is a highly complex process that requires both verbal and non-verbal communication. Nonverbal communication includes (but is not limited to) body language, facial expressions, eye contact, personal space, touch and body contact, formality of names, and time awareness.

Other factors that affect communication are volume of voice, tone, and acceptable greetings. Often clients communicate differently with family and friends than they do with health-care personnel. Nurses should be aware that in some cultures (e.g., those with a strong caste system, which involves a class structure) communication between those in the upper and lower classes may be affected by tradition. For example, some cultures hold the role of women in health care in high esteem, whereas other cultures may consider women in health care as the bottom rung on the ladder.

Nonverbal Responses

Nurses who work with non-English-speaking clients need to develop alternative ways to measure a client's understanding rather than depending only on a verbal response. Nurses must be cautious when interpreting the nonverbal responses from some cultural groups. Some cultures respond to all questions with the reply "yes," a nod, or a smile. This response, in the American culture, usually indicates understanding and **compliance.** However, particularly in Asian cultures, nodding and smiling can be signs of respect for the nurse's position or an attempt to avoid confrontation. The following is a classic example:

An English-speaking nurse gave a non-English-speaking Asian client preoperative instructions about how to prepare an abdominal surgical site. She thought that she had shown the client how the bottle of povidone-iodine, a powerful skin disinfectant, was to be used in scrubbing the area. The client smiled and nodded throughout the instruction. When asked whether he had any questions, he did not respond. The nurse took the silence to mean that he had no questions. When the nurse left the room, the client promptly drank the whole bottle of povidone-iodine. Fortunately, the error was discovered immediately, and no long-term complications occurred from the accident.

B o x 2 1 . 2

Guidelines for Communicating with Non-English-Speaking Clients

1. Use interpreters rather than translators. Translators just restate the words from one language to another. An interpreter decodes the words and provides the meaning behind the message.
2. Use dialect-specific interpreters whenever possible.
3. Use interpreters trained in the health-care field.
4. Give the interpreter time alone with the client.
5. Provide time for translation and interpretation.
6. Be aware that interpreters may affect the reporting of symptoms, insert their own ideas, or omit information.
7. Avoid the use of relatives who may distort information or not be objective.
8. Avoid using children as interpreters, especially with sensitive topics.
9. Use same-age and same-gender interpreters whenever possible. However, clients from cultures who have a high regard for the elderly may prefer an older interpreter.
10. Maintain eye contact with both the client and the interpreter to elicit feedback and read nonverbal clues.
11. Remember that clients can usually understand more than they express; thus, they need time to think in their own language. They are alert to the health-care provider's body language, and may forget some or all of their English in times of stress.
12. Speak slowly without exaggerated mouthing, allow time for translation, use active rather than passive tense, wait for feedback, and restate the message. Do not rush; do not speak loudly. Use a reference book with common phrases, such as *Roget's International Thesaurus* or *Taber's Cyclopedic Medical Dictionary*.
13. Use as many words as possible in the client's language and use nonverbal communication when unable to understand the language.
14. If an interpreter is unavailable, the use of a translator may be acceptable. The difficulty with translation is omission of parts of the message, distortion of the message, including transmission of information not given by the speaker, and messages not being fully understood.
15. Note that social class differences between the interpreter and the client may result in the interpreter's not reporting information that he or she perceives as superstitious or unimportant.

Source: Purnell, LD, and Paulanka, BJ: Transcultural Health Care. FA Davis, Philadelphia, 1998, pp 16–17, with permission.

> *Nurses who work with non-English-speaking clients need to develop alternative ways to measure a client's understanding rather than depending only on a verbal response.*

Speech Patterns

The use of silence by some cultural groups has led to misunderstandings in the health-care setting. For example, Asian-Americans consider silence to be a sign of respect, particularly for elders, whereas Arab-Americans and the English use silence to gain privacy. Among many people in Europe (e.g., the French, Russians, and Spanish), silence often indicates agreement.

Variations in communication style also account for misunderstandings and miscommunications. Factors such as loudness, intonation, rhythm, and speed of speech all are important in communication. Among certain cultural groups, American nurses have a reputation for speaking at a rapid rate and for using medical jargon. Some nurses also have a reputation for their tendency to increase the volume of their voices when communicating with clients who do not speak English, as if talking louder will increase understanding.

On the other hand, groups such as Native-Americans and Asian-Americans speak more softly and may be difficult to hear even when the nurse is standing at the bedside. These groups may misinterpret the louder, more forceful tone of the American nurse as an indication of anger. Arab-American groups are often noted for their dramatic communication styles. Nurses may misinterpret this behavior as hostility, when in reality they are merely trying to demonstrate a point using an emotional communication style. Nurses need to analyze their own speech patterns and consciously modify their tone and pace when working with different cultural groups to prevent misunderstandings.

Personal Matters

Nurses also need to recognize that certain groups are much less willing to disclose private matters or personal feelings than others. In general, clients from American or European origins tend to be less secretive about almost all issues, because the practice of sharing has been encouraged from an early age. However, many Asian cultures, particularly the Japanese, are highly reluctant to discuss personal topics with either family or health-care providers. Other groups, such as Mexican-Americans, discuss personal issues openly with friends and family members but are reluctant to do so with health-care providers who they do not know well.

Even within these groups there are wide variations. American women probably constitute one of the most open groups when it comes to expressing personal feelings, whereas American men tend to have much more difficulty with this type of communication.

Open-Ended Language

Nurses presume that all clients should trust them instantaneously just because they are nurses and should answer even the most personal questions immediately. As discussed earlier, it may be much more productive to start the communication process with small talk and general, nonthreatening questions to establish an atmosphere of trust. Often the use of open-ended questions and statements allows the client to express beliefs and opinions that would be difficult to discover through closed-end questions that the client can answer with a simple "yes" or "no."

As the level of trust increases, the client will be more likely to reveal important information in the more sensitive areas of the assessment. In addition, sensitivity to the nonverbal aspects of the communication process allows nurses to use behaviors that increase trust and to avoid gestures, facial expressions, or eye contact that may relay a message of superiority, hostility, anger, or disapproval.

Touch Misinterpreted

The touching of clients from different cultures in ways that they consider inappropriate is a leading cause of miscommunication. American nurses are taught early on in their first nursing classes, usually physical assessment or basic skill courses, that it is necessary to "lay on hands" in order to provide good care. Students who are reluctant to palpate the femoral pulses of their laboratory partner or remove a client's shirt to auscultate anterior heart and breath sounds may receive a failing grade for the course.

However, touching in other cultures conveys a number of alternative meanings, ranging from power, anger, and sexual arousal to affirmation, empathy, and cordiality. For example, it is generally not acceptable for men and women to touch in many Arab cultures, except in the privacy of the home and in the context of marriage. American women nurses who palpate pulses, listen to breath sounds, or palpate for tactile fremitus when assessing men from an Arab culture may be communicating a message that they never intended.

Some groups, such as Mexican-Americans or Italian-Americans, who frequently touch and hug family members and friends, are much less receptive to touching by strangers during health-care examinations, particularly if the health-care provider is of the opposite sex. In these situations, it would be extremely important for the nurse to explain what he or she is going to do and why it is important before the particular physical contact occurs. The nurse should also avoid any unnecessary contact, such as palpation of femoral pulses when the client has pneumonia.

Personal Space

Closely related to the issue of touch is the concept of personal space. Personal space is a zone that individuals maintain around themselves in most casual social situations. When a person's personal space is violated, it often creates a generalized feeling of discomfort or threat, which causes the person to move away from the offending individual. Nurses routinely violate clients' personal space when performing physical assessments or providing basic care.

The distance required to maintain a comfortable personal space varies widely from one culture to another. People who belong to the European, Canadian, or American cultures usually require between 18 and 22 inches of distance for a comfortable personal space when communicating with strangers or casual acquaintances. In contrast, individuals from the Jewish, Arab, Turkish, and Middle-Eastern cultures may require as little as 3 to 5 inches of personal space when talking with another person and often interpret physical closeness as a sign of acceptance. In addition, they prefer to stand face to face and maintain eye contact when they are talking.

It is easy to understand why misinterpretations in communication might arise. A client from a Middle-Eastern culture might judge an American nurse to be cold and aloof, although she is merely maintaining a comfortable personal space from the client. Likewise, an American nurse may feel physically threatened by the close communication style of a Turkish-American client and continually back away from the client in an attempt to re-establish his or her personal space.

Eye Contact

Similarly, eye contact communicates different messages to different cultures. Among American and many European cultures, making periodic eye contact during conversations indicates that the person is attentive to the communication and is a means of measuring the person's sincerity. Common sayings such as, "Look me in the eye and say that," or admonitions for public speakers to make eye contact with the audience emphasize the underlying positive value these cultures place on eye contact. Lack of eye contact may be interpreted as inattention, insincerity, or disregard.

In contrast, some Native-American cultures believe that the eyes are the windows of the soul and that direct eye contact by another may be interpreted as an attempt to "steal the soul" from the body. Between Native-American men, direct eye contact is a sign of challenge and aggression and may precipitate a violent, physical confrontation. Among some South-American cultures, sustained eye contact is a sign of disrespect, whereas in other cultural groups, particularly Mexican-Americans, eye contact with a child is believed to convey the *mal de ojo,* or "evil

eye." Many childhood and adult illnesses among these cultures are attributed to the effects of the evil eye, and practices such as tying red cloths or strings around the children's wrists are used to ward off the illnesses. Eye contact, a routine part of American culture, has diverse and powerful meanings to clients from other cultures.

The complexity and importance of communication should never be underestimated when working with clients from diverse cultures. Merely speaking a language does not encompass the entirety of communication. Awareness of the meanings of gestures, body positions, facial expressions, and eye movements is essential in culturally competent communication.

> *...touching in other cultures conveys a number of alternative meanings, ranging from power, anger, and sexual arousal to affirmation, empathy, and cordiality.*

LOOKING DEEPER

Several other elements must be considered for effective transcultural nursing, including passive obedience, cultural synergy, building on similarities, and conflict resolution. The term *passive obedience* refers to a type of behavior that develops when clients from a different culture believe that the nurse is an authority figure or expert in health-care matters. Although many cultures may display this type of behavior to some extent, it is most commonly seen among Asian-American groups. These cultures try to cope with the uncertainty of their health status and the threat of an authority figure by becoming passively obedient. Rather than asking questions they think will reveal their lack of knowledge or confusion about some health-care issue or that they believe may challenge the authority of the nurse, they become passively obedient and compliant.

Cultural Conflicts

It is inevitable that conflicts will arise from time to time when caring for clients of different cultures. It is important to recognize that the origins of many conflicts reside within the individual. Nurses may label clients from other cultures as noncompliant, when in reality the nurse has an incomplete understanding of the client's culture or unrealistic expectations for behavior.

Other common reasons for noncompliance among culturally diverse clients include the lack of external symptoms of disease, inconvenient or painful treatments, and lack of external support from family members or close friends.

Respect for Healing Traditions

The nurse first needs to ask the client what traditional treatments are used in dealing with this disease. In some cases, where the traditional treatments are similar to the ones used by the health-care facility, the nurse may be able to demonstrate this similarity to the client.

In other cases, the treatments may be very different. However, if culturally based alternative treatments do not interfere with the prescribed treatment plan or threaten the client's health, they can be used simultaneously with the standard medical treatments. For example, nurses who work in the

Native-American health-care system and hospitals have become accustomed to finding bone fragments, feathers, and leather medicine pouches in the beds of their clients.

> *...if culturally based alternative treatments do not interfere with the prescribed treatment plan or threaten the client's health, they can be used simultaneously with the standard medical treatments.*

Cultural Synergy

Nurses who work actively to develop cultural synergy tend to be more successful in the delivery of competent transcultural care. *Cultural synergy* is a term that implies that health-care providers make a commitment not only to learn about other cultures but also to immerse themselves in those cultures. Nurses achieve cultural synergy when they begin to selectively include values, customs, and beliefs of other cultures in their own worldviews. The first step in cultural synergy is the desire to know everything there is about another culture and to purposely establish relationships with individuals from other cultures.

More Alike Than Different

Closely related to cultural synergy is the recognition that cultures are much alike in many aspects. It seems that most books and publications written about cultural diversity present only the diversity of cultures and not the similarities. Although recognition of cultural differences is important, it should be just one step toward the ultimate realization that there are more similarities than differences among cultures.

Many colleges offer courses in comparative religions that identify the many similarities of the fundamental beliefs that underlie the major religions. However, many college courses on cultural diversity have not evolved past the point of identifying cultural differences. Perhaps this is due in part to the salad bowl approach to cultural communication that exists in current society. Perhaps a new approach to acculturation, based on the similarities between cultures rather than on the differences, needs to be developed.

Issues in Practice

Consider the following case study:

In 1990, Jose Bisigan, aged 87 years, and his wife Carmen, aged 85, sold their small restaurant and immigrated to Los Angeles from a small town in the Visayan region of the Philippines. They came to join their first-born daughter, nurse Felicia, aged 54, her husband, and their three children aged 10 to 18. Mr. Bisigan speaks limited English and is in a poststroke rehabilitation unit. Since the stroke, he has had mild aphasia, mild confusion, and bladder and bowel continence problems. His hypertension and long-standing diabetes are controlled with medication and diet. His wife, daughter, and grandchildren have been supportive of him during this first hospitalization experience. Mr. Bisigan's family has cooperated with the health team, often agreeing with minimal resistance to the prescribed treatment management. The rehabilitation team recommended subacute rehabilitation treatment as part of the discharge plan.

As a businessman and the elder in the family household, Mr. Bisigan is looked to for counsel by the immediate and extended family. Mr. Bisigan's status, however, has caused friction between Felicia and her husband, Nestor, an American-born Filipino who works as a machinist. Nestor has accused Felicia of giving excessive attention to her mother and father. Felicia's worries about her parents' health have made Nestor very resentful. He has increased his already daily "outings with the boys." Felicia maintains a full-time position in acute care and a part-time night shift position in a nursing home.

Mr. Bisigan's discharge is pending, and a decision must be made before Medicare coverage runs out. Felicia has to consider the possible choices available to her father and the family's circumstances and expectations. Mrs. Bisigan, who is being treated for hypertension, has always deferred decisions to her husband and is looking to Felicia to make the decisions. Because of her work schedule, the absence of a responsible person at home, her mother's health problems, and intergenerational friction, Felicia considers nursing home placement. She is, however, reluctant to broach the subject with her father, who expects to be cared for at home. Mrs. Bisigan disagrees with putting her husband in a nursing home and is adamant that she will care for her husband at home.

Felicia delayed talking to her father until the rehabilitation team requested a meeting. At the meeting, Felicia indicated that she could not bring herself to present her plan to put her father in a nursing home because of her mother's objection and her own fear that her father will feel rejected. Feeling very much alone in resolving the issue about nursing home placement, she requested the team to act as intermediary for her and her family.

- Identify cultural family values that contribute to the conflicts experienced by each family member.
- Identify a culturally competent approach the team can use when discussing nursing home placement with the Bisigans.

(continued)

Issues in Practice <small>continued</small>

- How might the rehabilitation program be presented to Mrs. Bisigan and still allow her to maintain her spousal role?
- Discuss at least three communication issues in the family that are culture-bound and suggest possible interventions.
- Identify psychocultural assessments that should be done by the rehabilitation team to have a greater understanding of the dynamics specific to this family.
- Identify health promotion counseling that might be discussed with the Bisigans' grandchildren.
- Identify and explain major sources of stress for each member of this household.

Source: Purnell, LD, and Paulanka, BJ: Transcultural Health Care. FA Davis, Philadelphia, 1998, pp 269–270, with permission.

INFORMATION SOURCES FOR TRANSCULTURAL NURSING

From a Conference . . .

The recent explosion of interest in cultural diversity and transcultural nursing has led to a proliferation of literature on the topic. The origins of the current transcultural movement can be traced back to 1974, when a transcultural conference on communication and culture was held at the University of Hawaii School of Nursing. Following the success of this conference, a series of transcultural conferences were planned over the next year to bring together nurses, sociologists, anthropologists, and other social scientists to discuss issues that would eventually form the basis for transcultural nursing.

Not long after the Hawaii conference, the Transcultural Nursing Society was organized. It was incorporated in 1981 and began publishing its semi-annual official journal, *Journal of Transcultural Nursing,* in 1989. It is now being published four times a year. In 1976, the American Nurses Association (ANA) recommended that multicultural content be included in nursing curricula. Since then, the ANA has organized the Council on Intercultural Nursing, which publishes the *Intercultural Nursing Newsletter.*

. . . to a Specialty

Since the 1980s, more and more universities and colleges have started offering graduate degrees in transcultural, cross-cultural, and international nursing. Graduates are now able to become certified transcultural nurses (CTNs) by completing oral and written examinations offered by the Transcultural Nursing Society. Nurses do not need to be from minority groups to obtain the CTN.

Society has not remained stagnant during this period of development and organization. Growing numbers of immigrants, changing governmental regulations, and grassroots movements all have contributed to the pressure placed on nursing to recognize and effectively care for clients from different cultures.

Conclusion

The major changes in U.S. demographics that began in the 1980s—and have been accelerating ever since—require nurses to provide culturally sensitive care. Based on the fundamental belief of professional nursing that all individuals are to be cared for with respect and dignity regardless of culture, beliefs, or disease process, nurses must actively seek multicultural education.

However, nurses need to keep in mind that cultural assessments and decisions about care are relative to the nurse's personal experiences, beliefs, and culture. There is a natural tendency to unconsciously stereotype individuals from other cultures on the basis of one's internal value system. There is also a tendency to batch all individuals from one culture into a single group, when in reality, there may be wide variations within the group.

It is a well-accepted belief that nurses who value cultural diversity will deliver higher-quality care. Nurses who have a high level of cultural knowledge and sensitivity maximize their nursing interventions when they become coparticipants and client advocates for individuals who might otherwise be lost in an impersonal health-care system. Only when nurses can understand the client's perspective, develop an open style of communication, become receptive to learning from clients of other cultures, and accept and work with the ambiguities inherent in the care of multicultural clients will they become truly culturally competent health-care providers.

Bibliography

Anderson, K: Teaching cultural competence using an exemplar from literal journalism. Nursing Education 43(6):253–260, 2004.

Aroian, K: Effective, efficient and equitable health care: What can cultural diversity teach us about sacred cows. J Prof Nurs 20(6):349–351, 2005.

Batnardi, M, and Perkel, L: Learning achievement programs: Fostering student cultural diversity. Nurse Educator 30(1):17–21, 2005.

Brenman, S: Cultural immersion through ethnography: The lived experience and group process. J Nurs Educ 43(6):285–288, 2004.

Briesacher, B, et al.: Racial and ethnic disparities in prescription coverage and medication use. Health Care Finance 25(2):63–76, 2004.

Carter, M: The ABCs of staffing decisions. Nursing Management 36(6):16, 2004.

Carol, R: Overcoming bias in the nursing workplace. Minority Nurse Winter, 28–33, 2005.

De Chesnay, M: Caring for the Vulnerable: Perspective in Nursing Theory, Practice and Research. Jones & Bartlett, Boston, 2005.

Flowers, D: Culturally competent nursing care: A challenge for the 21st century. Critical Care Nurse 24(4):46–50, 2004.

Health care disparities continue among minorities, the poor says HHS. Medical Ethics Advisor 20(2):13–16, 2004.

Johnson, L: The role of cultural competency in eliminating health disparities. Minority Nurse Winter, 52–55, 2005.

Leininger, M: Culture Care Diversity & Universality: A Worldwide Nursing Theory, ed. 2. Jones & Bartlett, Boston, 2005.

Leishman, J: Perspectives of cultural competence in health care. Nursing Standard 19(11):33, 2004.

Linnard-Palmer, L: Parents' refusal of medical treatment for cultural or religious beliefs: An ethnographic study of health care professionals' experiences. J Pediatr Oncol Nurs 22(1):48–57, 2005.

Nokes, K, et al.: Does service learning increase cultural competency, critical thinking and civil engagement? Nursing Education 44(2):65–71, 2005.

Marquand, B: On the case. Minority Nurse Winter, 34–38, 2005.

Purnell, LD, and Paulanka, BJ: Transcultural Health Care. FA Davis, Philadelphia, 1998.

Racial/ethnic and gender diversity in nursing education. Southern Regional Education Board, Council on Collegiate Education for Nursing, 2002.

Raiger, J: Applying a cultural lens to the concept of burnout. Journal of Transcultural Nursing 16(1):71–76, 2005.

Spector, R: Cultural Care: Guide to Heritage Assessment and Health Traditions, ed. 3. Prentice Hall, Englewood Cliffs, New Jersey, 2004.

Spector, R: Cultural diversity in health and illness, ed 6. Prentice Hall, Englewood Cliffs, New Jersey, 2004.

Terhone, C: From desegregation to diversity: How far have we really come? J Nurs Educ 43(5):195–196, 2004.

22

Developments in Current Nursing Practice

Barbara Bellfield

Learning Objectives:

After completing this chapter, the reader will be able to:

- Discuss the nurse's role in forensics, bioterrorism, disasters, case management, entrepreneurship, legal consulting, and case management.

- Discuss ways in which to develop a nurse-run business.

- Identify factors that indicate the need for case management.

- Discuss the importance of the nurse's early recognition of a bioterrorist attack.

- Give examples of organizations that nurses can become involved in to provide assistance in the event of a disaster.

NEW ROLES FOR THE NURSE

The profession of nursing is dynamic and ever-changing. Nursing roles evolve and develop in response to societal needs. This chapter will discuss the new and exciting practice roles in nursing. Included will be a discussion of forensic nursing, bioterrorism and disaster nursing, nurse entrepreneurs, nurse case managers, and legal nurse consultants.

FORENSIC NURSING

Forensic nursing is a newly emerging field that forms an alliance between nursing, law enforcement, and the forensic sciences. The term *forensic* means anything belonging to, or pertaining to, the law.

An Emerging Discipline

Forensic nursing, as defined by the International Association of Forensic Nurses (IAFN), is "the application of nursing science to public or legal proceedings; the application of the forensic aspects of healthcare combined with the bio-psycho-social education of the registered nurse in the scientific investigation and treatment of trauma and/or death of victims and perpetrators of abuse, violence, criminal activity and traumatic accidents." Forensic nurses provide a continuum of care to victims and their families beginning in the emergency room or crime scene and leading to participation in the criminal investigation and the courts of law.[1]

Nurses, particularly emergency room nurses, have long provided care to victims of domestic violence, rape, and other injuries resulting from criminal acts. They have collected, preserved, and documented legal evidence. This was often done without formal training. It was not until 1992 that the term *forensic nursing* was coined.

What Do You Think?

Do you know any nurses who are involved in forensic nursing? Is this a role that you might be interested in pursuing after graduation?

"Nurses, particularly emergency room nurses, have long provided care to victims of domestic violence, rape, and other injuries resulting from criminal acts."

The IAFN was founded in the summer of 1992. Seventy-four nurses, primarily sexual assault nurse examiners, came together in Minneapolis, Minnesota, to develop an organization of nurses who practice within the arena of the law. This very diverse group includes, but is not limited to, legal nurse consultants, forensic nurse death investigators, forensic psychiatric nurses, as well as forensic correctional nurses.

The organization's membership tripled within its first year. By 1999, the IAFN had more than 1800 members. The American Nurses Association (ANA) recognized forensic nursing as a subspecialty in 1995, and the Scope and Standards of Forensic Practice was established in 1997. As this is a new field, the definition of the forensic nurse role is continuing to evolve. With the formation of the IAFN and the designation of the forensic specialty, nurses were given an identity and recognition for a role they have long been performing.

Forensic nurses specialize in several diverse roles and are beginning to find employment in a variety of settings. These roles include the sexual assault nurse examiner (SANE), the forensic nurse death investigator, the forensic psychiatric nurse, the forensic correctional nurse, and the legal nurse consultant.

Sexual Assault Nurse Examiner

A SANE is a registered nurse trained in the forensic examination of sexual assault victims. A SANE has an advanced education and clinical preparation specialized in this area.

Sexually assaulted clients present with special medical, legal, and psychological needs. They require a competent collection of evidence that assists in both the investigation and prosecution of the incident. The SANE offers compassionate care that is often found to be lacking among law enforcement personnel. The care provided by SANEs has been designed to preserve the victim's dignity and reduce psychological trauma. Research data collected in recent years indicates that the SANE's comprehensive forensic evidence collection leads to more effective investigations and more successful prosecutions.[2]

Usually SANEs work in a hospital or emergency room with other members of a sexual assault response team (SART). The other team members may include physicians, law enforcement personnel, social workers, child/adult protective service workers, and therapists.

SANEs are specially trained to perform all aspects of the care of sexually assaulted clients. Their responsibilities include interviewing the victim, completing the physical exam, collecting specimens for forensic evidence, and documenting the findings. They also provide emotional support for victims and family members. When the case goes to court, the SANE serves as an expert legal witness.

To become a SANE, a registered nurse must complete an adult/adolescent SANE education program. These programs are available through a traditional university setting and on-line. The training includes either a minimum of 40 contact hours of instruction or three semester units of classroom instruction by an accredited school of nursing. Trainees also must have clinical supervision until they demonstrate competency in SANE practice. After successful

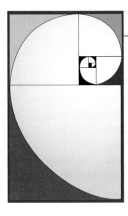

Issues in Practice

If You Were the Nurse on Duty, What Would You Do?

Below are scenarios that exemplify typical situations for the nurse in general practice. Identify your probable response. Critically analyze each situation in terms of what you know and do not know. What types of facts or skills are not part of your current knowledge base?

You are working on a maternity unit when a woman who is an inmate from a correctional institution is admitted in an advanced stage of labor. A correctional officer is in attendance; the woman is shackled at the feet and hands. As she is wheeled to the labor room, you note that the client has had 10 previous pregnancies and four live births.

- What factors make the care of this woman different from other pregnant women?
- Is she dangerous?
- How do you maintain confidentiality with this client?
- As an offender in custody, does she surrender any rights?

You work in a hospital setting that is experiencing an increase in violence in the workplace. Perpetrators of street, child, and domestic violence often follow their victims to the hospital setting and continue to pose a significant threat to the whole hospital community. It is important to assess the potential for violence.

- How will you contribute to the reduction of risk in the workplace?
- Identify risk factors and cues for violence.
- How would you implement strategies to assist violence management in the acute care setting?

A halfway house for paroled offenders is due to be constructed in your community. Residents are angry and afraid to have ex-convicts living in their neighborhood. A town meeting is scheduled in which the issue will be discussed. Does nursing have anything to contribute to the discussion?

- What do we know about mentally ill offenders, sex offenders, perpetrators of domestic violence, and others?
- What is the therapeutic outcome for those mentally ill offenders who have completed rehabilitation programs?
- What is the risk to the community?
- What stress management strategies are helpful to a community?

You work at a junior high school, providing sex education and health promotion programs for young teenagers. You notice that more and more young people are wearing gang colors and using gang-related language and hand signals.

- How does this affect your work?
- Does this change your priorities?
- Are there referrals or strategies that should be initiated because of the gang affiliations of your students?

completion of the program, the candidate is able to take the certification examination.

Legal Nurse Consultant

The legal nurse consultant is a licensed registered nurse who critically evaluates and analyzes health-care issues in medically related law suits. Because the legal system is involved, nurses acting as consultants are considered to be practicing forensics. Nurses uniquely combine their medical expertise with legal knowledge to assess compliance with accepted standards of health-care practice.

Legal nurse consultants work in collaboration with attorneys and other legal and health-care professionals. They may have independent practices, work in the hospital setting in risk management, or be employed by law firms or health insurance companies.

> *Legal nurse consultants work in collaboration with attorneys and other legal and health-care professionals. They may have independent practices, work in the hospital setting in risk management, or be employed by law firms or health insurance companies.*

The following is a list of activities performed by the legal nurse consultant that distinguishes their specialty practice:

1. Drafting legal documents under the supervision of an attorney
2. Interviewing witnesses
3. Providing education to attorneys and other involved parties on health-care issues and standards
4. Researching nursing literature, standards, and guidelines as they relate to issues within a particular case
5. Reviewing, analyzing, and summarizing medical records
6. Identifying and conferring with expert witnesses
7. Assessing causation and issues of damages as they relate to the case
8. Developing a case strategy in collaboration with other members of the legal team
9. Providing support during the legal proceedings
10. Educating and mentoring other registered nurses in the practice of legal nurse consulting[3]

Medical Examiner Nurse Death Investigator

The role of the death investigator is to advocate for the deceased. A death investigator is a professional with experiential and scientific knowledge who can accurately determine the cause of death. In other words, the forensic nurse death investigator is a registered nurse who is functioning in the death investigator's role.

The forensic nurse death investigator may assume several different titles such as forensic nurse investigator, death investigator, or deputy coroner. In some areas of the country, nurses actually practice as coroners. There are currently no required credentialing or education standards for nurse death investigators in the United States. Each region of the country specifies the requirements in its own jurisdictions.

The basic knowledge all nurses possess, such as pharmacology, anatomy, physiology, growth, and development, is a requirement for the death investigation role. This nursing knowledge allows the investigator to sort out factors involved in a death. Nurses also learn advanced communication skills and knowledge of the grief process during their education. These skills are required for notifying next of kin and interviewing witnesses.[4]

Forensic nurse death examiners have a number of responsibilities. They respond to scenes of deaths or accidents and work in collaboration with law enforcement. At the scene, the forensic nurse death examiner examines the body, pronounces death, and takes tissue and blood samples. They take pictures of the body and evidence at the scene. A nurse death investigator must be able to recognize and integrate other evidence, such patterns of injury as revealed during the investigation. They are responsible for record keeping and arrange for the transport of the body to the morgue or to the coroner's office for autopsy for further examination. The nurse death examiner works with the forensic pathologist to collect evidence in the lab during the autopsy.

What Do You Think?

Have you ever been involved in a court case or law suit? What was your role? How would being a nurse trained in legal issues have changed what you did or said?

Forensic Psychiatric Nurse

Forensic psychiatric nurses work with individuals who have mental health needs and who have entered the legal system. These nurses generally practice in state psychiatric institutions, jails, and prisons.

Nurses in this role perform physical and psychiatric assessments and develop plans of care for the clients entrusted to their care. At the most basic level, forensic psychiatric nurses assist clients with self-care, administer medical care and treatment, and monitor the effectiveness of the treatment. Psychiatric interventions are developed to promote coping skills and improve mental health in a therapeutic environment.[5]

Forensic psychiatric nurses may also have an advanced practice role. Registered nurses with a master's degree in psychiatric–mental health nursing practice as clinical nurse specialists or nurse practitioners. Nurses in this role are able to diagnose and treat individuals with psychiatric disorders and often are allowed to prescribe medications. They may function as primary care medical and mental health providers, psychotherapists, and consultants. Advanced practice forensic psychiatric nurses may practice independently, in mental health centers, state facilities, and HMOs.

Forensic Correctional Nurse

Correctional facilities reflect the demographics of the general population with an increasingly aging incarcerated population who have age-related health-care problems. Forensic correctional nurses provide health care for inmates in correctional facilities such as juvenile centers, jails, and prisons. They manage acute and chronic illness, develop health-care plans, dispense medications, and perform health screenings, and health education. Forensic correctional nurses conduct psychiatric assessments and respond to emergency situations. The role of the forensic correctional nurse offers a high level of autonomy compared with other nursing roles.

Evolving Requirements

There is no official certification as a forensic nurse in the United States except for the SANE certification. Many nurses working in forensic roles believe certification requirements will develop as the specialty of forensic nursing continues to evolve and becomes better defined. In the near future, nursing education will be required to develop classes that teach forensic nursing as a part of their curriculum.

> *The role of the forensic correctional nurse offers a high level of autonomy compared with other nursing roles.*

NURSE ENTREPRENEUR

Should You Be Your Own Boss?

An entrepreneur is someone who establishes and runs his or her own business. A nurse entrepreneur starts a business by combining nursing experience and knowledge with business knowledge. Starting a business can be risky financially and certainly is far different from the nurse's traditional role as an employee in an institution.

However, nurses are educated to think independently and are sometimes willing to take risks when it is for the benefit of their clients. As professionals who can translate their expertise and confidence into new arenas, nurses are capable of achieving personal and financial success running their own businesses.[6]

Historically, nurse-run businesses have usually focused on temporary staffing agencies, nursing education, or consultant roles. Nurse entrepreneurs can also include nurse attorneys, nurse case managers, nurse educators, nurse death investigators, nurse midwives, nurse paralegals, psychiatric nurses, legal nurse consultants, and sexual assault nurses.

Assess Your Nursing Skills

In making the decision to start a business, nurses need to first assess their nursing experience to determine what type of business would be appropriate for their skill and knowledge levels. For example, a sexual assault nurse examiner may contract services to emergency rooms or law enforcement agencies. A critical care nurse may start a home care agency offering high-tech services for clients in the home setting. Nurses may develop self-defense courses they can market to high-risk professions, such as forensic psychiatric and forensic correctional nurses.

After nurses determine what skills and knowledge they possess, they need to develop a plan on how to establish the business. A basic level of knowledge about finances and the business start-up process is essential for success. The hopeful entrepreneur needs to consider the customer who will be seeking his or her services, what customers need and desire, what start up costs might be, and who the competition may be. Answering these questions will allow the nurse to assess the potential success of the business.[7]

Any nurse can start a business. Generally, no advanced degrees are required unless the business requires the diagnosis and treatment of clients. Key qualities required for success are a high degree of self-motivation and passion for the business to succeed. Nurse entrepreneurs are limited only by their creativity and desire to succeed.

CASE MANAGEMENT

The Case Management Society of America (CMSA) defines case management as ". . . a collaborative process of assessment, planning, facilitation and advocacy for options and services to meet an individual's health needs through communication and available resources to promote quality, cost-effective

outcomes."[8] Effective collaboration among all members of the health-care team is essential to meet the needs of clients in today's complex heath-care system.

A Care Coordinator

Nurse case managers act as advocates for clients and their families by coordinating care and linking the client with the physician, other members of

What Do You Think?

Do you know any nurse with the title of "case manager?" Interview them and note what duties they perform as part of their roles.

the health-care team, resources, and the payer. The goal of the nurse case manager is to help the client obtain high-quality, cost-effective care while decreasing the duplication and fragmentation of care. Research data indicates that active participation by a nurse case manager in the care of a client positively affects the outcomes experienced by the client.

Nurses are uniquely prepared by virtue of their education and professional experiences to fulfill the role of case manager. The holistic health-care approach has been an underlying principle of nursing care since the time of Florence Nightingale. Nurses have experience in arranging referrals, providing client education and acting as a liaison between physicians and specialty care.

Any client who may face challenges regarding care and recovery can benefit from case management. This includes hospitalized clients, those with complex medical conditions, those requiring specialty care, and clients who have personal or psychological circumstances that may interfere with recovery. Factors that indicate the need for a nurse case manager include:

1. A complex treatment plan that requires coordination or a plan that is unclear
2. An injury or illness that may permanently prevent the client from returning to a previous level of health
3. A pre-existing medical condition that may complicate or prolong recovery
4. A need for assistance in accessing health-care resources
5. Environmental stressors that may interfere with recovery

Physicians Catch Up

The Case Management Society of American Standards of Practice for Case Management cites the physician and case manager collaboration as essential for successful case management.[9] Although recent research shows that clients benefit from case management, it has been underused by physicians. Case managers and physicians met in 2003 to identify barriers to the use of case management and to explore ways to increase the use of case managers. One result of this meeting was the development of the Consensus Paper of 2003 Physician and Case Management Summit: Exploring Best Practices in Physician & Case Management Collaboration to Improve Patient Care. This paper identified both barriers and ways to promote effective, collaborative use of case management by physicians (Box 22.1).

The research that attributes improved client outcomes directly to case management is compelling. It appears the nurse case managers will continue to expand their role in the health-care system of the future.

> " *Nurse case managers act as advocates for clients and their families by coordinating care and linking the client with the physician, other members of the health-care team, resources, and the payer.* "

Box 22.1

Collaboration of Case Managers and Physicians

Barriers to Use of Case Managers by Physicians

1. Lack of resources and financial incentives in medical practice to integrate case management
2. Resistance to change by physicians and time pressures imposed on physicians
3. Insufficient awareness of the role of the case manager among physicians and consumers
4. Insufficient promotion of their value by case managers
5. Lack of evidence of the value of case management

Facilitators of the Use of Case Managers by Physicians:

1. Recognizing, understanding, and utilizing case management
2. Standardizing the education of and definition of case managers
3. Educating physicians and consumers about case management
4. Compensation for doctors who utilize case manager services
5. Education of patients in accessing case management
6. Validated research on the effectiveness of case management
7. Recognizing the CMSA Standards of Practice for legitimacy and credibility of the nurse case manager role.

BIOTERRORISM

An Acute Health Issue

Bioterrorism is the use of microorganisms with the deliberate intent of causing infection to achieve political goals. Biological weapons are relatively easy and inexpensive to produce. The use of microorganisms is particularly effective because their release can go undetected for an extended period of time because their effects are not immediate. This allows for their person-to-person spread before they are detected.

Table 22.1 Epidemiological Clues to a Biological Attack

Presence of a large epidemic
Unusually severe disease or unusual routes of exposure
Unusual geographic area, unusual season, or absence of normal vector
Multiple simultaneous epidemics of different diseases
Outbreak of zoonotic disease
Unusual strains of organisms or antimicrobial-resistant patterns
Higher attack rates in persons exposed
Credible threat, as determined by authorities, of biological attack
Direct evidence of biological attack

The vulnerability of the United States to a biological attack became painfully apparent with the delivery of anthrax spores through the postal system as an infective agent after the 9/11 attacks.[10] The need to protect a vulnerable American population from further terrorist attacks became an acute public health issue. Also, the discovery of offensive biological weapons programs of the former Soviet Union and Iraq, as well as uncertainty about the whereabouts of weaponized biological agents produced in those programs, has increased the national anxiety level concerning bioterrorism. Since 1998 the ANA has worked in conjunction with the American College of Emergency Physicians (ACEP) to develop strategies for health-care providers to respond to nuclear, biological, and chemical incidents.

Early Recognition

For nurses and other clinicians, the key to an effective response is training in the early recognition of a bioterrorist attack. Recognizing and treating outbreaks early on is critical for rapid implementation of measures to prevent spread of disease. Response to bioterrorist attacks is similar to the traditional public health response to naturally occurring outbreaks of communicable diseases, but the focus needs to be on early detection. However, early

recognition is challenging in the case of weaponized biological agents that terrorists may use because the initial presentation of symptoms are highly variable.

Clinical Presentation

Nurses and other clinicians must be familiar with the specific symptoms and clinical syndromes caused by bioterrorism agents (Table 22.1). One of the first indications of a biological attack will be an increase in the number of individuals seeking care from primary care providers and emergency rooms. Hospitals, doctors, nurses, and public health professionals will be on the front lines of any attack. A heightened level of suspicion, plus knowledge of the relevant epidemiological clues, should help in the recognition of changes in illness patterns.[11]

> " *Since 9/11 the need to protect a vulnerable American population from further terrorist attacks became an acute public health issue.* "

Biological Agents

The Centers for Disease Control (CDC) developed a list of biological agents that are considered the

Table 22.2 Critical Biological Agent Categories for Public Health Preparedness

Category	Biological Agent	Disease
A: Highest immediate risk	*Variola major*	Smallpox
	Bacillus anthracis	Anthrax
	Yersinia pestis	Plague
	Clostridium botulinum (botulinum toxins)	Botulism
	Fancisella tularensis	Tularemia
	Filoviruses and arenaviruses (Ebola & Lassa virus)	Viral hemorrhagic fevers
B: Next highest risk	*Coxiella burnetii*	Q fever
	Brucella species	Brucellosis
	Burkholderia mallei	Glanders
	Burkholderia pheudomallei	Meliodosis
	Alphaviruses (VEE, EEE, WEE*)	Encephalitis
	Rickettsia prowazekii	Typhus fever
	Toxins (e.g., ricin, staphylococcal enterotoxin B)	Toxic syndromes
	Chlamydia psittaci	Psittacosis
	Food-safety threats (e.g., Salmonella species, *E. coli* 0157:H7	
	Water-safety threats (e.g., *Vibrio cholerae, Cryptosporidium parvum*)	
C: Potential, but not an immediate risk	Emerging-threat agents (e.g., Nipah virus, hantavirus)	EEE, eastern equine encephalitis; VEE, Venezuelan equine encephalitis; WEE, western equine encephalitis

most likely to be used in a bioterrorist attack (Table 22.2). Infective agents were included based on their ability to produce widely disseminated infections, high mortality rates, potential for major public health impact, ability to cause panic and social disruption. Those that require special action for public health preparedness were also included. Category A agents possess the highest immediate risk for use as biological weapons; category B agents pose the next highest risk. Category C agents pose a potential for use, but are not considered an immediate risk for use as biological weapons.

Effective Response

Identification and Management
In the event of a widespread bioterrorism attack, nurses in all levels and types of health-care settings have the potential to become involved. To develop a prompt and effective response, nurses and other health-care providers must know the modes of transmission, incubation periods, symptoms, and communicable periods of these diseases as outlined by the CDC.

Once a potential outbreak is detected, it must be brought to the attention of the appropriate health-care agencies or specialist in infective diseases. All nurses should have accurate around the clock information on the resources available for their geographic area. Once appropriate notifications have been made, nurses will use their skills of clinical evaluation and history taking to identify the infective organism, mode of transmission, and source of exposure. In addition, nurses play a critical role in managing post-exposure prophylaxis and its complications, as well as psychological and mental health problems brought on by the event.

Have you received any specialized training in disaster or bioterrorism preparedness? If you have, how does it make you better able to care for victims of disaster or bioterrorism? If you have not, why? Do you feel prepared to care for these victims?

Response Training

The American College of Emergency Physicians in alliance with the American Nurses Association submitted a list of recommendations to the Health and Human Services Office of Emergency Preparedness in April, 2001. Included was the recommendation that all basic nurse education programs include information on how to respond to mass casualty events. The task force also recommended that self-study modules and other types of specialty programs be developed for ER nurses that would contain more in-depth information on the detection and management of bioterrorism.

The ANA is actively involved in developing ways to better prepare nurses to respond to bioterrorist events. In collaboration with the Department of Health and Human Services, they established the National Nurses Response Team (NNRT). This joint effort was unveiled at the ANA's 2002 biennial convention.

Activation and Deployment

In the event that the president declares a bioterrorism state of disaster, the NNRT will be activated to respond by providing mass immunization or chemoprophylaxis to a population at risk. The NNRT, under the auspices of the Department of Health and Human Services, will be quickly deployed in response to a major national event.

The ANA and federal officials' goal is to recruit 10 regional teams of 200 nurses. The ANA is working to recruit these nurse teams and will provide ongoing education to the NNRT in disaster response. The Department of Health and Human Services is responsible for the screening and processing of potential nurse team members after they have been recruited by the ANA.

When the NNRT teams are deployed, the members become "federalized," and the federal government will pay their salaries, reimbursement for travel, and housing costs during the duty period. In case of a terrorism disaster, the deployment will be limited to two weeks to minimize the impact on the nurses' employers.

The nursing profession faces serious challenges in the response to threats of bioterrorism. The nation is counting on nurses to play a vital role in bioterrorism preparedness and response. The public depends on nurses to be the frontline responders and to protect them from the effects of bioterrorism. Nurses must be able to communicate medical information and educate the public quickly after a crisis. It is imperative that the nursing profession train nurses in appropriate, effective responses to ensure the best outcome in a frightening, unfamiliar event.

DISASTER NURSING

A disaster is a catastrophic event that leads to major loss. The American Red Cross defines a disaster as ". . . an occurrence such as a hurricane, tornado, storm, flood, high water, wind-driven water, tidal wave, earthquake, drought, blizzard, pestilence, famine, fire, explosion, building collapse, commercial transportation wreck, or other situations that cause human suffering or create human needs that the victims cannot alleviate without substantial assistance."[12]

Many Roles for the Nurse

Every disaster poses its own unique challenges. The role of the nurse in specific disaster care depends upon the nature of the particular disaster and the type and numbers of injuries.

Often in disaster situations, nurses function outside their usual practice setting and may assume a variety of roles in meeting the needs of the disaster victims. Nurses must be able to perform under stressful and sometimes physically dangerous conditions. Many times a nurse functions as a triage practitioner, assessing victims and prioritizing care for the best use of resources. Nurses also provide direct treatment, which may be brief, or they may be involved in more complex roles, such as mobile surgical units (Box 22.2).

The National Disaster Medical System (NDMS) is the agency responsible for mobilizing disaster relief and it works closely with local fire, police, and emergency medical services to provide comprehensive disaster relief. NDMS also uses volunteer disaster response teams known as IMSURTs (International Medical/Surgical Response Teams) in which nurses are an essential component. The IMSURTs

---

Box 22.2

Responsibilities of the Disaster Nurse

Short term:
1. Provide emergency medical assistance. Special attention is given to vulnerable groups, such as the handicapped, children, and the elderly.
2. Provide assistance in the mobilization of necessary resources such as food, shelter, medication, and water.
3. Work in collaboration with existing organizational structures and resources.

Long term:
1. Provide assistance with resettlement programs and psychological, economic, and legal needs.
2. Partner with independent, objective media, local and national branches of government, international agencies, and nongovernmental organizations.

---

provide emergency medical services any place in the world where there is a lack of resources.

Medical assistance is provided in hospitals, local clinics, or the field. Deployable Rapid Assembly Shelter Hospitals (DRASHs) are mobile shelters that can be used by the IMSURT team as a small independent hospital. The DRASH is designed with triage emergency care, intensive care units, and surgical rooms. The IMSURT program was designed to support emergency medical response systems in locations worldwide that have become overwhelmed by a major disaster.

> *Often in disaster situations, nurses function outside their usual practice setting and may assume a variety of roles in meeting the needs of the disaster victims. Nurses must be able to perform under stressful and sometimes physically dangerous conditions.*

Additional Disaster Relief

Other areas in which nurses can provide assistance during disasters include, but are not limited to:

- Disaster Medical Assistance teams. A Disaster Medical Assistance Team (DMAT) is a group of front-line medical personnel, including nurses, who provide health care after a disaster. These may include terrorist, natural, or environmental disasters.
- Medical Reserve Corps. This group is part of the USA Freedom Corp. The USA Freedom Corps was developed in 2002 in response to Americans' desire to volunteer and serve their communities in the wake of the September 11, 2001, terrorist attacks in the United States.
- American Red Cross. Registered nurses can join their local red cross and receive specialized training in disaster and bioterrorism preparedness.
- Commission Corps Readiness Force. The agency deploys teams to respond to public health emergencies.[13]

Conclusion

Florence Nightingale wrote in 1859 that "no man, not even a doctor, ever gives any other definition of what a nurse should be than this 'devoted and obedient.' This definition would do just as well for a porter. It might even do for a horse!"[14] The profession of nursing has come a long way since Nightingale made the first efforts to move it out of its position of servitude to physicians.

Nursing is constantly evolving and defining itself as it strives to include expanded roles of practice. Of the many new and exciting roles for nurses, forensic, bioterrorism, disaster, entrepreneur, case management, and legal consultant have developed in response to the needs of society.

The tragic events of September 11, 2001, in New York City, Washington, DC, and Pennsylvania revealed how poorly prepared the United States was to deal with disasters. In response, legislation was enacted on federal and state levels that began to address the many issues associated with terrorist acts. Large sums of funding also became available to train health-care works to be better able to deal with a variety of potential terrorist acts. Collaboration between groups that often had little to do with each other in the past became an essential component of these plans. The Department of Health and Human Services and the ANA have been working closely to educate nurses in disaster and bioterrorism responses.

Although nurses have practiced in these areas for many years, they are only now beginning to be recognized for the unique skills and qualities they bring to these roles. For example, emergency room nurses have long had as part of their job descriptions interviews and assessments of crime victims, collection and proper handling of evidence, and accurate and complete documentation of injuries and information provided by crime victims. In the role of client advocate, nurses have always been case managers through the assessment of client needs, coordination of referrals for specialized or long-term care, and the coordination of nonnursing services such as diet teaching and social services.

All nurses have the knowledge of anatomy, physiology, growth, and development that is required for the death examiner position. As more nurses seek the specialized training that is now available for many of these roles and obtain nationally recognized certification as a demonstration of their knowledge, they will gain acceptance as highly qualified and valuable members of these specialized health-care teams.

Issues in Practice

Authorization of Subspecialty Roles to Be Limited in Texas

Rethinking Advanced Practice

The Texas Board of Nurse Examiners is responsible for authorizing Advanced Practice Nurses (APNs) to practice as clinical nurse specialists or nurse practitioners in the state of Texas. The board bases its authorization on the individual's educational preparation. The board has expressed concerns regarding the increasing number of subspecialty areas in which nurses were seeking advanced practice authorization. Some of the areas of concern included ophthalmology, diabetes management, and forensics subspecialty. The primary concern cited by the board was that the educational preparation in the subspecialty areas may result in individuals who are not prepared to recognize a broad range of conditions and diseases because of the narrow focus of their training. They also expressed concerns that APNs may be unable to find employment because of the limitations of their training.

The board expressed its belief that subspecialty practices are valuable and should continue. They also believe, however, that it is in the best interest of the public that the APN have a broad-based foundation to enter into practice. The subspecialty training is to be considered an additional expertise and will not require further recognition by the board.

In April, 2003, the board requested that the Advanced Practice Nursing Advisory Committee (APNAC) review the APN titles that were currently recognized. They were to then advise the board of the titles that should continue to be recognized. The APNAC recommended that the board recognize only those titles for which there is a national certification examination specifically targeted to that role and to specialty areas that include broad-based educational preparation.

The committee also recommended a time-limited exception to these recommendations to individuals currently enrolled in an advanced practice education programs. These exceptions are for roles that were currently recognized by the board, but would not continue to be recognized in the future. Under these exceptions, nurses could practice in their specialty area but only in the state of Texas. In July of 2004, the board voted to propose amendments relating to advanced practice titles and published these proposals to notify the public.

A Public Hearing

A public hearing regarding these proposed amendments was held October 20, 2004. Testimony was heard from eleven organizations and five individuals. Among the organizations represented were the ANA, the Texas Nurses Association (TNA), and the National Association of Clinical Nurse Specialists (NACNS). The ANA expressed concerns that the nursing profession should not be wed to the idea that nurses should be generalists and not specialists. They believe that there are mechanisms already in place, such as defined scope and standards of practice, to protect patient consumers and ensure appropriate training of APNs. They also believe that proposed amendments could be construed as restraint of trade and hamper the recognition of APNs as accepted members of health-care delivery systems.

(continued)

Issues in Practice   _{continued}

Multiple concerns were expressed by other organizations attending the hearing. There were concerns that changes would have a negative economic impact on the state and discourage nurses from coming to Texas to practice. Some felt that enrollment numbers in nursing programs would decline. Concerns were expressed that the board was exceeding its authority. Others felt that the board had not adequately collaborated with national and state leaders in these roles before proposing the recommended changes. A number of the attendees expressed agreement with the proposed amendments. Each comment expressed by those present at the hearing was responded to by the board. A summary of the hearing can be found at www.sos.state.tx.us.

The initially proposed amendments were withdrawn January 27, 2005. The board integrated some of the proposed changes made during the October 20, 2004, meeting. The changes that were made do not change the limitations on the APN roles that the board will recognize. On February 11, 2005, the Texas Board of Nurse Examiners formally approved amendments to Chapter 21, Advanced Practice Nurses, 22 TAC 222.2 and 221.7. These changes are to become effective January 1, 2006.

Sources: American Nurses Association: Texas Board of Nurse Examiners: Restrictive Proposed Changes to Limit Advanced Practice Specialties, 2004. www.nursingworld.org/gova/state.htm. Texas Register: Proposed Rules: Board of Nurse Examiners 30(6):635–645, 2005.

Critical Thinking Exercises

Application of Human Rights

What information do you need to make a decision? The reader is encouraged to explore applications of human rights from the point of view of the victim and the perpetrator of the crime. Think about how the issue of human rights would be defined and protected in the following examples. What is the nurse's role?

- A married father of two, an upstanding member of the community, is accused of child molestation and is admitted to the unit for psychiatric evaluation and submission of tissue samples.
- A female inmate becomes pregnant in prison and does not want anyone to know who the father is.
- A young man has a history of substance abuse and mental illness. He refuses medication to control psychotic behavior and is confined in a forensic psychiatric facility because of the claim that he is incompetent to stand trial for car theft.
- A mother of an infant is being interviewed in a suspected child abuse case. She admits that she was sexually and physically abused as a child and throughout her marriage. The priority is to establish her role in the current charges involving injury of her 3-month-old infant.

References

1. Knight, K: The real CSI: Forensic nursing in the ED. Nursing Spectrum 8(19):8–9, 2004.
2. Seng, J: The first year as sexual assault nurse examiner: Role transition and role-related stress within a new SANE team. Journal of Emergency Nursing 30(2):126–133, 2004.
3. Barnet, D: Switching gears: Becoming a legal nurse consultant. Nursing Spectrum 16(16):6–7, 2004.
4. Kopishke, L: Forensics corner. Mitigation specialist: A natural role for the LNC. Journal of Legal Nurse Consultant 15(3):22–23, 2004.
5. Dale, C: Focus. High, medium, and low security care: Does the type of care make any difference to the role of the forensic mental health nurse? Nurs Res 9(3): 168–184, 2004.
6. Hoban, V: The nurse entrepreneurs. Nursing Times 100(29):20–22, 2004.
7. Dayhoff, N: CNS entrepreneurs: Innovators in patient care. Source Book Advanced Practice Nurses 6–8, 2005.
8. Case managers work on the unit with staff nurses: initiative improves patient care. Hospital Case Manager 12(5):68–69, 2004.
9. Collins, P: Are emergency department registered nurse case managers an option for your hospital? Care Management 10(5):29–31, 2004.
10. Henning, K: Health system preparedness for bioterrorism: Bringing the tabletop to the hospital. Infection Control Hospital Epidemiology 25(2):146–155, 2004.
11. Steed, C: Integrating bioterrorism education into nursing school curricula. J Nurs Educ 43(8):362–367, 2004.
12. Trossman, S: Nurses provide care during one hurricane after another. American Nurse 36(6):1, 7, 2004.
13. Reineck, C: The readiness estimate and deployability index: A self-assessment tool for emergency center RNs in preparation for disaster care. Topics in Emergency Medicine 26(4):349–356, 2004.
14. Goodnow, M: Outlines of Nursing History. W. B. Saunders, Philadelphia/London, 1935.

Bibliography

Bemis, P: Being your own boss: It's more than just a pipe dream. Nursing Spectrum, 2004. www.communitynursingspectrum.com/ Magazinearticles/articles.cfm?AID=9882.
Berkowitz, B: One year later: The impact and aftermath of September 11. Public Health Nursing Practice: Aftermath of September 11, 2001. Online Journal of Issues in Nursing 7(3), 2002. wwwnursingworld.org/ojin/topic19/ tcp19_4.htm.
Campbell, M: Nurse entrepreneur gives new face to care. Nursing Matters 15(5):14, 22, 2004.
Chang, P: The development of intelligent, triage-based, mass-gathering emergency medical service PDA support systems. J Nurs Res 12(3):227–235, 2004.

Cogar, S: The legal nurse consultant's role in defending law enforcement officers. Journal of Legal Nurse Consultant 15(1):3–6, 2004.
Cox, E: Disaster nursing: New frontiers for critical care. Critical Care Nurse 24(3):16–18, 20–24, 2004.
Hayward, M: Facing danger. Nursing Standard 19(3):20–21, 2004.
Heitkemper, M: Clinical nurse specialists: State of the profession and challenges ahead. Clinical Nurse Specialist 18(3):135–140, 2004.
Nash, D, et al.: Consensus paper of the 2003 Physician and Case Management Summit: Exploring Best Practices in Physician and Case Management Collaboration to Improve Patient Care. Case Management Society of America, 2003.
Pasqualone, G: Perspectives on the Future of Forensic Nursing. Online Forensic Nurse Magazine, 2005. www.forensicnursemag.com/articles/3b1cover.html.
Wessling, S: The Case for Forensic Nursing. Minority Nurse.Com, 2003. www.minoritynurse.com/
Young, C: Biological, chemical, and nuclear terrorism readiness: Major concerns and preparedness of future nurses. Disaster Management Response 2(4):109–114, 2004.

Associations and Web Sites

American Academy of Forensic Sciences: www.aafs.org
American Association of Legal Nurse Consultants: www.aalnc.org
American College of Forensic Examiners International: www.acfei.com
American Forensic Nurses: www.amrn.com
American Psychiatric Nurses Association: www.apna.org
Forensic Nurse Magazine: www.forensicnursemag.com
International Association of Forensic Nurses: www.forensicnurse.org; www.iafn.org
Legal Nurse Consultant Certificate Program: www.continuing-legal@udel.edu
National Alliance of Sexual Assault Coalitions: www.taasa.org
National Association of Correctional Nursing: www.correctionalnursing.org
National Association of Independent Nurses: www.independentrn.com
National Commission on Correctional Healthcare: www.ncchc.org
Nurse Entrepreneur Network: www.Nurse-Entrepreneur-Network.com
Nursing Entrepreneur: www.nursingentrepreneurs.com
National Nurses in Business Association: www.nnba.net
Office for Victims of Crime Resource Center: www.ncjrs.org
Office for Victims of Crime: www.ojp.usdoj.gov/ovc
Public Health Functions Projects: www.health.gov. phfunctions/public.htm
Rape, Abuse and Incest National Network (RAINN): www.rainn.org
Sexual Assault Resource Service (SARS): www.sane-sart.com
Violence Against Women Office: www.ojp.usdoj.gov/vawo

23

Nursing Research and Evidence-Based Practice

Mary Ann Remshardt

Learning Objectives

After completing this chapter, the reader will be able to:

- Discuss the necessity of nursing research as an essential component of comprehensive client care.

- Describe ways in which nursing research can be used to enhance communication and understanding between cultures.

- Demonstrate the ability to identify the basic similarities and differences related to qualitative and quantitative research designs.

- Identify at least four strategies that may help promote implementation of valid research findings in clinical settings.

- Define and describe the concept and utility of evidence-based practice.

- Discuss the research-practice gap as this relates to nursing research and identify some ideas for promoting change.

A UNIQUE BODY OF KNOWLEDGE

One characteristic that defines a profession is the creation of a unique body of knowledge and related skills to guide its practitioners. There are many ways of obtaining knowledge. In the nursing profession, the development of a distinct body of nursing knowledge is an ongoing process. Nursing has a long and dignified history as a service and caring profession. In contrast, nursing as a scientific discipline is just now taking its first unsteady steps. As with every profession, nursing continues to evolve to meet the needs of a changing society and rapidly developing health-care technology.

TRIAL AND ERROR

In the past, much of what constituted the practice of the profession of nursing was on the basis of the edicts of those in authority. Founded upon experiential learning, nursing focused on doing exactly what was prescribed by the person in charge, usually the physician. Prior nursing was considered a unique body of knowledge; it made sense for nurses to rely on the judgment of those who were considered by society to be authorities on health and illness and with whom nurses worked closely.

In the past, when skills used in the promotion of health and healing were developed, often through trial and error, they were then passed on by tradition. The trial and error method historically served as the primary source of health-care knowledge. Other approaches used in the care of the ill were discovered serendipitously.

Today the *search* for knowledge within what is *known* is being systematically replaced by *research* that reveals what is *best* in nursing practice. Research is the approach through which nursing knowledge, although not infallible, may be judged much more reliable and transferable than that afforded by authority, tradition, or past experiences. Nursing as a science depends on valid research evidence to support best practice. Research provides the crucial link between theory and practice.

> " *In theory, there is no difference between theory and practice. But, in practice, there is.* Jan L. van de Snepscheut "

This chapter presents an overview of pertinent issues regarding the critical nature of research as scientific support for the profession of nursing.

> " *If you can change your mind, you can change the world.* Joe Reimer "

NURSING RESEARCH DEFINED

Nursing research defines nursing as a profession and as such must be embraced by nursing professionals. As one of a number of professions involved in providing health care, nursing accepts responsibility for defining its own uniqueness. Scientific inquiry is the tool of choice for tasks related to professional clarification, justification, extension, and collaboration.

The Goals of Inquiry

Nurses are held accountable for their actions and must equip themselves to defend the interventions they initiate through strong empirical evidence. At the very minimum, nursing care must be safe. With contemporary cost-containment issues, nursing interventions are expected to demonstrate practicality as well as cost effectiveness. Research can show which approaches to nursing care are most effective and which do not work. The profession of nursing will not experience a true renaissance until scientific inquiry becomes as much a part of daily practice as caring interventions.

Nursing research is more than a method of inquiry. Nursing research is a systematic process for answering questions through the discovery of new information with the ultimate goal of improving client care.[1] The purpose of nursing research is "to

test, refine and advance the knowledge on which improved education, clinical judgment, and cost-effective, safe, ethical nursing care rests."[2]

Beyond Clinical Practice

Some authors would limit the scope of nursing research to the clinical practice of nursing. In its fullest meaning however, nursing research involves a systematic quest for knowledge designed to address questions and solve any problems relevant to the profession including issues related to nursing practice, nursing education, and nursing administration.[3] Nursing research should be conducted to expand and clarify the body of knowledge unique to the discipline of nursing.

Redefining the client. Nurses know that clients are more than just individuals receiving nursing care within selected clinical settings. Nursing clients are family units, communities, organizations, institutions, corporations, local and state agencies, and citizens of a country as well as the global community. Accurately measuring how effectively the nursing profession meets the needs of an expanding and diverse consumer base depends on its ability to successfully integrate an expanding and diverse body of scientific knowledge into the daily practice of nurses. Nurses must focus on promoting better understanding of the research process and encouraging their colleagues to seek the evidence needed to explain, modify, and improve nursing practice.

Setting priorities and directions. Clinical decisions and the resulting nursing interventions are justified by scientifically documented findings. Using nursing research, nurse investigators not only address issues related to cost, safety, quality, and accessibility of health care, but look ahead to establish priorities and to define the future direction of the nursing profession.

Crossing cultural boundaries. One modern requirement for the profession is to understand and address cultural issues involved in nursing care and to understand the various cultures within the communities where they practice. Nurses must also learn to look beyond perceptual and geographic boundaries to promote dialogue, investigation, and collaboration with many international nursing colleagues in the interest of culturally sensitive and global concerns. Culturally related issues provide many opportunities for nursing research (see Chapter 21).

DEVELOPMENT AND PROGRESSION OF RESEARCH IN NURSING

The Origin of Nursing Research

Florence Nightingale is viewed as the person who first elevated nursing to the status of a profession, as presented in her first book *Notes on Nursing* (1859).[4] Nightingale is also credited with introducing research to the profession. Nightingale believed in the importance of "naming nursing" by the use of observed data to support the need for health-care reforms, including those related to nursing education. Nightingale recognized the impact of combining strong logical thinking and empirical research in developing a sound scientific base upon which to build the practices of the profession of nursing.

Methodical Observation

As the first recognized nurse epidemiologist, Florence Nightingale systematically collected objective data and described environmental factors in 1855 that impacted health and illness. During the Crimean War, appalled by what she observed of the care of soldiers, Florence Nightingale was forward-thinking enough to implement and then demand scientific inquiry in the practice setting. She methodically gathered the facts that eventually supported her claims that lack of cleanliness, fresh air, proper rest, and nutrition contributed to high levels of disease and death seen in the front line "hospital" during the war.

As a result of her research, she petitioned forcefully for more supplies, better food, and cleaner conditions. As a result of her advocacy, the mortality rate among wounded soldiers dropped from 42 percent to 2 percent. Her work during the 1800s was not fully appreciated until more than a century later.[4]

The Development of Research

Even today, the full realization of how important this one woman's work was for the profession of nursing is still being evaluated. She had few professional role models, relatively little education, a military organization that doubted her value, and meager financial support. Her accomplishments, considering the challenge, were phenomenal. It is interesting to speculate about how much more progress would have been made in building the unique body of nursing knowledge if only other nurses of the time had heeded Nightingale's earliest call for research.

A Look at Nursing Education

During the 1940s, many studies concerning nursing education came to the forefront because of the tremendous demand for educated nurses during World War II. Nursing education practices were evaluated in a study commissioned by the National Nursing Council for War Service. Findings from this study and others at the time uncovered weaknesses in nursing education. This relatively new wave of research spawned several other studies that looked at nurses' functions, roles, attitudes, acceptance, and interactions with clients.

A Center for Nursing Research

Several events that occurred during the 1950s prompted those conducting nursing research to carve out an ever-expanding path for the profession of nursing that continues to widen today. Nurses with advanced degrees were increasing in numbers. A center for nursing research was formed at the Walter Reed Army Institute of Research.

Creation of the American Nurses' Foundation and *Nursing Research* (the journal) allowed publication of nursing research findings that gave both a face and a voice to the studies. Many of these studies became both the mirror and microscope through which nurses studied themselves. This self-appraisal was an unprecedented research approach for any profession.

A New Definition of Nursing

In the 1960s, phrases such as *conceptual framework, conceptual model,* and *nursing process* made their first appearances in textbooks and other nursing literature (see Chapter 4). Nursing leaders, now becoming more focused on theoretical support for nursing, continued to lament the relative lack of research.

Many professional nursing organizations set priorities for research during this time. It was also during this time that another visionary nurse heralded a call to the table of logical reasoning and empirical research. Virginia Henderson, one of the early nursing theorists, defined the role of nursing as "to assist individuals (sick or well) with those activities contributing to health, or its recovery or to a peaceful death, that they perform unaided, when they have the necessary strength, will, or knowledge; to help individuals carry out prescribed therapy and to be independent of assistance as soon as possible."

This definition was so conceptually clear that it was accepted by the International Council of Nurses (ICN) in 1960, and Henderson's work went on to identify many relevant research questions for the practice of professional nursing.

A Growth in Research Programs

In the 1970s, the number of graduate nursing programs experienced tremendous growth, and so did the number of nurses conducting research. Increases in the number of research studies being conducted pointed out the need for an improved means to give those studies voice, and three more research journals were developed: *Advances in Nursing Science, Research in Nursing and Health,* and the *Western Journal of Nursing Research.* During this time the research focus changed from the study of nurses to the study of client care needs. Clinical challenges were identified as having the highest priority for nursing research.

A Source of National Data

The 1980s witnessed another information explosion with the continued growth rate of research-trained, graduate school–educated nurses and the introduction of computers. Research and writing were both enhanced by electronic databases and the expanding World Wide Web. In 1983, the American Nurses' Association created the Center for Research for Nursing.

The mission of this center is to serve as a source of national data for the profession. In 1986, The National Center for Nursing Research (NCNR) at the National Institutes of Health was established by congressional mandate. The mission of this organization is to support clinical (applied) and basic research to create a scientific foundation for the care of individuals across the life-span. During the 1980s, a journal with the specific intention of providing research directed toward the practicing clinical nurse took form in *Applied Nursing Research.*

A New Focus on Practice

In 1993, the NCNR was awarded full institute status, and the National Institute of Nursing Research (NINR; www.nih.gov/ninr.org) came into being. In 1996, NINR had a reported $55 million budget, and it

was poised to promote and support research priorities established during that decade. Since the late 1990s, studies have become more focused on the practice of nursing, the outcomes of nursing and other health-care services, and the building of a stronger knowledge base by replicating previous research using a variety of settings and situations.

Evidence-Based Practice

Today, the movement to achieve cost-effective, high-quality care based on scientific inquiry generates the drive for nurses to achieve evidence-based practice (EBP). EPB is today's nursing issue of priority. Because of the volume of literature being published by all health-care professions, including nursing, it is important to develop skills of critical discernment. Critical discernment requires the nurse to understand the research process and to sift through and carefully assesses all available and credible research findings. Once the research has been analyzed and judged, recommendations can be made for using the best practice techniques based on best evidence.

Currently, nurses have not only been given the responsibility to conduct research but to evaluate, critique, and apply the research findings of other nurses and health-care professionals in their own practice. Understanding research is more than merely learning simple methods of inquiry.

> " *The future is here. It is just not widely distributed yet. William Gibson* "

THE RESEARCH PROCESS

Nursing students, long before graduation, often notice something in the clinical setting that grabs their attention. They may simply have wondered if a different intervention would work better in a particular situation or if the best technique was being used or what was the evidence that showed that a particular technique *is* the best one to use.

As neophytes, students may question interventions or solutions that seasoned nurses often take for granted. Students may see the experienced nurse's familiar world differently and their minds may be open to possibilities that others may not see. Questioning the status quo is a key first step in the research process. Employing critical thinking often leads to visualization of a research project, the development of a plan, the implementation of that plan, and finally, sharing of the findings with others. This process follows a logical progression from abstract ideas to concrete actions.

Research Designs

The word *design* implies both creativity and structure. The design for a research study can be seen as a road map or a recipe. It serves as a fairly flexible set of guidelines that will provide the researcher with answers to the questions of inquiry.

To choose a research design, the nurse must first develop a vision of the overall plan for a study, including a general idea of the type of data needed to answer the research question. The design is a critical link that connects the researcher's framework with appropriate types of data. The level of pre-existing knowledge in the area of inquiry also helps determine the research design. If little is known about a specific subject, an exploratory study may be the best method for uncovering new information. In exploratory research, there is usually more interest in looking at the qualitative characteristics of data. Hypotheses are not usually required for these studies.

If the researcher is looking at variables that are independent, objective, or demonstrate cause and effect, then a quantitative design is best. If the question invites discovery of meanings, perceptions, and the collection of subjective data, then qualitative designs should be used.

Quantitative versus Qualitative Research

Historically and in the tradition of scientific inquiry, quantitative experimental research designs were the most highly respected. These designs are guided by a somewhat rigid set of rules that gives the most importance to the *process* of inquiry. However, over the past decade there has been a growing interest in, and respect for, qualitative approaches in research, especially in the social sciences. Social researchers see human interactions as complex, highly contextual, and too intricate to be studied using a rigid framework or standard instrument. Also, attempting to conduct quantitative research on human subjects often produces serious ethical dilemmas.

Qualitative Designs

The purpose of qualitative inquiry is to gain an understanding of how individuals construct meaning in their world, visualize a situation, and make sense of that situation. For example, to nurses, the concept of "caring"

Box 23.1
Qualitative Research Designs

Phenomenology
Ethnography
Grounded Theory
Historical Studies
Case Studies

is very important, yet the nurse will probably perceive caring differently than the client. The nurse researcher wishing to measure "caring interventions" might find this concept very difficult to quantify, but a qualitative method could yield much useable information.

Because of the nature of nursing and the usual subject matter (human beings), qualitative designs are best suited to answer questions that interest nurses. The most commonly used of these designs are seen in Box 23.1.

Semistructured interviews using open-ended questions and observations are the most commonly used data collection methods in qualitative studies. Knowledge generated by qualitative research answers questions related to the meaning and understanding of human experiences.

> *Not everything that can be counted, counts and not everything that counts can be counted. Albert Einstein*

Quantitative Designs

Quantitative designs are approaches that seek to verify data through prescriptive testing, correlation, and sometimes description. These designs imply varying degrees of control over the research material or subjects. Control of the research design can range from very tight to somewhat loose.

The design in quantitative research becomes the means used for hypothesis testing. The design also optimizes control over the variables to be tested and provides the structure and strategy for answering the research question. More highly controlled quantitative designs try to demonstrate causal relationships, and more flexible designs address relationships between and among variables. Box 23.2 summarizes and classifies quantitative research designs.

Box 23.2
Research Designs

Experimental Designs	Nonexperimental Designs
Pre-test/post-test control group	Comparative studies
Post-test only control group	Correlational studies
Solomon four group	Developmental studies
	Evaluation studies
Quasi-experimental Designs	*Meta-analysis Studies*
Nonequivalent control group	Methodological studies
Time series	Needs-assessment studies
	Secondary analysis studies
Pre-experimental Designs	*Survey studies*
One group pre-test/post-test	One-shot case study

In quantitative experimental design, a comparison of two or more groups is required. The groups under study must be as similar as possible so that results can be credited to the treatment of the variables and not to differences between the groups. The independent variable is the one managed or manipulated by the researcher. The dependent variable *depends on,* or is altered as a direct result of, the researcher's manipulation.

In research, it is good to remember that neither the quantitative nor the qualitative research school is better. Each research approach is useful in different ways and both expand understanding of health care and the nursing profession. What is important is to choose the methodology that best addresses the questions the researcher is asking and collects the data that are most useful.

> *Statistics are no substitute for judgment. Henry Clay*

NARROWING THE RESEARCH–PRACTICE GAP

Two Different Cultures

More and more, nurses are becoming academically astute in the area of research. Unfortunately, education alone does not ensure transfer of what is learned into daily nursing practice. Like the basic but critical nursing skill of sterile asepsis, research will become a part of each nurses' practice only when it becomes a part of each nurse's ideology.

Academic and practice arenas are often, in reality, two entirely different cultures. The critical and creative thinking so valued and promoted in the academic environment may fall victim to time and budget constraints within the clinical setting. To support what is best for clients, clinical practice areas such as hospitals must find ways to ensure that research finds safe harbor in the culture of practice. The implementation of research in practice will depend on inquisitiveness, development of cognitive skills, the ability to question one's own practice, and professional discipline. Nurses must also understand that sometimes research findings may conflict with practices rooted in tradition.[5]

Barriers to Research in Practice

Experts are now asking, "Why generate more research when that which has already been generated has not been adapted to practice?" This research–practice gap remains a bewildering challenge to the nursing profession.

An Isolated Skill

A challenge to the use of research in practice is that research skills are often taught to nursing students in isolation from other nursing subjects. This may broaden the division between research and practice because it separates the two elements early on in the nurse's development and education. Unless ways are found to focus inquiry and link research findings to clinical practice early on in the education process, the research–practice gap will likely remain.

As the situation currently stands, even though there has been an emphasis on nursing research for more than two decades, there are few indications that nurses on the front lines of clinical practice actively use research as a way to improve their practice.

Lack of Understanding

There are a number of barriers to the implementation of research in the health-care setting. Often, nurses skilled in clinical nursing may not be skilled in conducting or obtaining research data. Nurses who attempt to use research studies to answer practice questions may feel that the research does not provide the practical solutions for which they are looking. This concern may be valid because some researchers do not have an understanding of practice issues from the bedside nurse's viewpoint.

Conversely, practicing clinical nurses may lack the knowledge to understand or interpret the language of research. Published research often appears so esoteric and complicated that the message cannot be found in the bottle. Researchers must find ways of packaging their conclusions so that practicing nurses can quickly find easily understood clinical solutions to the care issues they are facing. Also, the information should be easy to access by those who provide direct care to clients: clinical nurses.

Unquestioned Practices

Entrenched nursing practices present another challenge. In the not too distant past, traditional nursing practices appear to have had a half-life longer than uranium. A few nursing traditions remain so widely accepted as fact that they are never questioned, and they therefore evade the scrutiny of testing. Best practices may never become evident without testing of those older practices that are accepted as necessary, preeminent, and sacrosanct.

Lack of Incentive

With the very real challenges of time and budget limitations, very few hospitals or other agencies offer encouragement or rewards to nurses who *are* willing to seek out and use research findings in an effort to improve practice. One survey conducted to identify barriers to implementation of research from clinicians' perspectives revealed "insufficient authority

and insufficient time" as the two obstacles most often cited.[1]

Resistance from Managers

Some researchers suggest that unit managers may view an environment of updates and change as unfavorable to maintaining a committed and cohesive staff. Some describe change as a threat to the constancy necessary for safe and expeditious client care.[6] Nurses willing to incorporate best practice evidence into clinical protocols must have the confidence in their own professional judgment and the courage to stand against those nurses who find comfort in unchanging traditional practices.

Incorporating Best Practice

Several strategies can help nurses conduct and use research for the improvement of nursing care, such as attending conferences in which clinical research findings and ideas for practice are presented. Other strategies proposed include, but are not limited to:

1. Incorporating research findings in textbooks, basic and continuing nursing education programs, and clinical policy and procedure manuals
2. Explicitly connecting research use to institutional goals and objectives
3. Developing joint committees between colleges of nursing and hospital nursing departments
4. Inviting staff nurses to find and present summaries and abstracts during unit meetings and clinical case conferences in an effort to increase the interest of colleagues working on their units[7]

Several of the most widely read clinically focused nursing journals such as *American Journal of Nursing, Nursing 200_,* and *RN* are beginning to add research sections to increase the ease of access to research, to assure a wider distribution of current clinical research findings, and to promote the incorporation of best practices based on credible evidence into clinical settings. This mission serves the profession by simplifying some of the language of research and by giving voice to the importance and practical nature of clinical research.

> *No problem can be solved by the same consciousness that created it. We must see the world anew. Albert Einstein*

Issues in Practice

Short Staffing in an Emergency

Halley had been working on the medical-surgical unit since her graduation from an ADN nursing program 2 months ago. She had also had clinical rotations at the same unit while in nursing school and felt comfortable and confident with the unit's procedures and her own skills. One Sunday evening the house supervisor stopped her just before the beginning of her shift and explained that the RN on the eight-bed maternity unit had called to say that she was going to be late because of a family emergency. Because of the overall short staffing on weekends at this hospital, Halley would need to be pulled to the maternity unit for no more than 2 hours to cover the RN position and pass medications until the regular nurse could arrive for her shift. That would leave the medical-surgical unit short staffed, but it was relatively quiet and only about three-quarters full.

Halley hurried to the maternity unit and received an abbreviated report from the staff who were waiting to go home. All the patients were stable and the only potential problem was a patient in the emergency department (ED) who was 36 weeks pregnant and might be in the early stages of labor. Although they hadn't received report on the patient in the ED, the departing staff joked that it would probably be the next morning before "anything happened."

After conducting an abbreviated initial assessment of the patients on the maternity unit, Halley called the ED to receive report on their patient. The patient was a 36-year-old woman who had three children, ages 12, 9, and 2. The ED nurse also reported that the patient's old charts revealed that the patient had a history of "precipitous labor" (a very rapid labor with the sudden birth of the baby). Given the relatively short time since the pateint's last delivery and the patient's history, Halley recognized that she did not have the skills or experience to provide safe care for this client.

Halley called the nursing supervisor and explained that she would need a nurse more experienced in OB to help admit and care for this new patient. The supervisor responded that the whole hospital was short of nurses and she had no one she could send. Halley would just have to do her best until the regular maternity unit nurse arrived.

A few minutes later, the ED nurses brought the patient to the maternity unit. After she was transferred to a unit bed, Halley did an initial admission assessment with the following results: blood pressure 166/123; pulse 134; contractions 2 to 3 minutes apart, regular and strong, fetal heart rate (FHR) 166, faint but regular, amniotic fluid leaking from the vagina. After making her assessment, Halley again called the supervisor and demanded that she come to the maternity unit immediately to help with this patient, who Halley felt was going to deliver her baby very soon. The supervisor responded that she was in the middle of a code blue in the ICU and that Halley would just have to hang on for the half hour or so until the maternity nurse was due to arrive.

- What are the primary underlying ethical principles involved in this dilemma?
- How do individual nurse's ethical obligations differ from those of a hospital's administration?
- What type of research data would help resolve this issue?
- Do you think this case study reflects a realistic situation?

EVIDENCE-BASED PRACTICE

Improvement of client care is the primary reason for conducting nursing research. Nursing interventions must be supported by accurate information. The current philosophy in nursing and health care is that professionals must use research evidence when making decisions about the clinical management of clients. Health-care decisions can be logically based upon either primary research or systematic reviews of literature or both.

Systematic Reviews

Systematic reviews present reliable summaries of past research. The role of such reviews has become more important as the volume of health-care literature has expanded. Other factors include the inconsistent quality of the research produced, the increased number of possible health-care interventions resulting from the many health-care products and medications available on the market today, and the exponential growth of health-related technology.

Consideration of these factors has prompted the proposal that systematic reviews of existing literature replace primary research as the main source of evidence for clinical decision making. One review of this type could replace many individual studies and free those making clinical decisions from finding, interpreting, and evaluating a collection of published primary research reports and articles.

Some believe that systematic reviews would represent the "gold standard" in research summaries. However, those eager to jump on the review-only bandwagon need to be careful that methods currently used for literature review may not most accurately reflect some of the nursing research being reviewed. The challenge exists in the "narrowly defined concept of what constitutes good evidence."[8]

Primary Research

What about only using nursing research studies as a source of information? One recurring criticism of primary nursing research is that much of it is accomplished as single studies. Some nursing researchers believe that many excellent qualitative studies are not followed by rigorous quantification.[9] Other nursing leaders continue to urge nurse researchers to make replication studies a high research priority, particularly for research addressing clinical nursing issues. A single study is rarely adequate for making decisions regarding clinical practice.[10]

The Best of Practice

EBP is believed to constitute the best of practice and has garnered the attention of health-care administrators because of its potential to decrease the cost of health-care delivery. Standards of nursing practice, clinical guidelines, and routine performance audits seek to promote the use of research findings to some degree. The availability of electronic databases, emphasis on the teaching of research in nursing curricula, along with such support organizations as the Cochrane Collaboration (www.cochrane.org), Best Evidence (www.acponline.com), and the Centers for Health Evidence (www.cche.net) all endorse the expectation that nurses must be able and willing to use evidence to inform their practice.

How Useful Is It?

Successful implementation of EBP also depends on how practical and useful the information is to the practicing nurse. The usefulness of information requires evaluation of several factors by the nurse including potential benefits versus possible harm, cost-effectiveness, availability of ongoing support resources, and willingness of the health-care staff and clients to accept change.

With the emphasis on the urgency for implementing EBP, critical and creative thinking have become even more important because:

• Nurses must access, understand, evaluate, and disseminate a rapidly expanding body of nursing and other health-related information.
• Nurses must be able to recognize commonalities and uncover inconsistencies regarding the values of the profession, the values of the organization that employs them, the needs of clients for whom they advocate, and even the popular culture that exerts pressure on the public's ability to make safe choices.
• Nurses recognize that it takes critical and creative thought to support research into complex health-care issues and to promote successful implementation of changes in professional practice.

The goals of EBP include cost-effective practice on the basis of the data produced by research, the dissemination of data, and the implementation of best practice interventions into the nurse's practice. The following have been identified as essential features of EBP:

- EBP is problem-based and within the scope of the practitioner's experience.
- EBP narrows the research–practice gap by combining research with existing knowledge.
- EBP facilitates application of research into practice by including both primary and secondary research findings.
- EBP is concerned with quality of service and is therefore a quality assurance activity.
- EBP projects are team projects and therefore require team support and collaborative action.
- EBP supports research projects and outcomes that are cost effective.[11]

In summary, evidence-based researchers conduct systematic reviews of existing literature. These reviews are important because of the large amount of healthcare literature already in existence that has not been assimilated into practice. The mission of EBP researchers is to evaluate and present the evidence that is available on a specific topic in a clear and unbiased way. Clinical recommendations evolving from this process present nurses with sound decisions based on best evidence. Consequently, researchers will not only know what questions have been satisfactorily answered, but they will also be better able to identify where gaps in the knowledge still exist.

Networking: Where to Begin

As more evidence becomes available to guide practice, agencies and organizations are developing EBP guidelines. The Agency for Healthcare Research and Quality funds several EBP centers that are accessible through their Web site (www.ahrq.gov) and sponsors a National Guideline Clearinghouse where abstracts for EBP are available at www.guideline.gov. The American Pain Society (www.ampainsoc.org), the Oncology Nursing Society (www.ons.org), and the Gerontological Nursing Interventions Research Center are also available (www.nursing.uiowa.edu/gnirc). The Best Practices Network presents information from several organizations and is available at www.best4health.org.

Leaders and educators within the profession of nursing agree that there is a role for every nurse in research, regardless of level of education.

RESEARCH ROLES BY EDUCATIONAL LEVEL

Leaders and educators within the profession of nursing agree that there is a role for every nurse in research, regardless of level of education. A minimal requirement for all twenty-first century nurses is the ability to develop *and use* basic research skills. Nurses striving to improve their individual practice are increasingly committed to building a body of knowledge specific to nursing. Findings from scientific inquiry define the unique and valuable roles and the challenges of nursing.

Areas of Competency

One of the hallmarks of success in the field of research is the identification of research competencies for nurses at each educational level of preparation. In its classic document, *Commission on Nursing Research: Education for Preparation in Nursing Research,* the American Nurses Association (ANA) identified research competencies for each classification of nursing education program. It is presumed that professional nurses committed to lifelong learning will cultivate their research expertise throughout their careers. Following are the expected research roles by educational level:

Associate Degree Nursing Graduate

1. Demonstrates awareness of the value or relevance of research in nursing
2. Assists in identifying problem areas in nursing practice
3. Assists in collection of data within an established structured format

Associate degree nurses are expected to demonstrate an awareness of the value of research in nursing by becoming knowledgeable consumers of research information and by helping identify problems within their scope of nursing practice that may warrant exploration.

Baccalaureate Degree Nursing Graduate

1. Reads, interprets, and evaluates research for applicability to nursing practice
2. Identifies nursing problems that need to be investigated and participates in the implementation of scientific studies
3. Uses nursing practice as a means of gathering data for refining and extending practice
4. Applies established findings of nursing and other health-related research to practice
5. Shares research findings with colleagues

Nurses with a baccalaureate education are expected to be intelligent consumers of research by understanding each step of the research process to interpret, evaluate, and determine the credibility of research findings. The baccalaureate nurse is able to distinguish between findings that are merely interesting and findings backed by enough data to be included in the nurse's practice. Baccalaureate-prepared nurses also participate in one or more phases of research projects. These nurses must be alert to and uphold the ethical principles of any research involving human participants and oversee the protection of individual rights as specified in the ANA Code of Ethics.

Master's Degree in Nursing

1. Analyzes and reformulates nursing practice problems so that scientific knowledge and scientific methods can be used to find solutions
2. Enhances quality and clinical relevance of nursing research by providing expertise in clinical problems and by providing knowledge about the way in which these clinical services are delivered

3. Facilitates investigation of problems in clinical settings by contributing to a climate supportive of investigative activities, collaborating with others in investigations, and enhancing nurses' access to clients and data
4. Investigates for the purpose of monitoring the quality of the practice of nursing in a clinical setting
5. Assists others in applying scientific knowledge in nursing practice

Doctorate Degree in Nursing or a Related Discipline

1. Provides leadership for the integration of scientific knowledge with other types of knowledge for the advancement of practice
2. Conducts investigations to evaluate the contributions of nursing activities to the well-being of clients
3. Develops methods to monitor the quality of the practice of nursing in a clinical setting and to evaluate contributions of nursing activities to the well-being of clients

Graduate of a Research-Oriented Doctoral Program

1. Develops theoretical explanation of phenomena relevant to nursing by empirical research and analytic processes
2. Uses analytic and empirical methods to discover ways to modify or extend existing scientific knowledge so that it is relevant to nursing
3. Develops methods for scientific inquiry of phenomena relevant to nursing[12]

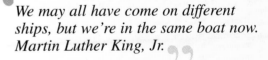

We may all have come on different ships, but we're in the same boat now.
Martin Luther King, Jr.

ETHICAL ISSUES IN RESEARCH

The Nuremberg Code

Although guidelines that govern human behavior have always been a part of recorded history, the need for ethical standards in research came to the public's attention in a dramatic way following World War II when evidence of the Nazi's experimentation and torture of selected groups of victims was revealed.

Box 23.3

Articles Adapted from The Nuremberg Code

1. The voluntary consent of human subjects is absolutely necessary.
2. The experiment should yield fruitful results for the good of society.
3. The experiment should be so designed and based on results of animal experimentation and knowledge of . . . the disease or problem under study that the anticipated results will justify performance of the experiment.
4. The experiment should be conducted so as to avoid all unnecessary physical and mental suffering and harm.
5. No experiment should be conducted where there is an a priori reason to believe that death or . . . injury will occur.
6. The degree of risk . . . should never exceed that determined . . . by the importance of the problem to be solved by the experiment.
7. Proper preparations should be made . . . to protect the experimental subject against even remote possibilities of injury, disability, or death.
8. Scientifically qualified people must only conduct the experiment. The highest degree of skill and care should be required through all stages of the experiment.
9. During the course of the experiment, the subject should be at liberty to bring the experiment to an end. . . .
10. During the course of the experiment, the scientist . . . must be prepared to terminate the experiment at any stage. . . .

Source: Modified from Trials of War Criminals before the Nuremberg Military Tribunals under Control Council Law No. 10, Vol. 2, pp. 181–182. Washington, DC, U.S. Government Printing Office, 1949.

During the trials of Nazi war criminals, the U.S. Secretary of State and Secretary of War discovered that the defense was trying to justify the atrocities committed by Nazi physicians as merely "medical research." As a result, the American Medical Association was asked to develop a code of ethics for research that would serve as a standard for judging the Nazi war crimes. This standard remains valid to this day and is known as the Nuremberg Code (Box 23.3).

National Research Act
Ethical issues are critical to all research, and researchers from all disciplines are bound by ethical principles that protect the rights of the public. One set of principles addressing the conduct of research came from the 1974 National Research Act. This act established the National Commission for Protection of Human Subjects in Biomedical and Behavioral Research.

Part of that act mandated the establishment of Institutional Review Boards (IRBs), whose primary responsibility is to safeguard, in every way, the rights of any individual participating in a research study.

IRBs are panels that review research proposals in detail to ensure that ethical standards are met in the protection of human rights. The mission of the IRB is to ensure that researchers do not engage in unethical behavior or conduct poorly designed research studies.

Every university, hospital, and agency that receives federal monies must submit assurances that they have established an IRB composed of at least five members. These members should reflect a variety of professional backgrounds, occupations, races, and cultures in an effort to uphold complete and unbiased project reviews.

Code of Ethics for Nurses
The profession of nursing also has its own code of ethics to which all nurses are legally and ethically bound. The development of this code was initiated by the ANA Board of Directors and the Congress on Nursing Practice in 1995. In June 2001, the ANA House of Delegates voted to accept a revised Code of Ethics, and in July 2001 the Congress of Nursing Practice and Economics voted to accept the new language, resulting in a fully approved Code of Ethics for Nurses with Interpretive Statements. A read-only

version of this document is available at www.nurs-ingworld.org/ethics/ecode.htm. Specific ANA position statements on selected ethics and human rights issues may be viewed at www.nursingworld.org/readroom/position/ethics (see Chapter 7).

The moral authority nurses possess by reason of their license and position in the health-care structure must be used to guard against those who may try to minimize the importance of that responsibility or, for a number of reasons, may attempt to convince nurses to set aside their responsibilities. Nursing research most often addresses the needs and behaviors of human beings. Embedded in nurses' professional code of ethics is the charge to protect every person from harm. This responsibility extends beyond *nursing* research to include any client-related issue and any type of behavioral or biomedical research or questionable procedure.

In nurses' position of trust with clients, nurses possess a great deal of influence over a population that is especially vulnerable because of health issues and needs. This unique position of trust gives nurses a higher responsibility to protect and defend those in their care.

In nurses' position of trust with clients, nurses possess a great deal of influence over a population that is especially vulnerable because of health issues and needs.

Informed Consent

Protection of human subjects underpins the conduct of research and implies that individuals have the information they need to make informed decisions. They have the right to be fully informed, not only about the care they receive but also about any research in which they participate. Informed consent is both an ethical and a legal requirement in the research process. The ethical principle of self-determination is central to the process.

Besides those with special health considerations, certain groups of individuals are considered particularly vulnerable owing, in part, to their lack of ability to give informed consent or their potential susceptibility to coercion. These groups include children, the mentally retarded, the elderly, those with terminal diseases, the homeless, and those who may have altered levels of consciousness as the result of condition, medication, or sedation.

Nurses are well aware of the need for informed consent and the provision of information prior to procedures. This knowledge can serve nurses well in their obligation to obtain informed consent prior to conducting research. The key elements of informed consent for research can be found in Box 23.4.

The language of the consent form must be clear and understandable, written in the primary language of the client, and with at most, an eighth grade reading level. Technical language should never be used. The Code of Federal Regulations states that subjects must never be asked to waive their rights or

Box 23.4

Key Elements of Informed Consent

1. Researcher is identified and credentials presented.
2. Subject selection process is explained.
3. Purpose of the research is described.
4. Study procedures are discussed.
5. Potential risks are identified.
6. Potential benefits are described.
7. Compensation, if any, is discussed.
8. Alternative procedures, if any, are disclosed.
9. Assurances regarding anonymity or confidentiality are explained.
10. The right to refuse participation or withdraw from the study at any time is assured.
11. An offer to answer all questions honestly is made.
12. The means of obtaining the study results is described.

Source: Nieswadomy, RM: Foundations of Nursing Research, 4th edition, copyright 2002. Adapted by permission of Pearson Education, Inc., Upper Saddle River, NJ.

Box 23.5

Guidelines for Critiquing the Ethical Features of Research

1. Was the study approved by an institutional review board (IRB)?
2. Was informed consent obtained from every subject?
3. Is there information regarding anonymity or confidentiality?
4. Were vulnerable subjects used?
5. Does it appear that any coercion may have been used?
6. Is it evident that potential benefits of participation outweigh the possible risks?
7. Were participants invited to ask questions about the study and told how to contact the researcher, should the need arise?
8. Were participants informed how to obtain results of the study?

Source: Nieswadomy, RM: Foundations of Nursing Research, 4th edition, copyright 2002. Adapted by permission of Pearson Education, Inc., Upper Saddle River, NJ.

to release the investigation from liability or negligence. It is important to note that various institutions and researchers, in an extended effort to protect research participants, include more than the 12 elements listed in Box 23.1.

Process Consent

In qualitative research, an important concept is process consent, which requires that the researcher renegotiate the consent if any unanticipated events occur.[13] An example of this might be a situation in which two parents with a small child in the hospital have given consent for the taping and study of "a day in the life of a hospitalized toddler."

During taping of the event, the parents are informed by the physician that a diagnosis is being questioned and their child must subsequently undergo an unexpected lumbar puncture. The parents may become visibly upset by this turn of events. In such a case the researcher should find a way of reconfirming the couple's ongoing interest in being part of the research study. When this family is given the opportunity to renegotiate the original agreement, the nurse researcher is confirming his or her role of advocate and proceeding in the best interest of all participants.

Detecting the Ethical Components of Written Research

It may be difficult to critique the ethical features of written research reports, but if there is evidence that permission to conduct the study was granted by an IRB, it is highly likely that the participants' rights were protected. Nurses have the responsibility of protecting the privacy and dignity of every individual, and the integrity of the nursing profession depends on doing what is right even when no one is looking.

Box 23.5 provides the guidelines for critiquing ethics in research.

> *There is no such thing as a minor lapse of integrity. Tom Peters*

IMPLEMENTING RESEARCH IN THE PRACTICE SETTING

Knowledge that is generated by research and then translated into policy and procedure becomes the ultimate guide to the scientific practice of nursing. A primary responsibility of every nurse conducting research is the distribution of the findings (evidence) that have application in the client care setting. Conversely, the professional responsibility of every nurse caring for clients requires that all nursing interventions be on the basis of reliable research findings.

Nursing research is of no value to the profession, or to the client, if the practice supported by the research is not used in the clinical setting. Unlimited opportunities for the generation and the dissemination of new knowledge exist in nursing, but the truly daunting task addresses the challenge of transforming that knowledge into practice.

The Call for Implementing Research

Research is becoming critical to the professional practice of nursing. The Joint Commission of the Association of Health Care Organizations (JCAHO) accreditation guidelines specify that client care intervention must be on the basis of information from scientifically valid and timely sources.

The mandate of the modern health-care system is that nurses make practice decisions based on the best scientific information available. Standard VII of the American Nurses Association (ANA) Standards of Clinical Nursing Practice states, "the nurse uses research findings in practice." Nurses may participate in research activities in a number of ways. They can conduct reviews of literature, critique research studies for the possibility of application to practice, or "[use] research findings in the development of policies, procedures and guidelines for client care."[14]

Approaches to Using Research

Nursing is not the only profession experiencing reluctance in transforming research into practice. Even though new knowledge is expanding at an exponential rate, every discipline seems to have some type of research–practice gap. Nurses are often hesitant to change current traditional practice to EBP. They often identify many difficulties involved in the changeover. Currently there are several models to help nurses apply research findings that support EBP. One model that appears both practical and relatively uncomplicated is found in Table 23.1.[15]

Promoting Change

It is often difficult for nurses to promote an environment conducive to change. In many hospitals, maintaining the status quo often appears to carry incen-

Table 23.1 Rosswurn and Larrabee Model for Application of Nursing Research

Assess the need for practice changes
(a) Involve all nurses that have a stake in the intervention or change
(b) Identify problems associated with the current practice
(c) Compare available information

Link the problem intervention and outcomes
(a) Identify possible interventions
(b) Develop outcome indicators

Produce best evidence for consideration
(a) Conduct a review of existing literature
(b) Compare and contrast the evidence found
(c) Determine feasibility (including cost in dollars and time)
(d) Consider benefits and risks

Design a proposed practice change.
(a) Define the anticipated change.
(b) Identify necessary resources
(c) Develop a plan based on desired outcomes

Implement and evaluate the proposed change.
(a) Conduct a pilot study.
(b) Assess the process and the outcomes.
(c) Make a decision to alter, accept, or reject the proposed change.

Support the change with ongoing evaluations of the outcomes.
(a) Communicate the desired change to those involved.
(b) Conduct in-service education sessions.
(c) Revise standards of practice (policy/procedures) reflecting the change
(d) Monitor the ongoing process and results.

tives that may intimidate even the most intuitive and confident change agent. The professional nurse committed to using the best evidence to provide the best care for clients can be most effective by using simple approaches that create an environment receptive to using research findings. Some tactics that may be helpful include:

• Reading clinical journals regularly but also critically. Nursing professionals are well informed and believe in the concept of lifelong learning.
• Attending clinically focused nursing conferences where the latest client care interventions are presented and discussed.

• Learning to look for evidence that clearly supports the effectiveness and the feasibility of widely used nursing interventions.
• Seeking work environments that promote the use of research findings and evidence-based care.
• Collaborating with a nurse researcher. Apprenticeship to one who masters a skill is an old but venerated means of learning that skill.
• Learning to critically scrutinize the status quo. Many worthwhile ideas for change come from those students and nurses "in the trenches" and at the bedside.

• Pursuing the possibility of a proposal and implementing the project. If the nurse finds a research-based idea for clinical care interesting, then taking the steps to research it can be productive.

All truth passes through three stages: Ridicule, opposition and then acceptance as being self-evident. Arthur Schopenhauer

Conclusion

Modern health care has become so complex and demanding that simple trial-and-error approaches will not provide the high-quality information required for the safe, effective, and economical care demanded by well-informed consumers. The nursing profession is beginning to move away from the "I do it because it's always been done this way" method of care to more scientifically rooted care practices based on research. As a result, the nurses are gaining increased recognition as a key member of the health-care team.

Also, nurses are now required to be able to analyze and evaluate research findings to determine which studies are high quality and which ones can be used as a guide for nursing practice. Similarly, nurses

are required to contribute to the body of nursing knowledge by participating in nursing research studies conducted at their facilities. It is presumed that nurses with advanced degrees will initiate and conduct high-quality research.

The ability of nurses to make thoughtful use of research is an important first step in the development of EBP. Society's call for cost containment, high-quality care, and documented outcomes of health-care services will continue to fuel the engine of positive health-care developments. As nursing looks to its future, research and EBP will increase in importance as factors that guide the day to day practice of nurses.

References

1. Fain, A: Reading, Understanding, and Applying Nursing Research. F.A. Davis Company, Philadelphia, 2004.
2. American Association of Colleges of Nursing, 1999, at www.aacn.nche.edu/Publications/positions/rscposst.htm.
3. Polit, D, and Hungler, B: Nursing Research Principles and Methods. Lippincott, Philadelphia/New York, 1999.
4. Goodnow, M: Outlines of Nursing History. W. B. Saunders, Philadelphia/London, 1935.
5. Seymour, B, et al: Valuing both critical and creative thinking in clinical practice: Narrowing the research-practice gap. J Adv Nurs 42(3):288–297, 2003.
6. Le-May, A, et al: Bridging the research-practice gap: Exploring the research cultures of practitioners and managers. J Adv Nurs 28:428–437, 1998.
7. Fain, A: Reading, Understanding, and Applying Nursing Research. F.A. Davis Company, Philadelphia, 2004.
8. Evans, D: Systematic reviews: Gatekeepers of nursing knowledge. Journal of Clinical Nursing 10(5):593–600, 2001.
9. Evers, G: Naming nursing: Evidence-based nursing. Nursing Diagnosis 12(4):137–142, 2001.
10. Nieswiadomy, R: Foundations of Nursing Research. Prentice Hall, Englewood Cliffs, NJ, 2002.
11. French, P: The development of evidence-based nursing. J Adv Nurs 29(1):72–79, 1999.
12. American Nurses' Association Commission on Nursing Research: Guidelines for the Investigative Function of Nurses. American Nurses' Association, Kansas City, MO, 1989.
13. Munhall, P: Ethical considerations in qualitative research. Western Journal of Nursing Research 10(2):150–162, 1988.
14. American Nurses Association Standards on Clinical Practice, 1991, p 16.
15. Rosswurm, M, and Larrabee, J: A model for change to evidence-based practice. Journal of Nursing Scholarship, 31(4):317–322, 1999.

Bibliography

Aroian, K: Effective, efficient and equitable health care: What can cultural diversity teach us about sacred cows. J Prof Nurs 20(6):349–351, 2005.

Ax, S, and Kincade, E: Nursing students' perceptions of research usefulness, implementation and training. J Adv Nurs 35(2):161–170, 2001.

Brink, P, and Wood, M: Basic Steps in Planning Nursing Research. Jones and Bartlett Publishers, Boston, 2001.

Brockopp, D, and Hastings-Tolsma, M: Fundamentals of Nursing Research. Jones and Bartlett Publishers, Boston, 2003.

Burns, N, and Grove, S, The practice of nursing research conduct, critique and utilization. Elsevier Saunders. St. Louis, Missouri, 2005.

Callister, M, et al: Inquiry in baccalaureate nursing education: Fostering evidence-based practice. Nursing Education 44(2):59–65, 2005.

Chesnay, M: Caring for the vulnerable: Perspectives in nursing theory, practice and research. Jones & Bartlett Publishers, Boston, 2005.

Dempsey, P, and Dempsey, A: Using nursing research. Lippincott, Philadelphia/New York, 2000.

Ellett, M, et al: Ethical and legal issues of conducting nursing research via the internet. J Prof Nurs 20(1):68–72, 2004.

Ferguson, L, and Day, R: Evidence-based nursing education: Myth or reality? Nursing Education 44(3):107–116, 2005.

Karigan, M: Ethics in clinical research: The Nursing Perspective. Am J Nurs 101(9):26–31, 2001.

Katz, J, et al: Essential qualifications for nursing students. Nursing Outlook 52(6):277–289, 2004.

Larrabee, J: Advancing quality improvement through using the best evidence to change practice. J Nurs Care Qual 19(1):10–13, 2004.

LoBiondo-Wood, G, and Haber, J: Nursing research methods, critical appraisal, and utilization. Mosby, St. Louis, 2002.

Long, K: Preparing nurses for the 21st century: Re-envisioning nursing education and practice. J. Prof Nurs 20(2):82–89, 2004.

Manojlovich, M: Predictors of professional practice behaviors in hospital settings. Nurs Res 54(1):41–47, 2005.

Mitchell, P: The "so what" question: The impact of nursing research. J Prof Nurs 20(6):347–249, 2005.

Pare, R, and Elovitz, L: Data warehousing: An aid to decision-making. T.H.E. Journal 43(9):32–34, 2005.

Streubert, H, and Carpenter, D: Qualitative research in nursing. Lippincott, Philadelphia, 1995.

Szirony, T, et al: Perceptions of nursing faculty regarding ethical issues in nursing research. Nursing Education 43(6):220–280, 2004.

GLOSSARY OF TERMS USED IN RESEARCH

Bias An influence that produces a distortion in the results of a research study.

Case studies An in-depth qualitative study of a selected phenomenon involving a person, a group of people, or an institution.

Causal relationship A relationship between variables in which the presence or absence of one variable (known as the "cause") will determine the presence or absence of the other variable (referred to as the "effect").

Collaboration A cooperative venture among those with a common goal.

Conceptual framework A framework of concepts that demonstrate their relationships in a logical manner. Although less well developed than a theoretical framework, this framework may be used as a guide for a study.

Conceptual model A set of abstract constructs that explains phenomena of interest.

Correlation The degree of association between two variables.

Empirical evidence Objective data gathered through use of the human senses.

Epidemiologist One who studies the distribution and determinants of health and illness and the application of findings as a means of promoting health and preventing illness.

Ethical standards Standards determined by principles of moral values and moral conduct.

Ethnography A qualitative research approach involving the study of cultural groups.

Evidence-based practice (EBP) The selective and practical use of the best evidence, as demonstrated by research, to guide health-care implementation and decisions.

Experimental research design A quantitative research design that meets all of the following criteria: an experimental variable that is manipulated, at least one experimental and one comparison group, and random assignments of participants to either the experimental or the comparison group.

GLOSSARY OF TERMS USED IN RESEARCH

Exploratory study The descriptive examination of available data to become as familiar as possible with the information.

Grounded theory An inductive approach to research using a systematic set of procedures to develop a theory that is then supported by, or "grounded" in, the data.

Historical studies Qualitative research involving the systematic collection and synthesis of data regarding people and events of the past.

Hypotheses A formal statement of the expected relationship between variables in a selected population

Informed consent Consent to participate in a study given by one who has full understanding of the study before the study begins. Informed consent is based on the principle of the right of each individual to self-determination.

Institutional review boards (IRB) Panels of individuals established at various agencies such as hospitals and universities to review all proposed research studies and to set standards for research involving human subjects.

Nonprobability sampling A sampling process in which a sample is selected from elements of a population through methods that are not random. Convenience, quota, and purposive sampling are examples of nonprobability sampling.

Nuremburg code A code of conduct that serves as one of the recognized guides in the ethical conduct of research.

Nursing research A process that permits nurses to ask questions directed at gaining new knowledge to improve the profession, including elements of patient care.

Phenomenology Qualitative research studies that examine lived experiences through descriptions of the meanings of such experiences by the individuals involved.

Primary research source A report or account of a research study written by the researcher(s) conducting the study. In historical research a primary source might be an original letter, diary, or other authenticated document.

Process consent A version of informed consent that is renegotiated when a situation originally consented to undergoes change.

Qualitative research design A systematic but subjective research approach implemented to describe life experiences and give them meaning.

Quantitative research design A systematic and objective process used to describe and test relationships and evaluate causal interactions among variables.

Quasiexperimental design A type of experimental design in which there is either no comparison group or no random assignment of participants.

Random sample A selection process that ensures that each member of a population has an equal probability of being selected.

Reliability The dependability or degree of consistency with which an instrument measures what it is intended to measure.

Replication study A research study designed to repeat or duplicate earlier research. A different sample or setting may be used while the essential elements of the original study are kept intact.

Research design A blueprint for conducting a research study.

Research process A process that requires the comprehension of a unique language and involves the ability to apply a variety of research processes.

Review of literature An exploration of available information to determine what is known and what remains unknown about a subject.

Sample A subset of a population selected to participate in a study as representative of that population.

Scientific inquiry A logical, orderly means of collecting data for the generation and testing of ideas.

Theoretical framework A framework based on propositional statements derived from one theory or interrelated theories.

Validity The ability of an instrument to measure the variables that it is intended to measure.

Variables Characteristics of individuals, objects, or situations that are susceptible to change and that may be manipulated or measured in quantitative research.

24

Alternative and Complementary Healing Practices

Lydia DeSantis

Learning Objectives

After completing this chapter, the reader will be able to:

- Compare the philosophy and objectives of alternative and complementary healing modalities with those of conventional Western medicine.

- List major reasons why a growing number of people use alternative and complementary healing modalities.

- Describe major types of alternative and complementary healing modalities.

- Summarize methods by which nurses and clients can obtain information about alternative and complementary healing modalities.

- Evaluate a client for use of alternative and complementary healing modalities.

- Identify the strengths and weaknesses of alternative and complementary healing modalities.

A DIFFERENT KIND OF HEALING

Complementary and alternative health-care practices are widely used by a large percentage of the population. Their popularity continues to increase dramatically with clients of all ages and backgrounds. It is important for nurses to have a good understanding of this type of health care to ensure their clients' safety and well-being and to be supportive of their practices.

According to the World Health Organization (WHO), 80 percent of the world's population uses what Americans call "alternative" practices as their primary source of health care. Because of the widely accepted use of these practices, WHO has officially sanctioned the incorporation of "safe and effective [alternative] remedies and practices for use in public and private health services." Currently, between 34 and 42 percent of Americans (60 to 83 million people) use alternative and complementary healing practices, as do 20 to 70 percent of people in Western Europe, 33 percent in Finland, and 49 percent in Australia.[1]

The trend toward alternative practices has continued to grow in the United States since the 1990s. Studies show that 40 percent of people have developed an increasingly positive attitude toward alternative practices, whereas only 2 percent had more negative opinions. Both the general public—72 percent—and health maintenance organizations (HMOs)—73 percent—expect consumer demand for this area of health care to remain moderate to strong. Few people—4 to 11 percent—rely solely on alternative practices to treat illness, but the number relying on conventional health care only is declining.[2]

" *The trend toward alternative practices has continued to grow in the United States since the 1990s.* "

What Do You Think?

Do you use any alternative health-care practices? What are they? Why do you use them?

_____

_____

_____

_____

_____

_____

_____

_____

_____

_____

_____

DEFINING ALTERNATIVE AND COMPLEMENTARY HEALING

Several definitions are used for alternative and complementary health-care practices. They are sometimes referred to as practices that are outside of conventional, science-based Western medicine and not sanctioned by the official health-scare system. A considerable range of practices and concepts is included in alternative and complementary healing. The glossary at the end of this chapter outlines many of these practices.

An Outdated Definition

There is no universally accepted definition. Many alternative health-care practices originated many years ago as a part of cultural belief systems and healing traditions. A commonly used definition in the United States for alternative and complementary modalities comes from the National Center for Complementary and Alternative Medicine (NCCAM), which is an agency of the National Institutes of Health. They define it as "those treatments and health care practices not taught widely in medical schools, not generally used in hospitals, and not usually reimbursed by medical insurance companies."

This definition is quickly becoming outdated. Many medical and nursing schools now include courses on alternative and complementary health-care practices. Also, the practice of alternative medicine is gradually becoming part of conventional health care. Physicians, nurses, and other health-care professionals are responding to the growing public use of these practices by incorporating selected ones into their own client care. Physicians have begun referring clients to a variety of alternative healers and using alternative therapies for their own health.

A Holistic Basis

In this chapter, alternative and complementary medicine is defined as the understanding and use of healing therapies not commonly considered to be part of Western biomedicine. The focus here is mainly on methods of self-care, wellness, self-healing, health promotion, and illness prevention. Therapies and practices are called *alternative* when used alone or with other alternative therapies and are called *complementary* when used with conventional therapies.

The use of the term *healing* is preferred to *medicine* because alternative and complementary modalities typically are based in holistic philosophies that go beyond treatment or cure of the physiological and psychological dimensions of care commonly associated with modern, scientific biomedicine. Holism refers to treatment of the whole person (body–mind– spirit) in that person's environmental context (physical, biological, social, cultural, and spiritual).

USE OF ALTERNATIVE AND COMPLEMENTARY THERAPIES

Who Uses Them

In most national studies of alternative therapy users, ethnic and racial minorities are underrepresented, particularly among persons who do not speak English. Such exclusions raise questions about whether the use rate of alternative therapies in the United States may exceed 42 percent, because the use of alternative therapies among immigrant populations and those with lower incomes tends to be high. Many such populations have grown up with these therapies as "folk" medicine, and they have worldviews that encompass different concepts of health, illness, and healing. Alternative health-care practices are most popular among women, people aged 35 to 49, people with higher educational levels (some graduate education), and those with annual incomes of more than $50,000.

Why Their Use Has Increased

Three general theories have been advanced to explain the growing use of alternative and complementary healing: (1) dissatisfaction with conventional health care, (2) a desire for greater control over one's health, and (3) a desire for cultural and philosophical congruence with personal beliefs about health and illness. Many other client-specific reasons have also been postulated, such as belief in the effectiveness of alternative therapies and the individual's health status (Box 24.1). The rising cost of conventional health care may play a role as well.

> *Three general theories have been advanced to explain the growing use of alternative and complementary healing: (1) dissatisfaction with conventional health care, (2) a desire for greater control over one's health, and (3) a desire for cultural and philosophical congruence with personal beliefs about health and illness.*

Dissatisfaction

The increasing use of alternative therapies is due in part to the feeling that that conventional health care is unable to deal with major health problems or improve a person's general health. People who have a high degree of distrust in conventional health care often rely primarily on alternative therapies. This lack of trust has increased recently for several reasons, including:

• Conflicting information from health-care related studies and clinical trials about risk prevention and health

Box 24.1

Reasons for Use of Alternative and Complementary Modalities

People use alternative therapies alone or together with conventional health care for a variety of reasons. There is no single predictor of use, and the reasons for use may vary from situation to situation. Persons who seem to benefit the most from the alternative approach are those who:

• Prefer a personal relationship with healers
• Refuse to give up hope and hopefulness, regardless of the illness or life-state
• Desire to focus on wellness, health promotion and maintenance, and illness prevention
• Are concerned with gentle alleviation and management of suffering and illness rather than aggressive management of the end-stage of life through technology, medications, surgery, and other invasive procedures
• Wish to participate actively in decision making about their health care
• Believe in the holistic aspects of existence rather than in the primacy of biological and physiological aspects
• Are "culture creatives"—persons at the leading edge of innovation and culture change and who have been exposed to alternative lifestyles and worldviews compatible with those from which alternative and complementary modalities and theories have arisen
• Share cultural and philosophical views similar to those from which alternative and complementary modalities have developed

Source: Austin, JA: Why patients use alternative medicine. JAMA 279:1548,1998. From Holistic Health Promotion & Complementary Therapies Manual 1st edition by ASPEN, 1998. Reprinted with permission of Delmar Learning.

promotion. For example, clients no longer know what to believe about salt intake, normal cholesterol levels, alcohol use, or hormone replacement therapy.

- Continuing emphasis of conventional health care on curative rather than preventive aspects of care. The lack of emphasis on illness prevention limits the ability of individuals to live long lives relatively free of disability from major chronic illnesses, such as arthritis, diabetes, cancer, and cardiovascular disease.

- Growing concern about costs, safety, and access to conventional health care. Many people are concerned about the increased incidence of hospital-acquired diseases, stories of the many deadly medication errors committed over the past few years, the ever-increasing number of invasive procedures, reports of antibiotic-resistant bacteria, and reliance on impersonal technology.

Desire for Control

Some people who use alternative therapies believe conventional care is too intolerant, authoritarian, and impersonal. They feel that some conventional health-care professionals lack sensitivity to the wishes of clients and their families when developing treatment plans. Clients believe they should be partners in and share in decision making about their care rather than just having decisions handed down to them.

In the United States, the majority of people report they are reluctant to tell conventional health-care professionals that they use alternative therapies. Although almost all (89 percent) who use alternative therapies do so under the supervision of an alternative healer, about half of this same group do not consult a conventional health-care professional before they begin. Fourteen percent of persons see both conventional health-care professionals and alternative healers. Similar patterns of self-care and nondisclosure to conventional health-care professionals are found throughout the industrialized world.[3]

Holistic Philosophy

Conventional health care is often faulted for its limited focus on the physiological dimension of health and curing to the exclusion of the unity of mind– body–spirit healing. Another negative characteristic of conventional health care is its excessive dependence on medicine, surgery, and technology rather than on the more natural and noninvasive alternative approach that focuses on self-care and self-healing.

What Do You Think?

Do you tell your physician or primary health-care provider that you use alternative therapies? What is their response?

Belief in Effectiveness

Clients who use alternative therapies do so because they believe those therapies will work, either alone or when combined with conventional treatments. Persons who consider their health to be poor or who have chronic illnesses report greater benefits from alternative than conventional health care and are more likely to try both at the same time. Referral from conventional health-care professionals, friends, or other users of alternative therapies is also a prominent reason for the simultaneous use of both systems. For many clients, alternative therapies simply make them feel better than conventional health care does.

Cost of Alternative Care

Estimated costs of alternative medicines (herbs and nutritional supplements), diet products, equipment, and books and courses totaled $14 billion in 2000. Sixty-seven percent of HMOs cover one or more alternative and complementary healing (ACH) modalities, but coverage is uneven and varies regionally. Chiropractic (65 percent) is the most common covered service, followed by acupuncture (31 percent), massage therapy (11 percent), and vitamin therapy (6 percent). HMOs expect to increase coverage for acupuncture to 36 percent, acupressure to 31 percent, massage therapy to 30 percent, and vitamin therapy to 27 percent. The most important reasons for adding coverage for these services are public demand, legislative mandate, and demonstrated clinical effectiveness.

CLASSIFYING ALTERNATIVE METHODS

The underlying goals of any type of health care include preventing illness, promoting and maintaining health, and caring for people while alleviating the suffering caused by illness. However, despite these common elements, health-care practices vary profoundly in their modalities (technologies), practitioner education and monitoring, underlying concepts (models) of health and illness, modes of care delivery, and social and legal mandates to provide care. Because of the large number of variables, a confusing array of health-care systems, practitioners, and healing modalities have developed. Two systems that can be used to help define and classify alternative and complementary therapies are the Healing Matrix, by Engebretson and Wardell, and the NCCAM classification.

The Healing Matrix
The Healing Matrix (Table 24.1) contrasts conventional and alternative modalities and practitioners.

The alternative modalities shown are (1) representative of those most commonly known by the general public, (2) sought in the United States and industrialized world, and (3) practiced most often by conventional health-care professionals, including nurses.

A Cross-Section of Care
Modalities in column 1 are technologies that cut across various healing systems. The technologies are arranged vertically from the most concrete to the most abstract. The remaining columns include various healing modalities from conventional, marginal, and alternative healing systems.

Physical Manipulation Technologies. These are also known as "bodywork therapies." They are administered by a therapist or by the clients themselves as part of a self-care program. They include health rituals and breathing exercises to better bring about the union of body–mind–spirit.

Ingested or Applied Substances. A number of substances, including herbs, vitamins and other nutritional supplements, and dietary regimens have the goal of helping the body heal itself, rid itself of toxins, and promote general health and wellness.

Table 24.1   The Healing Matrix

Technologies	Orthodox	Marginal	Alternative	
Physical manipulation	Surgery	Chiropractic	Rolfing	Craniosacral alignments
Ingested or applied substances	Physical therapy	Homeopathy	Feldenkrais	Massage therapy
Uses of energy	Pharmacology	Vitamin therapy	Naturopathic remedies	Yoga, Akido, Tai Chi
Mental	Laser surgery	Acupuncture	Herbs	Reflexology
Spiritual	Psychiatry	Acupressure	Flower remedies	Aromatherapy
		Secular or spiritual counseling	Reiki	Diet alternatives
		Established support groups (e.g., 12-step programs)	Magnetic or polarity healing	
		Therapeutic touch	Chakra balancing	
		Self-help groups	Radionics	
		Visualizations	Use of color, gems, and crystals	
		Affirmations	Psychic, spiritual, or intuitive healing	

Source: Adapted from Engebretson, J, and Wardell, D: A contemporary view of alternative healing modalities. Nurse Pract 18:51, 1993.

Energy Therapies. These modes of treatment maintain and/or restore health through the balancing of energy flow in the body. The goal is to restore the natural movement of vital forces, life essences, or other such vitalities that may have been disturbed by diseases or psychological factors.

Mental (Psychic) and Spiritual Therapies. Included in these therapies are group or individual counseling that helps the client develop or attain spiritual and personal growth. Examples include intuiting, revelations, visualization, astrological and other readings, and invoking the spirit world.

Conventional Health Care

The modalities listed in column 2 (orthodox [conventional]) are part of the official health-care system in the United States. They are based on knowledge rooted in scientific and biomedical principles.

Licensed Alternative Care

The modalities in column 3 (marginal) are generally learned through the study of the standard curricula in institutions of higher education. Alternative healers practicing such modalities are usually licensed by the state, and most have credentialing and a professional body that sets standards for their practice. They are not considered conventional therapies in the United States but may be part of conventional health-care systems in other nations.

For example, acupuncture is an essential mode of treatment in traditional Chinese medicine, which along with biomedicine, forms the conventional health-care system in the People's Republic of China. In 1997, The National Institutes of Health Consensus Panel on Acupuncture reviewed research studies and other information on its safety, efficacy, and effectiveness. The studies showed that there is sufficient evidence to approve acupuncture as an intervention for adult general and dental postoperative pain and to treat nausea and vomiting associated with chemotherapy.

Intuitively Based Care

The modalities presented in column 4 (alternative) are less physiological. They are based on a more intuitive type of knowledge. Most alternative healers practicing such modalities are self-taught, have learned through working with other more experienced practitioners, and/or have attended courses or

workshops on particular modalities. The alternative modalities in the bottom cell on the far right have the most intuitive knowledge base; that is, insights about the spiritual or physical self are gained through direct revelations or as interpreted by another. These include readers (e.g., astrologers or seers) or spiritual healers in touch with divine forces.

The NCCAM Classification

In 1992, Congress mandated the establishment of an Office of Alternative Medicine in the National Institutes of Health to enhance the study of ACH. In 1998, the Office became the National Center for Complementary and Alternative Medicine (NCCAM). Its mission is to conduct and support both basic and applied research and training and the dissemination of ACH information to conventional health-care professionals, alternative healers, and the public.

Complementary and alternative medicine (CAM) is defined by the NCCAM as those practices not commonly included in or used by conventional medicine. Seven major categories of CAM are defined and subdivided into practices that (1) fall under CAM, (2) are found in conventional health care but are classified as behavioral medicine, and (3) are overlapping—that is, they can fall in the domain of either CAM or behavioral medicine. Table 24.2 summarizes the NCCAM classification.

Table 24.2 Categories of Alternative Practice

I. Alternative Medical Systems
Traditional Oriental Medicine

Acupuncture	Herbal formulas
Diet	Massage and manipulation (Tui Na)
External and internal qi gong	Tai Chi

Traditional Indigenous Systems

Ayurvedic medicine	Traditional African medicine
Curanderismo	Traditional Aboriginal medicine
Central and South American	Unani-tibbi
Kampo medicine	SIDDHI
Native-American medicine	

Alternative Western Systems

CAM	Overlapping
Homeopathy	Anthroposophically extended medicine
Naturopathy	
Orthomolecular medicine	

II. Mind–Body Interventions
Mind–Body Methods

CAM	Behavioral Medicine	Overlapping
Yoga	Hypnosis	Art, music, and dance therapies
Tai Chi	Meditation	Humor
Internal qi gong	Biofeedback	Journaling

Religion and Spirituality

CAM		
Confession	Nontemporality	"Special" healers
Nonlocality	Soul retrieval	Spiritual healing

Social and Contextual Areas

CAM	Overlapping
Caring-based approaches (e.g., holistic nursing, pastoral care)	Community-based approaches (e.g., Native-American "sweat" rituals)
Intuitive diagnosis	Explanatory models
	Placebo

III. Biologically Based Therapies
Phytotherapy or Herbalism

Aloe vera	Echinacea	Ginseng	Mistletoe
Bee pollen	Evening primrose	Green tea	Peppermint oil
Biloba	Garlic	Hawthorne	Saw palmetto
Cat's claw	Ginger	Kava Kava	Witch hazel
Dong Quai	Ginkgo	Licorice root	Valerian

Special Diet Therapies

Atkins	McDougall	Fasting	Paleolithic
Diamond	Ornish	High fiber	Vegetarian
Kelly-Gonzalez	Pritikin	Macrobiotic	
Gerson	Wigmore	Mediterranean	
Livingston-Wheeler	Asian	Natural hygiene	

(continued)

Table 24.2   Categories of Alternative Practice (Continued)

Orthomolecular Therapies
Single Nutrients (Partial Listing)

Amino acids	Folic acid	Lysine	Niacinamide	Thiamine
Ascorbic acid	Glutamine	Manganese	Potassium	Tyrosine
Boron	Glucosamine sulfate	Magnesium	Selenium	Vanadium
Calcium	Iodine	Medium-chain triglycerides	Silicon	Vitamin A
Carotenes	Inositol	Melatonin	Glandular products	Vitamin D
Choline	Iron	Niacin	Riboflavin	Vitamin K
Fatty acids	Lipoic acid		Taurine	

Pharmacologic, Biologic, and Instrumental Interventions
Products

Antineoplastons	Cone therapy	Hyperbaric oxygen
Bee pollen	Enderlin products	Induced remission therapy
Cartilage	Enzyme therapies	Ozone
Cell therapy	Gallo immunotherapy	Revici system
Coley's toxins	H_2O_2	

Procedures/Devices

Apitherapy	Electrodiagnostics	Neural therapy
Bioresonance	Iridology	
Chirography	MORA device	

IV. Manipulative and Body-Based Methods
Chiropractic Medicine
Massage and Bodywork

Acupressure	Feldenkrais technique	Reflexology
Alexander technique	Osteopathic manipulative therapy (OMT)	Rolfing
Applied kinesiology	Pilates method	Swedish massage
Chinese Tui Na massage	Polarity	Trager bodywork
Craniosacral OMT		

Unconventional Physical Therapies

Colonics	Heat and electrotherapies	Light and color therapies
Diathermy	Hydrotherapy	

V. Energy Therapies
Biofield Therapies

External qi gong	Healing touch	Reiki
Healing science	Huna	Therapeutic touch

Bioelectromagnetic-Based Therapies

(Unconventional Use of Electromagnetic Fields)

Alternating and direct current fields	Magnetic fields	Pulsed fields

Source: Adapted from National Center for Complementary and Alternative Medicine: Classification of Alternative Medicine Practices. April 26, 2000. Available at: www.ccam.nih.gov/fcp/classify/index.html.

Category I

Category I includes alternative systems of theory and practice developed outside of Western biomedicine. For example, acupuncture and Oriental medicine are grounded in traditional Chinese medicine. Also included in this category are traditional indigenous systems, which include all medical systems other than acupuncture and Oriental medicine that developed outside of Western biomedicine. It also includes unconventional Western systems not classified elsewhere that were developed in the West but are not considered part of biomedicine, such as homeopathy.

Finally, this category includes naturopathy, which is an unconventional medical system that has gained prominence in the United States. This eclectic approach consists of a variety of natural systems, such as herbalism, lifestyle therapies, and diet as therapy.

Category II

Category II includes mind–body practices, religion and spirituality, and social and contextual areas. Mind–body medicine involves a variety of approaches to health care and contains three subcategories. Mind–body systems are seldom practiced alone but are usually combined with lifestyle interventions.

Mind–body methods may be part of a traditional medical system. They are sometimes used in conventional health-care practices; however they are characterized as CAM when used for conditions for which they are not normally prescribed. Religion and spirituality include treatments directed toward biological functions or clinical conditions. Social and contextual areas include treatment methods that are not included in other categories, such as cultural and symbolic interventions.

Category III

Biologically based therapies include products, interventions, and practices that are natural in origin and biologically based. They may or may not overlap with conventional medicine and its use of dietary supplements.

Phytotherapy, or herbalism, is the use of plant-derived products for purposes of prevention and treatment. Diet therapies use special diets to reduce risk factors or treat chronic diseases. Orthomolecular medicine is the use of nutritional products and food supplements that are not included in other categories for prevention and treatment of disease. Pharmacological, biological, and instrumental interventions are products and interventions not covered in other categories that are administered in an unconventional manner.

Category IV

Manipulative and body-based methods include body manipulation and/or body movement.

Category V

Energy therapies are based on manipulation of biofields with bioelectromagnetic-based therapies. Biofields include energy systems and energy fields internal and external to the body that are used for medical purposes. Bioelectromagnetics is the use of electromagnetic fields in an unconventional manner for medical reasons.

COMPARING CONVENTIONAL AND ALTERNATIVE PRACTICES

Many similarities exist between alternative and conventional health care. As they attempt to achieve similar goals, they may overlap in method, even though the methods are derived from different concepts of reality and different theoretical models. Table 24.3 summarizes characteristics often cited as common to alternative healing and contrasts them with those usually associated with conventional health care.

A Reductionist Philosophy

Focus on the Physical

In general, conventional medicine focuses on the physical or material part of the person, the body. It is concerned with the structure, function, and connections or communication between material elements that compose the body, such as bones, muscles, and nerves. Conventional medicine generally views all humans as being very similar biologically. Disease is seen as a deviation from what is generally considered to be a normal biological or somatic state.

Conventional medicine is sometimes considered reductionistic because it tends to reduce very complex entities (humans) to seemingly equal and more simple beings who are all anatomically and physiologically similar. From this perspective, it is believed that all individuals will respond in more or less the same ways to causative agents, such as bacteria and viruses, and respond similarly to common

Table 24.3 Contrasts Between Conventional and Alternative Health Care

Conventional	Alternative/Complementary
Chemotherapy	Plants and other natural products
Curing/treating	Healing/ministering care
Disease category	Unique individual
End-stage	Hope/hopefulness
Focus is on disease and illness	Focus is on health and wellness
Illness treatment	Health promotion and illness prevention
Individual is viewed as disease category	Individual is viewed as unique being
Nutrition is adjunct and supportive to treatment	Nutrition is the basis of health, wellness, and treatment
Objectivism: person is separate from disease	Subjectivism: person is integral to the illness
Client	Person
Practitioner as authority	Practitioner as facilitator
Practitioner paternalism/client dependency	Practitioner as partner/person empowerment
Positivism/materialism: data is physically measurable	Metaphysical: entity is energy system or vital force
Reductionistic	
Specialist care	Holistic
Symptom relief	Self-care
Somatic (body biologic and physiologic) model	Alleviation of causative factors
Science is only source of knowledge and truth	Behavioral-psycho-social-spiritual model
Technology/invasive	Multiple sources of knowledge and truth
	Natural/noninvasive

treatments, such as medicines and surgery. In other words, a person with measles, cirrhosis of the liver, or breast cancer will have a similar course of illness as other persons with those illnesses and will respond to treatments in basically the same manner.

Diagnosis by Category

Conventional medicine has developed extensive disease categories, and great emphasis is placed on diagnosis and cure based on the assessment of physical signs and symptoms. Most newly developed medications, when they are in the human-testing phase, are tested on men between the ages of 25 and 35 years old, with the presumption that they will work similarly in women, the elderly, and children. That presumption is not always accurate and there is a growing trend at pharmaceutical companies to human-test medications on groups of persons for whom they are more likely to be used.

Integration of Nonmaterial Factors

The physical body is the primary focus of conventional medicine. Because of this almost exclusive focus on the physical body, conventional medicine often does not consider or include the nonmaterialistic aspects of health and illness in diagnosis and treatment decisions. Thus, spiritual, psychological,

sociocultural, behavioral, and energy system aspects play little or no role in conventional medical treatment.

Conventional medicine does not generally view the client as an integrated person-body that is affected simultaneously by both material and nonmaterial factors during everyday life. The integration of these elements is not seen as important to the person's state of wellness or illness; therefore, therapies based on the concept of holism are not deemed to be important. Although the concept of a psychosocial body has gained some interest in Western practice, it has not been effectively incorporated into conventional care. The energetic and spiritual bodies are largely ignored.

> *Most newly developed medications, when they are in the human-testing phase, are tested on men between the ages of 25 and 35 years old, with the presumption that they will work similarly in women, the elderly, and children. That presumption is not always accurate.*

The Holistic Approach

The Multiple-Body View

In contrast, the alternative approach views the person-body as consisting of multiple, integrated elements that incorporate both the materialistic and nonmaterialistic aspects of existence. These elements include the physical (material), spiritual, energetic, and social bodies. This view allows for a variety of interpretations of how the various components of the person-body interact and function to affect health and illness, and respond to different therapeutic interventions.

The integration of multiple bodies into a unified but distinctly individual person-body results in the belief that the person-body responds as a whole to factors that affect its state of well-being. Although the signs and symptoms of illness for one person are similar to another person's, they may indicate different underlying causes on the basis of variable risk factors. From this viewpoint, diagnostic measures and interventions cannot be based on only one aspect of the person's being, but must be tailored to the person-body of each individual.

A Capacity for Self-Healing

A variety of alternative modalities are often needed to diagnose and treat each individual holistically. It often is not obvious when the health problems of the physical body correspond to the dynamics of the energetic body or when the energetic body merges with the spiritual body, and how they all are eventually integrated into the psychosocial body. The mediating role of the psychosocial body in the alternative approach emphasizes each person's capacity for self-healing. The importance of the mind-body interaction to elicit the placebo response, and the need for clients to participate actively in the monitoring and maintenance of their health and well-being, is a positive factor in the diagnosis and treatment of their illness.

The multiple-body view found in some alternative health-care practices requires an eclectic approach to health promotion and maintenance. The diagnosis and treatment of illness from a multiple body view requires more than dependence on a single healing tradition centered on a one-body concept or on a fixed set of diagnostic criteria. The alternative approach requires active participation of both well and ill persons to better promote health or diagnose and treat disorders rather than relying merely on their passive acceptance of a diagnosis and treatment plan from conventional health-care professionals.

Combining Modalities

The alternative philosophy includes both the material and nonmaterial aspects of the individual, stimulation of the self-healing forces, and the determination of a person's unique needs. It uses the concepts and treatment modalities of several healing traditions simultaneously. These modalities are based on different worldviews or concepts of reality and address the individual healing needs of each person.

For example, acupuncturists may also use massage and a variety of other types of bodywork and energy-system methods; chiropractors may incorporate diet, herbs, and other kinds of naturopathic methodologies into chiropractic spinal manipulations; and massage therapists may include mind–body techniques such as meditation, imagery, and visualization.

What Do You Think?

Name someone you know or know of who has gotten better after an illness although not expected to. Why do you think this happened?

The concept of a multiple-body individual is central to alternative and complementary healing. Healers function as facilitators in the promotion of health and healing (Box 24.2). In contrast, conventional therapy relies primarily on the concept of the physical-body individual, and conventional health-care providers function as experts in determining the meaning of physical signs and symptoms of health or

Box 24.2

Defining Alternative Healers

Alternative healers are those persons who practice one or more alternative or complementary modalities and who are not also licensed as conventional health-care professionals. Conventional health-care professionals who incorporate hands-on alternative and complementary modalities into their conventional patient care are termed *integrative practitioners*. They should undergo the same educational, certification, and licensing processes of both conventional and alternative healers for the modalities they use.

Keep in mind that creating a universally applicable definition of alternative healers is extremely difficult because of the wide variety of healing traditions in use and the number of specialized healing techniques contained within them. The difficulty is compounded by the fact that many alternative healers incorporate various modalities from different healing traditions into their practices. For example, chiropractors commonly use therapeutic touch, acupuncture, acupressure, massage therapy, and naturopathic or homeopathic therapies. Massage therapists may combine multiple types of massage (such as Alexander, Swedish, Trager, and sports) with therapeutic touch, aromatherapy, reflexology, nutritional supplements, and electromagnetic therapies. The growing use of alternative practices by conventional health-care professionals further complicates the task of defining and classifying alternative healers and their practices.

illness and prescribing interventions to promote health or cure illness. The concepts of wellness and holism, self-healing, energy systems, nutrition, and plant-based medicine can be used to compare and contrast alternative and conventional methods of healing.

> *The concept of a multiple-body individual is central to alternative and complementary healing. Healers function as facilitators in the promotion of health and healing.*

Wellness and Holism

Therapy from Outside

Wellness, from the perspective of conventional health care, tends to focus on individuals who are seen as being at risk for illness. Prevention often begins when signs or symptoms arise and is directed at alleviating them rather than treating or removing their underlying cause. At-risk individuals are permitted to engage in risky behaviors as long as conventional health care can find treatments or palliative measures for diseases it cannot prevent. From this perspective, health is often defined as the absence of disease and is considered synonymous with wellness.

The focus of conventional health care is reductionistic rather than holistic because treatment and diagnosis are frequently centered on the cellular, organ, or system levels of the body. It emphasizes the biological-physiological (body) dimension of the client and treats only the disease process for which signs and symptoms are already evident. The cause of illness is attributed to external forces or risk factors that "invade" the body from the surrounding physical, social, or biological environments.

From the biomedical view, treatment usually centers on identifying potentially dangerous or invading agents and then destroying, immobilizing, or extracting them from the person's body. Interventions consist mainly of chemotherapeutic agents (medications), surgery, or other externally imposed treatments aimed at preventing a person deemed to be at risk from becoming ill or to prevent signs and symptoms from becoming full-blown diseases.

> *The human spirit incorporates the values, perception of meaning, and purpose in life that can positively or negatively affect the ability to heal and achieve wellness.*

Therapy from Within

In contrast to conventional health care, the alternative model views wellness as a state in which individuals are in harmony or balance with their internal and external worlds. This approach is a common thread in nursing models or theories of health (see Chapter 4). Alternative modalities hold that most of the time wellness cannot be imposed upon a person by an outside entity or agency. Rather, wellness is achieved mainly by individuals through the process of self-care. The individual assumes responsibility for maintaining his or her own state of health or wellness. The individual, when ill, works to return to a state of wellness by restoring both the internal and external (environmental) state of balance and harmony.

External disruptions—such as work stress, personal tragedy, a troublesome interpersonal relationship, or illness of a parent, spouse, or child—are seen as capable of affecting internal harmony and producing signs and symptoms of physical, emotional, or spiritual illness. This provides a holistic view of individuals in which they are one with their internal and external environments, thereby requiring holistic care. Treatment must address the whole individual (body–mind–spirit) in an environmental (physical, biological, social, cultural, and spiritual) context.

Spirituality is an essential part of holistic treatment (see Chapter 20). The human spirit incorporates the values, perception of meaning, and purpose in life that can positively or negatively affect the ability to heal and achieve wellness. From this perspective, health (balance or harmony), or the absence of illness, is but one aspect of wellness.

Self-Care

In the alternative system, some examples of self-care measures for wellness include exercising, eating a well-balanced diet, praying, getting enough sleep, cleaning the house, using defensive driving measures, doing breast or testicular self-examinations, applying sunscreen at the beach, and practicing good hygiene. Other alternative measures require a high degree of specialist assistance such as acupuncture and energy therapies.

The next level of self-care requires seeking the assistance of others to achieve balance in self and the environment. This level includes getting help to find satisfying employment, seeking prenatal care or taking parenting classes when pregnant, going to community meetings to address environmental safety and citizen quality-of-life issues, undergoing routine health screening examinations (such as mammography and dental checkups), obtaining glasses to correct myopia, and getting vaccinations and keeping them up to date.

The third level of self-care requires a high degree of specialist assistance from alternative healers and others to deal with major disruptions in internal or external well-being. Measures from this level focus on the spiritual dimension and include searching for personal awakening, enlightenment, and self-actualization. Effective modalities to achieve this goal are often rooted in other systems of health care such as traditional Chinese medicine, Ayurveda, and spiritualism. In some cases, individuals may require the use of alternative modalities to deal with illnesses when conventional health care is no longer effective.

Self-Healing

Both alternative and conventional health care believe the body has the capacity to heal itself. The alternative system places self-healing as the central principle of its model and sees it as the basis of all healing. Thus, alternative healers focus on helping people determine why the cells of their body are sick and search for imbalances from a holistic perspective.

Conventional health care views the ability of the body to self-heal primarily through the normal process of replacing cells such as the physiological and biological processes involved in wound healing. It approaches the concept of body self-healing by questioning why the cells of the body are not replacing themselves and attempts to facilitate healing through external means, such as surgery, medications, or other invasive measures.

> *Conventional health care tends to dismiss the effects of healing after alternative modalities have been used by blaming it on the placebo response. They feel that healing takes place only because the individual believes the treatment is effective.*

The Placebo Response

Conventional health care tends to dismiss the effects of healing after alternative modalities have been used by attributing them to the placebo response. They feel that healing takes place only because the individual believes the treatment is effective. In conventional medicine, the term *placebo* has come to signify a type of sham treatment instituted to please difficult or anxious clients or a sugar pill given when conventional health-care professionals have nothing

more to offer the client. In biomedical clinical research, a placebo is a nontreatment given to the control group because it is assumed that it will not produce any changes in physiological responses and therefore prove the effectiveness of the active treatments.

What Do You Think?

What are the ethical issues involved in using placebos? If you were being given a placebo and you found out, how would you feel? What if you improved with the placebo? Would you still feel the same way?

The placebo response plays an important part in the testing of new drugs. The commonly used double-blind study requires that neither the researchers nor study participants know which group is receiving the study drug or which group is receiving an inert substance (placebo). At the conclusion of the study, researchers compare whether a higher percentage of the experimental group experienced the hoped-for results from the active medication than the control group received from the placebo. However, clinical studies have shown that some participants respond positively to placebo medications between 30 to 70 percent of the time. The clients with the highest positive results from placebos include those with:

• Pain from chronic disease, such as cancer pain, arthritis, back pain, angina pectoris, and gastrointestinal tract discomfort

- Autonomic nervous system disorders, such as phobias, psychoneuroses, depression, and nausea
- Neurohormonal disorders, such as asthma, other bronchial airflow conditions, and hypertension

How Does It Work?

Researchers do not have a good understanding of the mechanism by which the placebo response produces positive results. Some believe that the placebo effect is at work in all therapeutic intervention regardless of whether the intervention is an alternative or a conventional treatment. Four possible factors have been examined:

- An endorphin-mediated response
- Belief of the client
- Belief of the healer
- The client–healer relationship

" *Healers who believe in the therapeutic effectiveness of interventions and have the ability to convey that belief to their clients achieve more positive responses in clients than healers who remain skeptical about the interventions they are prescribing.* "

Endorphin-Mediated Response. Endorphins are the body's natural painkillers that, when released, reduce pain and bring about a degree of euphoria. Relaxation therapies and other types of stress-reducing and stress-controlling techniques are believed to promote the release of endorphins that produce pain relief. When experimental groups were give medications that block the release of endorphins, clients with postoperative dental pain reported an increase in pain because of blocking of the placebo effect. The placebo response changes the perception of the client but does not affect the underlying disease process.

Belief of the Client. A person's belief in the effectiveness of the therapy is an important factor to the success of the therapy and may be just as important as the therapy itself. Studies of client compliance in taking prescribed beta blocker heart medications in the first year after myocardial infarction showed that mortality rates were almost equal for those failing to take either the beta blocker or placebo. Mortality rates for both these groups were higher than the rates for those who faithfully took their prescribed medications or placebos.

Belief of the Healer. Healers who believe in the therapeutic effectiveness of interventions and have the ability to convey that belief to their clients achieve more positive responses in clients than healers who remain skeptical about the interventions they are prescribing. An attitude of caring and being in control tends to alleviate client anxieties and fears while increasing their hope and positive expectations.

Client–Healer Relationship. A trusting and close relationship between the client and healer has a positive psychological effect on clients and can become the mental catalyst they need for recovery. The ability of healers to communicate in an empathetic manner increases client satisfaction with care; increases compliance with mutually set goals, increases feelings of empowerment, self-confidence, and self-worth; and decreases depression and anxiety.

Although conventional health care considers many of these approaches as speculative, incomplete, or insufficient to explain the placebo response, alternative healers see the placebo response as measurable and reproducible evidence that the mind and body are intertwined. The placebo response is viewed as proof that feelings, thoughts, and beliefs can change the physiological and structural functioning of individuals.

Remembered Wellness. The term *remembered wellness* is used to describe the physiological response that occurs after positive therapeutic interventions. Remembered wellness includes the person's prior learning, experiences, environment, beliefs, and perceptions. It can also include biological and genetic factors.

Remembered wellness is triggered by memories of past events or times when good health and feelings of confidence, strength, hope, and peace were part of the person's life. Alternative therapies access these memories by stimulating relaxation, such as the quieting of the body and mind to promote healing. Clinical research has demonstrated relaxation to be effective in treating anxiety, pain, high blood pressure, and tachycardia and for stress management. Research studies have confirmed a close relationship between the central nervous system and the immune system and have shown that interaction occurs between the two mind–body pathways: the autonomic and neuroendocrine systems.

Much more research is required for a full scientific explanation of the how the mind and body interact to produce the placebo response and why remembered wellness produces the positive responses it often does. The placebo response remains an enigma to conventional health care and seems to imply an element of deceitfulness when used deliberately in client treatments. For alternative medicine, the placebo response and remembered wellness are forces that can be harnessed to bring about healing.

> *Alternative therapies refer to energy systems as fields, vital essences, balance, and flow that can be used by clients to prevent illness, promote health, and heal themselves. The basic concept is that external forces are not able to cause harm if the person is in the well state.*

Energy Systems

It has long been known scientifically that the human body is regulated by its own internal electrical energy system. Human beings cannot survive without the low levels of electricity that sustain and regulate life at the cellular and molecular levels. Electrical–chemical reactions are produced in the nervous system and help regulate other body systems; electrical impulses trigger heartbeats; and minute electrical currents regulate the production of hormones. The blood is composed largely of iron; therefore, magnetic forces exist in all parts of the body.

Conventional Uses of Energy

Conventional health care has long used various types of energy systems (e.g., electrical, magnetic, microwave, and infrared) for screening, diagnosis, and some types of treatment. Commonly used modalities include electrocardiograms, magnetic resonance imaging, electroencephalograms, electomyelograms, x-rays, radiation treatments for cancer, low-frequency

electric current to stimulate growth of bone cells (osteoblasts) to accelerate healing of fractures, types of electric shock therapy for cardiac arrest, cardioversions for cardiac arrhythmia, and pacemakers.

Conventional health care also uses bioenergy (body energy) to determine the degree of injury and estimate recovery times through the study of cells as they decompose, die, reproduce, and respond to pathogens and traumas. The majority of conventional treatments for many diseases are chemical (medications), surgical, and/or immobilization or manipulation of the affected body part. They are used primarily *after* the disease has been diagnosed.

Energy in Alternative Healing

Conventional medicine has been slow to recognize how the energy of the body can be used for health promotion and healing. Alternative therapies refer to energy systems as fields, vital essences, balance, and flow that can be used by clients to prevent illness, promote health, and heal themselves. The basic concept is that external forces are not able to cause harm if the person is in the well state. Alternative healers may be needed to assist individuals to manipulate the energy system primarily for self-protection or healing. Major alternative and complementary modalities using bioenergy and other energy fields are energy medicine, vital essences and balance, and external energy forces.

Energy Medicine

This therapy includes a number of techniques that use external energy sources to stimulate tissue regeneration or improve the immune system response. Relaxation of muscles through electrical stimulation is thought to promote general body relaxation, increase circulation, enhance waste removal, improve nutrition and oxygenation, and restore energy balance. Examples of energy medicine include electroacupuncture, biofeedback, magnet therapy, and sound and light therapy.

Vital Essences and Balance

In many alternative models, illness reflects blockage, loss, or imbalance of body energy or vital essence. Disturbance of internal body energy can result from external or internal factors. Treatment may be directed at removing the blockage of energy flow through such measures as acupuncture, acupressure, chiropractic adjustment, craniosacral therapy, or reflexology. It may also be directed at increasing the amount of energy and vital essence to restore balance in the body.

Ways that these changes are brought about include diet, herbs, exercises, and spiritual techniques, such as yoga, meditation, and internal qi gong. Therapies related to the creative arts, such as music, drawing, singing, chanting, and dancing are also used to restore balance and vital essences.

External Energy Forces
External energy forces, it is believed, have the capacity for healing. Some of these external energy forces are actual energy treatments. Other forces include mobilizing the healing energy of faith, spirituality, prayer, shamanism, crystals, and hand-mediated energetic healing techniques, such as therapeutic touch and healing touch (Box 24.3).

Nutrition
Nutrition and diet have long been recognized by both alternative and conventional healing systems as important in health promotion and illness treatment. They can also be risk factors for or even cause disease. In conventional health care, nutrition and diet are usually considered as adjuncts to biomedical treatment. In alternative systems, nutrition is commonly seen as a way of life and as a method of preventing illness.

Benefits of Natural Foods
Conventional health care commonly focuses on the need for food and a well-balanced diet without close regard to food production or processing. The safety of food sources in the contemporary diet has been called into question by both alternative healers and conventional health-care professionals because of increasing evidence of toxins in the food chain. These include:

- Pesticides used in agricultural production, lawn care, and pest control
- Industrial pollutants discharged into the air and water in which plants and animals live and obtain nutrients
- Chemicals added to food for preservation, to increase shelf life, or make food more aesthetically appealing and pleasing in texture and taste
- Irradiation used to kill organisms, retard sprouting, and preserve shelf life
- Antibiotics, hormones, and other drugs given to animals to improve their health and increase their size, weight, and speed of growth
- Alteration of nutrients during food processing
- Genetic alteration of foods for improved production rates and drought resistance

Box 24.3
Therapeutic Touch

Therapeutic touch (TT) and healing touch (HT) are two forms of hand-mediated energetic healing. TT refers to the Krieger-Kunz method, and HT to the techniques taught to health-care professionals and certified by the American Holistic Nurses' Association. HT relies on the ability of practitioners to choose appropriate energy healing techniques based on their interpretation of the patient's energy flow, whereas TT follows a set of rules and protocols based in traditional or ancient healing concepts of energy, such as aura (electromagnetic field), chakras, and prana (life-force or vital essence in Ayurvedic medicine).

No physical contact takes place between practitioner and client in either technique. The practitioner's hands are held, palms-down, 2 to 6 inches away from the client. Slow, rhythmic motions are made over the client from head to toe to detect blockage in the normal energy flow in the body. When energy blockages or imbalances are detected or sensed, they are rectified by transference of energy from the practitioner's hands to the client's energy field, replenishing the client's energy flow, removing energy obstructions, and releasing energy congestion. The transference of energy stimulates the healing powers of the body through the reduction of stress and anxiety, promotion of relaxation, and relief of pain. TT is also believed to relax crying babies, relieve asthmatic breathing, increase wound healing, and reduce fever, inflammation, headache, and postoperative pain.

Alternative modalities recommend only foods produced in a natural manner and in their natural environment. Emphasis on natural products can be attributed to four primary factors:

1. Concerns about food production and processing
2. The belief that the person-body, as both an energy system and a physical entity, is designed to live in a natural environment
3. The belief that what is eaten directly affects an individual's health
4. Increased consumption of nutrient-poor and energy-rich foods

Scientific evidence indicates that the more sedentary lifestyle and greater affluence experienced by many has resulted in excessive and unhealthy eating. The end result is a nation that has high rates of obesity, coronary artery disease, micronutrient deficiencies, congenital abnormalities, and cancer. Most alternative systems advocate consumption of plant-based, whole foods and complex carbohydrates. Increasing the amounts of food lower on the food chain helps decrease amounts of meat, saturated fats, and processed foods that dominate many diets. Examples of natural food diets include the macrobiotic and vegetarian diets.

> *Alternative systems, like conventional health care, consider nutritional supplements both as necessary to promote health through assurance of adequate dietary intake and as replacement therapy for conditions caused by nutrition deficiency.*

Dietary Supplements
The Food and Drug Administration (FDA) defines dietary supplements as "any product intended for ingestion as a supplement to the diet. This includes vitamins; minerals; herbs, botanical, and other plant-derived substances; and amino acids. . .and concentrates, metabolites, constituents and extracts of theses substances."

Supplements as Prevention
Conventional health-care professionals typically view nutritional supplements (vitamins and minerals) as replacement or preventive therapy for nutrition-deficient conditions. For example, rickets and osteoporosis can be prevented by adequate vitamin D and calcium intake; adequate ascorbic acid (vitamin C) intake prevents scurvy; neural tube defects in newborns can be prevented by sufficient maternal intake of folic acid (vitamin B_9) during the prenatal period. The FDA, based on research by the National Academy of Sciences, has established maximum recommended daily allowances (RDA) for vitamin and mineral intake. These levels are usually well above the amount at which deficiency diseases occur but below the level at which the client would experience toxic side effects.

Rethinking RDA levels. Studies indicate that approximately two-thirds of adults fail to consume the RDAs of fruits and vegetables. Also, some studies suggest that RDA levels may be too low for certain vitamins, minerals, and micronutrients to prevent the onset of chronic diseases in persons whose diets do not meet the recommended daily nutrient requirements. Especially susceptible are growing children, alcoholics, people with conditions preventing normal nutrient absorption, and pregnant, lactating, and post-menopausal women. Conventional health-care professionals consider general daily supplements, such as vitamin pills, sufficient to prevent deficiency diseases in persons with special dietary needs.

What Do You Think?

Should dietary supplements be considered medications? What are the advantages and disadvantages of classifying supplements as medications?

Alternative systems, like conventional health care, consider nutritional supplements both as necessary to promote health through assurance of adequate dietary intake and as replacement therapy for conditions caused by nutrition deficiency. Alternative systems also believe that orthomolecular therapy or megavitamin therapy (the administration of "megadoses" far in excess of RDAs for vitamins and minerals) is effective in curing diseases, increasing vitality, and enhancing overall well-being.

Regulation of Supplements

Concern about nutritional supplements also exists because, unlike drugs and most food additives, they are not regulated by the FDA. If manufacturers make no claims that they are effective against a disease, they do not need to be tested for safety and effectiveness before they are sold to the public. However, there has been a gradual increase in the regulation of these products over the past 20 years. The 1994 Dietary Supplement and Health Education Act (DSHEA) created a special category of 20,000 protected substances previously sold as supplements. The DSHEA defined supplements as including vitamins, minerals, amino acids, herbs, botanicals and other plant-derived products, and the extracts, metabolites, constituents, and concentrates of supplements.

The FDA can remove supplements from the market if it receives numerous reports of their adverse effects and then proves they are dangerous to consumers' health. The FDA issues public warnings when supplements are linked to safety concerns. The DSHEA also gave the FDA authority to improve and enforce product labeling, package inserts, and accompanying literature. To enhance product comparison, guidelines instituted in 1999 require a panel of "supplemental facts" or a "nutrition facts box" on labels, which include ingredients.

The U.S. Postal Service and the Federal Trade Commission (FTC) also regulate nutritional supplements and herbal products. The U.S. Postal Inspection Service monitors products purchased by mail and may intercept supplements shipped through the mail for false claims, such as stating that they can cure AIDS or cancer. The Office of Criminal Investigation can be contacted at (202) 268-2000.

The FTC has issued guidelines to ensure that advertising claims are substantiated by reliable scientific evidence. No longer acceptable are claims of effectiveness and safety on the basis of testimonials and other anecdotal evidence. Also outlawed are vague disclaimers, such as "results may vary." The term "traditional use" (e.g., folk remedy), which implies that the product is effective even without scientific evidence, has also been banned. The risks or qualifying information of any product must be prominently displayed and easily understood.

Plants as Medicine

Both alternative and conventional health care use plants as medicines. Herbalism, or "botanical medicine," also known as phytotherapy or phytomedicine in England and other parts of Europe, is the study and use of herbs or crude-based plant products for food, medicine, or prophylaxis. They can also be used to heal, treat, or prevent illness and improve the spiritual and physical quality of life.

Herbs may be angiosperms (flowering plants, trees, or shrubs), algae, moss, fungus, seaweed, lichen, or ferns. Herbs used as medicines come from some part of the plant (leaf, root, flower, fruit, stem, bark, or seed), its syrup-like exudates, or some combination of these. In some herbal traditions, nonplant products are used alone or in combination, with or without plants. They may include animal secretions and parts (such as bones, organs, or tissues), stones and gemstones, minerals and metals, shells, and insects and insect products.

Botanical healing in the form of herbal medicines was widely used in the United States until the early nineteenth century, when it was gradually displaced by the increasing prominence of the scientific method and labeled quackery. Phytomedicine continues to be a prominent branch of conventional health care in Europe. Botanicals are used by 40 percent of German and French physicians in their daily practices.

Scientists have yet to determine the pharmaceutical qualities of most plants, and little is known about what toxicities they can produce. The world supports an estimated 250,000 to 500,000 flowering plant species, but only 5,000 have been researched for their pharmacological effects.

Herbal Traditions

The use of herbal therapies varies according to culture and tradition. The three major groups of herbal therapies recognized throughout the world are from

Western medicine, traditional Chinese medicine, and Ayurvedic medicine.

Western Pharmacology

The Western herbal tradition relies primarily on the pharmacological action of herbs, most of which are derived from the plant kingdom. There are presently 119 plant-derived pharmaceutical medicines. Plant chemicals constitute about 25 percent of prescriptions by conventional health-care professionals, and another 30 percent are for medicines from plant products.

Chinese Medicine

Herbology is used in traditional Chinese medicine to enhance the flow and amount of chi, restore the harmonious balance of the complementary forces of yin and yang and balance the five elements (fire, earth, metal, water, and wood). In the Chinese system plants are prescribed based on their effects on the five elements and their corresponding body processes including organs, tissues, emotions, and temperatures (climates).

The Chinese believe that the five elements give rise to the five tastes that produce particular medicinal actions. Bitter-tasting herbs (fire) act to dry and drain. Sweet tasting herbs (earth) reduce pain and increase tone. Acrid herbs (metal) serve to disperse. Salty herbs (water) nourish the kidney. Sour herbs (wood) clean, helping preserve chi and nourish yin. Herbs are also symbolically classified according to temperature changes they are said to bring about in the body in the treatment of conditions: cold, cool, neutral, warm, and hot. The temperatures correspond to the symbolic climate qualities of the organs and the five elements.

Ayurvedic Medicine

Ayurvedic medicine also considers the taste or "essence" of the herb as an integral element in herbology. Ayurveda recognizes six essences (sweet, sour, salty, pungent, bitter, and astringent) and five elements (ether, water, fire, air, and earth). The elements are manifested as three doshas or humors (vata, pitta, and kapha) that govern body functioning and that must be kept in balance to maintain or restore a healthy state.

Vata, the principle of air, wind, or movement, is decreased by herbs that are sweet, sour, and salty, which exert a symbolic heating effect on the body. Vata is increased by herbs that are pungent, bitter, astringent, and cooling. Pitta, the principle of fire, is decreased by herbs that are sweet, bitter, astringent, and cooling and increased by those that are pungent, sour, salty, and heating. Kapha, the principle of water, is decreased by herbs that are pungent, bitter, astringent, and heating and increased by those that are sweet, sour, salty, and cooling.

Concerns About Herbal Therapies

There is growing concern in the United States about the use of herbal preparations by the general public without consultation with either conventional health-care professionals or alternative healers. Sales of herbal preparations have been growing tremendously. Another concern is the lack of licensing and standards for herbalists. Except for naturopaths, most herbalists have no foundation in phytochemistry or botanical medicine.

Also, in other cultural traditions, herbs are not prescribed based on the biological effects of their chemical ingredients. They are commonly prescribed based on the "doctrine of signatures" or their physical and taste characteristics. For example, herbs with heart-shaped leaves may be used to treat heart problems; those with red flowers or leaves may be used to control bleeding or blood disorders; and those with a sour taste may be given to decrease swelling or counteract the effects of "sugar" (diabetes mellitus).

Additional problems may arise because the public views most herbal remedies as natural products and therefore considers them to be pure, safe, relatively harmless, and more healthy than manufactured medicines. Recent problems with some natural products indicate that there is no guarantee of safety.

> *Nurses often feel uncomfortable with the use of herbal products and alternative therapies because of unclear definitions of various alternative and complementary practices and the widespread yet often unregulated use of alternative products and healers.*

THE PARADOX OF ALTERNATIVE HEALING PRACTICES

A Lack of Validation

Nurses often feel uncomfortable with the use of herbal products and alternative therapies because of unclear definitions of various alternative and complementary practices and the widespread yet often unregulated use of alternative products and healers. This paradox arises because most nursing knowledge comes from the biomedical sciences, but most alternative modalities (1) have not yet been scientifically validated or proven safe based on the scientific method and (2) are based in concepts of holism, self-care, and theoretical constructs that emanate from worldviews different from that of biomedicine and the scientific perspective.

In other words, for most alternative modalities, little is known about if or how they work, their side effects, or their interactions with conventional or other alternative modalities. Claims regarding their effectiveness come largely from testimonials of users or alternative healers rather than from evidence in scientific studies. Equally limited is valid knowledge about which conditions the various alternative modalities are effective against and about their short- and long-term effects.

The nursing profession has worked for many years to build its decision-making skills on knowledge derived from the scientific method and on using critical thinking and culture competence. Nurses promote self-care in clients by teaching them to make informed choices about their health-care options. Many of the alternative health-care practices in use today fly in the face of the nursing profession's movement toward evidence-based practice.

Few Regulatory Standards

The technical competence and knowledge of alternative healers are of considerable importance for nurses caring for clients who pursue alternative and complementary practices. Nurses and the general public are accustomed to determining the qualifications, assumed competency, and scope of practice of conventional health-care practitioners through externally regulated mechanisms. These external regulations include graduation from an accredited school, state-regulated licenses, credentialing, and attainment of specialty certifications from professional organizations or institutions of higher education. No such external processes or criteria exist to validate the competence and knowledge of most alternative practitioners.

The relative lack of regulatory standards makes selection of competent alternative practitioners exceedingly difficult. It is a major concern of the public, conventional health-care practitioners, and insurers, because clients may be subject to financial exploitation, ineffective therapies, and psychological and physical abuse.

A Challenge to Nurses

The challenge presented to nurses by alternative healing modalities relates to professional accountability. Nurses must learn about alternative modalities, their general safety and efficacy, and their use in specific health and illness conditions.

Human caring and cultural competence require that nurses be able to develop therapeutic partnerships with culturally diverse clients and empower them to take charge of their lives and health care. They need to preserve the client's right to self-determination and to practice alternative lifestyles as well as to pursue a variety of conventional or alternative therapies with or without consulting alternative healers or conventional health-care professionals. Nurses must keep an open mind while relying on sound evidence for recommendations about alternative practices and practitioners.

> *The challenge presented to nurses by alternative healing modalities relates to professional accountability. Nurses must learn about alternative modalities, their general safety and efficacy, and their use in specific health and illness conditions.*

Ask Questions

Some questions nurses need to ask when attempting to determine the quality and validity of information about an alternative modality are listed in Box 24.4. It is important to teach clients to ask similar questions as they are deciding on an alternative therapy and are attempting to sort out the often conflicting advice they receive from family, friends, conventional health-care professionals, alternative healers, and the media.

Box 24.4

Questions to Ask About Alternative Modalities

1. What evidence exists that the therapy is effective or harmful?

   - Is there experimental evidence? How effective is the alternative modality when examined experimentally?
   - Is there clinical practice evidence? How effective is the alternative modality when applied clinically?
   - Is there comparative evidence? How effective is the modality when compared with other treatments?
   - Is there summary evidence? Has the modality been evaluated and a consensus reached regarding its use and effectiveness for various health conditions?
   - Is there evidence of demand? Is the modality wanted by clients and/or practitioners?
   - Is there evidence of satisfaction? Does the alternative modality meet the expectations of clients and/or practitioners?
   - Is there cost evidence? Is the modality covered by health insurance? Is it cost effective?
   - Is the meaning evident? Is the modality the best and right one for the client?

2. How strong is the evidence? Is it based on testimonials, clinical observations, or scientific research?
3. Can the results be attributed to the placebo effect? Is the benefit from the placebo effect adequate to the client's needs?
4. Does evidence exist that the benefits of the therapy outweigh the risks?

   - Is the alternative modality potentially useful?
   - Is the modality essentially without value except for the potential placebo effect?
   - Is the modality potentially harmful?

5. Is there another way to obtain the same hoped-for results?
6. Who else has tried this alternative modality, and what was their experience?
7. Are there reputable (licensed and certified) alternative healers available? What has been their experience with this alternative modality?
8. What information do regulatory agencies have about the modality or the alternative healers?
9. What information is available in the popular media about the modality or alternative healers? Has it or can it be verified by clinical observations or research studies?

Sources: Barrocas, A: Complementary and alternative medicine: Friend, foe or OWA (other weird arrangements). J Am Diet Assoc 97:1373, 1997.
Kurtzweil, P: An FDA Guide to Dietary Supplements. January 1999. Available at: www.vm.cfsan.fda.gov/~dms/fdsupp.html.
Micozzi, MS (ed): Fundamentals of Complementary and Alternative Medicine. Churchill Livingstone, New York, 1996.
National Center for Complementary and Alternative Medicine: Considering CAM? March 1, 2000. Available at: www.nccam.nih.gov/nccam/fcp/faq/considercam.html.
National Center for Complementary and Alternative Medicine: NCCAM Clearinghouse. April 6, 2000. Available at: www.nccam.nih.gov/nccam/faq/clearinghouse/index.html.
Spencer, JC, and Jacobs, JJ: Complementary/Alternative Medicine: An Evidence-Based Approach. Mosby, St. Louis, 1999.

Many clients use alternative healing modalities without ever talking to a conventional health professional about it. They may fear a negative reaction. Others are not aware of the potential harm that may occur, especially when combining alternative therapies or alternative and conventional therapies. Some may consider the scientific evidence and conclude that most noninvasive and nondrug alternative therapies are harmless. Others may mistakenly assume that alternative therapies are regulated by the government and would not be available if they were dangerous.

Find Information

Lack of scientific information about alternative healing modalities is of concern to alternative healers, conventional health-care professionals, and clients. For nurses and their clients, the need to know where and how to find up-to-date, reliable information on alternative therapies is a must.

Information Resources

• The NCCAM offers one of the best general governmental resources for information on alternative modalities at the NCCAM Web site: www.nccam. nih.gov.

Several authoritative sources on herbal medicines are available for practitioners and clients.

• The FDA maintains a site for reporting and obtaining information about adverse effects and interactions of herbals through MedWatch (800-FDA-1088 or www.fda.gov/medwatch).
• FA Davis maintains a Web site on herbal medicines (www.DrugGuide. com) as does the United States Pharmacopeia (www.usp.org/information/ index.html).
• The American Botanical Society (512-926-4900) has a Web site (www. herbal gram.org) and publishes the *Herbalgram,* a newsletter on herbal medications.
• MICROMEDEX has an evidence-based series on herbal medicines and dietary supplements, toxicologies, clinical protocols, and client education (800-643-8116 or www.micomedex.com). It also links to the electronic database of herbal medicines from the Royal Pharmaceutical Society of Great Britain.
• Tyler's *The Honest Herbal* is one of the most reputable guides for the use of herbs.
• *The Physician's Desk Reference for Herbal Medicine* contains scientific findings on the efficacy, potential interactions, clinical trials, and case reports of herbs, as well as indexes on Asian, Ayurvedic, and homeopathic herbs.
• An English translation of *The Complete German Commission E Monographs: Therapeutic Guide to Herbal Medicine* is a compendium of monographs published by Commission E, a panel of experts responsible for regulating herbal products in

Germany, much as is done by the FDA in the United States. It contains information about the therapeutics of individual herbs, dosages, adverse effects, and pharmacology. The lack of regulatory standards for herbal products in the United States poses problems in applying findings from Commission E to herbal products manufactured in this country.

What Do You Think?

Does the facility where you do your clinical practice ask about alternative therapies during the admission assessment? Are you taught to assess for this information in your nursing program?

A growing number of clients and even professionals are turning to the Internet for information about alternative products and local practitioners of alternative therapies. Because information posted to the Internet is not regulated, this avenue of inquiry requires caution. Only one Web site is available with reputable information about ACH and specific modalities.

• Quackwatch (www.quackwatch.com/) offers fact sheets and reviews of specific alternative modalities, as well as those associated with certain illnesses. It also has sections on how to determine whether a Web site devoted to alternative modalities is trustworthy.

> *It is important to ask clients about their use of alternative therapies. Not doing so may place clients at risk for adverse health outcomes.*

Ask the Client

It is important to ask clients about their use of alternative therapies. Not doing so may place clients at risk for adverse health outcomes. When and how to assess for the use of ACH during the client-assessment process is a matter of judgment and should be guided by the nurse's knowledge of individual clients. An appropriate time is often after the chief complaint has been documented, because this is the time when questions are asked about the clients' reasons for seeking health care and what they have already done for their problem.

Discuss the use of alternative therapies tactfully and supportively. Keep complete and accurate documentation of all interactions with clients about alternative therapies and healers. And as much as possible, help direct clients toward the safest therapies and the most qualified practitioners.

Critical Thinking Exercises

- Contact three of the Web sites on alternative practices listed in this chapter. Evaluate them according to their quality, content, and usefulness to your practice.
- Identify a nurse practitioner or physician or other health-care provider in your area who uses alternative practices. Interview that person and arrange for a presentation to the class about alternative health-care practices.
- Select a client from your clinical experiences who is having pain. How might alternative practices help this client? Develop a care plan using both traditional and alternative methods for pain control.
- Identify and discuss three advantages of and three problems with alternative health-care practices.
- Select three nursing theories from Chapter 4 that use a holistic approach to nursing. Identify how and what alternative practices would work well with each one of these theories.

Conclusion

Alternative and nontraditional health-care practices are a growing part of health care in the United States. It is essential that nurses become aware of what these practices entail and how they may affect or interact with conventional therapies that the client is already receiving. Admission assessments for these practices, when clients enter the health-care system for whatever reason, should become a routine part of client evaluation. Nurses traditionally have approached health care from a holistic viewpoint that addresses all of the client's needs—mind, body, and spirit. As health care moves more toward alternative practices, nurses would be the logical choice to coordinate a comprehensive approach to health care that includes both traditional and alternative practices. Without this coordination, an already fragmented health-care system will become even more fragmented.

GLOSSARY OF TERMS FOR ALTERNATIVE AND COMPLEMENTARY HEALING

Inclusion of particular ideas or practices in this chapter implies no endorsement of them. Health-care practitioners and their clients must carefully evaluate the claims and qualifications of alternative and complementary healing practices and practitioners before making conclusions about them.

Acupressure From traditional Chinese medicine. Practitioner uses fingers or hands to apply pressure over acupuncture points on meridians to restore or enhance the flow of chi to maintain or restore balance.

Acupressure massage Practitioner uses massage techniques such as rubbing, kneading, percussion, and vibration over acupuncture points to improve circulation of chi.

Acupuncture From traditional Chinese medicine. Now commonly considered a complete treatment system on its own. The object of acupuncture is to reestablish the balance of energy in the body by inserting needles along meridian channels to alleviate blockage of chi. The points of insertion are believed to be linked to internal body organs.

Alexander technique A type of bodywork developed by Frederick Matthias Alexander to decrease muscle tension and fatigue, stress, and back and neck pain. Based on the belief that poor posture during daily activities contributes to physical and emotional problems. Use of body posture realignment through imaging and relaxation.

Allopathic medicine From the Greek words *allos* (other) and *pathos* (suffering). A synonym for conventional medicine. Practitioner uses medicines to counteract symptoms or heal by producing different effects or a second condition different from the one being treated.

Applied kinesiology Study of muscle activity and strength and health effects via the muscle-gland-organ link. Muscle dysfunction may be counteracted by nutrition, manual procedures (such as massage), applying pressure over muscle attachment points, and realignment.

Aromatherapy A type of herbal medicine. Uses odors of essential oils extracted from plants to treat various conditions, such as headaches, tension, and anxiety. Chemical composition of the oils provides pharmacological effects that include antibacterial, antiviral, antispasmodic, diuretic, vasodilatation, and mood-harmonizing actions. The oils may be applied via massage, inhaled, placed in baths and other forms of hydrotherapy, or taken internally.

Art therapy Use of artistic self-expression through drawing, sculpture, and painting to diagnose and treat behavioral or emotional problems.

Aura Magnetic field said to surround every person, plant, and animal. Adjustment of the field is said to affect health, emotions, spirit, and mind.

Auriculotherapy Also known as ear acupuncture and developed in France. Points on the external ear are believed to have neurological connections to other body areas. The points can be stimulated with acupuncture needles, massage, electronic stimulation, or infrared treatment.

Ayurvedic medicine From East Indian medicine. A personalistic, holistic, and naturalistic approach to health maintenance and treatment of illness. Maintains balance of the three doshas (bioenergies) of the body through diet and herbs, meditation, breathing exercises (pranayama), massage with medicated oils, yoga and other forms of vigorous exercise, and exposure to the sun for higher consciousness.

Bach flower essences Originated by Edward Bach, an English physician. Homeopathic preparations of oil concentrates extracted from flowers are administered to remedy emotional states rather than treating the signs and symptoms of physical illness. Specific concentrates or combinations of concentrates are associated with various emotional states. Each client is diagnosed individually because there is no corresponding psychological equivalent for every physical state.

Biofeedback Form of training that helps a person to consciously control or change normally unconscious body functions to improve overall health. Also refers to the method of immediately reporting back to the person information about a biological process that is being measured so the person can consciously alter or influence the process.

Bodywork General term used to describe various forms of massage therapy, energy balancing, deep-tissue manipulation, and movement awareness.

Botanical medicine Use of the entire plant or herb for treating illness or maintaining health.

Chakras Circles found along the midline of the body, in alignment with the spinal cord, that distribute energy throughout the body. If blocked, energy flow is inhibited.

Chelation therapy From the Greek word *chele* (to bind or to claw). Chelation uses minerals combined with amino acids, given intravenously or orally, to help cleanse the body of unnecessary or toxic minerals that block blood circulation.

Chi (Qi, Shi) From traditional Chinese medicine. Chi is the invisible life-force that circulates through the body along meridians, or channels. Maintaining or restoring the flow of chi restores and promotes health.

Chiropractic A Western medical system that postulates that partial joint dislocations (subluxations) cause the body to be misaligned. Removal or adjustment of subluxations balances the spinal–nervous system and restores and maintains health.

Craniosacral therapy *Cranio* refers to the cranium and *sacral* to the sacrum. In this therapy, the bones of the skull are manipulated to treat craniosacral dysfunctions caused by restriction in the flow of cerebrospinal fluid and misalignment of bones.

Crystal therapy Also called *gem therapy*. Quartz and other gemstones are believed to emit electromagnetic energy. Used frequently with light and color therapy.

Cupping From traditional Chinese and Ayurvedic medicines. Practitioner places a heated cup over the skin to draw out impurities, decrease blood pressure, increase circulation, and relieve muscle pain.

Curanderismo From the Spanish verb *to heal*. Healing tradition found in Mexican-American communities. Based in concepts of supernaturalism, balance, holism, and natural world illnesses.

Dance therapy Use of dance movement to enhance wellness and aid healing. Sharpens levels of awareness, enhances self-confidence, helps with motor coordination and physical skills, and assists with communication, especially with severely disturbed psychiatric clients.

Doshas Three (*vata, pitta,* and *kapha*) basic metabolic types, life-forces, or bioenergies in Ayurvedic medicine. Each has certain characteristics and tendencies that combine to determine a person's constitution. When in balance, mind and body are coordinated, resulting in vibrant health and energy. When out of balance, the body is susceptible to outside stressors, such as microorganisms, poor nutrition, and work overload.

Energy medicine Measurement of electromagnetic frequencies emitted by the body. The object is to diagnose energy imbalances that may cause or contribute to present or future illnesses and to use electromagnetic forces to counteract imbalances and restore the body's energy balance.

Environmental medicine Explores the role of environmental and dietary allergens in health and illness.

Feldenkrais method A type of bodywork or physical movement developed by Moshe Feldenkrais that stresses awareness through movement and helps the body work with gravity. Incorporates imaging, active moving, and forms of directed attention designed to re-educate the nervous system, teach subjects how to learn from their own kinesic feedback, and avoid movements that strain joints and muscles.

Gerson therapy Metabolic therapy developed by Max Gerson, a German physician. It is based on the belief that cancer results from metabolic dysfunctions in cells that can be countered by detoxification, a vegetarian diet, coffee enemas to stimulate excretion of liver bile, and the exclusion of sodium and an abundance of potassium.

Guided imagery A facilitated flow of thoughts that helps a person see, feel, taste, smell, hear, and touch something in the imagination. The power of the mind or imagination is used to stimulate positive physical responses and provide insight into health and an understanding of emotions as a cause of ill health.

Healing touch Healing tradition based on the belief in a universal energy system. Humans are seen as interpenetrating layers of energy systems just above and outside the body that are integrated with energy fields in the environment. Manipulation of such energy fields through touch can help restore a person's energy balance and health.

Hellerwork A type of bodywork developed by Joseph Heller as an outgrowth of Rolfing. It combines dialog, body movement education, and deep touch to achieve greater mind–body awareness and structural body alignment with gravitational forces. Therapy is individualized to different body types.

Herbal medicine The most ancient known form of health care. Also known as botanical medicine, phytotherapy, and phytomedicine. It uses the chemical makeup of herbs in much the same manner as conventional medicine uses pharmaceuticals. Herbal medicine is basic to traditional Chinese, Ayurvedic, and American Indian medical systems.

Homeopathy A Western medical system based on the principle "like cures like." Natural substances are prescribed in minute dilutions to cause the symptoms of the disease they are intended to cure, helping the body cure itself.

Humor therapy Deliberate use of laughter to improve quality of life by encouraging relaxation and stress reduction, distracting individuals from awareness of constant pain, and providing symptom relief.

Hydrotherapy Also known as "water cure." Use of hot, cold, or contrasting temperatures to maintain or restore health. Water, steam, or ice may be used in combination with baths, compresses, hot and cold packs, showers, and enemas or colonic irrigations.

Minerals, herbs, and oils may be added to enhance the therapeutic effects.

Hypnotherapy Use of hypnosis, power of suggestion, and trance-like states to access the deepest levels of the mind to bring about changes in behavior, treat health conditions, and manage medical and psychological problems.

Integrative medicine *Integrative* is synonymous with *complementary*. This is practiced by conventional health-care professionals who prescribe a combination of therapies from both systems.

Iridiology Iris diagnosis. In this belief system, each area of the body has a corresponding point on the iris of the eye. Thus, the state of health (balance) or disease (imbalance) can be diagnosed from the color, texture, or location of pigments in the eye.

Jin Shin Jyutsu A Japanese form of massage in which combinations of healing points on the body are held for a minute or more with the fingertips. The purpose is to enhance or restore the flow of chi.

Light and color therapy A method by which light is converted into electrical impulses, travels along the optic nerve to the brain, and stimulates the hypothalamus to send neurotransmitters to regulate the autonomic nervous system. Various colors of light are believed to stimulate different parts of the body.

Magnet therapy A type of electromagnetic therapy or energy medicine in which magnets are used to stimulate circulation, increase oxygen to cells, and facilitate healing by correcting disturbed or malfunctioning electromagnetic frequencies that the body emits.

Mantra A technique of Ayurvedic medicine used to reach a higher level of spiritual and mental functioning. It is a type of sound therapy used to change the "vibratory patterns of the mind" to release unconscious negative thoughts, psychological stress, and emotional distress. Often achieved by uttering a mystical word or phrase and associated with meditation.

Meditation Known as "mind-cure" or the use of contemplation to exercise the mind, which is an unseen force of healing. Thoughts and deep feelings are believed to be the primary arbiters of health through relaxation. Also known as a form of mental cleansing that enhances self-awareness and awareness of one's environment.

Megavitamin therapy A type of orthomolecular medicine in which diseases are prevented and cured by taking doses of vitamins larger than the normal or recommended amounts needed for general good health or prevention of deficiencies. The disease to be treated or prevented determines the type, dosage, and mode of administration of vitamins, minerals, and nutrient supplements.

Meridians From traditional Chinese medicine. Meridians are invisible channels by which chi flows through the body. Blockage along a meridian causes illness.

Mind–body medicine Healing based on the interconnectedness of the mind and body, individual responsibility for self-care, and the self-healing capabilities of the body. Uses a wide range of modalities, such as imaging, massage, hypnotherapy, meditation, yoga, concepts of balance, herbs, and diet.

Moxibustion From traditional Chinese medicine. Burning of *moxa* (dried or powered herbs) on or close to acupuncture points on the meridians to restore or improve the flow of chi.

Music therapy Use of music to enhance well-being and promote healing. Helps improve physical and mental functioning, alleviate pain, ease the psychological discomfort of illness, and improve quality of life, especially of terminally ill persons. Aids ability of mentally handicapped, autistic, and elderly persons with dementia to interact with others, learn, and relate to their environments.

Naturopathy A Western healing system. Heals through holism, use of natural substances, treating cause rather than symptoms (effects), empowering and motivating individuals to take responsibility for their own health, preventing disease through lifestyle and education, and doing no harm beyond using safe, natural therapies.

Neurolinguistic programming Focuses on how individuals learn, communicate, and change. *Neuro-* refers to how the brain works and the consistent and observable patterns that emanate from human thinking. *Linguistic* refers to the expression (verbal and nonverbal) of those patterns of thinking. *Programming* refers to how such patterns of thinking are interpreted and how they can be changed. Changing the patterns gives people the ability to make better choices for healthy behavior.

Orthodox Used as a synonym for conventional, Western, scientific, biomedicine, or official healthcare system.

Orthomolecular medicine *Ortho-* means normal or correct. This system treats physiological and psychological disorders by re-establishing, normalizing, or creating the optimal nutritional balance in the body by administering vitamins, minerals, amino acids, and other types of nutritional substances.

Osteopathy A Western system of medicine that considers the structural integrity of the body the most important factor in maintaining and restoring the person to health. The structural integrity or balance of the musculoskeletal system is maintained through physical therapy, joint manipulation, and postural re-education.

Oxygen therapy Use of various forms of oxygen to destroy pathogens and promote body healing. Includes hyperbaric, ozone, and hydrogen peroxide therapies.

Pharmacognosy Scientific study of the chemical properties of plants and natural products. A goal is to standardize herbal products to make sure they are free of harmful components and contain the identical amount of active ingredients.

Phytomedicine/phytotherapy A branch of botanical medicine especially prominent in Europe that includes the pharmaceutical study and therapeutic use of herbs, herbal derivatives, and herbal synthetics. Merges ancient herbal traditions with contemporary scientific investigation to standardize the active ingredients of herbal products.

Polarity therapy A combination of bodywork therapies and other hands-on techniques to restore the natural flow of energy through the body. Other therapies may include reflexology, hydrotherapy, and breathing techniques.

Prana From Ayurvedic medicine. Vital energy or life-force that runs through the body.

Qi Gong (Chi Kung, Chi Gong) From traditional Chinese medicine. Combines movement, meditation and deep relaxation, and regulation of breathing to enhance the flow of chi throughout the body to nourish vital organs.

Reflexology In this belief system, every part of the body has a corresponding area on the hands and feet. Thus, body parts can be stimulated by applying pressure to the appropriate sites on the hands or feet.

Reflexology is applied to relieve tension, improve circulation, promote relaxation, and restore energy balance by unblocking nerve impulses.

Reiki An ancient Buddhist version of healing touch practiced in Tibet and Japan. The word also means universal life-force. Energy is transferred to the person through the hands of the healer to restore energy balance in the body.

Relaxation response Physiological mechanism described by Herbert Benson in which body stress is reduced through regulation of internal activity, such as reduced metabolism and slowing of other physiological reactions.

Relaxation therapy Use of the relaxation response to reduce stress through release of physical and emotional tension. Various therapies are commonly included in other types of therapeutic programs. Examples are mind–body therapies such as biofeedback, hydrotherapy, imaging/visualization, meditation, qi gong, Tai Chi, and yoga.

Rolfing Developed by Ida Rolf. Technique of deep massage using the knuckles that is designed to counteract the effects of gravity on body balance. Fascia, connective tissue, and muscle are loosened and lengthened to help them return to their correct position.

Rosen technique A type of bodywork in which muscle tension is seen as repressed emotional conflicts. Deep and gentle pressure is applied as persons are questioned about what they are experiencing.

Shamanism Ancient healing approach found in most cultural systems. Shamans communicate with the spirit world via trances and other altered states of consciousness. They attempt to control spirits and effect change in the physical world. The belief is that the soul of the shaman separates from the body and explores the cosmos in search of cures for ill patients.

Sound therapy Elements of sound affect different parts of the brain, regulate corticosteroid hormone levels, and can affect the body's own rhythmic patterns.

Shiatsu Japanese form of massage whose literal meaning is *finger pressure*. Consists of firm pressure in a sequential and rhythmic manner. Pressure is exerted for 3 to 10 seconds on points along the body that correspond to acupuncture meridians. It is designed to "awaken the meridian."

Spiritual healing Cosmic healing energy is transferred or channeled from practitioner to client via laying on of the hands.

Swedish massage The most common form of massage, it focuses on superficial muscle layers. Practitioner uses kneading, friction, and long, gliding strokes to relieve muscle tension and promote relaxation.

Tai Chi From traditional Chinese medicine. Derived from qi gong but practiced at a much slower pace. Also one of the body–mind therapies. Combines contemplation (meditation) with movement or "moving meditation" and coordinated breathing.

Therapeutic massage Manipulation of soft tissues through a variety of techniques to affect the circulatory, lymphatic, and nervous systems.

Therapeutic touch A healing touch modality that does not involve actual touching of the patient's body. The therapist's hands are used to sense and interact with the client's energy field to redirect it, alleviate energy blockage, and restore balance.

Traditional Chinese medicine A complete system of healing based on the concept of the uninterrupted flow of chi or vital essence and the concept of balance (yin and yang), representing corresponding and interrelated elements in the internal world of the body and the external world. All illness is attributed ultimately to a disturbance of chi.

Trager therapy A method of bodywork developed by Milton Trager. Use of gentle, rhythmic touch and movement exercises to assist in the release of accumulated tensions. Uses sensory-motor feedback or mental gymnastics (mentastics) to learn how body moves. Purpose is to develop the ability to move more effortlessly.

Vibration medicine Healing systems that treat the body on an energy level. Cure is effected by ingestion of substances that adjust energy or rate of energy field vibration. Homeopathy is an example.

Visualization Also called guided imagery, centering, focusing, meditation, or distraction. Use of the imagination or power of the mind to get in touch with one's inner self. Involves all, several, or one of the senses to bridge the mind, body, and spirit.

Yin/yang Complementary but opposing phenomena or correspondents in Taoist philosophical thought that form the underpinning of traditional Chinese medicine. Yin and yang represent the interdependence of all elements of nature and body and mind. Yin represents the female force and passive, still, reflective aspects. Yang represents the male force and active, warm, moving aspects. For health to be maintained and wellness achieved, yin and yang must be in balance.

Yoga Means *union,* or the integration of mental, physical, and spiritual energies. Part of Ayurvedic medicine. The integration is accomplished through exercise in the form of assuming different body postures, meditation, and breathing.

References

1. Duryea, B: Marching to the beat of a different drummer: Complementary and alternative medicine. Imprint 52(2):54–57, 2005.
2. Schuster, T: Wellness lifestyles I: A theoretical framework linking wellness, health lifestyles, and complementary and alternative medicine. J Altern Complement Med 10(2):349–356, 2004.
3. Hill, F: Towards a new model for health promotion? An analysis of complementary and alternative medicine and models of health promotion. Health Education Journal 62(4):369–380, 2003.

Bibliography

Cassidy, C: What does it mean to practice an energy medicine? J Altern Complement Med 10(1):79–81, 2004.
Dosset, B: Florence Nightingale and holistic nursing. Imprint 52(2):58–60, 2005.
Honda, K: Use of complementary and alternative medicine among United States adults: The influences of personality, coping strategies, and social support. Prev Med 40(1):46–53, 2005.
Huebscher, R: Natural, Alternative, and Complementary Health Care Practices. Mosby, Inc., St. Louis, 2004.
Mariano, C: An overview of holistic nursing. Imprint 52(2):48–52, 2005.
National Center for Complementary and Alternative Medicine: Frequently Asked Questions. 2005 Available at: www.nccam.nih.gov/nccam/fcp/faq/index.html.
Savory-Posselius, M: Herbology. Home Health Care Management Practice 16(6):456–463, 2004.
Stretch, K: A survey of CAM approaches to obesity. Massage Today 5(1):1, 22, 2005.
Uzun, O: Nursing students' opinions and knowledge about complementary and alternative medicine therapies. Complementary Therapeutic Nurse Midwifery 10(4):239–244, 2004.
Walach, H: Homeopathic proving symptoms: Result of a local, non-local, or placebo process? A blinded, placebo-controlled pilot study. Homeopathy 93(4):179–185, 2004.
Weatherley-Jones, E: The placebo-controlled trial as a test of complementary and alternative medicine: Observations from research experience of individualised homeopathic treatment. Homeopathy 93(4):186–189, 2004.
World Health Organization: WHO's Policy and Activities on the Traditional Medicine. 2005. Available at: www.who.int/dap/trm0.html.
Yoon, S: Herbal product use by African American older women. Clinical Nursing Research 13(4):271–288, 2004.

abandonment Leaving a client without the client's permission; terminating the professional relationship without providing for appropriate continued or follow-up care by another equally qualified professional.

accountability Concept that each individual is responsible for his or her own actions and the consequence of those actions; professional accountability implies a responsibility to perform the activities and duties of the profession according to established standards.

accreditation Approval of a program or institution by a voluntary professional organization to provide specific education or service programs.

act Legislation that has become law.

active euthanasia Acts performed to help end a sick person's life.

acute-severe condition Health problem of sudden onset; a serious illness or condition.

adaptation Process of exchange between a person and the environment to maintain or regain personal integrity; the key principle in the Roy Model of Nursing.

administrative A governmental agency that implements legislation.

administrative rule or regulation An operating procedure that describes how a government agency implements the intent of a statute; state boards of nursing implement the nurse practice act.

advanced nursing education Master's- or doctoral-level education that provides knowledge and skills in areas such as research, education, administration, or clinical specialties.

advanced placement A process by which a student is given credit for a required course through transfer or examination rather than by enrolling in and completing the course.

advanced practice Extended role; increased responsibilities and actions undertaken by an individual because of additional education and experience; nurse practitioners are advanced practice nurses.

advocate One who pleads for a cause or proposal; one who acts on behalf of another.

affidavit Written, sworn statement.

affiliation agreement A formal agreement between an educational institution and another agency that agrees to provide clinical areas for student practice.

aggressiveness Harsh behavior that may result in physical or emotional harm to others.

ambulatory care center Type of primary care facility that provides treatment on an outpatient basis.

answer Document filed in the court by the defendant in response to the complaint.

anxiety Uneasiness or apprehension caused by an impending threat or fear of the unknown.

apathy Lack of interest.

appeal Request to a higher court to review a decision in the hopes of changing the ruling of a lower court.

appellant Person who seeks an appeal.

arbitrator Neutral third party who assesses facts independently of the judicial system.

articulation Type of education program that allows easy entry from one level to another; for example, many BSN programs have articulation for nurses with associate degrees.

artificial insemination Insertion of sperm into the uterus with a syringe.

assault Attempt or threat to touch.

assertiveness Ability to express thoughts, feelings, and ideas openly and directly without fear.

assessment Process of collecting information about a client to help plan care.

associate degree nursing program Type of nursing education program that leads to an associate degree with a major in nursing; usually located in a community or junior college, these programs nominally last 2 years.

audit Close review of records or documents to detect the presence or absence of specific information.

auscultation Assessment technique that requires listening with a stethoscope to various parts of the body to detect sounds produced by organs.

authoritarian Type of leadership style in which the leader gives orders, makes decisions for the group as a whole, and bears most of the responsibility for the outcomes. Also called autocratic, directive, or controlling.

autonomy State of being self-directed or independent; the ability to make decisions about one's future.

autopsy Examination of a body after death to determine the cause of death.

baccalaureate degree nursing program Type of nursing education program that leads to the bachelor's degree with a major in nursing; usually located in a college or university, the length of the program is 4 years.

bargaining agent Organization certified by a governmental agency to represent a group of employees for the purpose of collective bargaining.

baseline data Initial information obtained about a client that establishes the norms for comparison as the client's condition changes.

basic human rights Those considerations society deems reasonably expected for all people; right to self-determination, protection from discomfort and harm, dignity, fair treatment, and privacy.

battery Nonconsensual touching of another person that does not necessarily cause harm or injury.

behaviorism Psychological theory based on the belief that all behavior is learned over time through conditioning.

behavior modification Method to change behavior through rewards for positive behavior.

belief Expectations or judgments based on attitude verified by experiences.

beneficence Ethical principle based on the beliefs that the health-care provider should do no harm, prevent harm, remove existing harm, and promote the good and well-being of the client.

bereavement State of sadness brought on by the loss or death of a significant other.

bill Proposed law that is moving through the legislative process.

bill of rights List of statements that outline the claims and privileges of a particular group, such as the Client's Bill of Rights.

bioethical issues Issues that deal with the health, safety, life, and death of human beings, often arising from advances in medical science and technology.

biofeedback Ability to control autonomic responses in the body through conscious effort.

body substance isolation (BSI) Universal precautions; guidelines established by the Centers for Disease Control and Prevention (CDC) and the Occupational Safety and Health Administration (OSHA) to protect health-care professionals and the client from diseases carried in the blood and body fluids, such as HIV and hepatitis B; involves the use of gloves whenever one is in contact with blood or body fluids and the use of masks, gowns, and eye covers if a chance of aerosol contact with fluids exists.

brain death Irreversible destruction of the cerebral cortex and brain stem manifested by absence of all reflexes; absence of brain waves on an electroencephalogram.

breach of contract Failure by one of the parties in a contract to fulfill all the terms of the agreement.

burden of proof Requirement that the plaintiff submit sufficient evidence to prove a defendant's guilt.

burnout syndrome A state of emotional exhaustion that results from the accumulative stress of an individual's life, including work, personal, and family responsibilities.

cadaver donor Clinically or brain-dead individual who previously agreed to allow organs to be taken for transplantation.

capitated payment system System of reimbursement in which a flat fee is paid for health-care services for a prescribed period of time. Expenses incurred in excess of this fee are provider losses.

capricious Unpredictable; arbitrary.

career ladder Articulation of educational programs that permit advancement from a lower level to a higher level without loss of credit or repetition of coursework.

career mobility Opportunity for individuals in one occupational area to move to another without restrictions.

case management Health-care delivery in which a client advocate or health-care coordinator helps the client through the hospitalization to obtain the most appropriate care.

case manager Health-care provider who coordinates cost-effective quality care for individuals who are generally at high risk and require long-term complex services.

certification Official recognition of a degree of education and skills in a profession by a national specialty organization; recognition that an institution has met standards that allow it to deliver certain services.

challenge examination Examination that assesses levels of knowledge or skill to grant credit for previous learning and experience; passing a challenge examination gives the individual credit for a course not actually taken.

chart Legal document that contains all the pertinent information about a client who is in a hospital or clinic; usually includes medical and nursing history, medical and nursing diagnosis, laboratory test results, notes about the client's progress, physician's orders, and personal data.

charting Process of recording (written or computer-generated) specific information about the client in the chart or medical record.

civil law Law concerned with the violation of the rights of one individual by another; it includes contract law, treaty law, tax law, and tort law.

claims-made policy Type of malpractice insurance that protects only against claims made during the time the policy is in effect.

client More modern term for patient; an individual seeking or receiving health-related services.

client goal Statement about a desired change, outcome, or activity that a client should achieve by a specific time.

clinical education Hands-on part of a nursing program that allows the student to practice skills on actual clients under the supervision of a nursing instructor.

clinical forensic nurse Professional nurse who specializes in management of crime victims from trauma to trial through collection of evidence, assessment of victims, or making judgments related to client treatment associated with court-related issues.

clinical ladder Type of performance evaluation and career advancement in which nursing positions for direct client care have two or more progressive levels of required skill leading to advancement in salary and responsibility; it allows nurses to remain in direct client care while making career advancements rather than having to move into administration.

clinical pathways Case-management protocols used to enhance quality of care, encourage cost-effectiveness, and promote efficiency.

closed system System that does not exchange energy, matter, or information with the environment or with other systems.

code of ethics Written values of a profession that act as guidelines for professional behavior.

collective bargaining Negotiations for wages, hours, benefits, and working conditions for a group of employees.

collective bargaining unit Group of employees recognized as representatives of the majority, with the right to bargain collectively with their employer and to reach an agreement on the terms of a contract.

committee Group of legislators, in the House or Senate, assigned to analyze bills on a particular subject.

common law Law based on past judicial judgments made in similar cases.

comparable worth Method for determining employees' salaries within an organization so that the same salary is paid for all jobs that have equivalent educational requirements, responsibilities, and complexity regardless of external market factors.

competencies Behaviors, skills, attitudes, and knowledge that an individual or professional has or is expected to have.

competency-based education Courses or programs based on anticipated student outcomes.

complaint Legal document filed by a plaintiff to initiate a lawsuit, claiming that the plaintiff's legal rights have been violated.

compliance Voluntary following of a prescribed plan of care or treatment regimen.

computer technology Use of highly advanced technological equipment to store, process, and access a vast amount of information.

concept Abstract idea or image.

conceptual framework Concept, theory, or basic idea around which an educational program is organized and developed.

conceptual model Group of concepts, ideas, or theories that are interrelated but in which the relationship is not clearly defined.

confidentiality Right of the client to expect the communication with a professional to remain unshared with any other person unless a medical reason exists or unless the safety of the public is threatened.

consensus General agreement between two or more individuals or groups regarding beliefs or positions on an issue or finding.

consent Voluntary permission given by a competent person.

consortium Two or more agencies that share sponsorship of a program or an institution.

constitutional law Law contained within a federal or state constitution.

continuing care Nursing care generally provided in geriatric day care centers or in the homes of elderly clients.

continuing education Formal education programs and informal learning experiences that maintain and increase the nurse's knowledge and skills in specific areas.

continuing education unit (CEU) Specific unit of credit earned by participating in an approved continuing education program.

continuous quality improvement (CQI) Type of total quality management whose primary goal is the improvement of the quality of health care.

contract Legally binding agreement between two or more parties.

contractual obligation Duty to perform a service identified by a contract.

copayment Percentage of the cost of a medical expense that is not covered by insurance and must be paid by the client.

core curriculum Curriculum design that enables a student to leave a career program at various levels, with a career attained and with the option to continue at another higher level or career; it is organized around a central or core body of knowledge common to the profession.

coroner Elected public official, usually a physician, who investigates deaths from unnatural causes, including homicide, violence, suicide, and other suspicious circumstances.

correctional/institutional nurse Registered nurse who specializes in the health care of those in custody in secure settings such as jails or prisons.

credentialing Process whereby individuals, programs, or institutions are designated as having met minimal standards for the safety and welfare of the public.

crime Violation of criminal law.

criminal action Process by which a person charged with a crime is accused, tried, and punished.

criminal law Law concerned with violation of criminal statutes or laws.

criterion-referenced examination Test that compares an individual's knowledge with a predetermined standard rather than to the performance of others who take the same test.

critical thinking The intellectual process of rationally examining ideas, inferences, assumptions, principles, arguments, conclusions, issues, statements, beliefs, and actions for which all the relevant information may not be available. This process involves the ability to use the five types of reasoning (scientific, deductive, inductive, informal, practical) in application of the nursing process, decision making, and resolution of ambiguous issues.

curriculum Group of courses that prepare an individual for a specific degree or profession.

customary, prevailing, and reasonable charges The typical rate in a specific locale that payers traditionally reimburse physicians.

damages Money awarded to a plaintiff by a court in a lawsuit that covers the actual costs incurred by the plaintiff.

database Information collected by a computer program on a specific topic in a specified format.

defamation of character Communication of information that is false or detrimental to a person's reputation.

defendant Person accused of criminal or civil wrongdoing. A party to a lawsuit against whom the complaint is served.

delegation Assignment of specific duties by one individual to another individual.

democratic Type of leadership style in which the leader shares the planning, decision making, and responsibilities for outcomes with the other members of the group. Also called participative leadership.

deontology Ethical system based on the principle that the right action is guided by a set of unchanging rules.

dependent practitioner Provider of care who delivers health care under the supervision of another health-care practitioner; for example, a physician assistant is supervised by a physician, or an LPN is supervised by an RN.

deposition Sworn statement by a witness that is made outside the courtroom; sworn depositions may be admitted as evidence in court when the individual is unable to be present.

diagnosis Statement that describes or identifies a client problem and is based on a thorough assessment.

diagnosis-related groups (DRGs) Prospective payment method used by the U.S. government and many insurance companies that pay a flat fee for treatment of a person with a particular diagnosis.

differentiated practice Organizational process of defining nursing roles based on education, experience, and training.

dilemma Predicament in which a choice must be made between two or more equally balanced alternatives; it often occurs when attempting to make ethical decisions.

directed services Health-care activities that require contact between a health-care professional and a client.

discharge planning Assessment of anticipated client needs after discharge from the hospital and development of a plan to meet those needs before the client is discharged.

disease Illness; a functional disturbance resulting from an individual organism's inability to adapt to certain stressors; an abnormal physiologic state caused by microorganisms, cancer, or other conditions.

distributive justice Ethical principle based on the belief that the right action is determined by that which will provide an outcome equal for all persons and will also benefit the least fortunate.

due process Right to have specific procedures or processes followed before the deprivation of life, liberty, or property; the guarantee of privileges under the Fifth and Fourteenth Amendments to the U.S. Constitution.

duty Obligation to act created by a statute, contract, or voluntary agreement.

emerging health occupations Health-care occupations that are not yet officially recognized by government or professional organizations.

employee Individual hired for pay by another.

Employee Retirement Income Security Act (ERISA) Federal law that grants incentives to employers to offer self-funded health insurance plans to their employees.

employer Individual or organization that hires other individuals for pay to carry out specific duties during certain hours of employment.

empowerment Process in which the individual assumes more autonomy and responsibility for his or her actions.

endorsement Reciprocity; a state's acceptance of a license issued by another state.

end product Output of a system not reusable as input.

energy Capacity to do work.

entry into practice Minimal educational requirements to obtain a license for a profession.

environment Internal and external physical and social boundaries of humans; all those things that are outside a system.

essentials for accreditation Minimal standards that a program must meet to be accredited.

ethical dilemma Ethical situation that requires an individual to make a choice between two equally unfavorable alternatives.

ethical rights (moral rights) Rights that are based on moral or ethical principles but have no legal mechanism of enforcement.

ethical system System of moral judgments based on the beliefs and values of a profession.

ethics Principles or standards of conduct that govern an individual or group.

ethnic group Individuals who share similar physical characteristics, religion, language, or customs.

euthanasia Mercy killing; the act or practice of killing, for reasons of mercy, individuals who have little or no chance of recovery by withholding or discontinuing life support or by administering a lethal agent.

evaluation Fifth step in the nursing process; used to determine whether goals set for a client have been attained.

evaluation criteria Outcome criteria; desired behaviors or standards.

expanded role Extended role; increased responsibilities and actions undertaken by an individual because of additional education and experience.

expert witness Individual with knowledge beyond the ordinary person, resulting from special education or training, who testifies during a trial.

external degree Academic degree granted when all the requirements have been met by the student; a type of outcomes-based education in which credit is given when the individual demonstrates a certain level of knowledge and skill, regardless of how or when these skills are attained; challenge examinations are often used.

false imprisonment Intentional tort committed by illegally confining or restricting a client against his or her will.

family Two or more related individuals living together.

Federal Tort Claims Act Statute that allows the government to be sued for negligence of its employees in the performance of their duties; many states have similar laws.

feedback Reentry of output into a system as input that helps maintain the internal balance of the system.

fee for service Payment is expected each time a service is rendered. Includes physician office visits, diagnostic procedures (laboratory tests, x-rays), and minor surgical procedures.

fellowship Scholarship or grant that provides money to individuals who are highly qualified or highly intelligent.

felony Serious crime that may be punished by a fine of more than $1000, more than 1 year in jail or prison, death, or a combination thereof.

fidelity The obligation of an individual to be faithful to commitments made to self and others.

for-profit Health-care agencies in which profits can be used to raise capital to pay stockholders dividends on their investments. Also called proprietary agencies.

foreign graduate nurse Individual graduated from a school of nursing outside the United States. This individual is required to pass the U.S. NCLEX-RN CAT to become a registered nurse in the United States.

forensic nurse Registered nurse who specializes in the integration of forensic science and nursing science to apply the nursing process to individual clients, their families, and the community, bridging the gap between the health-care system and the criminal justice system.

forensic psychiatric nurse Registered nurse who specializes in application of psychosocial nursing knowledge linking offending behavior to client characteristics; nurse specializing in forensic psychological evaluation and care of offender populations with mental disorders.

forensic science Body of empirical knowledge used for legal investigation and evidence-based judgment in police or criminal cases.

fraud Deliberate deception in provision of goods or services; lying.

functional nursing Nursing care in which each nurse provides a different aspect of care; nurses are assigned a set of specific tasks to perform for all clients, such as passing medications.

general systems theory Set of interrelated concepts, definitions, and propositions that describe a system.

genetics Scientific study of heredity and related variations.

gerontology Study of the process of aging and of the effects of aging on individuals.

goal Desired outcome.

Good Samaritan Act Law that protects health-care providers from being charged with contributory neg-ligence when they provide emergency care to persons in need of immediate treatment.

grievance Complaint or dispute about the terms or conditions of employment.

group practice Three or more physicians or nurse practitioners in business together to provide health care.

health Complete physical, mental, and social well-being; a relative state along a continuum ranging from severe illness to ideal state of being; the ability to adapt to illness and to reach the highest level of functioning.

health-care consumer Client or patient; an individual who uses health-care services or products.

health-care team Group of individuals of different levels of education who work together to provide help to clients.

health insurance purchasing cooperative (HIPCs) Large groups of people or employers who band together to buy insurance at reduced costs. HIPCs may be organized by private groups or the government.

health maintenance organization (HMO) Prototype of the managed health-care system; method of payment for a full range of primary, secondary, and tertiary health-care services; members pay a fixed annual fee for services and a small deductible when care is given.

health policy Goals and directions that guide activities to safeguard and promote the health of citizens.

health practitioner Individual, usually licensed, who provides health-care services to individuals with health-care needs.

health promotion Interventions and behaviors that increase and maintain the level of well-being of persons, families, groups, communities, and society.

health systems agency (HSA) Local voluntary organization of providers and consumers that plans for the health-care services of its geographic region.

hearsay Evidence not based on personal knowledge of the witness and usually not allowed in courts.

holistic Treatment of the total individual, including physical, psychological, sociologic, and spiritual elements, with emphasis on the interrelatedness of parts and wholes.

home health care Health-care services provided in the client's home.

hospice care Alternative way of providing care to terminally ill clients in which palliative care is used; the major goals of hospice care are control of pain, provision of emotional support, promotion of social interaction, and preparation for death; family support measures and anticipatory grief counseling are also used if appropriate.

hospital privileges Authority granted by a hospital, usually through its medical board, for a health-care practitioner to admit and supervise the treatment of clients within that hospital.

hypothesis Prediction or proposition related to a problem, usually found in research.

ideal role image Projection of society's expectations for nurses that clearly delineates the obligations and responsibilities, as well as the rights and privileges those in the role can lay claim to. Is often unrealistic.

illness Disease; a functional disturbance resulting from an individual organism's inability to adapt to certain stressors; an abnormal physiologic state caused by microorganisms, cancer, or other conditions.

implementation Fourth step in the nursing process, in which the plan of care is carried out.

incidence Number of occurrences of a specific condition or event.

incident report Document that describes an accident or error involving a client or family member that may or may not have resulted in injury; the purpose of the incident report is to track incidents and to make changes in the situations that caused them; the incident report is not part of the chart.

incompetency Inability of an individual to manage personal affairs because of mental or physical conditions; the inability of a professional to carry out professional activities at the expected level of functioning because of lack of knowledge or skill or because of drug or alcohol abuse.

indemnity insurance Health insurance in which the contractual agreement is between the consumer and the insurance company. Providers are not involved in these arrangements, and rates are not pre-established.

independent nurse practitioner Nurse who has a private practice in one of the expanded roles of nursing.

independent practice association (IPA) Type of HMO usually organized by physicians that requires fee-for-service payment.

independent practice organization (IPO) Type of IPA in which a group of providers deals with more than one insurer at a time.

independent practitioner Health-care provider who delivers health care independently with or without supervision by another health-care practitioner.

indirect services Health-care actions that do not require direct client contact but that still facilitate care, such as the supply and distribution department of a hospital.

informed consent Permission granted by a person based on full knowledge of the risks and benefits of participation in a procedure or surgery for which the consent has been given.

injunction Court order specifying actions that must or must not be taken.

input Matter, energy, or information entering a system from the environment.

inquest Formal inquiry about the course or manner of death.

institutional licensure Authority for an individual health-care provider to practice that is granted by the individual's employing institution; the institution determines the educational preparation, training, and functions of each category of provider it employs; no longer legally permitted, unlicensed assistive personnel (UAPs) act under a form of de facto institutional licensure.

intentional tort A willful act that violates another person's rights or property and may or may not cause physical injury.

interrogatories Written questions directed to a party in a lawsuit by the opposing side as part of the discovery process.

intervention Nursing action taken to meet specific client goals.

invasion of privacy Type of quasi-intentional tort that involves (1) an act that intrudes into the seclusion of the client, (2) intrusion that is objectionable to a reasonable person, (3) an act that intrudes into private facts or published as facts or pictures of a private nature, and (4) public disclosure of private information.

Joint Commission on Accreditation of Healthcare Organizations (JCAHO) Organization that performs accreditation reviews for health-care agencies.

judgment Decision of the court regarding a case.

jurisdiction Authority of a court to hear and decide lawsuits.

justice Fairness; giving people their due.

Kardex Portable card file that contains important client information and a care plan.

laisseze-faire Type of leadership style in which the leader does little planning, sets few goals, avoids decision making, and fails to encourage group members to participate. Also called permissive or nondirective leadership.

law Formal statement of a society's beliefs about interactions among and between its citizens; a formal rule enforced by society.

legal complaint Document filed by a plaintiff against a defendant claiming infringement of the plaintiff's legal rights.

legal obligations Obligations that have become formal statements of law and are enforceable under the law.

legal rights (welfare rights) Rights that are based on a legal entitlement to some good or benefits and are enforceable under the legal system with punishment for violations.

legislator Elected member of either the House of Representatives or the Senate.

legislature Body of elected individuals invested with constitutional power to make, alter, or repeal laws.

liable Obligated or held accountable by law.

libel Written defamation of character.

license Permission to practice granted to an individual by the state after he or she has met the requirements for that particular position; licensing protects the safety of the public.

licensed practical nurse (LPN) Licensed vocational nurse; technical nurse licensed by any state, after completing a practical nursing program, to provide technical bedside care to clients.

licensing board Government agency that implements the statutes of a particular profession in accordance with the Professions Practice Act.

licensure Process by which an agency or government grants an individual permission to practice; it establishes a minimal level of competency for practice.

licensure by endorsement Method of obtaining a license to practice by having a state acknowledge the individual's existing comparable license in another state.

licensure by examination Method of obtaining a license to practice by successfully passing a state board examination.

living will Signed legal document in which individuals make known their wishes about the care they are to receive if they should become incompetent at a future date; it usually specifies what types of treatments are permitted and what types are to be withheld.

lobbyist Person who attempts to influence political decisions as an official representative of an organization, group, or institution.

locality rule standard of care Legal process that holds an individual nurse accountable both to what is an acceptable standard within his or her local community and to national standards as developed by nurses throughout the nation through the American Nurses Association (ANA), national practice groups, and health-care agencies.

malfeasance Performance of an illegal act.

malpractice Negligent acts by a licensed professional based on either omission of an expected action or commission of an inappropriate action resulting in damages to another party; not doing what a reasonable and prudent professional of the same rank would have done in the same situation.

managed care System of organized health-care delivery systems linked by provider networks; health maintenance organizations are the primary example of managed care.

mandatory licensure Law that requires all who practice a particular profession to have and to maintain a license in that profession.

manslaughter Killing of an individual without premeditated intent; different degrees of manslaughter exist, and most are felonies.

mediation Legal process that allows each party to present their case to a mediator, who is an independent third party trained in dispute resolution.

medical examiner Coroner; a physician who investigates deaths that appear to be from other than natural causes.

Medicaid State health-care insurance program, supported in part by federal funds, for health-care services for certain groups unable to pay for their own health care; amount and type of coverage vary from state to state.

medically indigent Individuals who cannot personally pay for health-care services without incurring financial hardship.

Medicare Federally run program that is financed primarily through employee payroll taxes and covers any individual who is 65 years of age or older as well as blind and disabled individuals of any age.

Medicare Utilization and Quality Peer Review Organization (PRO) Organization that reviews the quality and cost of Medicare services.

Medigap policies Health insurance policies that are purchased to cover expenses not paid by Medicare.

midwife Individual experienced in assisting women during labor and delivery; they may be lay midwives, who have no official education, or certified nurse midwives, who are RNs in an expanded role, having received additional education and passed a national certification examination.

misdemeanor Less serious crime than a felony; punishable by a fine of less than $1000 or a jail term of less than 1 year.

model Hypothetical representation of something that exists in reality. The purpose of a model is to attempt to explain a complex reality in a systematic and organized manner.

morality Concept of right and wrong.

moral obligations Obligations based on moral or ethical principles but *not* enforceable under the law.

morals Fundamental standards of right and wrong that an individual learns and internalizes during the early stages of childhood development, based primarily on religious beliefs and societal norms.

mores Values and customs of a society.

mortality Property or capacity to die; death.

motivation Internal drive that causes individuals to seek achievement of higher goals; desire.

multicompetency technician Allied health-care provider who has skills in two or more areas of practice through the process of cross-training.

multiskilled practitioner Health-care professional who has skills in more than one area of health care, such as an RN who has training in physical therapy.

national health insurance Proposed system of payment for health-care services whereby the government pays for the costs of the health care.

negative entropy Tendency toward increased order in a system.

negligence Failure to perform at an expected level of functioning or the performance of an inappropriate function resulting in damages to another party; not doing what a reasonable and prudent person would do in a similar situation.

no-code order Do not resuscitate (DNR) order; an order by a physician to withhold cardiopulmonary resuscitation and other resuscitative efforts from a client.

nonfeasance Failure to perform a legally required duty.

nonmaleficence Ethical principle that requires the professional to do no harm to the client.

nontraditional education Methods of education that do not follow the traditional lecture and clinical practice methods of learning; may include computer-simulated learning, self-education techniques, or other creative methods.

nonverbal A type of communication that uses any methods except written and spoken messages and constitutes 93 percent of the communication between individuals. It includes body language, gestures, facial expression, tone, pace, personal space, etc.

normative ethics Questions and dilemmas requiring a choice of actions where there is a conflict of rights or obligations between the nurse and the client, the nurse and the client's family, or the nurse and the physician.

norm-referenced examination Examination scored by comparison with standards established on the performance of all others who took the same examination during a specific time; the NLN achievement examinations are norm referenced.

not-for-profit (nonprofit) agencies Agencies in which all profits must be used in the operation of the organization.

nurse clinician Registered nurse with advanced skills in a particular area of nursing practice; if certified by a professional organization, a nurse clinician may also be a nurse practitioner, but more often this designation refers to nurses in advanced practice roles such as nurse specialists.

nurse practice act Part of state law that establishes the scope of practice for professional nurses, as well as educational levels and standards, professional conduct, and reasons for revocation of licensure.

nurse practitioner Nurse specialist with advanced education in a primary care specialty, such as community health, pediatrics, or mental health, who is prepared independently to manage health promotion and maintenance and illness prevention of a specific group of clients.

nurse specialist (clinical nurse specialist) Nurse who is an expert in providing care focused on a specialized field drawn from the range of general practice, such as cardiac nurse specialist.

nurse theorist Nurse who analyzes and attempts to describe what the profession of nursing is and what nurses do through nursing models or nursing theories.

nursing assessment Systematic collection and recording of client data, both objective and subjective, from primary and secondary sources using the nursing history, physical examination, and laboratory data, for example.

nursing diagnosis Statements of a client's actual or potential health-care problems or deficits.

nursing order Statement of a nursing action selected by a nurse to achieve a client's goal; may be stated as either the nurse's or the client's expected behavior.

nursing process Systematic, comprehensive decision-making process used by nurses to identify and treat actual and potential health problems.

nursing research Formal study of problems of nursing practice, the role of the nurse in health care, and the value of nursing.

nursing standards Desired nursing behaviors established by the profession and used to evaluate nurses' performance.

obligations Demands made on individuals, professions, society, or government to fulfill and honor the rights of others. Obligations are often divided into two categories–moral and legal (welfare).

occurrence policy A type of malpractice insurance that protects against all claims that occurred during the policy period regardless of when the claim is made.

omission Failure to fulfill a duty or carry out a procedure recognized as a standard of care; often forms the basis for claims of malpractice.

oncology Area of health care that deals with the treatment of cancer.

open curriculum Educational system that allows a student to enter and leave the system freely; often uses past education and experiences.

open system System that can exchange energy, matter, and information with the environment and with other systems.

ordinance Local or municipal law.

outcome criteria Standards that measure changes or improvements in clients' conditions.

out-of-pocket expenses Amount the client is responsible for paying for a health-care service.

output Matter, energy, or information released from a system into the environment or transmitted to another system.

palliative Type of treatment directed toward minimizing the severity of a disease or illness rather than curing it; for example, for a client with terminal cancer, relief of pain is the main goal (palliative), rather than cure.

panel of approved providers A list of physicians, nurse practitioners, pharmacies, and other health-care providers that are approved by an insurance plan and to whom reimbursement will be made by the insurer.

patient Client; an individual seeking or receiving health-care services.

patient day Client day; the 24-hour period during which hospital services are provided that forms the basis for charging the patient, usually from midnight to midnight.

pediatrics Study and care of problems and diseases of children younger than the age of 18.

peer review Evaluation against professional standards of the performance of individuals with the same basic education and qualifications; formal process of review or evaluation by coworkers of an equal rank.

perceived role image The individual's own definition of the role, which is usually more realistic than the ideal role, involving rejection or modification of some of the norms and expectations of society.

percussion Physical examination involving the tapping of various parts of the body to determine density by eliciting different sounds.

performed role image The duties performed by the practitioner of a role. Often produces reality shock in new graduate nurses.

perjury Crime committed by giving false testimony while under oath.

permissive licensure Law that allows individuals to practice a profession as long as they do not use the title of the profession; no states now have permissive licensure.

phenomenology Philosophical approach that holds that consciousness determines reality in space and time.

plaintiff Individual who charges another individual in a court of law with a violation of the individual's rights; the party who files the complaint in a lawsuit.

point-of-service plans Insurance plans in which consumers can select providers outside of a prescribed provider panel if they are willing to pay an additional fee.

political action Activities on the part of individuals that influence the actions of government officials in establishing policy.

political involvement Group of activities that, individually or collectively, increase the voice of nursing in the political or health-care policy process.

politics Process of influencing the decisions of others and exerting control over situations or events; includes influencing the allocation of scarce resources.

practical nursing program Vocational nursing program; a program of study leading to a certificate in practical nursing, usually 12 to 18 months in length; these programs are located in a vocational or technical school or in a community or junior college; after passing the NCLEX-LPN CAT examination, students become licensed practical nurses (LPNs).

precedent Decision previously issued by a court that is used as the basis for a decision in another case with similar circumstances.

preceptor Educated or skilled practitioner who agrees to work with a less-educated or less-trained individual to increase the individual's knowledge and skills; often staff nurses who work with student nurses during their senior year.

precertification Approval for reimbursement of services prior to their being rendered.

preferred provider organization (PPO) Method of payment for employee health-care benefits in which employers contract with a specific group of health-care providers for a lower cost for their employees' health-care services but require the employee to use the providers listed.

premium Amount paid on a periodic basis for health insurance or HMO membership.

prescriptive authority Legal right to write prescriptions for medications, granted to physicians, veterinarians, dentists, and advanced practice nurses.

preventive care Well care; nursing care provided for the purpose of maintaining health and preventing disease or injury, often through community health clinics, school nursing services, and storefront clinics.

primary care Type of health care for individuals and families in which maintenance of health is emphasized; first-line health care in hospitals, physicians offices, or community health clinics that deal with acute conditions.

primary care nurse Hospital staff RN assigned to a primary care unit to provide nursing care to a limited number of clients who are followed by the same nurse from admission to discharge.

primary intervention Health promotion, illness prevention, early diagnosis, and treatment of common health problems.

private-duty nurse Nurse in private practice; nurse self-employed for providing direct client care services either in the home or the hospital setting.

privileged communication Information imparted by a client to a physician, lawyer, or clergyman that is protected from disclosure in a court of law. Communication between a client and a nurse is not legally protected, but nurses can participate in privileged communication when they overhear information imparted by the client to the physician.

profession Nursing; an occupation that meets the criteria for a profession, including education, altruism, code of ethics, public service, and dedication.

professional review organization Multilevel program to oversee the quality and cost of federally funded medical care programs.

professionalism Behaviors and attitudes exhibited by an individual that are recognized by others as the traits of a professional.

prospective payment system (PPS) System of reimbursement for health-care services that establishes the payment rates before hospitalization based on certain criteria, such as diagnostic-related groups (DRGs).

protocol Written plan of action based on previously identified situations; standing orders are a type of protocol often used in specialty units that have clients with similar problems.

provider Person or organization who delivers health care including health promotion and maintenance and illness prevention and treatment.

provider panel Health-care providers selected to render services to a group of consumers within a managed-care plan.

proximate cause Nearest cause; the element in a direct cause-and-effect relationship between what is done by the professional and what happens to the client. As, for instance, when a nurse fails to raise the side rails on the bed of a client who has received a narcotic medication, and the client falls out of bed and breaks a hip as a result.

public policy Decision made by a society or its elected representatives that has a material effect on citizens other than the decision makers.

quality Level of excellence based on pre-established criteria.

quality assurance Activity conducted in health-care facilities that evaluates the quality of care provided to ensure that it meets pre-established quality standards.

quasi-intentional tort A violation of a person's reputation or personal privacy.

reality shock (transition shock) A sudden and sometimes traumatic realization on the part of the new graduate that the ideal or perceived roles do not match the actual performed role.

recertification Periodic renewal of certification by examination, continuing education, or other criteria established by the accrediting agency.

reciprocity Endorsement; a state's acceptance of a license issued by another state.

registration Listing of a license with a state for a fee.

registry Published list of those who are registered; the agency that publishes the list of individuals who are registered.

regulations Rules or orders issued by various regulatory agencies, such as a state board of nursing, which have the force of law.

rehabilitation Restoration to the highest possible level of performance or health of an individual who has suffered an injury or illness.

relative intensity measures (RIMs) Method for calculating nursing resources needed to provide nursing care for various types of clients; helps determine the number and type of staff required based on client acuity and needs.

respondent superior Legal doctrine that holds the employer or supervisor responsible for the actions of the employees or of those supervised; for example, under this doctrine, RNs are held responsible for the actions of unlicensed assistive personnel under their supervision.

responsibility Accountability; the concept that all individuals are accountable for their own actions and for the consequences of those actions.

restorative care Curative care; nursing care that has as its goal cure and recovery from disease.

resume Curriculum vitae; a summary of an individual's education, work experience, and qualifications.

retrospective payment system Payment system for health care in which reimbursement is based on the actual care rendered rather than on preset rates.

right Just claim or expectation that may or may not be protected by law; legal rights are protected by law, whereas moral rights are not.

risk management Evaluating the risk of clients and staff for injuries and for potential liabilities and implementing corrective and preventive measures.

secondary care Nursing care usually provided in short-term and long-term care facilities to clients with commonly occurring conditions.

secondary intervention Acute care designed to prevent complications or resolve health problems.

secured settings Any institutional setting imposing restriction of movement, confinement, and limitations to activity and access; jails, locked units or locked mental institutions, prisons.

service insurance Health insurance in which services are provided for a prescribed fee that is established between the providers and the insurance company.

sexual assault nurse examiner (SANE) A registered nurse specializing in care of victims of sexual assault, performing physical and psychosocial examination, collection of physical evidence, and therapeutic interventions to minimize trauma.

significant other Individual who is not a family member but is emotionally or symbolically important to an individual.

slander Oral defamation of character.

sliding-scale fees Fees for services that are based on the client's ability to pay.

slow-code order Physician's order that the efforts for resuscitation of a client who is terminally ill should be initiated and conducted at a leisurely pace; the goal of a slow-code order is to allow the client to die during an apparent resuscitation, Slow-code orders are not acceptable practice and do not meet standards of care.

staff nurse Nurse generalist who works as an employee of a hospital, nursing home, community health agency, or some other organization providing primary and direct nursing care to clients.

standards Norms; criteria for expected behaviors or conduct.

standard of best interest A type of decision made about an individual's health care when he or she is unable to make the informed decision for his or her own care; based on what the health-care providers and/or the family decide is best for that individual.

standards of care Written or established criteria for nursing care that all nurses are expected to meet.

standards of practice Written or established criteria for nursing practice that all professional nurses are expected to meet.

standing order Written order by physician for certain actions or medication administration to be initiated or given in certain expected circumstances; similar to protocols.

statute Law passed by a government's legislature and signed by its chief executive.

statute of limitations Specific time period in which a lawsuit must be filed or a crime must be prosecuted; most nursing or medical lawsuits have a 2-year statute of limitations from the time of discovery of the incident.

statutory law Law passed by a legislature.

stereotype Fixed or predetermined image of or attitude toward an individual or group.

stress Crisis situation that causes increased anxiety and initiation of the flight-or-fight mechanism.

stressor Internal or external force to which a person responds.

structure criteria Physical environmental framework for client care.

subpoena Court document that requires an individual to appear in court and provide testimony; individuals who do not honor the subpoena can be held in contempt of court and jailed or fined.

subsystem Smaller system within a large system.

summary judgment Decision by a judge in cases in which no facts are in dispute.

sunset law Law that automatically terminates a program after a pre-established period of time unless that program can justify its need for existence.

support system Environmental factors and individuals who can help an individual in a crisis cope with the situation.

systems theory Theory that stresses the interrelatedness of parts in any system in which a change in one part affects all other parts; often, the system is greater than the sum of its parts.

taxonomy Classification system.

team nursing Method of organizing nursing care in which each client is assigned a team consisting of RNs, LPNs, and nursing assistants to deliver nursing care.

technician Individual who carries out technical tasks.

technology Use of science and the application of scientific principles to any situation; often involves the use of complicated machines and computers.

teleology Utilitarianism; an ethical system that identifies the right action by determining what will provide the greatest good for the greatest number of persons. This system has no set, unchanging rules; rather, it varies as the situation changes.

tertiary care Nursing care usually provided in long-term care and rehabilitation facilities for chronic diseases or injuries requiring long recovery.

tertiary intervention Provision of advanced and long-term health-care services to acutely ill clients, including the use of advanced technology, complicated surgical procedures, rehabilitation services, and care of the terminally ill.

testimony Oral statement of a witness under oath.

theory Set of interrelated constructs (concepts, definitions, or propositions) that presents a systematic view of phenomena by specifying relations among variables with the purpose of explaining and predicting phenomena.

third-party payment Payment for health-care services by an insurance company or a government agency rather than directly by the client.

third-party reimburser Organization other than the client, such as an employer, insurance company, or governmental agency that assumes responsibility for payment of health-care charges for services rendered to the client.

throughput Matter, energy, or information as it passes through a system.

tort Violation of the civil law that violates a person's rights and causes injury or harm to the individual. Civil wrong independent of an action in contract that results from a breach of a legal duty; a tort can be classified as unintentional, intentional, or quasi-intentional.

tort-feasor Person who commits a tort.

total quality management (TQM) Method for monitoring and maintaining the quality of health care being delivered by a particular institution or health-care industry.

trial Legal proceedings during which all relevant facts are presented to a jury or judge for legal decision.

Tri-Council Nursing group composed of the American Nurses Association (ANA), National League for Nursing (NLN), American Association of Colleges of Nursing (AACN), and American Organization of Nurse Executives (AONE).

two plus two (2 + 2) program Nursing education program that starts with an associate (2-year) degree and then moves the individual to a baccalaureate degree with an additional 2 years of education.

Uniform Anatomical Gift Act Legislation providing for a legal document signed by an individual indicating the desire to donate specific body organs or the entire body after death.

unintentional tort A wrong occurring to a person or that person's property even though it was not intended; negligence.

universal health-care coverage Health-care reimbursement benefits for all U.S. citizens and legal residents.

universal precautions Body substance isolation; guidelines established by the Centers for Disease Control and Prevention (CDC) and the Occupational Safety and Health Administration (OSHA) to protect health-care professionals and clients from diseases carried in the blood and body fluids, such as HIV and hepatitis B; involves the use of gloves whenever in contact with blood or body fluids and masks, gowns, and eye covers if a chance exists of contact with aerosol fluids.

upward mobility Movement toward increased status and power in an organization through promotion.

utilitarianism Teleology; an ethical system that identifies the right action by determining what will provide the greatest good for the greatest number of persons. This system has no set, unchanging rules; rather, it varies as the situation changes.

utilization guidelines Guidelines that stipulate the amount of services that can be delivered by a health-care provider.

value Judgment of worth, quality, or desirability based on attitude formed from need or experience; a strong belief held by individuals about something important to them.

values clarification Process by which individuals list and prioritize the values they hold most important.

veracity The principle of truthfulness. It requires the health-care provider to tell the truth and not intentionally deceive or mislead clients.

verbal A type of communication based on written or spoken messages that constitute approximately 7 percent of the total communication between individuals.

veto Signed refusal by the president or a governor to enact a bill into law. If the president vetoes a bill, the veto may be overridden by a two-thirds vote of the membership of both the House and Senate.

vicarious liability Imputation of blame on a person for the actions of the other.

victimization Experience of physical, emotional, or psychological trauma in which the individual suffers injury, fear, self-blame, and/or other dysfunction.

vocational nursing program Licensed practical nursing program in Texas and California; a program of study leading to a certificate in vocational nursing, usually 12 to 18 months in length; these programs are located in vocational and technical schools and community and junior colleges; after passing the NCLEX-LPN CAT examination, students become licensed vocational nurses (LVNs).

Specialty Nursing Organizations

Academy of Medical-Surgical Nurses (AMSN)
North Woodbury Road, Box 56
Pitman, NJ 08071
Phone: (609) 589-6677
Fax: (609) 589-7463
• **www.medsurgnurse.org**

American Academy of Ambulatory Care Nursing (AAACN)
North Woodbury Road, Box 56
Pitman, NJ 08071
Phone: (609) 582-9617
Fax: (609) 589-7463
• **www.aaacn.org**

American Association of Critical-Care Nurses (AACN)
101 Columbia
AlisoViejo, CA 92656-1491
Phone: (800) 899-2226/(949) 362-2000
Fax: (949) 362-2020
• **www.aacn.org**

American Association of Diabetes Educators (AADE)
444 N. Michigan Avenue
Suite 1240
Chicago, IL 60611-3901
Phone: (312) 664-2233/(800) 644-2233
Fax: (312) 644-4411
• **www.aadenet.org**

American Association of Neuroscience Nurses (AANN)
224 N. Des Plaines #601
Chicago, IL 60661
Phone: (312) 993-0043
• **www.aann.org**

American Association of Nurse Anesthetists (AANA)
222 South Prospect Avenue
Park Ridge, IL 60068-4001
Phone: (847) 692-7050
Fax: (847) 692-6968
• **www.aana.com**

American Association of Occupational Health Nurses (AAOHN)
50 Lenox Pointe
Atlanta, GA 30324
Phone: (404) 262-1162
Fax: (404) 262-1165
• **www.aaohn.org**

American Association of Spinal Cord Injury Nurses (AASCIN)
75-20 Astoria Boulevard
Jackson Heights, NY 11370-1177
Phone: (718) 803-3782
Fax: (718) 803-0414
• **www.aascin.org**

American College of Nurse-Midwives (ACNM)
1522 K Street, N.W., Suite 1000
Washington, DC 20005
Phone: (202) 289-0171
Fax: (202) 289-4395
• **www.acnm.org**

American Nephrology Nurses Association (ANNA)
North Woodbury Road, Box 56
Pitman, NJ 08071
Phone: (609) 589-2187
Fax: (609) 589-7463
• **www.inurse.com/anna**

American Psychiatric Nurses' Association (APNA)
6900 Grove Road
Thorofare, NJ 08086
Phone: (609) 848-7990
Fax: (609) 848-5274
• **www.apna.org**

American Society of Anesthesiologists (ASA)
520 North Northwest Highway
Park Ridge, IL 60068
Phone: (847) 825-5586
Fax: (847) 825-1692
• **www.asahq.org**

American Society of Ophthalmic Registered
Nurses, Inc. (ASORN)
655 Beach Street
P.O. Box 193030
San Francisco, CA 94119
Phone: (415) 561-8513
Fax: (415) 561-8575
• **http://webeye.ophth.uiowa.edu/asorn**

American Society of Pain Management Nurses (ASPMN)
7794 Grow Drive
Pensacola, FL 32514-7072
Phone: (888) 34-ASPMN
Fax: (850) 484-8762
• **www.aspmn.org**

American Society of Plastic and Reconstructive Surgical Nurses, Inc. (ASPRSN)
North Woodbury Road, Box 56
Pitman, NJ 08071
Phone: (609) 589-6247
Fax: (609) 589-7463

American Society of Post Anesthesia Nurses (ASPAN)
11512 Allecingie Parkway
Richmond, VA 23235
Phone: (804) 379-5516
Fax: (804) 379-1386
• **www.aspan.org**

American Urological Association Allied, Inc. (AUAA)
11512 Allecingie Parkway
Richmond, VA 23235
Phone: (804) 379-1306
Fax: (804) 379-1386

Association for Practitioners in Infection Control (APIC)
505 E. Hawley Street
Mundelein, IL 60060
Phone: (708) 949-6052
Fax: (708) 566-7282

Association of Perioperative Registered Nurses (AORN)
2170 S. Parker Road, Suite 300
Denver, CO 80231-5711
Phone: (303) 755-6300/(800) 755-2676
Fax: (303) 750-2927
• **www.aorn.org**

Association of Pediatric Oncology Nurses (APON)
11512 Allecingie Parkway
Richmond, VA 23235
Phone: (804) 379-9150
Fax: (804) 379-1386
• **www.apon.org**

Association of Rehabilitation Nurses (ARN)
5700 Old Orchard Road, First Floor
Skokie, IL 60077-1057
Phone: (708) 966-3433
Fax: (708) 966-9418
• **www.rehabnurse.org**

Association of Women's Health, Obstetric and Neonatal Nurses (AWHONN)
2000 L Street, N.W., Suite 740
Washington, DC 20036
Phone: (800) 673-8499
Fax: (202) 728-0575
• **www.awhonn.org**

Dermatology Nurses' Association (DNA)
North Woodbury Road, Box 56
Pitman, NJ 08071
Phone: (609) 582-1915
Fax: (609) 589-7463
• **www.dna.inurse.com**

Emergency Nurses Association (ENA)
915 Lee Street
Des Plaines, IL 60016-6569
Phone: (800) 243-8362
Fax: (847) 460-4001
• **www.ena.org**

Federated Ambulatory Surgery Association (FASA)
700 N. Fairfax Street, #306
Alexandria, VA 22314
Phone: (703) 836-8808
Fax: (703) 549-0976
• **www.fasa.org**

International Society of Nurses in Genetics, Inc. (ISONG)
University of North Dakota
Department of Pediatrics/Genetics
501 Columbia Road
Grand Forks, ND 58203
Phone; (701) 777-4243

Intravenous Nurses Society, Inc. (INS)
Two Brighton Street
Belmont, MA 02178
Phone: (617) 489-5205
Fax: (617) 484-6992

National Association of Nurse Massage Therapists (NANMT)
6851 Yumuri Street, #8
Coral Gables, FL 33146
Phone: (305) 667-6821
• **www.nanmt.org**

National Association of Nurse Practitioners in Reproductive Health (NANPRH)
2401 Pennsylvania Avenue, N.W., #350
Washington, DC 20037-1718
Phone: (202) 466-4825
Fax: (202) 466-3826

National Association of Orthopaedic Nurses (NAON)
North Woodbury Road, Box 56
Pitman, NJ 08071
Phone: (609) 582-0111
Fax: (609) 589-7463

National Association of Pediatric Nurse Associates and Practitioners (NAPNAP)
1101 Kings Highway North, Suite 206
Cherry Hill, NJ 08034
Phone: (609) 667-1773
Fax: (609) 667-7187
• **www.napnap, org**

National Association of School Nurses, Inc. (NASN)
P.O. Box 1300
Scarborough, ME 04070-1300
Phone: (207) 883-2117
Fax: (207) 883-2683
• **www.nasn.org**

National Federation for Specialty Nursing Organizations (NFSNO)
East Hully Avenue, Box 56
Pitman, NJ 08071
Phone: (856) 256-2333
Fax: (856) 589-7463
• **www.inurse.com/nfsno**

National Flight Nurses Association (NFNA)
6900 Grove Road
Thorofare, NJ 08086-9447
Phone: (609) 384-6725
Fax: (609) 848-5274
• **www.astna.org**

National Nurses Society on Addictions (NNSA)
5700 Old Orchard Road, First Floor
Skokie, IL 60077-1057
Phone: (708) 966-5010
Fax: (708) 966-9418

Oncology Nursing Society (ONS)
501 Holiday Drive
Pittsburgh, PA 15220-2749
Phone: (412) 921-7373
Fax: (412) 921-6565
• **www.ons.org**

Society of Ambulatory Anesthesiologists (SAMBA)
520 N. Northwest Highway
Park Ridge, IL 60068-2573
Phone: (847) 825-5586
• **www.sambahq.org**

Society of Critical Care Medicine (SCCM)
701 Lee Street, Suite 200
Des Plaines, IL 60016
Phone: (847) 827-6869
Fax: (847) 827-6886
• **www.sccm.org**

Society of Gastroenterology Nurses and Associates, Inc. (SGNA)
1070 Sibley Tower
Rochester, NY 14604
Phone: (716) 546-7241
Fax: (716) 546-5141
• **www.sgna.org**

Society of Otorhinolaryngology and Head-Neck Nurses, Inc. (SOHN)
116 Canal Street, Suite A
New Smyrna Beach, FL 32168-7004
Phone: (904) 428-1695
Fax: (904) 423-7566
• **www.sohnnurse.com**

American Association of Nurse Attorneys (TAANA)
720 Light Street
Baltimore, MD 21230
Phone: (410) 752-3318
Fax: (410) 752-8295
• **www.taana.org**

American Holistic Nurses Association (AHNA)
4101 Lake Boone Trail, Suite 201
Raleigh, NC 27607
Phone: (919) 787-5181
Fax: (919) 787-4916
• **www.ahna.org**

National Association of GCRC Nurse Managers (NAGCRCNM)
Clinical Research Center
The Center for Health Sciences

27-066 CHS 169747
10833 Le Conte Avenue
Los Angeles, CA 90024-169747
Phone: (310) 825-5225
Fax: (310) 206-9440

National Association for Health Care Recruitment (NAHCR)
P.O. Box 5769
Akron, OH 44372
Phone: (216) 867-3088
Fax: (216) 867-1630
• **www.nahcr.com**

National Student Nurses' Association, Inc. (NSNA)
555 West 57th Street
New York, NY 10019
Phone: (212) 581-2211
Fax: (212) 581-2368
• **www.nsna.org**

Nursing Organization Liaison Forum (NOLF)
600 Maryland Avenue, S.W.
Suite 100 West
Washington, DC 20024
Phone: (202) 554-4444

Page numbers followed by *b* indicate boxes; page numbers followed by *f* indicate figures; page numbers followed by *t* indicate tables.

A

Abandonment of client, 167
Abortions, 135–137
    elective, 136, 139
    self-selected, 136
    therapeutic, 136
    use of fetal tissue, 139–140
Abuse, child, 153–154
Accident, unavoidable, 172
Accountability
    in increasing power in nursing, 17
    in nursing informatics, 348
    professional train in nursing, 6
Accreditation, 42, 45
Achievement, in Johnson Behavioral System Model, 71
Acquired immunodeficiency syndrome (AIDS), 152
Act utilitarianism, 125
Action-oriented critical thinking, 105
Active euthanasia, 149
Active listening, 251
Activities of daily living (ADLs), 66
Acupuncture, 470
Adaptation, Roy Adaptation Model, 62, 63*t*
Administrator, 315
Advance directives, 146, 150*f*
    common questions about, 175*b*
    nurse's role in, 175
    Patient Self-Determination Act, 173–175
Advanced placement, 90
Advanced practice nurses (APNs), 12, 42, 253
    education for, 94
    licensure, 41
Advocate, 136
Affidavit, 170
Agency shop, 310
Aggressive behavior/communication, 55, 278
AIDS (acquired immunodeficiency syndrome), 152
Alinsky's rules for radicals, 374–374*b*
Alliance for the Mentally Ill, 337
Alternative and complementary healing (ACH), 468
Alternative and complementary healing practices, 80, 465–495
    categories, 471–472*t*
    comparing to conventional medicine, 473–484, 474*t*
    defining alternative healers, 476*b*
    definition of, 466
    energy systems, 480–481
    finding information about, 487
    glossary of terms for, 490–495
    Healing Matrix, 469, 469*t*
    NCCAM classification of, 470–473
    nutrition, 481
    paradox of, 485–488
    plants as medicine, 483
    questions to ask about, 485–487, 486*b*
    self-healing, 475
    wellness and holism, 440–476
Alternative healers, 476*b*
Altruistic activities, 9
Ambulatory care centers, 78
American Association of Colleges of Nursing (AACN), 12, 45, 49, 85
American Association of Critical-Care Nurses (AACN), 42
    standards of care, 176
American Cancer Society, 337
American Heart Association, 337
American Holistic Nurses' Association (AHNA), 404*b*
American Journal of Nursing, 33, 387
American Medical Association (AMA), 9
American Nurse, 387
American Nurses Association (ANA), 9
    addressing and defining delegation phenomenon, 291
    Code of Ethics, 9, 118, 127, 128*b*, 252, 298
    Council of State Boards of Nursing, 40
    definition of forensic nursing, 432
    definition of nursing informatics, 346
    definition of nursing supervisor, 314
    on education for nurses, 83–86
    efforts for self-governance, 315
    history of, 32
    membership in, 45
    opposition to assisted suicide, 152
    Political Action Committee, 46
    political and economic activities of, 46
    position on DNR decisions, 175
    power of professional unity, 16
    purposes of, 45
    relations with specialty organizations, 49
    standards of care, 176
    support of collective bargaining, 306
American Nurses Credentialing Center (ANCC), 12, 42, 346
American Red Cross, 27, 32, 48
    critical incident stress debriefing teams, 236
American Society of Superintendents of Training Schools for Nurses, 32

Anger, effect on ability to communicate, 269–270
Answer (lawsuit), 163, 169
Anxiety, client, caused by genetic information, 138
Apathy, 235
Appeal (legal issue), 171
Appellant, 171
Arbitration
   in contract negotiations, 311
   dispute resolution in legal matters, 172
Arbitrator, 172
Army Nurse Corps, 27
Articulation, 90, 347
Artificial insemination, 139
Assault and battery, 166
Assertive communication, 274–278, 277b
   aggressive communication versus, 278
   personal risks of, 276
Assertiveness, 273
   assessing self-assertiveness, 275, 277b
   rules for, 275
Assisted suicide, 144, 149–152
Associate degree in nursing (ADN), 29, 41, 87–88
Assumption of risk, 171
Assumptions, identification and challenging of, 106
Asymmetric information, 344
Author credentials, 7
Authoritarian leadership style, 248t, 249–250
   benevolent, 249
   dictatorial, 249
Authority, 314
Autonomy, 358
   as key concept in ethics, 118
   nurse's relationship to physician, 10
Ayurveda, 478, 484

B

Baccalaureate education, 10, 84, 88–89
Bachelor of Science in Nursing (BSN), 89
Bargaining
   best-practice, 307
   collective. *See* Collective bargaining
Baseline data, 62
Basic Guide to Safe Delegation (ANA), 300
Basic human rights, 124
Battery, 166
Behavior modification, 273
Beneficence, 119, 123, 147, 154
Best-practice bargaining, 307
Bias, 104
   on Web sites, 7–8
Bill of Rights, of U.S. Constitution, 123
Bioelectromagnetic-based therapy, 472t
Bioethical issues, 124, 135–160. *See also* Ethics
   abortion, 135–137
   acquired immunodeficiency syndrome, 152
   assisted suicide, 149–152
   euthanasia, 149–152
   fetal tissue research, 139
   genetics and genetic research, 137–139
   involving children, 153–157
   organ transplantation, 140–141
   right to die, 144–149
   scarce resources used to prolong life, 141–144
Biofeedback, 471t
   for stress reduction, 269
Biofield therapy, 472t, 473

Biological agents, 438–439, 439t
Biopsychosocial relationships, 56
Bioterrorism, 438–441
Bipartisan tactics, 388
Board of directors, 315
Board of Nursing Model, of governance, 316
Board of trustees, 315
Bodyworks, 469
Bolton Nurse Training Act, 28
Botanical medicine, 483
Brain death, 140, 142b
Breach of confidentiality, 168
Breach of contract, 312b
Breach of duty, 164, 165b
Burden of proof, 163
Burnout syndrome, 234–235
   spiritual perspective of, 409
   symptoms of, 235, 235b

C

Cadaver donors, 140
California Nurses Association, 48
Canada Health Act (CHA), 327
Canadian Nurses Association, Code of Ethics, 128
Capitated payment system, 329
Capricious behavior, of physician toward nurses, 105
Cardiopulmonary resuscitation (CPR), 144, 172
Care delivery models, 259–261
   functional nursing, 259, 260t
   modular nursing, 259, 260t
   primary care nursing, 259, 260t
   team nursing, 259, 260t
Career ladder, 90
Career mobility, 90
Caring, 70
   Watson Model of Human Caring, 63t, 68–70
Case management, 82, 436
   ANCC and, 13
   protocols of, 331
Case Management Society of America (CMSA), 436, 437
Case managers, 12–13, 82, 437b
Categorical imperative, 126
Caucuses
   legislative, 379
   in mediation, 172
Certification, 37, 42–44
   individual, 42
   organizational, 42–44
Certified nurse's assistants (CNAs), 41
Certified registered nurse anesthetist (CRNA), 94
Certified transcultural nurses (CTN5), 429
Chakras, 402
Challenge examinations, 91
Change
   external, 257
   internal, 257
   motivating people to make changes, 257–258, 257b, 259t
   planned, 257
   reactive change, 257
   unplanned, 257
Character, defamation of, 167
Charge nurse, 259, 260t
Chart, 177
Charting
   correction of errors in, 169
   by exception, 177

chi (human energy system), 401
Child abuse, 153–154
Child neglect, 153
Children
    age for rational decision making, 156
    ethics involving, 153–157
    informed consent issues, 140, 153, 154–156
    as organ donors, 140, 154–155
Chiropractic care, 472*t*
Chronicity of illness, effect on health-care delivery system, 324
Civil law 162*b*, 163
Claims-made insurance policy 179, 180*b*
Client
    abandonment of, 167
    aggressive behavior in, 55
    communication with, 268
    education level of, 80
    finding information on Internet, 357
    goals of, 55
    in Johnson Behavioral System Model, 70–72
    in King Model of Goal Attainment, 63*t*, 67
    knowledge of, 178–179
    in Neuman Health-Care Systems Model, 63*t*, 72
    non-English-speaking, 424, 424*b*
    in nursing models, 56
    in Orem Self-Care Model, 63*t*, 65
    rapport with, 178
    in Roy Adaptation Model, 62, 63*t*
    stress for, 269
    in Watson Model of Human Caring, 63*t*, 68
Client records. *See* Medical records
Client/consumer-driven health-care system, 83
Clinical forensic nursing, 431
Clinical ladder, 233*b*
Clinical nurse specialist (CNS), 12, 94, 177
Clinical pathways, 82, 331
Clinical psychologists, 11*t*
Closed shop, 310
Closed system, 61
Code of ethics, 117
    American Nurses Association, 9, 118, 128*b*, 252, 298
    Canadian Nurses Association, 128
    nursing, 127–129, 135
Coercive power, 14–16
Cognitive dissonance, 223
Collaborative practice, 81
Collective bargaining, 46, 303–322
    bargaining unit for use in hospitals, 306*b*
    contract negotiations, 311–312
    divisiveness of, 309–310
    ethical issues in, 309
    goals of, 306–307
    governance and, 314–318
    interest-based, 307
    legislative development of, 304–306
    nurses' questions about, 308–311
    participation by nursing supervisor, 313
    perspective on, 304–308
    professionalism and, 308
    representation, 312–313
    threat to job security, 310
Common law, 162, 162*b*
Communication, 266–289
    aggressive style, 278–279
    assertive style, 274–277, 277*b*
    barriers to clear, 274*b*

benefits of clear, 274*b*
characteristics of organizer, 389, 389*b*
conflict management, 281
coping skills related to, 284–286
with difficult people, 283–284
effect of anger on, 269–270
effect of change on, 267
effect of competition on, 271
effect of diversity on, 279–281
effect of stress on, 268
group dynamics, 270–271
nonverbal, 273, 423
principles of, 286*b*
problem solving, 281
submissive style, 278
transcultural, 423–426
understanding, 273–274
verbal, 273
working environment and, 272
Community health centers, 334
Community health nurses, 83
Comparable worth, 309
Comparative negligence, 171
Compassion, 396
Competency, 9
Competency-based education, 90
Competition, effect on ability to communicate, 271–272
Complaint, 105
    legal, 169
Complementary healing practices. *See* Alternative and complementary healing practices
The Complete German Commission E Monograph: Therapeutic Guide to Herbal Medicine, 487
Compliance, 423
Computer system, 331. *See also* Nursing informatics
Concepts, common to nursing models, 56–59
Conceptual framework, 60
Conceptual model, 55
Conference committee, 379
Confidentiality, 104
    breach of, 168
    of genetic screening, 138
Conflict management, 281–283
    confronting the conflict, 282
    ignoring the conflict, 282
    postponing the conflict, 282
Congregational nurses. *See* Parish nurses
Congressional shared governance model, 317
Conservatives, 376
Constituent-specific legislation, 381
Contextual awareness, 106
Continuing education units (CEUs), 42, 357
Continuing nursing education, 178, 252
Continuous quality improvement (CQI), 298, 330, 352
Contract
    breach of, 312*b*
    elements of good, 312*b*
Contract negotiations, 311–312
Contracting for nursing services model, of governance, 316–317
Contributory negligence, 171
Conventional health care, comparing to alternative and complementary healing, 470
Coping skills, of leader, 255
Correctional/institutional nursing, 435
Council of National Representatives, 48
Courage, as leadership quality, 252–254

Cover letter, sent with resume, 227*b*, 228
CPR (cardiopulmonary resuscitation), 144, 172
Creative thinking, 100, 107
Credentials
    author, 7
    of health-care team members, 11*t*
Credibility, 349
Crime, 162
Criminal action, 163
Criminal law, 162*b*, 162–163
Criterion-reference examination, 202
Critical incident stress debriefing (CISD) team, 236–237
Critical thinking, 99–112
    characteristics of, 100–105
    in decision making, 107–108
    as leadership behavior, 251
    nurses of the future, 79–82
    skills, 105–107
Cross-training, 100, 260
Cultural assessment, 421–423, 421*b*
Cultural awareness
    development of, 419–423
Cultural belief systems, 419–420
Cultural competence, 423
    providing culturally competent care, 417
    Purnell's Model of Cultural Competence, 421, 421*b*
Cultural conflicts, 426–427
Cultural diversity, 413–430
    increases in, 80
    melting pot versus salad bowl, 415–417
    providing culturally competent care, 423–426
    transcultural communication, 423–426
    U.S. ethnic population trends, 417
Cultural meaning-centered nursing model, 73
Cultural relativism, 416
Cultural synergy, 427
Culture
    concepts of, 415
    definition of, 413–415
    diversity in. *See* Cultural diversity

D
Dalai Lama, 403
Damages, liability for, 163
Data, definition of, 345
Data gathering, 105–106, 130
Data interpretation, 130
Database, 83
Death, criteria for, 140
Death investigation, 434
Deathbed visions, 403
Decentralized care, 224
Decision-making process
    critical thinking in, 107
    ethical, 115, 124, 130*f*, 156
Decoding, 273
Decompression, establishing daily routine for, 240
Deductive reasoning, 101
Defamation of character, 167
Defendant, 163
Defense of the fact, 172
Delegation, 290
    barriers to effective, 297*b*
    decision tree for, 297*b*
    developing delegation skills, 295–298
    direct, 300

    five rights of, 296*b*
    improper delegation of tasks, 165*b*, 168*b*
    indirect, 300
    legal issues in, 298
    nursing responsibilities when delegating, 291–295
    supervision versus, 290–291
Democratic leadership style, 248–249, 248*t*
Demographics
    affecting health-care delivery system, 323–324
    changes in, 80
Deontological system
    advantages of, 126–127
    disadvantages of, 127
    ethical precepts, 126
    rule, 126
Dependency, 71
Dependent children. *See* Children
Dependent practitioners, 298
Deposition, 170
    giving, 170*b*
Developmental crisis theory, 394
Diagnosis-related groups (DRGs), 329
Dietary supplements, 482
Difficult people, 283
Diploma schools, 86–87
Direct delegation, 300
Disaster Medical Assistance Team (DMAT), 442
Disaster nursing, 441
Disaster response, 30
Discharge planning, 82
Disciplinary hearing, 181
Discovery (lawsuit), 169
Disease, 56
Dispute resolution, alternative forums of, 172
Distributive justice, 120, 145
Diversity, 415
    cultural. *See* Cultural diversity
    effect on communication, 279–281
Do-not-resuscitate (DNR) orders, 144, 149, 150, 175
Dock, Lavinia Lloyd, 32
Doctor of education (EdD), 93
Doctor of nursing (DN, ND), 93
Doctor of nursing education (DNEd), 93
Doctor of nursing science (DNSc), 93
Doctor of philosophy (PhD), 93
Doctor of science in nursing (DSN), 93
Doctoral degree, 91–94
Downskilling, 48
Due process, 169
Durable power of attorney (DPOA), 147
Durable power of attorney for health care (DPOAHC), 121, 130–131, 174, 174*b*
Duty (legal), 164, 165*b*
    breach of, 164, 165*b*

E
Economic globalization, 80
Education. *See* Nursing education
Elected office, nurses holding, 386
Elective abortions, 136, 139
Electronic medical records, 352–354
Eliminative behavior, 71
Emerging health occupations, 78
Emotional distress, intentional infliction of, 167
Employees, 226
Employers, 226

Employment, in today's job market, 225
Encoding process, in communication, 273
End product, 61
Endorphins, 479
Energy
    conventional uses of, 480
    as leadership quality, 254
    in open and closed systems, 60–61
Energy forces, external, 481
Energy medicine, 480
Energy systems, human, 401
    alternative practices and, 480
    therapeutic touch, 406–408
Energy therapies, 470, 472*t*
Environment
    concept in nursing models, 58
    in Johnson Behavioral System Model, 63*t*, 71
    in King Model of Goal Attainment, 63*t*, 67
    in Neuman Health-Care Systems Model, 63*t*, 73
    in Orem Self-Care Model, 63*t*, 65
    in Roy Adaptation Model, 62, 63*t*
    in Watson Model of Human Caring, 63*t*, 70
Ergonomics, 350
Ethical decision making, 115, 124, 130*f*, 156
Ethical dilemma, 117
    involving living wills, 147–149
Ethical rights, 123
Ethical systems, 124–127
Ethics. *See also* Bioethical issues
    application of ethical theories, 127–129
    of collective bargaining, 309
    definitions in, 115–117
    key concepts in, 117–124
    normative, 124
    in nursing, 115–134
Ethics committees, 124
Ethnic groups, organizations focusing on, 49
Euthanasia, 144, 149–152
    active, 149
    passive, 149
Evidence-based practice (EBP), 6, 54, 348
Evil eye, 426
Executive branch, of government, 377, 377*b*,
    378*f*
Expanded role, 94
Expert power, 14
Expert witness, 165
External change, 257
External degree program, 89
Extraordinary treatment, 144
Eye contact, 426

F

Fallacy, 101, 102
False imprisonment, 166
Family members, nurse caring for relatives, 15
Family nurse practitioner (FNP), 94
Federal government, 440
Federal Tort Claims Act, 179
Federal Trade Commission (FTC), regulation of dietary
    supplements, 483
Fee-for-service model, 316
Feedback loop, 61–62
Feeding tube, removal of, 143
Fellowships, 226
Felonies, 162

Fetal tissue research, 139
Fidelity, 119
Fletcher, Joseph, 125
Food and Drug Administration (FDA), regulation of dietary
    supplements, 482
Forensic nursing, 431–435
    definition of, 431–432
    evolving requirements, 435
    specialties in, 432
Forensic psychiatric nursing, 435
Formalistic system. *See* Deontological system
Freedom of choice, 136
Functional nursing, 259, 260*t*
Funding, legislative, 381

G

General systems theory, 59–62
Genetic engineering, ethical issues about, 137
Genetic research, ethical issues about, 137
Genetic screening, 137
Geriatric nurse practitioner (GNP), 92
Goals
    of client, 55
    of collective bargaining, 306–307
    of nurse, 237–239
Goal setting, 237
Good Samaritan Act, 171, 172
Goodrich, Annie W., 33, 39
Governance, 314–318
    board of nursing model of, 316
    collective bargaining and, 317–318
    contracting for nursing services model of,
        316–317
    definition of, 314
    nurses' role in, 315
    shared governance, 317
Government
    executive branch of, 377, 377*b*, 378*f*
    health-care regulations and policies, 81
    judicial branch of, 377, 377*b*, 378*f*
    legislative branch of, 377, 377*b*, 378*f*
    politics and, 372
    structure of, 377, 377*b*, 378*f*
Governors, 315
Grassroots organizations, 48
Greatest good, determination of, 155, 155*b*
Grievance procedures, 308, 312*b*
Group dynamics
    in communication, 270–271
    leadership and management and, 258

H

Healing Matrix, 469, 469*t*
Health
    concept in nursing models, 56–58
    in Johnson Behavioral System Model, 63*t*, 71
    in King Model of Goal Attainment, 63*t*, 67–68
    in Neuman Health-Care Systems Model, 63*t*, 72
    in Orem Self-Care Model, 63*t*, 65
    in Roy Adaptation Model, 62, 63*t*
    in Watson Model of Human Caring, 63*t*, 70
Health care, consumer demands, 37
Health-care costs
    effect of nursing shortage on, 337
    out-of-control, 81
    scarce resources used to prolong life, 141

Health-care delivery system, 323–342
  assisted living centers, 335
  care delivery models, 259–261
  community health centers, 334
  continuous quality improvement in, 330
  demographics affecting, 323–324
  hospice care, 336
  long-term care facilities, 334
  luxury health-care centers, 368–369
  managed care, 329
  nurse-run health centers, 337, 436
  parish nurses, 336–337, 404*b*
  paying for, 329
  public health departments, 333
  rural health care, 335–336
  school-based health care, 333
  voluntary health agencies, 337
  workplace health centers, 334
Health-care information
  access to, 349
Health-care insurance
  genetic screening and, 137–138
  private, 332*b*
  universal health-care coverage, 144, 145
Health-care practices, questioning of, 104
Health-care team, 82
  members of, 10–13, 11*t*
Health-care trends, 80–81
Health informatics, 344. *See also* Nursing informatics
Health Insurance Portability and Accountability Act (HIPAA), 168, 355
Health insurance purchasing cooperatives (HIPCs), 336
Health maintenance activities, of nurse, 240
Health maintenance organizations (HMOs), 344, 465
Hearsay, 170
Henry Street Settlement, 33
Herbalism, 471*t*, 484
Herzberg Motivation-Hygiene Theory, of management, 256
Hierarchy of Needs Theory, applied to nursing management, 256
Hippocrates, 25, 115
HIV (human immunodeficiency virus), 152
Holism, 56, 466
Home health care
  home-health-care nursing, 83
  telehealth systems, 336
Homicide, 149
The Honest Herbal, 487
Hope, 396
Hospice care, 143, 336
House of Representatives, U.S.
  Appropriations Committee, 382
  Commerce Committee, 382
  committees of, 382
  Ways and Means Committee, 382
Human energy fields. *See* Energy systems, human
Human engineering, 350
Human factors, effect on nursing informatics, 350–352
Human Genome Project, 80, 138
Human immunodeficiency virus (HIV), 152, 324
Human interaction theory, of management, 255–256
Hygiene factors, 256
Hypnosis, 471*t*
Hypothesis, 54

I

Ideal role image, 222
Ideology, political, 376

Incident reports, 169, 272
Incompetency, 166
Incompetent clients, right to self-determination, 174–175
Indemnity insurance, 179
Independent nurse practitioners, 74, 94
Independent thinking, 103
Indirect delegation, 300
Individual certification, 42
Individual differences, acknowledgment and respect for, 251
Individual responsibility, professional traits in nursing, 6
Inductive reasoning, 101, 106
Informatics. *See* Nursing informatics
Information, definition of, 345
Informed consent, 147
  children and, 140, 152, 154–156
  exceptions to, 173
  failure to obtain, 166
  genetic screening and, 138
  issues in health-care litigation, 173
Ingested or applied substances, 469, 469*t*
Initiative, as leadership quality, 254
Input, in systems theory, 61
Institutional licensure, 41, 368
Integrity, as leadership quality, 252
Intellectual functioning, professional traits in nursing, 5
Intentional infliction of emotional distress, 167
Intentional torts, 166
Intercultural Nursing Newsletter, 429
Interest-based bargaining, 307
Intergovernmental Regulatory Reform Commission (IRRC), 384
Internal change, 257
International Association of Forensic Nurses (IAFN), 431, 432
International Center for the Integration of Health and Spirituality (ICIHS), 405*b*
International Council of Nurses (ICN), 47
Internet, 357. *See also* Web sites
Internship, 226
Interpersonal systems, 67
Interrogatories, 169
Interventions, nursing, taxonomy of, 56, 57*b*
Interviews, 229–234
  fashion do's and don'ts, 232*b*
  follow-up letter, 234, 234*b*
  interview mistakes, 233*b*
  questions that indicate interest in institution, 233, 233*b*
Intuition, 101
Invasion of privacy, 168
In vitro fertilization, source for fetal tissue, 139
Iowa Intervention Project, 56, 57*b*

J

Job, definition of, 4
Job market, 225
Job security, collective bargaining as threat to, 310
Johnson & Johnson Company, "Discover Nursing" ad campaign, 78*b*
Johnson Behavioral System Model, 63*t*, 70–72
Johnson v. Women's Hospital, 167
Joint Commission on Accreditation of Healthcare Organizations (JCAHO), 42, 176, 330
Journal of Transcultural Nursing, 429
Journals, health-care, 349
Judicial branch, of government, 377, 377*b*, 378*f*
Jurisdiction, 170
Jury selection, 170
Justice, distributive, 120, 145

K

Kevorkian, Dr. Jack, 149
ki (human energy system), 401
King, Imogene M., 67
King Model of Goal Attainment, 63*t*, 67–68
  cultural meaning-centered theory, 73
Knowledge, definition of, 345

L

Labor Management Relations Act (LMRA), 306
Ladder programs, 90–91
Laissez-faire leadership style, 248, 248*t*
Laws, 116–117
  civil law, 162*b*, 163
  common law, 162, 162*b*
  constitutional law, 136
  criminal law, 162, 162*b*
  divisions of, 162–169, 162*b*
  sources of, 161–162, 162*b*
  statutory law, 38, 161–162, 162*b*
  tort law, 163
Lawsuits, 161
  common issues in health-care litigation, 173–177
  facing, 169–171
  prevention of, 177–179
Leadership, 247–265
  group dynamics, 258
  key behaviors, 251–252, 252*b*
  key qualities, 252–255, 252*b*
  leadership style theory, 248, 248*t*
  management versus, 261
  recent theories, 251–252
  relationship-task orientation theory of, 250
  situational theory of, 251
  trait theory of, 247, 248*b*
  transformational theory of, 251
Legal complaint, 169
Legal issues, in delegation, 298–300
Legal nurse consultant, 434
Legal obligations, 123
Legal rights. *See* Welfare rights
Legislation
  development of collective bargaining, 304–306
  drafting legislation, 389–390
  introduction of legislation, 381
  issues driving development of legislation, 381
Legislative branch, of government, 377, 377*b*, 378*f*
Legitimate power, 16
Liability
  for damages, 163
  legal issues in delegation, 298–300
  vicarious, 300
Liability insurance, 179, 180*b*
  indemnity insurance, 179
  occurrence policy, 179, 180*b*
Libel, 167
Liberals, 376
Libertarians, 376
Licensed practical nurses (LPNs), 3, 12, 28, 90, 239
  registered nurse delegating tasks to, 298
Licensed vocational nurses (LVNs), 3, 28, 90
  registered nurse delegating tasks to, 298
Licensure, 9, 40–41
  early attempts at, 39
  institutional, 41, 368

mandatory 41
mutual recognition model for, 40
need for, 38
permissive, 40
for practical/vocational nurses, 90
reciprocity in, 41
registered nurse, 168*b*
registration versus, 40–41
revocation of nursing license, 39*b*, 179–181
as statutory law, 161–162
Licensure examinations, 77
Living will, 130, 146, 146*b*, 173, 174*b*
  checklist for evaluation of, 146*b*
  ethical difficulties of, 147–149
Lobbying, 381, 388
Locality rule standards of care, 176
Logical thinking, 101
Long-term care facilities, 334
Long-term goals, of nurse, 237
Luxury health-care centers, 368–369

M

Magnet hospitals, 369
Majority leader, 379
Majority whip, 379
Malfeasance, 162
Malpractice, 164, 165*b*, 181
  defenses to suit, 171–171
Man-Living-Health Model, 73
Managed care, 81
  organization, 329, 331*b*
  preferred provider organizations, 332*b*
  preoccupation with profit, 48
Management, 255–257
  group dynamics, 258
  Hierarchy of Needs Theory applied to, 256
  human interaction theory of, 255–256
  leadership versus, 261
  making changes successfully, 257–258, 257*b*, 259*t*
  Motivation-Hygiene Theory of, 256
  motivational theory of, 256
  time-motion theory of, 255
Mandated staffing ratios, 19–20, 338
Mandatory licensure, 41
Manslaughter, 150
Maslow, Abraham, 256
Master's degree, 91–94
Master's of science in nursing (MSN), 92
Master's of science with a major in nursing (MS Nursing), 92
Media. *See* News media
Mediation
  in contract negotiations, 311
  dispute resolution in legal matters, 172
Medicaid, 67, 120, 332*b*
Medical equipment design, 351*b*
Medical errors, 121, 351
Medical examiner, 434
Medical informatics, 344. *See also* Nursing informatics
Medical records
  defamation lawsuits and, 167
  paper, 352*b*
  in prevention of lawsuits, 177–178, 178*b*
Medical Unit, Self-Contained Transportable (MUST) hospital, 29
Medicare, 67, 332*b*
Medication research project, 50
Meditation, 409

Meditative prayer, 404
Medline database, 349
Mercy killing, 150
Micronutrients, dietary supplements, 482
Mind-body medicine, 471*t*, 473
Minority leader, 379
Misdemeanors, 162
Mobile Army Surgical Hospital (MASH) unit, 29
Model. *See also* Nursing models
    definition of, 55
Modular nursing, 259, 260*t*
Montague, Mildred, 87
Moore, Thomas, 401
Moral obligations, 123
Moral rights. *See* Ethical rights
Morals, 116
Mores, 116
Mosaic Code, 25
Motivational theory, of management, 256
Motivation-Hygiene Theory, of management, 256
Multitasking, 239, 410
Mutual gains bargaining, 307
Mutual Recognition Model for Nursing Licensure, 40
Mystics, 403

N

National Association of Hispanic Nurses, 49
National Association of Pediatric Nurse Associates and
        Practitioners (NAPNAP), 42
National Black Nurses Association, 49
National Center for Complementary and Alternative Medicine
        (NCCAM), 470–473
National Council Licensure Examination (NCLEX), 183–221
    computer skills required for, 213
    examination format, 209–214
    example of computer examination question, 209*b*
    handling anxiety about, 203
    history of, 40
    logistic scale, 213*b*
    obtaining exam results, 216
    pass-fail basis, 215
    study strategies
        formal NCLEX reviews, 218
        group study 216–217
        individual study tips, 217–218
        review books, 216
    test plan, 202–209
        client health needs, 204
        integrated concepts and processes, 207
        levels of cognitive ability, 205–207
    test-taking strategies, 186–197
National Easter Seal Society for Crippled Adults and
        Children, 337
National Labor Relations Act (NLRA), 304, 314
National Labor Relations Board (NLRB), 304–306, 308
National League for Nursing (NLN), 9, 32, 42, 45, 87
National League for Nursing Accrediting Commission (NLNAC),
        45, 87, 99
National League for Nursing Testing Division, 40
National Nursing Accrediting Service, 87
National Organization of Public Health Nursing, 32
National Student Nurses' Association (NSNA), 46
Natural food diets, 481–482
Navy Nurses, 27
Near-death experience, 402–403
Needs dissatisfiers, 256

Needs motivators, 256
Negative feedback, 62
Neglect, child, 153
Negligence, 164
    comparative, 171
    contributory, 171
Neonatal nurse practitioner (NNP), 94
Networking, 17
Neuman Health-Care Systems Model, 63*t*, 72–73
New York Nurse Practice Act, nurse practitioner amendment,
        94–95
News media, political influence of, 380
Nightingale, Florence, 3, 29, 31, 39, 84, 398
Nightingale School of Nursing, 86
"Nocebo effect," 405
Non-English-speaking clients, 424, 424*b*
Non sequitur, 101–102
Noncode orders, 128
Nonfeasance, 164
Nonmaleficence, 119, 147, 152
Nontraditional education, 360
Nonverbal communication, 273, 423
Norm-referenced examination, 202
Normative ethics, 124
North American Nursing Diagnosis Association (NANDA), 400
Notes on Nursing, 399
Nurse clinician, 177
Nurse manager, 261–262
Nurse midwife, 42, 94
Nurse practice acts, 162, 176–177
    development of, 38
Nurse practitioners (NPs), 12, 94
    independent, 74
Nurse-run health centers, 436
Nurse specialist, 94
Nurse-to-client staffing ratios. *See* Staffing ratios
Nurses
    origin of term, 25–26
    parish, 336
    politically active, 367–392
    responsibilities when delegating, 291–295
    role in governance, 315
    spiritual wellness in, 408–410
    of the future, 79–83
    transition from student to nurse, 222–224
Nurses Associated Alumnae of the United States and Canada, 32, 39
Nurses of Pennsylvania (NPA), 48
Nursing
    as profession, 5–9
    concept in nursing models, 59
    disaster nursing, 441
    ethics in, 115–134
    failing short of criteria for profession, 9–10
    functional, 259, 260*t*
    in Johnson Behavioral System Model, 63*t*, 72
    keeping nursing skills current, 178
    in King Model of Goal Attainment, 63*t*, 67
    modular, 259, 260*t*
    in Neuman Health-Care Systems Model, 63*t*, 73
    in Orem Self-Care Model, 63*t*, 65
    origins of, 23–27
    primary care, 259, 260*t*
    in Roy Adaptation Model, 62, 63*t*
    team, 259, 260*t*
    transcultural, 423, 429
    in Watson Model of Human Caring, 63*t*, 70

Nursing administration, 317
Nursing administrators, 315
Nursing and Health Care, Washington Focus, 387
Nursing board of directors, 316
Nursing diagnosis, 177
Nursing education
  for advanced practice, 94–95
  American Nurses Association position paper on, 83–86
  associate degree nursing, 87–88
  baccalaureate degree, 84, 88–89
  continuing education, 178, 252
  diploma schools, 86–87
  "Discover Nursing" ad campaign, 78*b*
  ladder programs, 90–91
  masters and doctoral programs, 91–94
  for nurses of future, 82
  paradigm shifting in, 79, 83
  Pew Health Professions Commission Report, 69–70, 79
  practical/vocational nursing, 89–90
  transition from student to nurse, 222–224
Nursing informatics, 343–364
  areas of focus in, 346
  confidentiality in, 354–357
  definition of, 344–346
  electronic medical records, 352–354
  ethical issues in, 354–357
  future technologies, 360
  human factors that affect, 350–352
  security in, 354–357
  smart devices, 359
  technology and communication, 343–344
  telehealth and, 358–361
  uses of Internet, 357–358
Nursing Interventions Classification (NIC), 56
Nursing Minimum Data Set (NMDS), 348
Nursing models. *See also specific models*
  concepts common to, 56–59
  conceptual models, 55
  differences between theory and model, 54–56
  major models, 62–73, 63*t*
  trends for the future, 73–74
Nursing organizations, 44–49
Nursing process, 64
  assessment plase of, 64, 207
  evaluation phase of, 208–209
  implementation phase of, 66–67, 208
  intervention phase of, 208
    primary interventions, 73
    secondary interventions, 73
  nursing diagnoses, 64, 177
  problem solving, 281
  questions of NCLEX, 207–209
Nursing research, 81, 348
"Nursing science," 6
Nursing shortage, 81, 224–225
  effect on health-care costs, 337–340
  use of foreign nurses, 368
Nursing supervisor, in collective bargaining, 313–314
Nursing theory
  differences between theory and model, 54–56
  general systems theory, 59–62
  major theories, 62–73, 63*t*
  spirituality and religion in, 399
  trends for the future, 73–74
Nutrition, alternative and complementary healing practices, 481
Nutritional supplements. *See* Dietary supplements

O
Obedience, passive, 426
Obligations, 123
  legal, 123
  moral, 123
Obstetrics-gynecology nurse practitioner, 94
Occupation, definition of, 4
Occurrence insurance policy, 179, 180*b*
Office of Alternative Medicine (OAM), 404*b*
Old boy system, 17
Omission of an act, 164
Omnibus Budget Reconciliation Act (OBRA), 123, 147
OncoLink, 357
Open curriculum, 91
Open shop, 310
Open system, 60–61
Optimism, as leadership quality, 252*t*, 254
Option rights, 124
Ordinances, 162
Orem, Dorothea E., 65
Orem Self-Care Model, 63*t*, 65
Organ donor, 140, 142*b*
  child as, 140, 154–155
Organ recipient, selection of, 141, 142*b*
Organ transplantation, 140–141, 142*b*
Orthomolecular medicine, 471–472*t*
Out-of-pocket expenses, 166
Outcome criteria, 87
Output, in systems theory, 61

P
Palliative care, 80, 143
Parish nurses, 336, 404*b*
Passive euthanasia, 149
Passive obedience, 426
Paternalism, 123
Patient Self-Determination Act, 173–175
Pediatric nurse practitioner (PNP), 92
Pediatrics, ethical concerns in, 153–157
Peer evaluation, 271
Peer review, 316
  of Web sites, 7
Perceived role image, 222
Performed role image, 222
Perjury, 170
Permissive licensure, 40
Perseverance, as leadership quality, 254
Personal space, 425–426
Personal systems, 67
Personal values, 106*b*
Pew Health Professions Commission Report, 69–70, 79
Pharmacists, 11*t*
Phenomenology, 395
Physical manipulation technologies, 469
Physical therapists, 11*t*
Physician assistants, 11*t*
The Physician's Desk Reference for Herbal Medicine, 487
Physicians
  case managers and, 437*b*
  as health-care team member, 11*t*
Phytomedicine, 483
Phytotherapy, 471*t*
Placebo response, 121, 405, 478
Plaintiff, 163
Planned change, 258

Pocket veto, 383
Political action
    definition of, 373
    increasing power in nursing, 16
Political campaign
    resources needed for, 385
    volunteers in, 385
Political capital, 383
Politically active nurse, 367–392
    activity at state level, 371
    Alinsky's rules for tactics, 374–375*b*
    characteristics of organizer, 389, 389*b*
    definitions of politics, political action, and related concepts, 373–376
    drafting legislation, 389–390
    formation of political alliances, 390
    government and politics, 372
    how to be politically active, 384–389
    how to organize, 388–389
    key players in policy formation and legislative process, 377–380
    political process, 381–384
    reasons to be active, 373
    structure of government, 377, 377*b*, 378*f*
    tactics of, 387–388
    understanding the issues, 367
    what one nurse can do, 385–389
Politics, government and, 372
Population-based care, 80–81
Populists, 376
Position, definition of, 4
Positive feedback, 61
Post-traumatic stress disorder (PTSD), 236
Postal Service, U.S., regulation of dietary supplements, 483
Power
    coercive, 14–16
    collective, 16
    empowerment in nursing, 13–18
    expert, 14
    legitimate, 16
    nature of, 13
    origins of, 13
    referent, 13–14
Power approach, to defining a profession, 4–5
Power of rewards, 14
Practical nursing education, 89–90
prana (human energy system), 401
Prayer, 404, 409
Precedent, 162
Preceptorships, 225
Preferred provider organizations (PPOs), 332*b*, 344
Prejudice, on Web sites, 7–8
Prejudice-free thinking, 104
Prescriptive authority, 94
Presentation, of information on Web sites, 8
Primary care, 79
Primary care nursing, 259, 260*t*
Primary interventions, 73
Priority setting, 240
Privacy
    invasion of, 168
    right to, 136, 152, 154
Privileged communication, 167–168
Problem solving, 281
    identification of underlying problem, 105
    as leadership behavior, 251
    strategies for, 239–241

Process approach, to defining a profession, 4
Procrastination, 239
Profession
    approaches to defining, 4
    development of, 3–22
    nursing as, 5–6
Professional, definition of, 4
Professional development, 10
Professional identity, 10
Professionalism
    definition of, 4
    in increasing power in nursing, 17
Professional standards review organizations (PSROs), 328
Professional unity, 16
Program issues, requiring legislation, 381
Prospective payment system (PPS), 329, 344
Protocols, 106
Proximate cause, 164
Psychiatric nurse practitioner, 94
Public demand, for legislation, 381
Public health departments, 333
Public policy, 373
Public service function, of nursing, 9
Purnell's Model of Cultural Competence, 421, 421*b*

Q

Quackwatch, 487
Quaker Society of Protestant Sisters of Charity, 27
Quality assurance, 330–331
Quasi-intentional torts, 167

R

Radicals, 376
Rapport with clients, 178
Reality shock, in workplace, 222–243
Reasoning
    deductive, 101
    inductive, 101, 106
Recertification, 42
Reciprocity in licensure, 41
Recommended daily allowances (RDAs), 482
References, 227
Referent power, 13–14
Registered nurses (RNs), 12
    delegation of tasks, 291
    licensure, 41, 168*b*
Registration, 40
    licensure versus, 40–41
Rehabilitation nurse practitioner (RNP), 94
Reiki, 401, 469*t*
Relationship-centered nursing care, 82
Relationship-task orientation theory, of leadership, 250
Relative intensity measures (RIMs), 260
Relatives, nurse caring for family members, 15
Relaxation response, 406
Religion
    in nursing theory, 397
    spirituality and, 397
Remembered wellness, 405, 479
Respiratory therapists, 11*t*
Respondent superior, 300
Restorative care, 56
Resume, 226, 227*b*
Resuscitation, of terminally ill client, 130
Retreat, 409
Revocation of nursing license, 39b, 179–181

Rewards, power of, 14
Right to care, 152
Right to die, 144–149
Right to 1ife, 136
Right to privacy, 136, 152, 154
Right to work laws, 310
Rights, 123–124
    basic human, 124
    ethical, 123
    option, 124
    welfare, 123
Rights-in-trust, 155
Risks, assumption of, 171
Robb, Isabel Adams Hampton, 31–32
Roe v. Wade, 136
Role image
    ideal, 222
    perceived, 222
    performed, 222
Roy, Sister Callista, 62
Roy Adaptation Model, 62, 63*t*
Rule deontology, 126
Rule utilitarianism, 125
Rules for Radicals, 384
Rural health care, 335–336
    telehealth systems, 336, 358

S

Sai Baba, 403
Satisfiers, 256
Schessler v. Keck, 167
School-based health care, 333
Science of Unitary Human Beings, 400, 406
Secondary interventions, 73
Security, 71
    in nursing informatics, 354–357
Self-assertiveness, 275, 277*b*
Self-care
    universal, 65
    for wellness, 477–478
Self-care model of nursing, 63*t*, 65
Self-determination, 136, 138, 144, 151, 154
    right of incompetent client, 174–175
Self-governance, 315
Self-healing, 475
Self-interest, in politics, 373
Self-knowledge, as leadership quality, 255
Self-protection, 71
Self-restoration, 409
Self-selected abortions, 136
Senate, U.S.
    Appropriations Committee, 382
    committees of, 382
    Finance Committee, 382
    Labor and Human Relations Committee, 382
Service Employees International Union, 306
Sexual assault nurse examiner (SANE), 432
Sexual assault response team (SART), 432–434
Sexual behavior, 71
Shared governance model, 317
    congressional shared governance model, 317
    unit-based shared governance model, 317
Short-term goals, of nurse, 237–238
Sigma Theta Tau, 48
Sisters of Charity, 27
Situation ethics, 125

Situational theory of leadership, 251
Slander, 167
Slow-code order, 130
Smart devices, 359
Social globalization, 80
Social systems, 67
Social workers, 11*t*
Soul, 401
Specialized nursing knowledge, 6
Spiritual care, 405
Spiritual questions, 396*b*
Spiritual wellness, 408–410
Spirituality, 393–412
    definition of, 396
    manifestation of, 398
    nature of, 396–398
    parish nursing, 404*b*
    practices in health and illness, 403–408
    tradition of, in nursing, 398–403
    wellness and nursing practice, 408–410
Staffing ratios, mandated, 19–20
Standard of best interest, 123
Standards of care, 176
    locality rule, 176
stare decisis, principle of, 162
State boards of nursing (SBNs), 38, 41
    revocation of nursing license by, 39*b*, 179–181
State government, 371
State nurses associations (SNAS), in collective bargaining, 306, 312
Statute, 162
Statute of limitations, 169
Statutory laws, 38, 161–162, 162*b*
Stem cell research, 139
Stereotype, 104
Storefront clinic, funding for, 50
    critical incident debriefing team, 236–237
Stress management, 235–238
    identification of own problems, 238
    problem-solving strategies, 239–241
    setting personal goals, 237–238
Stress reduction techniques, 269
Stressors, 73
Strike, by nurses, 306, 309, 312, 319–320
Submissive behavior/communication, 278
Subpoenas, 170
Subsystems, 71
Suggestions for Thought, 398
Suicide, assisted, 144, 149–152
Summary judgment, 171
Supervision
    delegation versus, 290–291
    inadequate, 165*b*, 168*b*
Support system, 409
Synergy, cultural, 427
Systems theory, 59–62

T

Taft-Hartley Act, 306, 314
Taking in, 71
Taxonomy, of nursing interventions, 56, 57*b*
Team building, 258
Team nursing, 259
Technician, 90
Technology, communication and, 343–344
Technology explosion, 80
Telehealth, 358–360

Telemedicine, 358
Terminally ill clients, 149
    resuscitation of, 130
    using scarce resources to prolong life, 141–144
Tertiary care, 73
Testimony, 170
Tests, taking and passing. *See* National Council Licensure
        Examination (NCLEX)
Theory. *See also* Nursing theory
    definition of, 54–55
Therapeutic abortions, 136
Therapeutic relationship skills, 82
Therapeutic touch (TT), 406, 481*b*
Third-party reimbursers, 360
Thomas v. Corso, 184
Throughput, 61
Time management, 239
Time-motion theory, of management, 255
Timeliness, of information on Web sites, 8
Tort, 163
    intentional, 166–167
    quasi-intentional, 167–169
    unintentional, 164–166
Tort-feasor, 163
Tort law, 163
Total quality management (TQM). *See* Continuous quality
        improvement
Touching, in different cultures, 425
Trait approach, to defining a profession, 5
Trait theory, of leadership, 247, 248*b*
Transcultural communication, 423–426
Transcultural nursing, 429
Transcultural Nursing Society, 429
Transformational theory, of leadership, 251
Transition shock, 222
Transplantation, organ, 140–141, 142*b*
Trial, 170–171
Trustees, 315
Tube feeding, 143
Two plus two (2 + 2) programs, 91

U

Unavoidable accident, 172
Unfair labor practices, 307
Unified Nursing Language System (UNLS), 347
Unintentional torts, 164–166
Union membership, 303
Unit-based shared governance model, 317
Unit service assistants, 260
United Network of Organ Sharing, 142*b*
Universal health-care coverage, 145

Universal self-care, 65
Unlicensed assistive personnel (UAP), 12, 41
    in modular nursing, 260
    registered nurse delegating tasks to, 291
Unplanned change, 257
Upward mobility, 90
Usability engineering, 350
Utilitarianism
    advantages of, 125
    disadvantages of, 125–126
    ethical precepts, 125

V

Value conflicts, 116
Value system, 106
Values, 70, 73, 116
    personal, 106*b*
Values clarification, 106
Ventilator, 144
Veracity, 121
Verbal communication, 273
Veto, 383
Vicarious liability, 300
Visualization, 406
Vital essences, 480
Vocational nursing education, 89–90
Voluntary health agencies, 337

W

Wald, Lillian, 32, 39
Web sites, 7–8
    disease-specific, 357
    information on herbal medicine, 487
Welfare rights, 123
Wellness
    holism and, 476
    remembered, 405, 479
    spiritual, 408–410
Well-roundedness, as leadership quality, 254
Western Interstate Commission for
        Higher Education, 49
Whistle-blower protection, 129
World Health Organization (WHO), 465
Win-win bargaining, 303
Workplace, reality shock in, 222–243
Workplace Advocacy Initiative, 306
Workplace health centers, 334
Write once, read many (WORM) programs, 357

Y

Yoga, 469*t*, 481